ANESTHESIA
A Comprehensive Review

ANESTHESIA
A Comprehensive Review

SIXTH EDITION

Brian A. Hall, MD
Assistant Professor of Anesthesiology
College of Medicine, Mayo Clinic
Rochester, Minnesota

Robert C. Chantigian, MD
Associate Professor of Anesthesiology
College of Medicine, Mayo Clinic
Rochester, Minnesota

ELSEVIER

Elsevier
1600 John F. Kennedy Blvd.
Ste 1800
Philadelphia, PA 19103-2899

ANESTHESIA: A COMPREHENSIVE REVIEW, SIXTH EDITION

ISBN: 978-0-323-56719-0

Notice

Practitioners and researchers must always rely on their own experience and knowledge in evaluating and using any information, methods, compounds or experiments described herein. Because of rapid advances in the medical sciences, in particular, independent verification of diagnoses and drug dosages should be made. To the fullest extent of the law, no responsibility is assumed by Elsevier, authors, editors or contributors for any injury and/or damage to persons or property as a matter of products liability, negligence or otherwise, or from any use or operation of any methods, products, instructions, or ideas contained in the material herein.

Previous editions copyrighted: 2015, 2010, 2003, 1997, 1992

Library of Congress Control Number: 2019941294

Senior Content Strategist: Sarah E. Barth
Content Development Specialist: Angie Breckon
Publishing Services Manager: Shereen Jameel
Project Manager: Radhika Sivalingam
Design Direction: Bridget Hoette

Printed in India

Last digit is the print number: 9 8 7 6 5 4

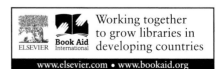

Preface

Numerous changes have occurred in medicine in general, and in anesthesia specifically, since work started on the first edition more than three decades ago. What has not changed, however, is the utility and learning value in working through questions and understanding the principles behind the correct answer. This exercise tests one's knowledge and challenges the reader.

As with all earlier editions, the aim of this work is to help the reader identify areas that require more study as well as reinforce previously acquired knowledge. This book is not intended to replace textbooks but to serve as an aid to them. The mere act of reading questions and thinking about possible answers often results in acquisition of new facts. The practice of weighing, deliberating over, and processing information can result in long-term retention of the material. Similarly, answering a question incorrectly also has inherent learning value, particularly if the reader studies the explanation and realizes where he or she erred.

All questions have been reviewed, at the very least, by one additional author. Often, vetting has included review by multiple physicians, particularly if there is a controversial aspect to the question or possibility for misinterpretation.

This book has stood the test of time and, in fact, the parents of some of the present-day contributors participated in writing earlier editions of the book an entire generation earlier.

All the authors, contributors, and proofreaders hope that this book will prove enjoyable, prove intellectually stimulating, and add valuable pearls to the "intellectual database" of all those who read it.

Brian A. Hall
Robert C. Chantigian

List of Contributors

Paul Carns, MD
Assistant Professor of Anesthesiology
College of Medicine
Mayo Clinic
Rochester, Minnesota

Paula D.M. Chantigian, MD
Assistant Professor of Obstetrics
College of Medicine
Mayo Clinic
Rochester, Minnesota

Robert C. Chantigian, MD
Associate Professor of Anesthesiology
Mayo Clinic
Rochester, Minnesota

Brian A. Hall, MD
Assistant Professor of Anesthesiology
Mayo Clinic
Rochester, Minnesota

Keith A. Jones, MD
Professor of Anesthesiology
University of Alabama School of Medicine
Birmingham, Alabama

Allan Klompas, MB, ChB, BAO
Instructor of Anesthesiology
College of Medicine
Mayo Clinic
Rochester, Minnesota

Julian Naranjo, DO
Instructor in Anesthesiology
College of Medicine
Mayo Clinic
Rochester, Minnesota

Kent H. Rehfeldt, MD, FASE
Associate Professor of Anesthesiology
College of Medicine
Mayo Clinic
Rochester, Minnesota

Francis X. Whalen, MD
Assistant Professor of Anesthesiology
Department of Anesthesiology
and Critical Care Medicine
College of Medicine
Mayo Clinic
Rochester, Minnesota

The large and diverse body of information contained in the sixth edition of *Anesthesia: A Comprehensive Review* is more extensive than ever before and required input and consultation from numerous participants. Great care has gone into vetting all questions to ensure they are scientifically sound and provide useful information to the reader. Recent editions of anesthesia textbooks, publications from anesthesia journals, websites for specialty guidelines, and so on, all served as sources or references for the multiple choice questions.

In addition to the co-authors, the authors wish to express their gratitude to Drs. Martin Abel, Dorothee Bremerich, Jonathan Charnin, David Danielson, Niki Dietz, William Lanier, Troy Seelhammer, Juraj Sprung, Mathew Warner, Denise Wedel, Toby Weingarten, Roger White, and Tara Hall, RRT. Several Mayo Clinic anesthesia residents checked textbook references and citations and proofread the chapters before production was carried out. The authors are grateful to the following physicians:

Kaitlyn Brennan, D.O., MPH
Layne Bettini, M.D., J.D.
Ashley Dahl, M.D.
Paul Davis, M.D.
Lindsay Hunter Guervara, M.D.
Jeffrey Huang, MD
Megan Hamre, M.D.
Melissa Kenevin, M.D.
Matthew Moldan, M.D.
Daniel Plack, M.D.
MacKenzie Quale, M.D.
Torunn Sivesind, M.D.
Lindsay Warner, M.D.
Danielle Zheng, M.D., Ph.D.

Harvey Johnson and Liana Johnson were instrumental in typing, arranging, and organizing all the questions.

Lastly the authors are grateful for the expertise of the many skillful people at Elsevier, without whose help publication would not have been possible. Special thanks to Sarah Barth, Senior Content Strategist, Angie Breckon, Content Development Specialist, and Radhika Sivalingam, Project Manager.

Brian A. Hall, MD
Robert C. Chantigian, MD

Contents

PART 1

Basic Sciences

CHAPTER 1

Anesthesia Equipment and Physics

DIRECTIONS (Questions 1 through 90): Each question or incomplete statement in this section is followed by answers or by completions of the statement, respectively. Select the ONE BEST answer or completion for each item.

1. A 75-year-old patient in the intensive care unit (ICU) is extubated after recovering from acute respiratory distress syndrome (ARDS). He has a history of previous myocardial infarction, congestive heart failure, and pneumonia. He has an A-line, pulmonary artery (PA) catheter and is receiving oxygen by nasal cannula. Which of the following techniques is **LEAST** accurate for assessing an intravascular fluid challenge?
A. Central venous pressure (CVP)
B. PA occlusion pressure
C. Transesophageal echocardiography (TEE)
D. Measurement of pulse pressure variation (PPV)

2. Select the correct statement regarding color Doppler imaging.
A. It is a form of M-mode echocardiography
B. The technology is based on continuous wave Doppler
C. By convention, motion toward the ultrasound probe is red and motion away from the probe is blue
D. Two ultrasound crystals are used: one for transmission of the ultrasound signal and one for reception of the returning wave

3. When the pressure gauge on a size "E" compressed-gas cylinder containing N_2O begins to fall from its previous constant pressure of 750 psi, approximately how many liters of gas will remain in the cylinder?
A. 200 L
B. 400 L
C. 600 L
D. Cannot be calculated

4. What percent desflurane is present in the *vaporizing chamber* of a desflurane vaporizer (pressurized to 1500 mm Hg and heated to 23° C)?
A. Nearly 100%
B. 85%
C. 65%
D. 45%

5. If the internal diameter of an intravenous catheter were doubled, flow through the catheter would be
A. Decreased by a factor of 2
B. Decreased by a factor of 4
C. Increased by a factor of 8
D. Increased by a factor of 16

6. A size "E" compressed-gas cylinder completely filled with N_2O contains how many liters?
A. 1160 L
B. 1470 L
C. 1590 L
D. 1640 L

7. Which of the following methods can be used to detect all leaks in the low-pressure circuit of all contemporary anesthesia machines?
A. Negative-pressure leak test
B. Common gas outlet occlusion test
C. Traditional positive-pressure leak test
D. None of the above

8. Which of the following valves prevents transfilling between compressed-gas cylinders?
A. Fail-safe valve
B. Check valve
C. Pressure-sensor shutoff valve
D. Adjustable pressure-limiting valve

9. The driving force of the ventilator (Datex-Ohmeda 7000, 7810, 7100, and 7900) on the anesthesia workstation is accomplished with
A. Compressed oxygen
B. Compressed air
C. Electricity alone
D. Electricity and compressed oxygen

10. The pressure gauge on a size "E" compressed-gas cylinder containing O_2 reads 1600 psi. How long could O_2 be delivered from this cylinder at a rate of 2 L/min?
  A. 90 minutes
  B. 140 minutes
  C. 250 minutes
  D. 320 minutes

11. A 25-year-old healthy patient is anesthetized for a femoral hernia repair. Anesthesia is maintained with isoflurane and N_2O 50% in O_2, and the patient's lungs are mechanically ventilated. Suddenly, the "low-arterial saturation" warning signal on the pulse oximeter gives an alarm. After the patient is disconnected from the anesthesia machine, he undergoes ventilation with an Ambu bag with 100% O_2 without difficulty, and the arterial saturation quickly improves. During inspection of your anesthesia equipment, you notice that the bobbin in the O_2 rotameter is not rotating. This most likely indicates
  A. Flow of O_2 through the O_2 rotameter
  B. No flow of O_2 through the O_2 rotameter
  C. A leak in the O_2 rotameter below the bobbin
  D. A leak in the O_2 rotameter above the bobbin

12. The O_2 pressure-sensor shutoff valve requires what O_2 pressure to remain open and allow N_2O to flow into the N_2O rotameter?
  A. 10 psi
  B. 30 psi
  C. 50 psi
  D. 100 psi

13. A 78-year-old patient is anesthetized for resection of a liver tumor. After induction and tracheal intubation, a 20-gauge arterial line is placed and connected to a transducer that is located 20 cm below the level of the heart. The system is zeroed at the stopcock located at the wrist while the patient's arm is stretched out on an arm board. How will the arterial line pressure compare with the true blood pressure (BP)?
  A. It will be 20 mm Hg higher
  B. It will be 15 mm Hg higher
  C. It will be the same
  D. It will be 15 mm Hg lower

14. The second-stage O_2 pressure regulator delivers a constant O_2 pressure to the rotameters of
  A. 4 psi
  B. 8 psi
  C. 16 psi
  D. 32 psi

15. You are called to assist a colleague who notes a large gas leak in the anesthesia circuit. Very high oxygen flows (15 L/minute) are being used, but the ventilator bellows do not fill during the ventilator cycle. You then attempt to manually ventilate the patient, but the reservoir bag does not fill. You then disconnect the patient from the anesthesia machine and attempt to ventilate the patient with an anesthesia bag (connected to separate oxygen source), but high oxygen flows are still required to achieve even a low positive pressure for ventilation. The most appropriate step would be
  A. Deflate cuff and reinflate until there is a good seal
  B. Pull out nasogastric tube
  C. Reintubate the patient
  D. Reconnect the endotracheal tube to the anesthesia machine circuit with 15 L/minute flow O_2 plus 15 L/flow air

16. A sevoflurane vaporizer will deliver an accurate concentration of an unknown volatile anesthetic if the latter shares which property with sevoflurane?
  A. Molecular weight
  B. Oil/gas partition coefficient
  C. Vapor pressure
  D. Blood/gas partition coefficient

17. A 58-year-old patient has severe shortness of breath and "wheezing." On examination, the patient is found to have inspiratory and expiratory stridor. Further evaluation reveals marked extrinsic compression of the midtrachea by a tumor. The type of airflow at the point of obstruction within the trachea is
  A. Laminar flow
  B. Turbulent flow
  C. Undulant flow
  D. Stenotic flow

18. Concerning the patient in Question 17, administration of 70% helium in O_2 instead of 100% O_2 will decrease the resistance to airflow through the stenotic region within the trachea because
  A. Helium decreases the viscosity of the gas mixture
  B. Helium decreases the friction coefficient of the gas mixture
  C. Helium decreases the density of the gas mixture
  D. Helium increases the Reynolds number of the gas mixture

19. A 56-year-old patient is brought to the operating room (OR) for elective replacement of a stenotic aortic valve. An awake 20-gauge arterial catheter is placed into the right radial artery and is then connected to a transducer located at the same level as the patient's left ventricle. The entire system is zeroed at the transducer. Several seconds later, the patient raises both arms into the air until his right wrist is 20 cm above his heart. As he is doing this the BP on the monitor reads 120/80 mm Hg. What would this patient's true BP be at this time?
   A. 140/100 mm Hg
   B. 135/95 mm Hg
   C. 120/80 mm Hg
   D. 105/65 mm Hg

20. An admixture of room air in the waste gas disposal system during an appendectomy in a paralyzed, mechanically ventilated patient under general volatile anesthesia can best be explained by which mechanism of entry?
   A. Positive-pressure relief valve
   B. Negative-pressure relief valve
   C. Soda lime canister
   D. Ventilator bellows

21. Automated noninvasive blood pressure (ANIBP) devices calculate which of the following using proprietary algorithms?
   A. Systolic BP
   B. Diastolic BP
   C. Mean arterial BP
   D. Both systolic and diastolic BPs

22. Currently, the commonly used vaporizers (e.g., GE-Datex-Ohmeda Tec 4, Tec 5, Tec 7; Dräger Vapor 19.n and 2000 series) are described as having all of the following features **EXCEPT**
   A. Agent specificity
   B. Variable bypass
   C. Bubble through
   D. Temperature compensated

23. For any given concentration of volatile anesthetic, the splitting ratio is dependent on which of the following characteristics of that volatile anesthetic?
   A. Vapor pressure
   B. Molecular weight
   C. Specific heat
   D. Minimum alveolar concentration (MAC) at 1 atmosphere

24. On Monday morning the absorbent granules in your anesthesia machine, which was not used in the last 48 hours, are violet. In addition to rebreathing CO_2 when exhausted, this form of absorbent also carries the risk of
   A. Channeling
   B. Fire
   C. Compound A formation
   D. Carbon monoxide production

25. During the pre-anesthesia checkout (PAC) of the anesthesia delivery system, the mounted oxygen E cylinder is shown to have a pressure of 1200 psi. Before proceeding with the next case, the most appropriate action would be:
   A. Leave cylinder valve open and proceed with case
   B. Close cylinder valve and proceed with case
   C. Replace the cylinder, open valve to check pressure, then close and proceed with case
   D. Replace the cylinder, open valve to check pressure, and proceed with case

26. ECG monitors utilize high- and low-frequency filters to reduce noise (artifact). Which of the following are reduced with low-frequency filtering?
   A. Muscle fasciculation
   B. Respirations
   C. Tremor
   D. Electromagnetic interference from other devices

27. If the anesthesia machine is discovered Monday morning to have run with 5 L/min of oxygen all weekend long, the most reasonable course of action before administering the next anesthetic would be to
   A. Administer 100% oxygen for the first hour of the next case
   B. Place humidifier in line with the expiratory limb
   C. Avoid use of sevoflurane
   D. Change the CO_2 absorbent

28. According to National Institute for Occupational Safety and Health (NIOSH) regulations, the highest concentration of volatile anesthetic contamination allowed in the OR atmosphere when administered in conjunction with N_2O is
   A. 0.5 ppm
   B. 2 ppm
   C. 5 ppm
   D. 25 ppm

29. The device on anesthesia machines that most reliably detects delivery of hypoxic gas mixtures is the
   A. Fail-safe valve
   B. O_2 analyzer
   C. Second-stage O_2 pressure regulator
   D. Proportion-limiting control system

30. A ventilator pressure-relief valve stuck in the closed position can result in
   A. Barotrauma
   B. Hypoventilation
   C. Hyperventilation
   D. Low breathing circuit pressure

31. A mixture of 1% isoflurane, 70% N_2O, and 30% O_2 is administered to a patient for 30 minutes. The expired isoflurane concentration measured is 1%. N_2O is shut off, and a mixture of 30% O_2 and 70% N_2 with 1% isoflurane is administered. The expired isoflurane concentration measured 1 minute after the start of this new mixture is 2.3%. The best explanation for this observation is
    A. Intermittent back pressure (pumping effect)
    B. Diffusion hypoxia
    C. Concentration effect
    D. Effect of N_2O solubility in isoflurane

32.

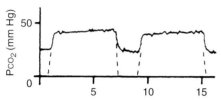

(From van Genderingen HR et al: Computer-assisted capnogram analysis, J Clin Monit 3:194–200, 1987, with kind permission of Kluwer Academic Publishers.)

The capnogram waveform above represents which of the following situations?
    A. Kinked endotracheal tube
    B. Bronchospasm
    C. Incompetent inspiratory valve
    D. Incompetent expiratory valve

33. Select the **FALSE** statement.
    A. If a Magill forceps is used for a nasotracheal intubation, the right nares is preferable for insertion of the nasotracheal tube
    B. Extension of the neck can convert an endotracheal intubation to an endobronchial intubation
    C. Bucking signifies the return of the coughing reflex
    D. Postintubation pharyngitis is more likely to occur in female patients

34. Gas from an N_2O compressed-gas cylinder enters the anesthesia machine through a pressure regulator that reduces the pressure to
    A. 60 psi
    B. 45 psi
    C. 30 psi
    D. 15 psi

35. Eye protection for OR staff is needed when laser surgery is performed. Clear wraparound goggles or glasses are adequate with which kind of laser?
    A. Argon laser
    B. Nd:YAG (neodymium:yttrium-aluminum-garnet) laser
    C. CO_2 laser
    D. None of the above

36. Which of the following systems prevents attachment of gas-administering equipment to the wrong type of gas line?
    A. Pin index safety system
    B. Diameter index safety system
    C. Fail-safe system
    D. Proportion-limiting control system

37. A 59-year-old pacemaker-dependent patient comes to surgery with the pacemaker programmed in the DDD mode. Extracorporeal shock wave lithotripsy (ESWL) is scheduled for fragmentation of several 3- to 5-mm kidney stones. What preparation is needed before undertaking ESWL in this setting to avoid inappropriate firing of the lithotripter?
    A. Program pacemaker to DVI
    B. Program pacemaker to VVI
    C. Program pacemaker to DOO
    D. Proceed with the case

38. The dial of an isoflurane-specific, variable bypass, temperature-compensated, flowover, out-of-circuit vaporizer (i.e., modern vaporizer) is set on 2%, and the infrared spectrometer measures 2% isoflurane vapor from the common gas outlet. The flowmeter is set at a rate of 700 mL/min during this measurement. The output measurements are repeated with the flowmeter set at 100 mL/min and 15 L/min (vapor dial still set on 2%). How will these two measurements compare with the first measurement taken?
    A. Output will be less than 2% in both cases
    B. Output will be greater than 2% in both cases
    C. Output will be 2% at 100 mL/min O_2 flow and less than 2% at 15 L/min flow
    D. Output will be less than 2% at 100 mL/min and 2% at 15 L/min

39. Which of the following would result in the greatest decrease in the arterial hemoglobin saturation (SpO_2) value measured by the dual-wavelength pulse oximeter?
    A. Intravenous injection of indigo carmine
    B. Intravenous injection of indocyanine green
    C. Intravenous injection of methylene blue
    D. Elevation of bilirubin

40. A 45-year-old patient recovering in the ICU after a motor vehicle accident is continuously being assessed with transcutaneous O_2 and CO_2 monitoring. Compared with conventional arterial blood gas values, those for transcutaneous oxygen ($PtcO_2$) and transcutaneous carbon dioxide ($PtcCO_2$) would likely be
    A. Higher (both)
    B. $PtcO_2$ lower, $PtcCO_2$ higher
    C. $PtcO_2$ higher, $PtcCO_2$ lower
    D. Lower (both)

41. Which of the following combinations would result in delivery of a lower-than-expected concentration of volatile anesthetic to the patient?
    A. Sevoflurane vaporizer filled with desflurane
    B. Isoflurane vaporizer filled with sevoflurane
    C. Sevoflurane vaporizer filled with isoflurane
    D. All of the above would result in less than the dialed concentration

42. At high altitudes, the flow of a gas through a rotameter will be
    A. Greater than expected
    B. Less than expected
    C. Less than expected at high flows but greater than expected at low flows
    D. Greater than expected at high flows but accurate at low flows

43. A patient presents for knee arthroscopy and tells his anesthesiologist that he has a VDD pacemaker. Select the true statement regarding this pacemaker.
    A. It senses and paces only the ventricle
    B. It paces only the ventricle
    C. Its response to a sensed event is always inhibition
    D. It is not useful in a patient with atrioventricular (AV) nodal block

44. All of the following would result in less trace gas pollution of the OR atmosphere **EXCEPT**
    A. Use of a high gas flow in a circular system
    B. Tight mask seal during mask induction
    C. Use of a scavenging system
    D. Allow patient to breathe 100% O_2 as long as possible before extubation

45. The greatest source for contamination of the OR atmosphere is leakage of volatile anesthetics
    A. Around the anesthesia mask
    B. At the vaporizer
    C. At the CO_2 absorber
    D. At the endotracheal tube

46. Uptake of sevoflurane from the lungs during the first minute of general anesthesia is 50 mL. How much sevoflurane would be taken up from the lungs between the 16th and 36th minutes?
    A. 25 mL
    B. 50 mL
    C. 100 mL
    D. 500 mL

47. Which of the drugs below would have the **LEAST** impact on somatosensory evoked potentials (SSEPs) monitoring in a 15-year-old patient undergoing scoliosis surgery?
    A. Midazolam
    B. Propofol
    C. Isoflurane
    D. Vecuronium

48. Which of the following is **NOT** found in the low-pressure circuit on an anesthesia machine?
    A. Oxygen supply failure alarm
    B. Flowmeters
    C. Vaporizers
    D. Vaporizer check valve

49. Frost develops on the outside of an N_2O compressed-gas cylinder during general anesthesia. This phenomenon indicates that
    A. The saturated vapor pressure of N_2O within the cylinder is rapidly increasing
    B. The cylinder is almost empty
    C. There is a rapid transfer of heat to the cylinder
    D. The flow of N_2O from the cylinder into the anesthesia machine is rapid

50. The **LEAST** reliable site for central temperature monitoring is the
    A. PA
    B. Skin on the forehead
    C. Distal third of the esophagus
    D. Nasopharynx

51. Of the following medical lasers, which laser light penetrates tissues the most?
    A. Argon laser
    B. Helium–neon laser (He–Ne)
    C. Nd:YAG laser
    D. CO_2 laser

52. Which of the following supraglottic airway devices features a built-in bite block, a channel for nasogastric suctioning, and a cuff modified to extend to the posterior surface of the mask?
    A. LMA Fastrach
    B. LMA Supreme
    C. Air-Q
    D. I-Gel

53. The maximum F_{IO_2} that can be delivered by a nasal cannula is
    A. 0.30
    B. 0.35
    C. 0.40
    D. 0.45

54. General anesthesia is administered to an otherwise healthy 38-year-old patient undergoing repair of a right inguinal hernia. During mechanical ventilation, the anesthesiologist notices that the scavenging system reservoir bag is distended during inspiration. The most likely cause of this is
A. An incompetent pressure-relief valve in the mechanical ventilator
B. An incompetent pressure-relief valve in the patient's breathing circuit
C. An incompetent inspiratory unidirectional valve in the patient's breathing circuit
D. An incompetent expiratory unidirectional valve in the patient's breathing circuit

55. Which color of nail polish would have the greatest effect on the accuracy of dual-wavelength pulse oximeters?
A. Red
B. Yellow
C. Blue
D. Green

56. The minimum macroshock current required to elicit ventricular fibrillation is
A. 1 mA
B. 10 mA
C. 100 mA
D. 500 mA

57. The line isolation monitor
A. Prevents microshock
B. Prevents macroshock
C. Provides electric isolation in the OR
D. Sounds an alarm when grounding occurs in the OR

58. Kinking or occlusion of the transfer tubing from the patient's breathing circuit to the closed scavenging system interface can result in
A. Barotrauma
B. Hypoventilation
C. Hypoxia
D. Hyperventilation

59. The reason a patient is not burned by the return of energy from the patient to the ESU (electrosurgical unit, Bovie) is that
A. The coagulation side of this circuit is positive relative to the ground side
B. Resistance in the patient's body attenuates the energy
C. The exit current density is much less than…?
D. The exit current density is much less than that at the handpiece

60. Select the **FALSE** statement regarding noninvasive arterial BP monitoring devices.
A. If the width of the BP cuff is too narrow, the measured BP will be falsely lowered
B. The width of the BP cuff should be 40% of the circumference of the patient's arm
C. If the BP cuff is wrapped around the arm too loosely, the measured BP will be falsely elevated
D. Frequent cycling of automated BP monitoring devices can result in edema distal to the cuff

61. When electrocardiogram (ECG) electrodes are placed for a patient undergoing a magnetic resonance imaging (MRI) scan, which of the following is true?
A. Electrodes should be as close as possible and in the periphery of the magnetic field
B. Electrodes should be as close as possible and in the center of the magnetic field
C. Placement of electrodes relative to field is not important as long as they are far apart
D. ECG cannot be monitored during an MRI scan

62. Which of the reasons below best accounts for the capnography tracing depicted in this figure?

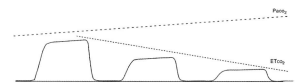

(Adapted from Szocik J, Teig M, Tremper K. Anesthetic monitoring. In: Basics of Anesthesia, ed 7, Pardo M, Miller R (Eds). Elsevier; 2018.)

A. Severe obstructive airways disease
B. Exhausted CO_2 absorbent
C. Ruptured cuff
D. Pulmonary embolism

63. The most frequent cause of mechanical failure of the anesthesia delivery system to deliver adequate O_2 to the patient is
A. Attachment of the wrong compressed-gas cylinder to the O_2 yoke
B. Improperly assembled O_2 rotameter
C. Fresh-gas line disconnection from the anesthesia machine to the in-line hosing
D. Disconnection of the O_2 supply system from the patient

64. The esophageal detector device
A. Uses a negative-pressure bulb
B. Is especially useful in children younger than 1 year of age
C. Requires a cardiac output to function appropriately
D. Is reliable in morbidly obese patients and parturients

65. The reason CO_2 measured by capnometer is less than the arterial Pa_{CO_2} value measured simultaneously is
  A. Use of ion-specific electrode for blood gas determination
  B. Alveolar capillary gradient
  C. One-way values
  D. Alveolar dead space

66. Which of the following arrangements of rotameters on the anesthesia machine manifold is safest with left-to-right gas flow?
  A. O_2, CO_2, N_2O, air
  B. CO_2, O_2, N_2O, air
  C. Air, CO_2, O_2, N_2O
  D. Air, CO_2, N_2O, O_2

67. A Datex-Ohmeda Tec 4 vaporizer is tipped over while being attached to the anesthesia machine but is placed upright and installed. The soonest it can be safely used is
  A. After 30 minutes of flushing with dial set to "off"
  B. After 6 hours of flushing with dial set to "off"
  C. After 30 minutes with dial turned on
  D. Immediately

68. In the event of misfilling, what percent sevoflurane would be delivered from an isoflurane vaporizer set at 1%?
  A. 0.6%
  B. 0.8%
  C. 1.0%
  D. 1.2%

69. How long would a vaporizer (filled with 150 mL volatile) deliver 2% isoflurane if total flow is set at 4.0 L/min?
  A. 2 hours
  B. 4 hours
  C. 6 hours
  D. 8 hours

70. Raising the frequency of an ultrasound transducer used for line placement or regional anesthesia (e.g., from 3 MHz to 10 MHz) will result in
  A. Higher penetration of tissue with lower resolution
  B. Higher penetration of tissue with higher resolution
  C. Lower penetration of tissue with higher resolution
  D. Higher resolution with no change in tissue penetration

71. The fundamental difference between microshock and macroshock is related to
  A. Location of shock
  B. Duration
  C. Voltage
  D. Lethality

72. Intraoperative awareness under general anesthesia can be eliminated by closely monitoring
  A. Electroencephalogram
  B. BP/heart rate
  C. Bispectral index (BIS)
  D. None of the above

73. A mechanically ventilated patient is transported from the OR to the ICU using a portable ventilator that consumes 2 L/min of oxygen to run the mechanically controlled valves and drive the ventilator. The transport cart is equipped with an "E" cylinder with a gauge pressure of 2000 psi. The patient receives a tidal volume (V_T) of 500 mL at a rate of 10 breaths/min. If the ventilator requires 200 psi to operate, how long could the patient be mechanically ventilated?
  A. 20 minutes
  B. 40 minutes
  C. 60 minutes
  D. 80 minutes

74. A 135-kg man is ventilated at a rate of 14 breaths/min with a V_T of 600 mL and positive end-expiratory pressure (PEEP) of 5 cm H_2O during a laparoscopic banding procedure. Peak airway pressure is 50 cm H_2O, and the patient is fully relaxed with a nondepolarizing neuromuscular blocking agent. How can peak airway pressure be reduced without a loss of alveolar ventilation?
  A. Increase the inspiratory flow rate
  B. Take off PEEP
  C. Reduce the I:E ratio (e.g., change from 1:3 to 1:2)
  D. Decrease V_T to 300 and increase rate to 28

75. The pressure and volume per minute delivered from the central hospital oxygen supply are
  A. 2100 psi and 650 L/min
  B. 1600 psi and 100 L/min
  C. 75 psi and 100 L/min
  D. 50 psi and 50 L/min

76. During normal laminar airflow, resistance is dependent on which characteristic of oxygen?
  A. Density
  B. Viscosity
  C. Molecular weight
  D. Temperature

77. If the oxygen cylinder were being used as the source of oxygen at a remote anesthetizing location and the oxygen flush valve on an anesthesia machine were pressed and held down, as during an emergency situation, each of the items below would be bypassed during 100% oxygen delivery **EXCEPT**
  A. O_2 flowmeter
  B. First-stage regulator
  C. Vaporizer check valve
  D. Vaporizers

78. After induction and intubation with confirmation of tracheal placement, the O_2 saturation begins to fall. The O_2 analyzer shows 4% inspired oxygen. The oxygen line pressure is 65 psi. The O_2 tank on the back of the anesthesia machine has a pressure of 2100 psi and is turned on. The oxygen saturation continues to fall. The next step should be to
A. Exchange the tank
B. Replace pulse oximeter probe
C. Disconnect O_2 line from hospital source
D. Extubate and start mask ventilation

79. The correct location for placement of the V_5 lead is
A. Midclavicular line, third intercostal space
B. Anterior axillary line, fourth intercostal space
C. Midclavicular line, fifth intercostal space
D. Anterior axillary line, fifth intercostal space

80. The diameter index safety system refers to the interface between
A. Pipeline source and anesthesia machine
B. Gas cylinders and anesthesia machine
C. Vaporizers and refilling connectors attached to bottles of volatile anesthetics
D. Both pipeline and gas cylinders interface with anesthesia machine

81. Each of the following is cited as an advantage of calcium hydroxide lime (Amsorb Plus, Drägersorb) over soda lime **EXCEPT**
A. Compound A is not formed
B. CO is not formed
C. More absorptive capacity per 100 g of granules
D. It does not contain NaOH or KOH

82.

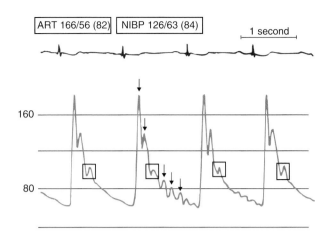

(From Mark JB: Atlas of Cardiovascular Monitoring, New York, Churchill Livingstone, 1998, Figure 9-4.)

The arrows in the figure above indicate
A. Respiratory variation
B. An underdamped signal
C. An overdamped signal
D. Atrial fibrillation

83. During a laparoscopic cholecystectomy, exhaled CO_2 is 6%, but inhaled CO_2 is 1%. Which explanation could **NOT** account for the 1% inhaled CO_2?
A. Channeling through soda lime
B. Faulty expiratory valve
C. Exhausted soda lime
D. Absorption of CO_2 through peritoneum

DIRECTIONS (Questions 84 through 86): Please match the color of the compressed-gas cylinder with the appropriate gas.

84. Helium

85. Nitrogen

86. CO_2

A. Black
B. Brown
C. Orange
D. Gray

DIRECTIONS (Questions 87 through 90): Match the figures below with the correct numbered statement. Each lettered figure may be selected once, more than once, or not at all.

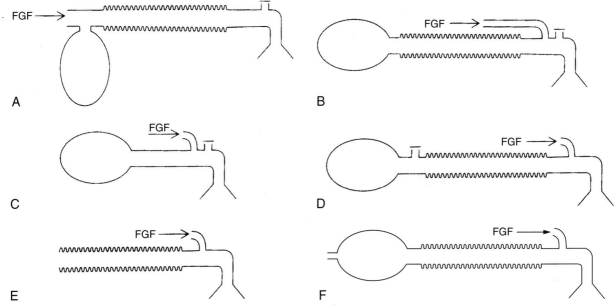

(Modified from Willis BA, Pender JW, Mapleson WW: Rebreathing in a T-piece: volunteer and theoretical studies of Jackson-Rees modification of Ayre's T-piece during spontaneous respiration, Br J Anaesth 47:1239–1246, 1975. © The Board of Management and Trustees of the British Journal of Anesthesia. Reproduced by permission of Oxford University Press/British Journal of Anesthesia.)

87. Best for spontaneous ventilation

88. Best for controlled ventilation

89. Bain system is modification of

90. Jackson-Rees system

Anesthesia Equipment and Physics
Answers, Explanations, and References

1. (D) Cardiac output is determined by four main factors: preload, afterload, myocardial contractility, and heart rate. An intravascular fluid challenge is frequently used to increase preload and cardiac output. Preload refers to the amount of stretch of the cardiac muscle at the start of systole and is indirectly determined by the pressure in the ventricle (an increase in pressure usually means increase to stretch, unless there is a cardiac tamponade, which prevents the heart from filling). Afterload refers to the resistance in blood flow from the ventricle as determined by the aortic valve or arterial resistance. Contractility refers to the measurement of force the cardiac muscle can generate.

A PA catheter is often placed to measure the CVP, PA pressure, and wedge pressure, and can determine the cardiac output (usually by thermodilution). The CVP measures the filling pressure for the right ventricle, and the PA occlusion or wedge pressure measures the filling pressure for the left ventricle. TEE can be used to look at the size of the ventricular chambers and how well they contract (e.g., ejection fraction).

When a patient is receiving positive pressure ventilation, measurement of PPV or systolic pressure variation (SPV) can be done. When positive pressure is applied to the lungs during mechanical ventilation (i.e., during inspiration), venous return to the right side of the heart and right ventricle stroke volume is reduced, decreasing cardiac output and systolic BP. Pulse pressure is the difference between systolic and diastolic BPs. PPV is defined as the pulse pressure between breaths (PPmax) minus the pulse pressure during positive pressure ventilation (PPmin) divided by the mean pulse pressure (PPmax + PPmin/2) times 100%. For example, if the PPmax is 90 (systolic BP 160, diastolic 70) and the PPmin is 70 (systolic BP 130, diastolic 60) then the PPV = (90 - 70)/80 = 25%. Patients are considered fluid responsive (i.e., an increase in BP or cardiac output) if the PPV is >15% and not fluid responsive if the PPV is <7%. Alternatively, SPV, which is the difference in systolic BP during inspiration (positive intrathoracic pressure) and expiration, can be determined, with normal values of 7 to 10 mm Hg. Hypovolemic patients have an elevation in SPV. Patients with an SPV >10 mm Hg are fluid responsive, whereas those with an SPV <5 mm Hg are not fluid responsive.

For both SPV and PPV the patient must be mechanically ventilated and in a regular rhythm (not in atrial fibrillation) for the calculations. Measurements of BP are with an arterial line. This patient has been extubated, so measurement of PPV or SPV cannot be performed. *(Miller: Basics of Anesthesia, ed 7, pp 352–357; Miller: Miller's Anesthesia, ed 8, pp 1359–1361).*

2. (C) **Color Flow**. This Doppler modality is an application of pulsed wave Doppler technology that allows determination of velocity at a specific location. Velocity is color coded and superimposed over a two-dimensional image. However, like pulsed wave Doppler, color Doppler is limited by signal aliasing. Fluid or tissue that moves toward the probe causes compression of sound waves and an increase in the received frequency, whereas motion away from the probe leads to a reduced frequency. Although ultrasound machine color maps can often be adjusted, by convention flow toward the probe is coded red, whereas flow away from the probe is coded blue (BART: Blue Away Red Toward).

Continuous wave Doppler. Continuous wave Doppler uses two dedicated ultrasound crystals, one for continuous transmission and a second for continuous reception of ultrasound signals. This permits measurement of very high frequency Doppler shifts or velocities. The "cost" is range ambiguity. In other words, the precise location of the peak velocity along the length of the Doppler cursor is not definitely known. Instead, the clinician must infer the location of the highest velocity, such as a stenotic aortic valve. Continuous wave Doppler is used for measuring very high velocities (e.g., stenosis of a valve or prosthesis).

Pulsed Doppler. In contrast to continuous wave Doppler, which records the signal along the entire length of the ultrasound beam, pulsed wave Doppler permits sampling of blood flow velocities from a specific region, known as the sample volume. This modality is particularly useful for assessing the relatively low velocity flows associated with transmitral or transtricuspid blood flow, pulmonary venous flow, and left atrial appendage flow. To permit this, a pulse of ultrasound is transmitted by a single piezoelectric crystal, and then the receiver "listens" during a subsequent interval defined by the distance from the transmitter and the sample site. This transducer mode of transmit-wait-receive is repeated at an interval termed the pulse-repetition frequency (PRF). The PRF is therefore depth dependent, being greater for near regions and lower for distant or deeper regions. The position of the sample volume is varied by adjusting the length of the transducer "receive" interval. In contrast to continuous wave Doppler, which is sometimes performed without two-dimensional guidance, pulsed Doppler is always performed with two-dimensional guidance to determine the sample volume position. Because pulsed wave Doppler echo repeatedly samples the returning signal, there is a maximum limit to the frequency shift or velocity that can be measured unambiguously. Thus the maximum detectable frequency shift, or Nyquist limit, is one half the PRF. If the velocity of interest exceeds the Nyquist limit, "wraparound" of the signal occurs, first into the reverse channel and then back to the forward channel; this is known as aliasing. *(Barash: Clinical Anesthesia, ed 8, p 743).*

3. (B) The pressure gauge on a size "E" compressed-gas cylinder containing liquid N_2O shows 750 psi when it is full and will continue to register 750 psi until approximately three fourths of the N_2O has left the cylinder (i.e., liquid N_2O has all been vaporized). A full cylinder of N_2O contains 1590 L. Therefore when 400 L of gas remain in the cylinder, the pressure within the cylinder will begin to fall *(Miller: Basics of Anesthesia, ed 7, p 223; Barash: Clinical Anesthesia, ed 8, p 658).*

4. (D) Desflurane is unique among the current commonly used volatile anesthetics because of its high vapor pressure of 664 mm Hg. Because of the high vapor pressure, the vaporizer is pressurized to 1500 mm Hg and electrically heated to 23° C to give more predictable concentrations: 664/1500 = about 44%. If desflurane were used at 1 atmosphere, the concentration would be about 88% [664 mm Hg/760 mm Hg = 88]. *(Barash: Clinical Anesthesia, ed 8, p 461).*

5. (D) Factors that influence the rate of laminar flow of a substance through a tube are described by the Hagen-Poiseuille law of friction. The mathematical expression of the Hagen-Poiseuille law of friction is as follows:

$$\dot{V} = \frac{\pi r^4 (\Delta P)}{8 L \mu}$$

where $\dot{V}$ is the flow of the substance, r is the radius of the tube, ΔP is the pressure gradient down the tube, L is the length of the tube, and μ is the viscosity of the substance. Note that the rate of laminar flow is proportional to the radius of the tube to the fourth power. If the diameter of an intravenous catheter is doubled, flow would increase by a factor of two raised to the fourth power (i.e., a factor of 16) *(Ehrenwerth: Anesthesia Equipment: Principles and Applications, ed 2, pp 377–378; Barash: Clinical Anesthesia, ed 8, pp 365–366).*

6. (C) The World Health Organization requires that compressed-gas cylinders containing N_2O for medical use be painted blue. Size "E" compressed-gas cylinders completely filled with liquid N_2O contain approximately 1590 L of gas. See table from Explanation 10 *(Barash: Clinical Anesthesia, ed 8, p 658).*

7. (D) Anesthesia machines should be checked each day before their use. For most machines, three parts are checked before use: calibration for the oxygen analyzer, the low-pressure circuit leak test, and the circle system. Many consider the low-pressure circuit the area most vulnerable for problems because it is more subject to leaks. Leaks in this part of the machine have been associated with intraoperative awareness (e.g., loose vaporizer filling caps) and hypoxia. To test the low-pressure part of the machine, several tests have been used. For the positive-pressure test, positive pressure is applied to the circuit by depressing the oxygen flush button and occluding the Y-piece of the circle system (which is connected to the endotracheal tube or the anesthesia mask during anesthetic administration) and looking for positive pressure detected by the airway pressure gauge. A leak in the low-pressure part of the machine or the circle system will be demonstrated by a decrease in airway pressure. With many newer machines, a check valve is positioned downstream from the flowmeters (rotameters) and vaporizers but upstream from the oxygen flush valve, which would not permit the positive pressure from the circle system to flow back to the low-pressure circuit. In these machines with the check valve, the positive-pressure reading will fall only with a leak in the circle part, but a leak in the low-pressure circuit of the anesthesia machine will not be detected. In 1993 use of the U.S. Food and Drug Administration universal negative-pressure leak test was encouraged, whereby the machine master switch and the flow valves are turned off, and a suction bulb is collapsed and attached to the common or fresh gas outlet of the machine. If the bulb stays fully collapsed for at least 10 seconds, a leak did not exist (this needs to be repeated for each vaporizer, each one opened at a time). Of course, when the test is completed, the fresh gas hose is reconnected to the circle system. Because machines continue to be developed and to differ from one another, you should be familiar with each manufacturer's machine preoperative checklist. For example, the negative-pressure leak test is recommended for Ohmeda Unitrol, Ohmeda 30/70, Ohmeda Modulus I, Ohmeda Modulus II and II plus, Ohmeda Excel series, Ohmeda CD, and

Datex-Ohmeda Aestiva. The Dräger Narkomed 2A, 2B, 2C, 3, 4, and GS require a positive-pressure leak test. The Fabius GS, Narkomed 6000, and Datex-Ohmeda S5/ADU have self-tests (Miller: Miller's Anesthesia, ed 8, pp 752–755; Barash: Clinical Anesthesia, ed 8, p 654).

Negative Pressure Leak Test

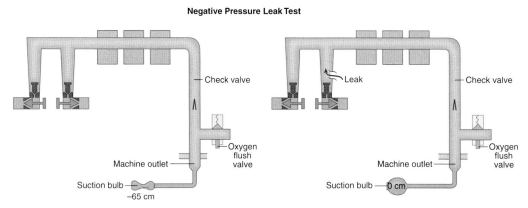

(Reprinted with permission from Andrews JJ: Understanding anesthesia machines. In: 1988 Review Course Lectures, Cleveland, International Anesthesia Research Society, 1988, p 78.)

8. (B) Check valves permit only unidirectional flow of gases. These valves prevent retrograde flow of gases from the anesthesia machine or the transfer of gas from a compressed-gas cylinder at high pressure into a container at a lower pressure. Thus these unidirectional valves will allow an empty compressed-gas cylinder to be exchanged for a full one during operation of the anesthesia machine with minimal loss of gas. The adjustable pressure-limiting valve is a synonym for a pop-off valve and can be adjusted to allow varying degrees of pressure to be transmitted to the patient. A fail-safe valve is a synonym for a pressure-sensor shutoff valve. The purpose of a fail-safe valve is to discontinue the flow of N_2O (or proportionally reduce it) if the O_2 pressure within the anesthesia machine falls below 30 psi *(Miller: Miller's Anesthesia, ed 8, p 756; Barash: Clinical Anesthesia, ed 8, p 657).*

9. (A) The control mechanism of standard anesthesia ventilators, such as the Ohmeda 7000, uses compressed oxygen (100%) to compress the ventilator bellows and electric power for the timing circuits. Some ventilators (e.g., North American Dräger AV-E and AV-2+) use a Venturi device, which mixes oxygen and air. Still other ventilators use sophisticated digital controls that allow advanced ventilation modes. These ventilators use an electric stepper motor attached to a piston (Miller: Miller's Anesthesia, ed 8, p 757; Ehrenwerth: Anesthesia Equipment: Principles and Applications, ed 2, pp 160–161; Barash: Clinical Anesthesia, ed 8, p 684).

10. (C) U.S. manufacturers require that all compressed-gas cylinders containing O_2 for medical use be painted green. A compressed-gas cylinder completely filled with O_2 has a pressure of approximately 2000 psi and contains approximately 625 L of gas. According to Boyle's law, the volume of gas remaining in a closed container can be estimated by measuring the pressure within the container. Therefore, when the pressure gauge on a compressed-gas cylinder containing O_2 shows a pressure of 1600 psi, the cylinder contains 500 L (1600 psi /2100 psi = 0.77 and 0.77 times 650 = 500) of O_2. At a gas flow of 2 L/min, O_2 could be delivered from the cylinder for approximately 250 minutes (Ehrenwerth: Anesthesia Equipment: Principles and Applications, ed 2, p 4; Butterworth: Barash: Clinical Anesthesia, ed 8, p 657).

CHARACTERISTICS OF COMPRESSED GASES STORED IN "E" SIZE CYLINDERS THAT MAY BE ATTACHED TO THE ANESTHESIA MACHINE

Characteristics	Oxygen	N₂O	CO₂	Air
Cylinder color	Green*	Blue	Gray	Yellow*
Physical state in cylinder	Gas	Liquid and gas	Liquid and gas	Gas
Cylinder contents (L)	625	1590	1590	625
Cylinder weight empty (kg)	5.90	5.90	5.90	5.90
Cylinder weight full (kg)	6.76	8.80	8.90	5.90
Cylinder pressure full (psi)	2000	750	838	1800

*The World Health Organization specifies that cylinders containing oxygen for medical use be painted white, but manufacturers in the United States use green. Likewise, the international color for air is white and black, whereas cylinders in the United States are color-coded yellow.
From Miller RD: Basics of Anesthesia, ed 6, Philadelphia, Saunders, 2011, p 201, Table 15-2.

11. (B) Given the description of the problem, no flow of O_2 through the O_2 rotameter is the correct choice. In a normally functioning rotameter, gas flows between the rim of the bobbin and the wall of the Thorpe tube, causing the bobbin to rotate. If the bobbin is rotating, you can be certain that gas is flowing through the rotameter and that the bobbin is not stuck *(Ehrenwerth: Anesthesia Equipment: Principles and Applications, ed 2, pp 43–45; Barash: Clinical Anesthesia, ed 8, pp 661–662).*

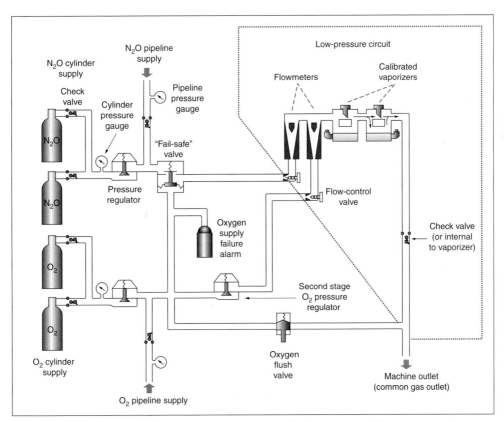

(Modified from American Society of Anesthesiologists (ASA): Check-out: A Guide for Preoperative Inspection of an Anesthesia Machine, Park Ridge, IS, ASA, 1987. A copy of the full text can be obtained from the ASA at 520 N. Northwest Highway, Park Ridge, IL 60068-2573.)

12. (B) Fail-safe valve is a synonym for pressure-sensor shutoff valve. The purpose of the fail-safe valve is to prevent the delivery of hypoxic gas mixtures from the anesthesia machine to the patient resulting from failure of the O_2 supply. Most modern anesthesia machines, however, would not allow a hypoxic mixture, because the knob controlling the N_2O is linked to the O_2 knob. When the O_2 pressure within the anesthesia machine decreases below 30 psi, this valve discontinues the flow of N_2O or proportionally decreases the flow of all gases. It is important to realize that this valve will not prevent the delivery of hypoxic gas mixtures or pure N_2O when the O_2 rotameter is off, because the O_2 pressure within the circuits of the anesthesia machine is maintained by an open O_2 compressed-gas cylinder or a central supply source. Under these circumstances, an O_2 analyzer will be needed to detect the delivery of a hypoxic gas mixture *(Ehrenwerth: Anesthesia Equipment: Principles and Applications, ed 2, pp 37–40; Barash: Clinical Anesthesia, ed 8, p 656).*

13. (C) It is important to zero the electromechanical transducer system with the reference point at the approximate level of the heart. This will eliminate the effect of the fluid column of the transducer system on the arterial BP reading of the system. In this question, the system was zeroed at the stopcock, which was located at the patient's wrist (approximate level of the ventricle). The BP expressed by the arterial line will therefore be accurate, provided the stopcock remains at the wrist and the transducer is not moved once zeroed. Raising the arm (e.g., 15 cm) decreases the BP at the wrist but increases the pressure on the transducer by the same amount (i.e., the vertical tubing length is now 15 cm H_2O higher than before) (Ehrenwerth: Anesthesia Equipment: Principles and Applications, ed 2, pp 276–278; Miller: Miller's Anesthesia, ed 8, pp 1354–1355; Barash: Clinical Anesthesia, ed 8, p 714).

14. (C) O_2 and N_2O enter the anesthesia machine from a central supply source or compressed-gas cylinders at pressures as high as 2200 psi (O_2) and 750 psi (N_2O). First-stage pressure regulators reduce these pressures to approximately 45 psi. Before entering the rotameters, second-stage O_2 pressure regulators further reduce the pressure to approximately 14 to 16 psi. (Miller: Miller's Anesthesia, ed 8, p 761; Barash: Clinical Anesthesia, ed 8, pp 660–661).

15. (B) This patient has a huge air leak. Before switching to an anesthesia bag connected to a separate oxygen source, possible reasons to consider include disconnected hoses (inspiratory limb or expiratory limb) from the circle system, disconnection of the Y piece from the anesthesia circuit to the endotracheal tube (ETT) tube, failure to close the CO_2 absorber or a crack in the CO_2 absorber system, check valve or anesthesia pressure limiting valve (pop-off valve) malfunction, flowmeter or vaporizer leak, disconnection in the oxygen analyzer, disconnection from the fresh gas flow to the circle system, and pipeline pressure below 50 psi causing a failure in the oxygen supply pressure to give oxygen flow. Most of these should have been evaluated in the preoperative check of the machine before inducing anesthesia. When the same problem with ventilation occurs with an anesthesia bag connected to a separate oxygen source, the anesthesia machine is not the problem. Rarely would the leak from an underinflated ETT or an esophageal intubation cause that much of an air leak; however, when an NG tube inadvertently enters the trachea instead of the GI tract and the suction connected to the NG tube is turned on, you quickly deflate the lung and will not be able to adequately ventilate the patient. Resolution of the air leak will occur when NG suction is turned off or when the NG tube is removed from the trachea. (Miller: Miller's Anesthesia, ed 8, pp 752–817).

16. (C) Agent-specific vaporizers, such as the Sevotec (sevoflurane) vaporizer, are designed for each volatile anesthetic. However, volatile anesthetics with identical saturated vapor pressures can be used interchangeably, with accurate delivery of the volatile anesthetic. Although halothane is no longer used in the United States, that vaporizer, for example, may still be used in developing countries for administration of isoflurane (Ehrenwerth: Anesthesia Equipment: Principles and Applications, ed 2, pp 72–73; Barash: Clinical Anesthesia, ed 8, pp 668-669, 672).

VAPOR PRESSURES

Agent	Vapor Pressure mm Hg at 20° C
Halothane	243
Sevoflurane	160
Isoflurane	240
Desflurane	669

17. (B) Turbulent flow occurs when gas flows through a region of severe constriction such as that described in this question. Laminar flow occurs when gas flows down parallel-sided tubes at a rate less than critical velocity. When the gas flow exceeds the critical velocity, it becomes turbulent. (*Barash: Clinical Anesthesia, ed 8, p 366*).

18. (C) During turbulent flow, the resistance to gas flow is directly proportional to the density of the gas mixture. Substituting helium for oxygen will decrease the density of the gas mixture, thereby decreasing the resistance to gas flow (as much as threefold) through the region of constriction (Ehrenwerth: Anesthesia Equipment: Principles and Applications, ed 2, pp 230–234; Barash: Clinical Anesthesia, ed 8, pp 365–366).

19. (C) Modern electronic BP monitors are designed to interface with electromechanical transducer systems. These systems do not require extensive technical skill on the part of the anesthesia provider for accurate use. A static zeroing of the system is built into most modern electronic monitors. Thus after the zeroing procedure is accomplished, the system is ready for operation. The system should be zeroed with the reference point of the transducer at the approximate level of the aortic root, eliminating the effect of the fluid column of the system on arterial BP readings (Ehrenwerth: Anesthesia Equipment: Principles and Applications, ed 2, pp 276–278; Barash: Clinical Anesthesia, ed 8, pp 713–714).

20. (B) Waste gas disposal systems, also called scavenging systems, are designed to decrease pollution in the OR by anesthetic gases. These scavenging systems can be passive (waste gases flow from the anesthesia machine to a ventilation system on their own) or active (anesthesia machine is connected to a vacuum system, then to the ventilation system). Positive-pressure relief valves open if there is an obstruction between the anesthesia machine and the disposal system, which would then leak the gas into the OR. A leak in the soda lime canisters would also vent to the OR. Given that most ventilator bellows are powered by oxygen, a leak in the bellows will not add air to the evacuation system. The negative-pressure relief valve is used in active systems and will entrap room air if the pressure in the system is less than −0.5 cm H_2O. (Ehrenwerth: Anesthesia Equipment: Principles and Applications, ed 2, pp 101–103; Miller: Miller's Anesthesia, ed 8, p 802; Barash: Clinical Anesthesia, ed 8, pp 693–694).

21. (D) The standard method for BP measurements introduced by NS Korotkoff in 1905 was by auscultation, which measures the systolic (first sounds heard when the BP cuff is deflated) and diastolic BP (significantly muffled or disappearance of sounds with further deflation of the cuff), but not the mean arterial blood pressure (MAP). MAP is calculated using the following formula:

$$MAP = [(2 \text{ times the diastolic BP}) + \text{systolic BP}]/3$$

The reason the diastolic BP is multiplied by 2 is that the diastolic portion of the cardiac cycle is usually twice as long as the systolic portion of the cardiac cycle.

ANIBP measurements are based on oscillometry, with small changes in cuff pressure during cuff deflation used to estimate mean arterial BP. Both systolic and diastolic pressures are calculated according to proprietary algorithms by each manufacturer and are therefore less reliable than the values for MAP. Typically systolic BP corresponds to a pressure where escalating pulsations reach 25% to 50% of maximum. Diastolic pressure is the most unreliable calculation and is derived when the pulse amplitude is a small fraction of the peak amplitude. (*Miller: Anesthesia, ed 8, pp 1347–1348*).

22. (C) Because volatile anesthetics have different vapor pressures, the vaporizers are agent specific. Vaporizers are described as having variable bypass, which means that some of the total fresh gas flow (usually less than 20%) is diverted into the vaporizing chamber, and the rest bypasses the vaporizer. Tipping the vaporizers (which should not occur) may cause some of the liquid to enter the bypass circuit, leading to a high concentration of anesthetic being delivered to the patient. The gas that enters the vaporizer flows over (does not bubble through) the volatile anesthetic. The older (now obsolete) Copper Kettle and Vernitrol vaporizers were not agent specific, and oxygen (with a separate flowmeter) was bubbled through the volatile anesthetic; then, the combination of oxygen with volatile gas was diluted with the fresh gas flow (oxygen, air, N_2O) and administered to the patient. Because vaporization changes with temperature, modern vaporizers are designed to maintain a constant concentration over clinically used temperatures (20° C to 35° C) (*Barash: Clinical Anesthesia, ed 8, pp 668–678*).

23. (A) Vaporizers can be categorized into variable-bypass and measured-flow vaporizers. Measured-flow vaporizers (nonconcentration calibrated vaporizers) include the obsolete Copper Kettle and Vernitrol vaporizers. With measured-flow vaporizers, the flow of oxygen is selected on a separate flowmeter to pass into the vaporizing chamber, from which the anesthetic vapor emerges at its saturated vapor pressure. By contrast, in variable-bypass vaporizers, the total gas flow is split between a variable bypass and the vaporizer chamber containing the anesthetic agent. The ratio of these two flows is called the splitting ratio. The splitting ratio depends on the anesthetic agent, the temperature, the chosen vapor concentration set to be delivered to the patient, and the saturated vapor pressure of the anesthetic. (*Barash: Clinical Anesthesia, ed 8, pp 668–678*).

24. (A) Most anesthesia machines have a circle absorption system, which includes a canister of carbon dioxide (CO_2) absorbent that can effectively absorb exhaled CO_2. This allows the anesthesia machines to use lower fresh gas flows, decreasing the amount of expensive inhaled anesthetics used. CO_2 absorbents use the principle of neutralizing an acid ($CO_2 + H_2O$ produces carbonic acid $= H_2CO_3$) with a base (mostly calcium hydroxide $= Ca(OH)_2$). Some natural hydration of the granules is essential to allow the chemical reactions to occur. The end product of the reaction is calcium carbonate, water, and heat.

$$H_2CO_3 + Ca(OH)_2 \text{ produces calcium carbonate } (CaCO_3) + H_2O + Heat$$

Soda Lime contains: 76% to 81% $Ca(OH)_2$, 14% to 19% H_2O, 4% $NaOH$, and 1% KOH. $NaOH$ and KOH serve as an effective catalyst for the chemical reactions to occur. Unfortunately, these catalysts degrade sevoflurane to the nephrotoxic called compound A, and degrade desflurane as well as isoflurane to produce clinically significant amounts of carbon monoxide (CO) when the granules are desiccated.

The catalyst used in Amsorb Plus and Litholyme does not degrade sevoflurane to compound A and does not produce CO from volatile anesthetics when the granules are desiccated.

Amsorb Plus contains; >80% $Ca(OH)_2$, 13% to 18% H_2O, and 4% $CaCl_2$

Litholyme contains; >75% $Ca(OH)_2$, 12% to 19% H_2O, and 3% $LiCl$

The indicator dye used in soda lime that changes from off-white to violet can change back to the original white color when the granules dry. In contrast, the indicator dye for Amsorb Plus and Litholyme changes from off-white to violet but does not change back to off-white.

The absorptive capacity of Litholyme is similar to soda lime and slightly better than Amsorb Plus. In addition, there is less heat produced with the chemical reaction with Amsorb Plus and Litholyme compared with soda lime.

Channeling can occur with any absorbent type, and frank fire has only been reported with Baralyme, which is no longer available (*Miller: Basics of Anesthesia, ed 7, pp 233–236; Miller: Miller's Anesthesia, ed 8, pp 660–663, 787*).

25. (B) Recommendations for Pre-Anesthesia Checkout (PAC) Procedures (2008) made by the subcommittee of the American Society of Anesthesiologists (ASA) Committee on Equipment and Facilities clearly state, "the anesthesia care provider is ultimately responsible for proper function of all equipment used to provide anesthesia care."

Most anesthesia delivery systems have two sources of oxygen, a pipeline supply of oxygen (with a pressure >50 psi) and a backup oxygen cylinder in case there is a problem with the anesthesia pipeline supply. Item #5 of the ASA PAC refers to an adequate amount of pressure on the spare oxygen cylinder mounted on the anesthesia machine. Because of the increasing complexity of anesthesia delivery systems, the operating manuals should be understood. In general, the oxygen cylinder is used only when there is a failure of the pipeline oxygen supply. If there is no pipeline supply, then the oxygen cylinder must supply oxygen for the entire anesthetic. Although the ASA's 2008 checkout guidelines do not specify an exact pressure, manufacturer's manuals often recommend an oxygen cylinder pressure of >1000 psi.

After the tank is checked and found to have an adequate oxygen pressure, the tank's valve should be closed. The reason for closing the valve is to allow the activation of the machine's oxygen pressure alert when the pipeline pressure drops below a specific pressure. If activated, the provider becomes aware of the failure in pipeline supply of oxygen and then opens the valve to use the oxygen cylinder, knowing that the backup oxygen source is now being used. If the valve is left open and the pipeline supply fails, then the oxygen pressure alert will become activated only when the oxygen tank is also empty *(American Society of Anesthesiology – Recommendations for Pre Anesthesia Checkout Procedures (2008) in asahq.org; Miller: Miller's Anesthesia, ed 8, pp 804–817).*

26. (B) To improve signal quality, electrocardiographic monitors use filters to narrow the signal bandwidth to reduce environmental artifacts. These filters can be either low frequency (for distortion by patient movement such as those produced by breathing) or high frequency (for distortion from muscle fasciculations, tremors, or electrical equipment). Because the frequency filters can distort the ECG and produce false positive recordings (e.g., the ST segment or T wave changes), manufacturers have several filter modes, including a diagnostic mode that removes the filters. So if the ECG monitor looks different from the preoperative ECG, it may be best to turn off the filters and use the diagnostic mode *(Miller: Basics of Anesthesia, 7th ed, pp 345–346; Miller: Miller's Anesthesia, ed 8, pp 1434–2435).*

27. (D) CO can be generated when volatile anesthetics are exposed to CO_2 absorbers that contain NaOH or KOH (e.g., soda lime) and have sometimes produced carboxyhemoglobin levels of 35%. Factors that are involved in the production of CO and formation of carboxyhemoglobin include (1) the specific volatile anesthetic used (desflurane $\geq$ enflurane $>$ isoflurane $\gg$ sevoflurane $=$ halothane), (2) high concentrations of volatile anesthetic (more CO is generated at higher volatile concentrations), (3) high temperatures (more CO is generated at higher temperatures), (4) low fresh gas flows, and especially (5) dry soda lime (dry granules produce more CO than do hydrated granules). Soda lime contains 15% water by weight, and only when it gets dehydrated to below 1.4% will appreciable amounts of CO be formed. Many of the reported cases of patients experiencing elevated carboxyhemoglobin levels occurred on Monday mornings, when the fresh gas flow on the anesthesia circuit was not turned off and high anesthetic fresh gas flows ($>$5 L/min) for prolonged periods of time (e.g., >48 hours) occurred. Because of some resistance of the inspiratory valve, retrograde flow through the CO_2 absorber (which hastens the drying of the soda lime) will develop, especially if the breathing bag is absent, the Y-piece of the circuit is occluded, and the adjustable pressure-limiting valve is open. Whenever you are uncertain as to the dryness of the CO_2 absorber, especially when the fresh gas flow was not turned off the anesthesia machine for an extended or indeterminate period of time, the CO_2 absorber should be changed. This CO production occurs with soda lime and occurred more so with Baralyme (which is no longer available), but it does not occur with Amsorb Plus or Drägersorb Free (which contains calcium chloride and calcium hydroxide and no NaOH or KOH) *(Miller: Miller's Anesthesia, ed 8, pp 789–792; Barash: Clinical Anesthesia, ed 8, pp 681–683).*

28. (A) NIOSH mandates that the highest trace concentration of volatile anesthetic contamination of the OR atmosphere when administered in conjunction with N_2O is 0.5 ppm. *(Barash: Clinical Anesthesia, ed 8, p 691).*

29. (B) The O_2 analyzer is the last line of defense against the inadvertent delivery of hypoxic gas mixtures. It should be located in the inspiratory (not expiratory) limb of the patient's breathing circuit to provide maximum safety. Because the O_2 concentration in the fresh-gas supply line may be different from that of the patient's breathing circuit, the O_2 analyzer should not be located in the fresh-gas supply line *(Ehrenwerth: Anesthesia Equipment: Principles and Applications, ed 2, pp 209–210; Barash: Clinical Anesthesia, ed 8, pp 652–653).*

30. (A) The ventilator pressure-relief valve (also called the spill valve) is pressure controlled via pilot tubing that communicates with the ventilator bellows chamber. As pressure within the bellows chamber increases during the inspiratory phase of the ventilator cycle, the pressure is transmitted via the pilot tubing to close the pressure-relief valve, thus making the patient's breathing circuit "gas tight." This valve should open during the expiratory phase of the ventilator cycle to allow the release of excess gas from the patient's breathing circuit into the waste-gas scavenging circuit after the bellows has fully expanded. If the ventilator pressure-relief valve were to stick in the closed position, there would be a rapid buildup of pressure within the circle system that would be readily transmitted to the patient. Barotrauma to the patient's lungs would result if this situation were to continue unrecognized *(Barash: Clinical Anesthesia, ed 8, p 687).*

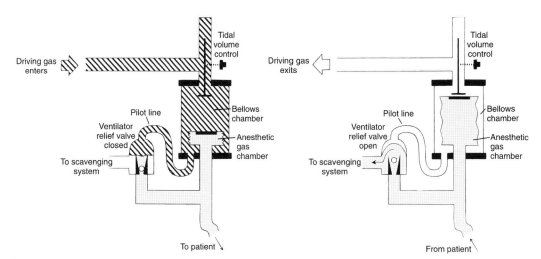

Tidal volume control

Driving gas enters

Pilot line

Ventilator relief valve closed

To scavenging system

Bellows chamber

Anesthetic gas chamber

To patient

Tidal volume control

Driving gas exits

Pilot line

Ventilator relief valve open

To scavenging system

Bellows chamber

Anesthetic gas chamber

From patient

(From Andrews JJ: Understanding your anesthesia machine and ventilator. In: 1989 Review Course Lectures, Cleveland, International Anesthesia Research Society, 1989, p 59.)

31. (D) Vaporizer output can be affected by the composition of the carrier gas used to vaporize the volatile agent in the vaporizing chamber, especially when N_2O is either initiated or discontinued. This observation can be explained by the solubility of N_2O in the volatile agent. When N_2O and oxygen enter the vaporizing chamber, a portion of the N_2O dissolves in the liquid agent. Thus the vaporizer output transiently decreases. Conversely, when N_2O is withdrawn as part of the carrier gas, the N_2O dissolved in the volatile agent comes out of solution, thereby transiently increasing the vaporizer output. *(Miller: Miller's Anesthesia, ed 8, pp 769–771).*

32. (D) The capnogram can provide a variety of information, such as verification of exhaled CO_2 after tracheal intubation, estimation of the differences in $Paco_2$ and $Petco_2$, abnormalities of ventilation, and hypercapnia or hypocapnia. The four phases of the capnogram are inspiratory baseline, expiratory upstroke, expiratory plateau, and inspiratory downstroke. The shape of the capnogram can be used to recognize and diagnose a variety of potentially adverse circumstances. Under normal conditions, the inspiratory baseline should be 0, indicating that there is no rebreathing of CO_2 with a normal functioning circle breathing system. If the inspiratory baseline is elevated above 0, there is rebreathing of CO_2.

If this occurs, the differential diagnosis should include an incompetent expiratory valve, exhausted CO_2 absorbent, or gas channeling through the CO_2 absorbent. However, the inspiratory baseline may be elevated when the inspiratory valve is incompetent (e.g., there may be a slanted inspiratory downstroke). The expiratory upstroke occurs when the fresh gas from the anatomic dead space is quickly replaced by CO_2-rich alveolar gas. Under normal conditions, the upstroke should be steep; however, it may become slanted during partial airway obstruction, if a sidestream analyzer is sampling gas too slowly, or if the response time of the capnograph is too slow for the patient's respiratory rate. Partial obstruction may be the result of an obstruction in the breathing system (e.g., by a kinked endotracheal tube) or in the patient's airway (e.g., chronic obstructive pulmonary disease [COPD] or acute bronchospasm). The expiratory plateau is normally characterized by a slow but shallow progressive increase in CO_2 concentration. This occurs because of imperfect matching of ventilation and perfusion in all lung units. Partial obstruction of gas flow either in the breathing system or in the patient's airways may cause a prolonged increase in the slope of the expiratory plateau, which may continue rising until the next inspiratory downstroke begins. The inspiratory downstroke is caused by the rapid influx of fresh gas, which washes the CO_2 away from the CO_2 sensing or sampling site. Under normal conditions, the inspiratory downstroke is very steep. The causes of a slanted or blunted inspiratory downstroke include an incompetent inspiratory valve, slow mechanical inspiration, slow gas sampling, and partial CO_2 rebreathing *(Ehrenwerth: Anesthesia Equipment: Principles and Applications, ed 2, p 248; Barash: Clinical Anesthesia, ed 8, pp 711–712; Miller: Basics of Anesthesia, ed 7, 342–347).*

33. (B) The complications of tracheal intubation can be divided into those associated with direct laryngoscopy and intubation of the trachea, tracheal tube placement, and extubation of the trachea. The most frequent complication associated with direct laryngoscopy and tracheal intubation is dental trauma. If a tooth is dislodged and not found, radiographs of the chest and abdomen should be taken to determine whether the tooth has passed through the glottic opening into the lungs. Should dental trauma occur, immediate consultation with a dentist is indicated. Other complications of direct laryngoscopy and tracheal intubation include hypertension, tachycardia, cardiac dysrhythmias, and aspiration of gastric contents. The most common complication that occurs while the endotracheal tube is in place is inadvertent endobronchial intubation. Flexion, not extension, of the neck or a change from the supine position to the head-down position can shift the carina upward, which may convert a midtracheal tube placement into a bronchial intubation. Extension of the neck can cause cephalad displacement of the tube into the pharynx. Lateral rotation of the head can displace the distal end of the endotracheal tube approximately 0.7 cm away from the carina. The right naris is preferable because the laryngoscope is in the left hand. The complications associated with extubation of the trachea can be immediate or delayed; of the immediate complications associated with extubation of the trachea, the two most serious are laryngospasm and aspiration of gastric contents. Laryngospasm is most likely to occur in patients who are lightly anesthetized at the time of extubation. If laryngospasm occurs, positive-pressure bag and mask ventilation with 100% O_2 and forward displacement of the mandible may be sufficient treatment. However, if laryngospasm persists, succinylcholine should be administered intravenously or intramuscularly. Pharyngitis is another frequent complication after extubation of the trachea. It occurs most commonly in female individuals, presumably because of the thinner mucosal covering over the posterior vocal cords in comparison with male individuals. This complication usually does not require treatment and spontaneously resolves in 48 to 72 hours. Delayed complications associated with extubation of the trachea include laryngeal ulcerations, tracheitis, tracheal stenosis, vocal cord paralysis, and arytenoid cartilage dislocation. *(Miller: Miller's Anesthesia, ed 8, p 1655).*

34. (B) Gas leaving a compressed-gas cylinder is directed through a pressure-reducing valve, which lowers the pressure within the metal tubing of the anesthesia machine to 45 to 55 psi *(Ehrenwerth: Anesthesia Equipment: Principles and Applications, ed 2, pp 27–34; Miller: Miller's Anesthesia, ed 8, p 756; Barash: Clinical Anesthesia, ed 8, p 657).*

35. (C) CO_2 lasers can cause serious corneal injury, whereas argon, Nd:YAG, ruby, or potassium titanyl phosphate lasers can burn the retina. Use of the incorrect filter provides no protection! Clear glass or plastic lenses are opaque for CO_2 laser light and are adequate protection for this beam (contact lenses are not adequate protection). For argon or krypton laser light, amber-orange filters are used. For Nd:YAG laser light, special green-tinted filters are used. For potassium titanyl phosphate:Nd:YAG laser light, red filters are used. *(Miller: Miller's Anesthesia, ed 8, pp 2604–2605).*

36. (B) The diameter index safety system prevents incorrect connections of medical gas lines. This system consists of two concentric and specific bores in the body of one connection, which correspond to two concentric and specific shoulders on the nipple of the other connection *(Ehrenwerth: Anesthesia Equipment: Principles and Applications, ed 2, pp 20, 27–28; Barash: Clinical Anesthesia, ed 8, p 657).*

37. (B) Lithotripsy is a noninvasive treatment using ultrasonic shock waves to break apart kidney stones. There are three main components of lithotripters; an energy source, a system to focus the shock wave, and fluoroscopy or ultrasound to visualize and localize the stone in focus. Because most lithotripters are triggered by the R wave of the ECG and can be fired inappropriately by the atrial-pacing artifact (with the potential of producing serious cardiac dysrhythmias), pacemakers should be changed to a mode that does not pace the atrium. Thus the lithotripter has no possibility of misinterpreting the atrial spike as an R wave. In addition, the shock waves can interfere with pacemaker function, and some devices can be damaged, so an alternative means of pacing should be available. After the lithotripter procedure, the pacemaker should be reactivated to the patient's original mode (in this case DDD) and checked for proper functioning. If the patient has an automatic implanted cardioverter-defibrillator (AICD), the AICD needs to be turned off during the treatment and reactivated after the treatment. *(Miller: Miller's Anesthesia, ed 8, pp 1474, 2235–2237).*

38. (A) The output of the vaporizer will be lower at flow rates less than 250 mL/min because there is insufficient pressure to advance the molecules of the volatile agent upward. At extremely high carrier gas flow rates (>15 L/min), there is insufficient mixing in the vaporizing chamber. *(Miller: Miller's Anesthesia, ed 8, pp 777-778; Barash: Clinical Anesthesia, ed 8, p 671).*

39. (C) Pulse oximeters estimate arterial hemoglobin saturation (SaO_2) by measuring the amount of light transmitted through a pulsatile vascular tissue bed. Pulse oximeters measure the alternating current component of light absorbance at each of two wavelengths (660 and 940 nm) and then divide this measurement by the corresponding direct current component. Then the ratio (R) of the two absorbance measurements is determined by the following equation:

$$R = \frac{AC_{660} / DC_{660}}{AC_{940} / DC_{940}}$$

Using an empiric calibration curve that relates arterial hemoglobin saturation to R, the actual arterial hemoglobin saturation is calculated. Based on the physical principles outlined above, the sources of error in SpO_2 readings can be easily predicted. Pulse oximeters can function accurately when only two hemoglobin species, oxyhemoglobin and reduced hemoglobin, are present. If any light-absorbing species other than oxyhemoglobin and reduced hemoglobin are present, the pulse oximeter measurements will be inaccurate. Fetal hemoglobin has a minimal effect on the accuracy of pulse oximetry because the extinction coefficients for fetal hemoglobin at the two wavelengths used by pulse oximetry are very similar to the corresponding values for adult hemoglobin. In addition to abnormal hemoglobins, any substance present in the blood that absorbs light at either 660 or 940 nm, such as intravenous dyes used for diagnostic purposes, will affect the value of R, making accurate measurements of the pulse oximeter impossible. These dyes include methylene blue and indigo carmine. Methylene blue has the greatest effect on SaO_2 measurements because the extinction coefficient is so similar to that of oxyhemoglobin. *(Ehrenwerth: Anesthesia Equipment: Principles and Applications, ed 2, pp 261–262; Miller: Miller's Anesthesia, ed 8, pp 1547–1548).*

40. (B) Direct measurement of arterial blood gases is the standard for monitoring arterial oxygen and carbon dioxide levels but only provides values for a specific point in time. Transcutaneous noninvasive measurements (Ptc) for oxygen ($PtcO_2$) and carbon dioxide ($PtcCO_2$) are based on the diffusion of O_2 and CO_2 through the skin. In order to get reliable transcutaneous readings, the skin must be warmed to facilitate gas diffusion. This, however, allows for some metabolism of oxygen and production of carbon dioxide by the skin. The net result is a lower $PtcO_2$ level and a higher $PtcCO_2$ level. (Miller: Miller's Anesthesia, ed 8, p 1574).

41. (B) Saturated vapor pressures depend on the physical properties of the liquid and the temperature. Vapor pressures are independent of barometric pressure. At 20° C the vapor pressures of halothane (243 mm Hg) and isoflurane (240 mm Hg) are similar, and at 1 atmosphere the concentration in the vaporizer for these drugs is 240/760, or about 32%. Similarly, the vapor pressures for sevoflurane (160 mm Hg) and enflurane (172 mm Hg) are similar, and at 1 atmosphere the concentration in the vaporizer for these drugs is 160/760, or about 21%. If desflurane (vapor pressure of 669 mm Hg) is placed in a 1-atmosphere pressure vaporizer, the concentration would be 669/760 = 88%. Because the bypass flow is adjusted for each vaporizer, putting a volatile anesthetic with a higher saturated vapor pressure would lead to a higher-than-expected concentration of anesthetic delivered from the vaporizer, whereas putting a drug with a lower saturated vapor pressure would lead to a lower-than-expected concentration of drug delivered from the vaporizer. (Barash: Clinical Anesthesia, ed 8, pp 668–678).

VAPOR PRESSURE AND MINIMUM ALVEOLAR CONCENTRATION

	Halothane	Enflurane	Sevoflurane	Isoflurane	Desflurane	Methoxyflurane
Vapor pressure 20° C mm Hg	243	172	160	240	669	23
MAC 30-55 yr	0.75	1.63	1.8	1.17	6.6	0.16

MAC, minimum alveolar concentration.

42. (D) Gas density decreases with increasing altitude (i.e., the density of a gas is directly proportional to atmospheric pressure). Atmospheric pressure will influence the function of rotameters because the accurate function of rotameters is influenced by the physical properties of the gas, such as density and viscosity. The magnitude of this influence, however, depends on the rate of gas flow. At low gas flows, the pattern of gas flow is laminar. Atmospheric pressure will have little effect on the accurate function of rotameters at low gas flows because laminar gas flow is influenced by gas viscosity (which is minimally affected by atmospheric pressure), not by gas density. However, at high gas flows, the gas flow pattern is turbulent and is influenced by gas density. At high altitudes (i.e., low atmospheric pressure), the gas flow through the rotameter will be greater than expected at high flows but accurate at low flows *(Ehrenwerth: Anesthesia Equipment: Principles and Applications, ed 2, pp 43–45, 230–231; Miller: Miller's Anesthesia, ed 8, p 2691).*

43. (B) Pacemakers have a three- to five-letter code that describes the pacemaker type and function. Given that the purpose of the pacemaker is to send electric current to the heart, the first letter identifies the chamber(s) paced: A for atrial, V for ventricle, and D for dual chamber (A + V). The second letter identifies the chamber where endogenous current is sensed: A, V, D, and O for none sensed. The third letter describes the response to sensing: O for none, I for inhibited, T for triggered, and D for dual (I + T). The fourth letter describes programmability or rate modulation: O for none and R for rate modulation (i.e., faster heart rate with exercise). The fifth letter describes anti-tachycardia function: A, V or D (A + V), or O. A VDD pacemaker is used for patients with AV node dysfunction but intact sinus node activity. (Miller: Miller's Anesthesia, ed 8, pp 1467-1468; Barash: Clinical Anesthesia, ed 8, pp 1724–1725).

44. (A) Although controversial, it is thought that chronic exposure to low concentrations of volatile anesthetics may constitute a health hazard to OR personnel. Therefore removal of trace concentrations of volatile anesthetic gases from the OR atmosphere with a scavenging system and steps to reduce and control gas leakage into the environment are required. High-pressure system leakage of volatile anesthetic gases into the OR atmosphere occurs when gas escapes from compressed-gas cylinders attached to the anesthetic machine (e.g., faulty yokes) or from tubing delivering these gases to the anesthesia machine from a central supply source. The most common cause of low-pressure leakage of anesthetic gases into the OR atmosphere is the escape of gases from sites located between the flowmeters of the anesthesia machine and the patient, such as a poor mask seal. The use of high gas flows in a circle system will not reduce trace gas contamination of the OR atmosphere. In fact, this could contribute to the contamination if there is a leak in the circle system (Miller: Miller's Anesthesia, ed 8, pp 3232–3234).

45. (A) Although there is insufficient evidence that chronic exposure to low concentrations of inhaled anesthetics may pose a health hazard to those in the OR, precautions are made to decrease the pollution of inhalation anesthetics there. This includes ventilating the room adequately (air in the OR should be exchanged at least 15 times an hour), maintenance of anesthetic scavenging systems to remove anesthetic vapors, and a tight anesthetic seal with no leakage of gas into the OR atmosphere. Although periodic equipment maintenance should be performed to make sure the anesthetic equipment is operating properly, leakage around an improperly sealed face mask as well as the face mask not applied to the face during airway manipulations (placement of an airway) poses the greatest risk of OR contamination from inhaled anesthetics (Miller: Miller's Anesthesia, ed 8, pp 3232–3234).

46. (C) The amount of volatile anesthetic taken up by the patient in the first minute is equal to the amount taken up between the squares of any two consecutive minutes (square root of time equation). Thus, if 50 mL is taken up in the first minute, 50 mL will be taken up between the first (1 squared) and fourth (2 squared) minutes. Similarly, between the fourth and ninth minutes (2 squared and 3 squared), another 50 mL will be absorbed. In this example, we are looking for the uptake between the 16th (4 squared) and 36th (6 squared) minutes, which would be 2 consecutive minutes squared, or 2 × 50 mL = 100 mL. (Miller: Miller's Anesthesia, ed 8, pp 650–651).

47. (D) In evaluating SSEPs, one looks at both the amplitude or voltage of the recorded response wave and the latency (time measured from the stimulus to the onset or peak of the response wave). A decrease in amplitude (>50%) and/or an increase in latency (>10%) is usually clinically significant. These changes may reflect hypoperfusion, neural ischemia, temperature changes, or drug effects. All of the volatile anesthetics and the barbiturates cause a decrease in amplitude as well as an increase in latency. Propofol affects both latency and amplitude and, like other intravenous agents, has a significantly less effect than "equipotent" doses of volatile anesthetics. Etomidate causes an increase in latency and an increase in amplitude. Midazolam decreases the amplitude but has little effect on latency. Opioids cause small and not clinically significant increases in latency and a decrease in amplitude of the SSEPs. Muscle relaxants have no effect on SSEPs (Miller: Miller's Anesthesia, ed 8, pp 1514–1517; Barash: Clinical Anesthesia, ed 8, p 1011).

48. (A) The anesthesia machine, now more properly called the anesthesia workstation, has two main pressure circuits. The higher-pressure circuits consist of the gas supply from the pipelines and tanks, all piping, pressure gauges, pressure reduction regulators, check valves (which prevent backward gas flow), the oxygen pressure-sensor shutoff valve (also called the oxygen failure cutoff or fail-safe valve), the oxygen supply failure alarm, and the oxygen flush valve—or, simplistically, everything up to the gas flow control valves and the machine common gas outlet. The low-pressure circuit starts with and includes the gas flow control valves, flowmeters, vaporizers, and vaporizer check valve and goes to the machine common gas outlet. See also figure for explanation to Question 12. (Barash: Clinical Anesthesia, ed 8, pp 652–679).

49. (D) Vaporization of a liquid requires the transfer of heat from the objects in contact with the liquid (e.g., the metal cylinder and surrounding atmosphere). For this reason, at high gas flows, atmospheric water will condense as frost on the outside of compressed-gas cylinders. (Miller: Basics of Anesthesia, ed 7, p 224).

50. (B) Temperature measurements of the PA, esophagus, axilla, nasopharynx, and tympanic membrane correlate with central temperature in patients undergoing noncardiac surgery. Skin temperature does not reflect central temperature and does not warn adequately of malignant hyperthermia or excessive hypothermia. (Miller: Miller's Anesthesia, ed 8, pp 1643–1644).

51. (C) Laser refers to Light Amplification by the Stimulated Emission of Radiation. Laser light differs from ordinary light in three main ways. First, laser light is monochromic (possesses one wavelength or color). Second, laser light is coherent (the photons oscillate in the same phase). Third, laser light is collimated (exists in a narrow parallel beam). Visible light has a wide spectrum of wavelengths in the 385- to 760-nm range. Argon laser light, which can penetrate tissues to a depth of 0.05 to 2.0 mm, is either blue (wavelength 488 nm) or green (wavelength 514 nm) and is often used for vascular pigmented lesions because it is intensively absorbed by hemoglobin. Helium–neon laser light is red, has a frequency of 632 nm, and is often used as an aiming beam because it has very low power and presents no significant danger to OR personnel. Nd:YAG laser light is the most powerful medical laser and can penetrate tissues from 2 to 6 mm. Nd:YAG laser light is in the near infrared range, with a wavelength of 1064 nm, has general uses (e.g., prostate surgery, laryngeal papillomatosis, coagulation), and can be used with fiberoptics. CO_2 laser light is in the far infrared range, with a long wavelength of 10,600 nm. Because CO_2 laser light penetrates tissues poorly, it can vaporize superficial tissues with little damage to underlying cells (Miller: Miller's Anesthesia, ed 8, pp 2598–2601; Barash: Clinical Anesthesia, ed 8, p 1392).

52. (B) There are four methods of administering anesthetic gases to a patient; mask, supraglottic airway, endotracheal tube, and a surgical airway (tracheostomy). The first supraglottic airway (laryngeal mask airway or LMA) was used in 1988. The LMA is basically an airway tube with a distal elliptical inflatable mask that has an anterior aperture. The LMA is inserted blindly into the pharynx, and the mask is inflated to obtain a seal around the glottis opening. The original LMA had two small, narrow bar-like structures to cover the distal opening. Because of the bar-like structures, you cannot pass an endotracheal tube through the airway tube of the LMA. The LMA Fastrach (Intubating LMA or ILMA) does not have the bar-like structures so that an endotracheal tube can be passed through the LMA into the trachea; then the LMA could be removed, leaving the endotracheal tube in the trachea. One disadvantage of the original LMA is the inability to empty the stomach. The reusable LMA Proseal and the single-use LMA Supreme were designed with the mask modified to extend the posterior surface for an improved seal, a built-in bite block to decrease the chance of an obstructed airway lumen, and a second lumen that allows for a suction catheter to pass through the LMA into the stomach. The Air-Q is another second-generation supraglottic airway, with a shorter airway tube, a bite block, and a removable circuit connector that more easily allows one to pass a standard endotracheal tube through the LMA into the trachea. The I-Gel is another second-generation supraglottic airway that was designed as a noninflatable supraglottic airway with a soft, gel-like seal. The I-Gel has a gastric channel that runs from the distal tip to an outlet lateral to the airway connector and allows for the insertion of a gastric tube. Suctioning of the stomach is not possible with the LMA Fastrach or Air-

Q supraglottic airways. (Barash: Clinical Anesthesia, ed 8, pp 775–778; Miller: Basics of Anesthesia, ed 7, pp 248–250; Miller: Miller's Anesthesia, ed 8, pp 1661–1665)

53. (D) The FIO_2 delivered to patients from low-flow systems (e.g., nasal prongs) is determined by the size of the O_2 reservoir, the O_2 flow, and the patient's breathing pattern. As a rule of thumb, assuming a normal breathing pattern, the FIO_2 delivered by nasal prongs increases by approximately 0.04 for each L/min increase in O_2 flow up to a maximal FIO_2 of approximately 0.45 (at an O_2 flow of 6 L/min). In general, the larger the patient's V_T or the faster the respiratory rate, the lower the FIO_2 for a given O_2 flow. (Miller: Miller's Anesthesia, ed 8, pp 2933–2934).

54. (A)

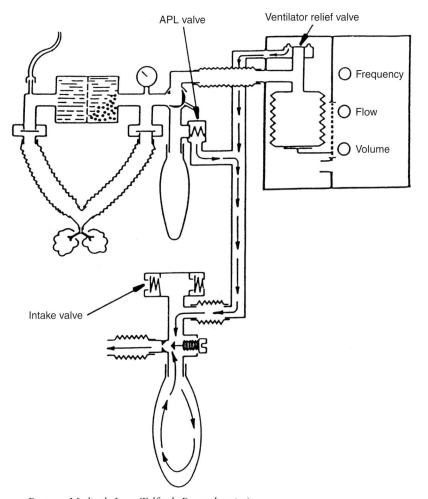

(Courtesy Draeger Medical, Inc., Telford, Pennsylvania.)

In a closed scavenging system interface, the reservoir bag should expand during expiration and contract during inspiration. During the inspiratory phase of mechanical ventilation, the ventilator pressure-relief valve closes, thereby directing the gas inside the ventilator bellows into the patient's breathing circuit. If the ventilator pressure-relief valve is incompetent, there will be a direct communication between the patient's breathing circuit and the scavenging circuit. This will result in delivery of part of the mechanical ventilator V_T directly to the scavenging circuit, causing the reservoir bag to inflate during the inspiratory phase of the ventilator cycle *(Ehrenwerth: Anesthesia Equipment: Principles and Applications, ed 2, pp 130–132; Miller: Miller's Anesthesia, ed 8, pp 2933–2934; Pardo: Basics of Anesthesia, ed 7, p 233).*

55. (C) The accurate function of dual-wavelength pulse oximeters is altered by nail polish. Because blue nail polish has a peak absorbance similar to that of adult deoxygenated hemoglobin (near 660 nm), it has the greatest effect on the SpO_2 reading. Nail polish causes an artifactual and fixed decrease in the SpO_2 reading as shown by these devices. Turning the finger probe 90 degrees so the light shines sidewise through the finger is useful when there is nail polish on the patient's fingernails (Miller: Miller's Anesthesia, ed 8, p 1547).

56. (C) Leakage electric currents less than 1 mA are imperceptible to touch. The minimal ventricular fibrillation threshold of current applied to the skin is about 100 mA. If the current bypasses the high resistance of the skin and is applied directly to the heart via pacemaker, central line, etc. (microshock), currents as low as 100 μA (0.1 mA) may be fatal. Because of this, the American National Standards Institute has set the maximum leakage of electric current allowed through electrodes or catheters in contact with the heart at 10 μA (Miller: Miller's Anesthesia, ed 8, p 3226; Barash: Clinical Anesthesia, ed 8, pp 111–112).

57. (D) The line isolation monitor gives an alarm when grounding occurs in the OR or when the maximum current that a short circuit could cause exceeds 2 to 5 mA. The line isolation monitor is purely a monitor and does not interrupt electric current. Therefore the line isolation monitor will not prevent microshock or macroshock (Brunner: Electricity, Safety, and the Patient, ed 1, p 304; Miller: Miller's Anesthesia, ed 8, pp 3221–3223.)

58. (A)

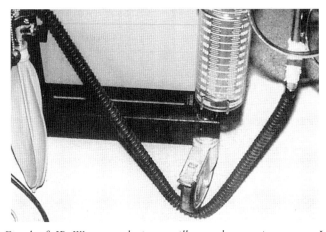

(From Azar I, Eisenkraft JB: Waste anesthetic gas spillage and scavenging systems. In Ehrenwerth J, Eisenkraft JB, editors: Anesthesia Equipment: Principles and Applications, St Louis, Mosby, 1993, p 128.)

A scavenging system with a closed interface is one in which there is communication with the atmosphere through positive-pressure and negative-pressure relief valves. The positive-pressure relief valve will prevent transmission of excessive pressure buildup to the patient's breathing circuit, even if there is an obstruction distal to the interface or if the system is not connected to wall suction. However, obstruction of the transfer tubing from the patient's breathing circuit to the scavenging circuit is proximal to the interface. This will isolate the patient's breathing circuit from the positive-pressure relief valve of the scavenging system interface. Should this occur, barotrauma to the patient's lungs can result *(Ehrenwerth: Anesthesia Equipment: Principles and Applications, ed 2, pp 130–137).*

59. (C) Electrocautery units, or electrosurgical units (ESUs), were invented by Professor W. T. Bovie and were first used in 1926. They operate by generating ultra-high frequency (0.1-3 MHz) alternating electric currents and are commonly used today for cutting and coagulating tissue. Whenever a current passes through a resistance such as tissue, heat is generated and is inversely proportional to the surface area through which the current passes. At the point of entry to the body from the small active electrode or cautery tip, a fair amount of heat is generated. For the current to complete its circuit, the return electrode plate or dispersive pad (incorrectly but commonly called the ground pad) has a large surface area, where very little heat develops. The dispersive pad should be as close as is reasonable to the site of surgery. If the current from the ESU passes through an artificial cardiac pacemaker, the pacemaker may misinterpret the current as cardiac activity and may not pace, which is why a magnet placed over the pacemaker will turn off the pacemaker sensor, putting the pacemaker in the asynchronous mode, and should be available (if the pacemaker's sensory mode is not turned off preoperatively). In addition, automatic implantable cardioverter-defibrillators (AICDs) may misinterpret the electric activity as ventricular fibrillation and defibrillate the patient. AICDs should be turned off before use of an ESU. *(Barash: Clinical Anesthesia, ed 8, pp 125–127).*

60. (B) ANIBP devices provide consistent and reliable arterial BP measurements. Variations in the cuff pressure resulting from arterial pulsations during cuff deflation are sensed by the device and are used to calculate MAP. Then, values for systolic and diastolic pressures are derived from formulas that use the rate of change of the arterial pressure pulsations and the MAP (oscillometric principle). This method provides accurate measurements of arterial BP in neonates, infants, children, and adults. The main advantage of ANIBP devices is that they free the anesthesia provider to perform other duties required for optimal anesthesia care. Additionally, these devices provide alarm systems to draw attention to extreme BP values, and they have the capacity to transfer data to automated trending devices or recorders. Improper use of these devices can lead to erroneous measurements and complications. The width of the BP cuff should be approximately 40% of the circumference of the patient's arm. If the BP cuff is too narrow or if the BP cuff is wrapped too loosely around the arm, the BP measurement by the device will be falsely elevated. Frequent BP measurements can result in edema of the extremity distal to the cuff. For this reason, cycling of these devices should not be more frequent than every 1 to 3 minutes. Other complications associated with improper use of ANIBP devices include ulnar nerve paresthesia, superficial thrombophlebitis, and compartment syndrome. Fortunately, these complications are rare. *(Miller: Miller's Anesthesia, ed 8, pp 1347–1348; Barash: Clinical Anesthesia, ed 8, pp 1287; 715–717).*

61. (B) ECG monitoring is often not used during MRI scans because artifacts are very common (abnormalities in T waves and ST waves), and heating of the wires during the scan would potentially burn the patient. However, ECG can be used if the electrodes are placed close together and toward the center of the magnetic field and the wires are insulated from the patient's skin and straight. In addition, the wires should not be wound together in loops (because this can induce heating of the wires), and worn or frayed wires should not be used. *(Miller: Miller's Anesthesia, ed 8, p 2655; Barash: Clinical Anesthesia, ed 8, p 888).*

62. (D) The capnography tracing provides a great deal of information. After intubation the mere presence of CO_2 is very reassuring. During the procedure, other data can be gleaned like presence of COPD, exhausted absorbent, stuck anesthesia circuit valves, and more. The tracing above depicts a scenario in which the patient's lungs are receiving progressively less blood flow. Such a tracing could come from a number of causes such as exsanguination, cardiac failure, and pulmonary embolism.

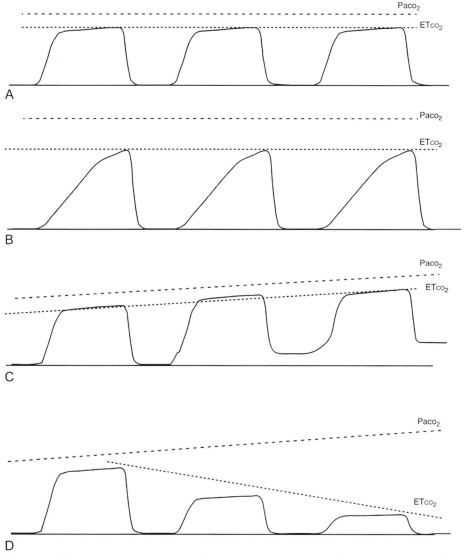

(From Szocik J, Teig M, Tremper K. Anesthetic monitoring. In: Basics of Anesthesia, ed 7, Pardo M, Miller R (Eds). Elsevier; 2018.)

63. (D) Failure to oxygenate patients adequately is an important cause of anesthesia-related morbidity and mortality. All of the choices listed in this question are potential causes of inadequate delivery of O_2 to the patient; however, the most frequent cause is inadvertent disconnection of the O_2 supply system from the patient (e.g., disconnection of the patient's breathing circuit from the endotracheal tube) *(Ehrenwerth: Anesthesia Equipment: Principles and Applications, ed 2, p 121; Miller: Miller's Anesthesia, ed 8, pp 780–781).*

64. (A) The esophageal detector device (EDD) is essentially a bulb that is first compressed and then attached to the endotracheal tube after the tube is inserted into the patient. The pressure generated is about −40 cm of water. If the endotracheal tube is placed in the esophagus, then the negative pressure will collapse the esophagus, and the bulb will not inflate. If the endotracheal tube is in the trachea, then the air from the lung will enable the bulb to inflate (usually in a few seconds, but sometimes more than 30 seconds). A syringe that has a negative pressure applied to it has also been used. Although initial studies were very positive about the use of the EDD, more recent studies show that up to 30% of correctly placed endotracheal tubes in adults may be removed because the EDD has suggested esophageal placement. Misleading results have been noted in patients with morbid obesity, late pregnancy, status asthmaticus, and copious endotracheal secretion, wherein the trachea tends to collapse. Its use in children younger than

1 year of age has shown poor sensitivity and poor specificity. Although a cardiac output is needed to get CO_2 to the lungs for a CO_2 gas analyzer to function, a cardiac output is not needed for an EDD. (Miller: Miller's Anesthesia, ed 8, p 1654).

65. (D) The capnometer measures the CO_2 concentration of respiratory gases. Today this is most commonly performed by infrared absorption using a sidestream gas sample. The sampling tube should be connected as close as possible to the patient's airway. The difference between the end-tidal CO_2 ($ETCO_2$) and the arterial CO_2 ($PaCO_2$) is typically 5 to 10 mm Hg and is due to alveolar dead space ventilation. Because nonperfused alveoli do not contribute to gas exchange, any condition that increases alveolar dead space ventilation (i.e., reduces pulmonary blood flow, as by pulmonary embolism or cardiac arrest) will increase dead space ventilation and the $ETCO_2$-to-$PaCO_2$ difference. Conditions that increase pulmonary shunt result in minimal changes in the $PaCO_2$–$ETCO_2$ gradient. CO_2 diffuses rapidly across the capillary-alveolar membrane (Miller: Miller's Anesthesia, ed 8, pp 1551–1553; Barash: Clinical Anesthesia, ed 8, pp 711–712).

66. (D) The last gas added to a gas mixture should always be O_2. This arrangement is the safest because it ensures that leaks proximal to the O_2 inflow cannot result in the delivery of a hypoxic gas mixture to the patient. With this arrangement (O_2 added last), leaks distal to the O_2 inflow will result in a decreased volume of gas, but the FIO_2 of anesthesia will not be reduced. (Ehrenwerth: Anesthesia Equipment: Principles and Applications, ed 2, pp 43–45; Miller: Basics of Anesthesia, ed 7, p 223; Barash: Clinical Anesthesia, ed 8, pp 661–664).

67. (C) Most modern Datex-Ohmeda Tec or North American Dräger Vapor vaporizers (except desflurane) are variable-bypass, flowover vaporizers. This means that the gas that flows through the vaporizers is split into two parts, depending on the concentration selected. The gas goes through either the bypass chamber on the top of the vaporizer or the vaporizing chamber on the bottom of the vaporizer. If the vaporizer is tipped, which might happen when a filled vaporizer is switched out or moved from one machine to another machine, part of the anesthetic liquid in the vaporizing chamber may get into the bypass chamber. This could result in a much higher concentration of gas than that dialed. With the Datex-Ohmeda Tec 4 or the North American Dräger Vapor 19.1 series, it is recommended to flush the vaporizer at high flows with the vaporizer set at a low concentration until the output shows no excessive agent (this usually takes 20-30 minutes). The Dräger Vapor 2000 series has a transport (T) dial setting. This setting isolates the bypass from the vaporizer chamber. The Aladin cassette vaporizer does not have a bypass flow chamber and has no tipping hazard (Miller: Miller's Anesthesia, ed 8, p 771; Barash: Clinical Anesthesia, ed 8, pp 672–673).

68. (A) Accurate delivery of volatile anesthetic concentration is dependent on filling the agent-specific vaporizer with the appropriate (volatile) agent. Differences in anesthetic potencies further necessitate this requirement. Each agent-specific vaporizer uses a splitting ratio that determines the portion of the fresh gas that is directed through the vaporizing chamber versus that which travels through the bypass chamber.

VAPOR PRESSURE, ANESTHETIC VAPOR PRESSURE, AND SPLITTING RATIO

	Halothane	Sevoflurane	Isoflurane	Enflurane
Vapor pressure at 20° C	243 mm Hg	160 mm Hg	240 mm Hg	172 mm Hg
VP/(BP − VP)	0.47	0.27	0.47	0.29
Splitting ratio for 1% vapor	1:47	1:27	1:47	1:29

BP, blood pressure; VP, vapor pressure.

The table shows the calculation (fraction) that when multiplied by the quantity of fresh gas traversing the vaporizing chamber (affluent fresh gas in mL/min) will yield the output (mL/min) of anesthetic vapor in the effluent gas. When this fraction is multiplied by 100, it equals the splitting ratio for 1% for the given volatile agent. For example, when the isoflurane vaporizer is set to deliver 1% isoflurane, one part of fresh gas is passed through the vaporizing chamber while 47 parts travel through the bypass chamber. One can determine on inspection that when a less soluble volatile agent like sevoflurane (or the obsolete volatile agent enflurane, for the sake of example) is placed into an isoflurane (or halothane) vaporizer, the output in volume percent will be less than expected; how much less can be determined by simply comparing their splitting ratios 27/47 or 0.6. Halothane and enflurane are no longer used in the United States, but old halothane and enflurane vaporizers can be (and are) used elsewhere in the world to accurately deliver isoflurane and sevoflurane, respectively *(Ehrenwerth: Anesthesia Equipment: Principles and Applications, ed 2, pp 72–73; Miller: Miller's Anesthesia, ed 8, pp 771–774).*

69. (C) Two percent of 4 L/min will be 80 mL of isoflurane per minute.

VAPOR PRESSURE PER MILLILITER OF LIQUID

	Halothane	Enflurane	Isoflurane	Sevoflurane	Desflurane
mL vapor per mL liquid at 20° C	226	196	195	182	207

Given that 1 mL of isoflurane liquid yields 195 mL of anesthetic vapor and by applying the calculation (195 mL vapor/1 mL liquid isoflurane) × (150 mL isoflurane liquid) = 29,250 mL isoflurane vapor, it follows that (29,250 mL ÷ 80 mL/min = 365 minutes). 365 minutes is around 6 hours *(Ehrenwerth: Anesthesia Equipment: Principles and Applications, ed 2, pp 65–70; Barash: Clinical Anesthesia, ed 8, pp 668–673).*

70. (C) The human ear can perceive sound in the range of 20 Hz to 20 kHz. Frequencies above 20 kHz, inaudible to humans, are ultrasonic frequencies (ultra = Latin for "beyond" or "on the far side of"). In regional anesthesia, ultrasound is used for imaging in the frequency range of 2.5 to 10 MHz. Wavelength is inversely proportional to frequency (i.e., λ = C/f [λ = wavelength, C = velocity of sound through tissue or 1540 m/sec, f = frequency]). Wavelength in millimeters can be calculated by dividing 1.54 by the Doppler frequency in megahertz. Penetration into tissue is 200 to 400 times wavelength, and resolution is twice the wavelength. Therefore a frequency of 3 MHz (wavelength 0.51 mm) would have a resolution of 1 mm and a penetration of up to 100 to 200 mm (10-20 cm), whereas 10 MHz (wavelength 0.15 mm) corresponds to a resolution of 0.3 mm but a penetration depth of no more than 60 to 120 mm (6-12 cm) *(Miller: Miller's Anesthesia, ed 8, pp 1398–1405; Miller: Basics of Anesthesia, ed 7, p 305).*

71. (A) *Microshock* refers to electric shock located in or near the heart. A current as low as 100 μA passing through the heart can produce ventricular fibrillation. Pacemaker electrodes, central venous catheters, PA catheters, and other devices in the heart are necessary prerequisites for microshock. Because the line isolation monitor has a threshold of 2 mA (2000 μA) for alarming, it will not protect against microshock *(Miller: Miller's Anesthesia, ed 8, p 3226; Barash: Clinical Anesthesia, ed 8, p 123).*

72. (D) Intraoperative awareness or recall during general anesthesia is rare (overall incidence is 0.2%, for obstetrics 0.4%, for cardiac 1%-1.5%) except for major trauma, which has a reported incidence as high as 43%. With the electroencephalogram, trends can be identified with changes in the depth of anesthesia; however, the sensitivity and specificity of the available trends are such that none serve as a sole indicator of anesthesia depth. Although using the BIS monitor may reduce the risk of recall, it, like the other listed signs as well as patient movement, does not totally eliminate recall. *(Miller: Miller's Anesthesia, ed 8, pp 1527–1528).*

73. (D) The minute ventilation is 5 L (0.5 L per breath at 10 breaths/min) and 2 L/min to drive the ventilator for a total O_2 consumption of 7 L/min. A full oxygen "E" cylinder contains 625 L. Ninety percent of the volume of the cylinder ($\approx$ 560 L) can be delivered before the ventilator can no longer be driven. At a rate of 7 L/min, this supply would last about 80 minutes *(Ehrenwerth: Anesthesia Equipment: Principles and Applications, ed 2, pp 29–33, 37; Miller: Basics of Anesthesia, ed 7, pp 221–223).*

74. (C) After eliminating reversible causes of high peak airway pressures (e.g., occlusion of the endotracheal tube, mainstem intubation, or bronchospasm), adjusting the ventilator can reduce the peak airway pressure. Increasing the inspiratory flow rate would cause the airway pressures to go up faster and would produce higher peak airway pressures. Removing PEEP would lower peak pressure at the expense of alveolar ventilation. Changing the I:E ratio from 1:3 to 1:2 will permit 8% (25% inspiratory time to 33% inspiratory time) more time for the V_T to be administered and will result in lower airway pressures. Decreasing the V_T to 300 and increasing the rate to 28 would give the same minute ventilation but not the same alveolar ventilation. Recall that alveolar ventilation equals (frequency) times (V_T minus dead space), and because dead space is the same (about 2 mL/kg ideal weight), alveolar ventilation would be reduced, in this case to a dangerously low level. Another option is to change from volume-cycled to pressure-cycled ventilation, which produces a more constant pressure over time instead of the peaked pressures seen with fixed V_T ventilation *(Miller: Miller's Anesthesia, ed 8, pp 3064–3074).*

75. (D) The central hospital oxygen supply to the ORs is designed to give enough pressure and oxygen flow to run the three oxygen components of the anesthesia machine (patient fresh gas flow, anesthesia ventilator, and oxygen flush valve). The oxygen flowmeter on the anesthesia machine is designed to run at an oxygen pressure of 50 psi, and for emergency purposes the oxygen flush valve delivers oxygen at 35 to 75 L/min *(Miller: Basics of Anesthesia, ed 7, pp 221–224).*

76. (B) Within the respiratory system, both laminar and turbulent flows exist. At low flow rates, the respiratory flow tends to be laminar, like a series of concentric tubes that slide over one another with the center tubes flowing faster than the more peripheral tubes. Laminar flow is usually inaudible and is dependent on gas viscosity. Turbulent flow tends to be faster, is audible, and is dependent on gas density. Gas density can be decreased by using a mixture of helium with oxygen. *(Barash: Clinical Anesthesia, ed 8, pp 365–366).*

77. (B) Anesthesia workstations have high-pressure, intermediate-pressure, and low-pressure circuits (see figure in the explanation for Question 11). The high-pressure circuit is from the oxygen cylinder to the oxygen pressure regulator (first-stage regulator), which takes the oxygen pressure from a high of 2200 psi to 45 psi. The intermediate-pressure circuit consists of the pipeline pressure of about 50 to 55 psi and goes to the second-stage regulator, which then lowers the pressure to 14 to 26 psi (depending on the machine). The low-pressure circuit then consists of the flow tubes, vaporizer manifold, vaporizers, and vaporizer check valve to the common gas outlet. The oxygen flush valve is in the intermediate-pressure circuit and bypasses the low-pressure circuit *(Ehrenwerth: Anesthesia Equipment: Principles and Applications, ed 2, pp 34–36; Miller: Miller's Anesthesia, ed 8, p 759; Barash: Clinical Anesthesia, ed 8, pp 652, 667–668).*

78. (C) Two major problems should be noted in this case. The first obvious problem is the inspired oxygen concentration of 4%, a concentration that is not possible if the gases going to the machine are appropriate unless the oxygen analyzer is faulty. Given the dire consequences of a hypoxic gas mixture, one must assume the oxygen analyzer is correct and work on the premise that the O_2 pipeline is supplying a gas other than oxygen. Second, the oxygen line pressure is 65 psi. The pipeline pressures are normally around 50 to 55 psi, whereas the pressure from the oxygen cylinder, if the cylinder is turned on, is reduced to 45 psi. For the oxygen tank to deliver oxygen to the patient, the pipeline pressure needs to be less than 45 psi, which in this case will occur only when the pipeline is disconnected. Although we rarely think of problems with hospital gas lines, a survey of more than 200 hospitals showed about 33% had problems with the pipelines. The most common pipeline problems were low pressure, followed by high pressure and, very rarely, crossed gas lines *(Ehrenwerth: Anesthesia Equipment: Principles and Applications, ed 2, p 34; Miller: Miller's Anesthesia, ed 8, p 756; Barash: Clinical Anesthesia, ed 8, p 656).*

79. (D) There are many ways to monitor the electric activity of the heart. The five-electrode system using one lead for each limb and the fifth lead for the precordium is commonly used in the OR. The precordial lead placed in the V_5 position (anterior axillary line in the fifth intercostal space) gives the V_5 tracing, which, combined with the standard lead II, is the most common tracing used to look for myocardial ischemia *(Miller: Miller's Anesthesia, ed 8, pp 1429–1434; Barash: Clinical Anesthesia, ed 8, p 1710).*

80. (A) See also Question 36. The diameter index safety system provides threaded, noninterchangeable connections for medical gas pipelines through the hospital as well as to the anesthesia machine. The pin index safety system has two metal pins in different arrangements around the yoke on the back of anesthesia machines, with each arrangement for a specific gas cylinder. Vaporizers often have keyed fillers that attach to the bottle of anesthetic and the vaporizer. Vaporizers not equipped with keyed fillers occasionally have been misfilled with the wrong anesthetic liquid *(Barash: Clinical Anesthesia, ed 8, pp 656–659; Miller: Basics of Anesthesia, ed 7, p 221–223).*

81. (C) Calcium hydroxide lime does not contain the monovalent hydroxide bases that are present in soda lime (namely, NaOH and KOH). Sevoflurane in the presence of NaOH or KOH is degraded to trace amounts of compound A, which is nephrotoxic to rats at high concentrations. Soda lime normally contains about 13% to 15% water, but if the soda lime is desiccated (water content <5%—which has occurred if the machine is not used for a while and the fresh gas flow is left on) and is exposed to current volatile anesthetics (isoflurane, sevoflurane, and especially desflurane), CO can be produced. Neither compound A nor CO is formed when calcium hydroxide lime is used. With soda lime and calcium hydroxide lime, the indicator dye changes from white to purple as the granules become exhausted. The two major disadvantages of calcium hydroxide lime are the expense and the fact that its absorptive capacity is about half that of soda lime (10.2 L of CO_2/100 g of calcium hydroxide lime versus 26 L of CO_2/100 g of soda lime). (*Miller: Miller's Anesthesia, ed 8, pp 787–789; Barash: Clinical Anesthesia, ed 8, pp 681–683; Miller: Basics of Anesthesia, ed 7, 233–236*).

82. (B) The aim of direct invasive monitoring is to give continuous arterial BPs that are similar to the intermittent noninvasive arterial BPs from a cuff, as well as to give a port for arterial blood samples. The displayed signal reflects the actual pressure and the distortions from the measuring system (i.e., the catheter, tubing, stopcocks, and amplifier). Although the signal is usually accurate, at times we see an underdamped or an overdamped signal. In an underdamped signal, as in this case, exaggerated readings are noted (widened pulse pressure). In an overdamped signal, readings are diminished (narrowed pulse pressure). However, the mean BP tends to be accurate in both underdamped and overdamped signals (*Miller: Miller's Anesthesia, ed 8, pp 1347–1359; Barash: Clinical Anesthesia, ed 8, pp 714–715*).

83. (D) Rebreathing of expired gases (e.g., stuck open expiratory or inspiratory valves), faulty removal of CO_2 from the CO_2 absorber (e.g., exhausted CO_2 absorber, channeling through a CO_2 absorber, or having the CO_2 absorber bypassed—an option in some older anesthetic machines), or addition of CO_2 from a gas supply (rarely done with current anesthetic machines) can all increase inspired CO_2. The absorption of CO_2 during laparoscopic surgery when CO_2 is used as the abdominal distending gas will increase absorption of CO_2 but will not cause an increase in inspired CO_2. (*Miller: Miller's Anesthesia, ed 8, pp 1551–1559*).

84. (B) (*Miller: Basics of Anesthesia, ed 7, pp 221–223; Ehrenwerth: Anesthesia Equipment: Principles and Applications, ed 2, p 7*).

85. (A) (*Miller: Basics of Anesthesia, ed 7, pp 221–223; Ehrenwerth: Anesthesia Equipment: Principles and Applications, ed 2, p 7*).

86. (D) Medical gas cylinders are color coded, but the colors may differ from one country to another. In the United States if there is a combination of two gases, the tank would have both corresponding colors; for example, a tank containing oxygen and helium would be green and brown. The only exception to the mixed gas color scheme is O_2 and N_2 in the proportion of 19.5% to 23.5% O_2 mixed with N_2, which is solid yellow (air) (*Ehrenwerth: Anesthesia Equipment: Principles and Applications, ed 2, p 7; Miller: Basics of Anesthesia, ed 7, pp 221–223*).

GAS COLOR CODES

Gas	United States	International
Air	Yellow	White and black
CO_2	Gray	Gray
Helium	Brown	Brown
Nitrogen	Black	Black
N_2O	Blue	Blue
Oxygen	Green	White

Data from Ehrenwerth J, Eisenkraft JB, Berry JM: Anesthesia Equipment: Principles and Applications, *ed 2, Philadelphia, Saunders, 2013.*

87. (A) *(Miller: Miller's Anesthesia, ed 8, pp 780–781; Miller: Basics of Anesthesia, ed 7, pp 225–229).*

88. (D) *(Miller: Miller's Anesthesia, ed 8, pp 780–781; Miller: Basics of Anesthesia, ed 7, pp 225–229).*

89. (D) *(Miller: Miller's Anesthesia, ed 8, pp 780–781; Miller: Basics of Anesthesia, ed 7, pp 225–229).*

90. (F) There are six types of Mapleson breathing circuits (designated A through F). These circuits vary in arrangement of the fresh-gas-flow inlet, tubing, mask, reservoir bag, and unidirectional expiratory valve. These systems are lightweight, portable, and easy to clean; they offer low resistance to breathing, and, because of high fresh gas inflows, they prevent rebreathing of exhaled gases. In addition, with these breathing circuits, the concentration of volatile anesthetic gases and O_2 delivered to the patient can be accurately estimated. The reservoir bag enables the anesthesia provider to provide assisted or controlled ventilation of the lungs. The unidirectional expiratory valve functions to direct fresh gas into the patient and exhaled gases out of the circuit. In the Mapleson A breathing circuit, the unidirectional expiratory valve is near the patient, and the fresh-gas-flow inlet is proximal to the reservoir bag. This arrangement is the most efficient for elimination of CO_2 during spontaneous breathing. However, because the unidirectional expiratory valve must be tightened to permit production of positive airway pressure when the gas reservoir bag is manually compressed, this breathing circuit is less efficient in preventing rebreathing of CO_2 during assisted or controlled ventilation of the lungs. The structure of the Mapleson D breathing circuit is similar to that of the Mapleson A breathing circuit except that the positions of the fresh-gas-flow inlet and the unidirectional expiratory valve are reversed. The placement of the fresh-gas-flow inlet near the patient produces efficient elimination of CO_2, regardless of whether the patient is breathing spontaneously or with controlled ventilation. The Bain anesthesia breathing circuit is a coaxial version of the Mapleson D breathing circuit, except that the fresh gas enters through a narrow tube within the corrugated expiratory limb of the circuit. The Jackson-Rees breathing circuit is a modification of the Mapleson E breathing circuit and is called a Mapleson F breathing circuit. In the Jackson-Rees breathing circuit, the adjustable unidirectional expiratory valve is incorporated into the reservoir bag, and the fresh-gas-flow inlet is close to the patient. This arrangement offers the advantage of ease of instituting assisted or controlled ventilation of the lungs, as well as monitoring ventilation by movement of the reservoir bag during spontaneous breathing *(Ehrenwerth: Anesthesia Equipment: Principles and Applications, ed 2, pp 109–117; Miller: Miller's Anesthesia, ed 8, pp 780–781; Miller: Basics of Anesthesia, ed 7, p 225–229).*

CHAPTER 2

Respiratory Physiology and Critical Care Medicine

DIRECTIONS (Questions 91 through 168): Each of the questions or incomplete statements in this section is followed by answers or by completions of the statement, respectively. Select the ONE BEST answer or completion for each item.

91. A 29-year-old man is admitted to the intensive care unit (ICU) after a drug overdose. The patient is placed on a ventilator with a set tidal volume (V_T) of 750 mL at a rate of 10 breaths/min. The patient is making no inspiratory effort. The measured minute ventilation is 6 L, and the peak airway pressure is 30 cm H_2O. What is the compression factor for this ventilator delivery circuit?
    A. 2 mL/(cm H_2O)
    B. 3 mL/(cm H_2O)
    C. 4 mL/(cm H_2O)
    D. 5 mL/(cm H_2O)

92. A 65-year-old patient is mechanically ventilated in the intensive care unit (ICU) after an open nephrectomy. How far should the suction catheter be inserted into the endotracheal tube for suctioning?
    A. To the midlevel of the endotracheal tube
    B. To the tip of the endotracheal tube
    C. Just proximal to the carina
    D. Past the carina

93. Maximizing which of the following lung parameters is the most important factor in prevention of postoperative pulmonary complications?
    A. Tidal volume (V_T)
    B. Inspiratory reserve volume
    C. Vital capacity
    D. Functional residual capacity (FRC)

94. An 83-year-old woman is admitted to the ICU after coronary artery surgery. A pulmonary artery catheter is in place and yields the following data: central venous pressure (CVP) 5 mm Hg, cardiac output (CO) 4.0 L/min, mean arterial pressure (MAP) 90 mm Hg, mean pulmonary artery pressure (PAP) 20 mm Hg, pulmonary artery occlusion pressure (PAOP) 12 mm Hg, and heart rate 90. Calculate this patient's pulmonary vascular resistance (PVR).
    A. 40 dyne-sec/cm^5
    B. 80 dyne-sec/cm^5
    C. 160 dyne-sec/cm^5
    D. 200 dyne-sec/cm^5

95. A 72-year-old man with a history of myocardial infarction 12 months earlier is scheduled to undergo elective repair of a 6-cm abdominal aortic aneurysm under general anesthesia. When would this patient be at highest risk for another myocardial infarction?
    A. During placement of the aortic cross-clamp
    B. Upon release of the aortic cross-clamp
    C. 24 hours postoperatively
    D. On the third postoperative day

96. Calculate the body mass index (BMI) of a man 200 cm (6 feet 6 inches) tall who weighs 100 kg (220 lb).
    A. 20
    B. 25
    C. 30
    D. 35

97. The normal FEV_1/FVC ratio is
    A. 0.99
    B. 0.80
    C. 0.60
    D. 0.50

98. Direct current (DC) cardioversion is not useful and, therefore, **NOT** indicated in an unstable patient with which of the following?
    A. Supraventricular tachycardia in a patient with Wolff-Parkinson-White syndrome
    B. Atrial flutter
    C. Multifocal atrial tachycardia (MAT)
    D. New-onset atrial fibrillation

99. During the first minute of apnea, the Pa_{CO_2} will rise
    A. 2 mm Hg/min
    B. 4 mm Hg/min
    C. 6 mm Hg/min
    D. 8 mm Hg/min

100. Potential complications associated with total parenteral nutrition (TPN) include all of the following **EXCEPT**
  A. Ketoacidosis
  B. Hyperglycemia
  C. Hypoglycemia
  D. Hypophosphatemia

101. O_2 requirement for a 70-kg adult is
  A. 150 mL/min
  B. 250 mL/min
  C. 350 mL/min
  D. 450 mL/min

102. The FRC is composed of the
  A. Expiratory reserve volume and residual volume
  B. Inspiratory reserve volume and residual volume
  C. Inspiratory capacity and vital capacity
  D. Expiratory capacity and V_T

103. Which of the following statements correctly defines the relationship between minute ventilation ($\dot{V}_E$), dead space ventilation ($\dot{V}_D$) and $Paco_2$?
  A. If $\dot{V}_E$ is constant and $\dot{V}_D$ increases, then $Paco_2$ will increase
  B. If $\dot{V}_E$ is constant and $\dot{V}_D$ increases, then $Paco_2$ will decrease
  C. If $\dot{V}_D$ is constant and $\dot{V}_E$ increases, then $Paco_2$ will increase
  D. If $\dot{V}_D$ is constant and $\dot{V}_E$ decreases, then $Paco_2$ will decrease

104. A 22-year-old patient who sustained a closed head injury is brought to the operating room (OR) from the ICU for placement of a dural bolt. Hemoglobin has been stable at 15 g/dL. Blood gas analysis immediately before induction reveals a Pao_2 of 120 mm Hg and an arterial saturation of 100%. After induction, the Pao_2 rises to 150 mm Hg and the saturation remains the same. How has the oxygen content of this patient's blood changed?
  A. It has increased by 10%
  B. It has increased by 5%
  C. It has increased by less than 1%
  D. Cannot be determined without $Paco_2$

105. Inhalation of CO_2 increases $\dot{V}_E$ by
  A. 0.5 L/min/mm Hg increase in $Paco_2$
  B. 1 to 1.5 L/min/mm Hg increase in $Paco_2$
  C. 2 to 2.5 L/min/mm Hg increase in $Paco_2$
  D. Greater than 3 L/min/mm Hg increase in $Paco_2$

106. The RIFLE criteria are designed to predict mortality from
  A. Renal failure
  B. Sepsis
  C. Hepatic failure
  D. Acute respiratory distress syndrome

107. Each of the following will cause erroneous readings by dual-wavelength pulse oximeters **EXCEPT**
  A. Carboxyhemoglobin
  B. Methylene blue
  C. Fetal hemoglobin
  D. Methemoglobin

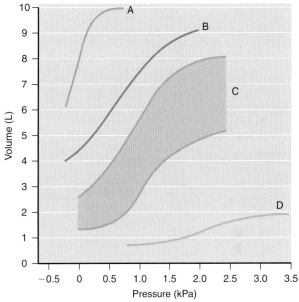

(From Miller RD: Miller's Anesthesia, ed 7, Philadelphia, Saunders, 2011, Figure 15-4. Courtesy the editor of the BMJ series: Respiratory Measurement.)

108. In the diagram above, curve "D" represents
  A. Emphysema
  B. Chronic bronchitis
  C. Normal lungs
  D. Fibrotic lungs

109. The P_{50} for normal adult hemoglobin is approximately
  A. 15 mm Hg
  B. 25 mm Hg
  C. 35 mm Hg
  D. 45 mm Hg

110. During a normal V_T (500-mL) breath, the transpulmonary pressure increases from 0 to 5 cm H_2O. The product of transpulmonary pressure and V_T is 2500 cm H_2O-mL. This expression of the pressure-volume relationship during breathing determines what parameter of respiratory mechanics?
  A. Lung compliance
  B. Airway resistance
  C. Pulmonary elastance
  D. Work of breathing

111. Select the true statement regarding palliative care
  A. It increases in-hospital cost
  B. It is reserved for patients with life expectancy less than 6 months
  C. It is not appropriate for patients in the ICU
  D. It can be used in conjunction with "aggressive" care

112. The normal vital capacity for a 70-kg man is
  A. 1 L
  B. 2 L
  C. 5 L
  D. 7 L

113. A 32-year-old man is found unconscious by the fire department in a room where he has inhaled 0.1% carbon monoxide for a prolonged period. His respiratory rate is 42 breaths/min, but he is not cyanotic. Carbon monoxide has increased this patient's minute ventilation by which of the following mechanisms?
  A. Shifting the O_2 hemoglobin dissociation curve to the left
  B. Increasing CO_2 production
  C. Causing lactic acidosis
  D. Decreasing Pa_{O_2}

114. An acute increase in Pa_{CO_2} of 10 mm Hg will result in a decrease in pH of
  A. 0.01 pH unit
  B. 0.02 pH unit
  C. 0.04 pH unit
  D. 0.08 pH unit

115. A 22-year-old college student with a history of complex regional pain syndrome (CRPS) in the left foot and ankle after a football injury is anesthetized for laparoscopic cholecystectomy. He reports allergy to penicillin and is treated for chronic pain with paroxetine (Paxil) and gabapentin (Neurontin) and indomethacin prn. He received fentanyl as the primary narcotic during his operation to facilitate early discharge. In the PACU he is shivering and has BP 183/98 mm Hg with pulse 121. He receives 15 mg meperidine; shivering persists. He reports minimal 3/10 pain. The best option at this juncture would be
  A. Repeat meperidine
  B. Labetalol
  C. Lorazepam (Ativan)
  D. Dantrolene

116. The following blood gases would best be explained by which disorder?
  pH 7.18, Pa_{CO_2} 25 mm Hg, HCO_3^- 11 mEq/L
  A. Aspirin overdose
  B. Nasogastric suction
  C. Chloride wasting diarrhea
  D. Hyperaldosteronism

117. The diagram below depicts which mode of ventilation?

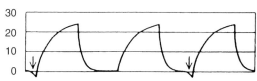

  A. Spontaneous ventilation
  B. Controlled ventilation
  C. Assisted ventilation
  D. Assisted/controlled ventilation

118. A 78-year-old man with a 125-pack-year smoking history is brought to the ICU after total laryngectomy for treatment of his laryngeal squamous cell carcinoma. In the ICU his tracheostomy tube becomes totally occluded and cannot be cleared with suctioning. The most appropriate course of action while waiting for the ENT surgeon would be
  A. Bag mask or laryngeal mask airway until help arrives
  B. Attempt to intubate with GlideScope or direct laryngoscopy
  C. Oral or nasal fiberoptic intubation
  D. Remove tracheostomy tube and intubate laryngectomy stoma with an endotracheal tube

119. The P_{50} of sickle cell hemoglobin is
  A. 19 mm Hg
  B. 26 mm Hg
  C. 31 mm Hg
  D. 35 mm Hg

120. Data from the ARDS network trial (ARDSNet) showed increased mortality from
  A. Atelectrauma
  B. Volutrauma
  C. Barotrauma
  D. Inhaled nitric oxide

121. Which of the following is the correct mathematical expression of Fick's law of diffusion of a gas through a lipid membrane ($\dot{V}$ = rate of diffusion, D = diffusion coefficient of the gas, A = area of the membrane, P1 − P2 = transmembrane partial pressure gradient of the gas, T = thickness of the membrane)?

  A. $\dot{V} = D \times \dfrac{A \times T}{P_1 - P_2}$

  B. $\dot{V} = \dfrac{A \times T}{D(P_1 - P_2)}$

  C. $\dot{V} = D \times \dfrac{A(P_1 - P_2)}{T}$

  D. $\dot{V} = D \times \dfrac{T(P_1 - P_2)}{A}$

122. Each of the following is decreased in elderly patients compared with their younger counterparts **EXCEPT**
A. Closing volume
B. FEV_1
C. Ventilatory response to hypercarbia
D. Vital capacity

123. Calculate the V_D/V_T ratio (physiologic dead space ventilation) based on the following data: $PaCO_2$ 45 mm Hg, mixed expired CO_2 tension ($PECO_2$) 30 mm Hg.
A. 0.1
B. 0.2
C. 0.3
D. 0.4

124. Which of the following statements concerning the distribution of O_2 and CO_2 in the upright lungs is **TRUE**?
A. PaO_2 is greater at the apex than at the base
B. $PaCO_2$ is greater at the apex than at the base
C. Both PaO_2 and $PaCO_2$ are greater at the apex than at the base
D. Both PaO_2 and $PaCO_2$ are greater at the base than at the apex

125. Which of the following acid-base disturbances is the least well-compensated?
A. Metabolic alkalosis
B. Respiratory alkalosis
C. Increased anion gap metabolic acidosis
D. Normal anion gap metabolic acidosis

126. What is the (calculated) PaO_2 of a patient on room air in Denver, Colorado? (Assume a barometric pressure of 630 mm Hg, respiratory quotient of 0.8, and $PaCO_2$ of 34 mm Hg.)
A. 80 mm Hg
B. 90 mm Hg
C. 100 mm Hg
D. 110 mm Hg

127. A venous blood sample from which of the following sites would correlate most reliably with PaO_2 and $PaCO_2$?
A. Jugular vein
B. Subclavian vein
C. Antecubital vein
D. Vein on posterior surface of a warmed hand

128. Which of the following pulmonary function tests is **LEAST** dependent on patient effort?
A. Forced expiratory volume in 1 second (FEV_1)
B. Forced vital capacity (FVC)
C. FEF 800 to 1200
D. FEF 25% to 75%

129. A 33-year-old woman with 20% carboxyhemoglobin is brought to the ER for treatment of smoke inhalation. Which of the following is **LEAST** consistent with a diagnosis of carbon monoxide poisoning?
A. Cyanosis
B. PaO_2 105 mm Hg, oxygen saturation 80% on initial room air arterial blood gases (ABGs)
C. 98% oxygen saturation on dual-wavelength pulse oximeter
D. Oxyhemoglobin dissociation curve shifted far to the left

130. The $PAO_2 - PaO_2$ of a patient breathing 100% O_2 is 240 mm Hg. The estimated fraction of the cardiac output shunted past the lungs without exposure to ventilated alveoli (i.e., transpulmonary shunt) is
A. 5%
B. 12%
C. 17%
D. 20%

131. Each of the following will alter the position or slope of the CO_2-ventilatory response curve **EXCEPT**
A. Hypoxemia
B. Fentanyl
C. N_2O
D. Ketamine

132. Which of the following statements concerning the distribution of alveolar ventilation ($\dot{V}_A$) in the upright lungs is **TRUE**?
A. The distribution of $\dot{V}_A$ is not affected by body posture
B. Alveoli at the apex of the lungs (nondependent alveoli) are better ventilated than those at the base
C. All areas of the lungs are ventilated equally
D. Alveoli at the base of the lungs (dependent alveoli) are better ventilated than those at the apex

133. In the resting adult, what percentage of total body O_2 consumption is due to the work of breathing?
A. 2%
B. 5%
C. 10%
D. 20%

134. The anatomic dead space in a 70-kg man is
A. 50 mL
B. 150 mL
C. 250 mL
D. 500 mL

135. The most important buffering system in the body is
A. Hemoglobin
B. Plasma proteins
C. Phosphate
D. $[HCO_3^-]$

136. A decrease in pH of 0.1 unit will result in
   A. A decrease in serum potassium concentration $[K^+]$ of 0.1 mEq/L
   B. A decrease in $[K^+]$ of 1.0 mEq/L
   C. An increase in $[K^+]$ of 1.0 mEq/L
   D. An increase in $[K^+]$ of 2.0 mEq/L

137. A 45-year-old man is rescued from a house fire and brought to the ER. He is noted to have major burns involving 45% of his body, with singed skin on the forehead and tip of his nose and painful burned hands. His blood pressure is 185/90 mm Hg, and his heart rate is 130. He complains of phlegm in his throat, has trouble phonating, and is coughing dark black material. The greatest need for this patient is
   A. Fluids to preserve renal function
   B. Beta blockade and analgesics
   C. Oxygen therapy with humidification
   D. Securing the airway

138. A 28-year-old, 70-kg woman with ulcerative colitis is receiving a general anesthetic for a colon resection and ileostomy. The patient's lungs are mechanically ventilated with the following parameters: V_E 5000 mL and respiratory rate 10 breaths/min. Assuming no change in V_E, how would V_A change if the respiratory rate were increased from 10 to 20 breaths/min?
   A. Increase by 500 mL
   B. Increase by 1000 mL
   C. Decrease by 750 mL
   D. Decrease by 1500 mL

139. Each of the following will shift the oxyhemoglobin dissociation curve to the right **EXCEPT**
   A. Volatile anesthetics
   B. Decreased Pa_{O_2}
   C. Decreased pH
   D. Increased temperature

140. The half-life of carboxyhemoglobin in a patient breathing 100% O_2 is
   A. 5 minutes
   B. 1 hour
   C. 2 hours
   D. 4 hours

141. A disadvantage of using propofol for prolonged sedation (days) of intubated patients in the ICU is potential
   A. Alkalosis
   B. Hypokalemia
   C. Hypolipidemia
   D. Bradycardia

142. A 17-year-old type 1 diabetic with history of renal failure is in the preoperative holding area awaiting an operation for acute appendicitis. Arterial blood gases are obtained with the following results: Pa_{O_2} 88 mm Hg, Pa_{CO_2} 32 mm Hg, pH 7.2, $[HCO_3^-]$ 12, $[Cl^-]$ 115 mEq/L, $[Na^+]$ 138 mEq/L, and glucose 251 mg/dL. The most likely cause of this patient's acidosis is
   A. Renal tubular acidosis
   B. Lactic acidosis
   C. Diabetic ketoacidosis
   D. Aspirin overdose

143. Methods to decrease the incidence of central venous catheter infections include all of the following **EXCEPT**
   A. Changing the central catheter every 3 to 4 days over a guidewire
   B. Using minocycline/rifampin impregnated catheters over chlorhexidine/silver sulfadiazine impregnated catheters for suspected long-term use
   C. Using the subclavian over the internal jugular route for access
   D. Using a single lumen over a multilumen catheter

144. Signs of Sarin nerve gas poisoning include all of the following **EXCEPT**
   A. Diarrhea
   B. Urination
   C. Mydriasis
   D. Lacrimation

145. Which of the following conditions would be associated with the **LEAST** risk of venous air embolism during removal of a central line?
   A. Spontaneous breathing, head up
   B. Spontaneous breathing, flat
   C. Spontaneous breathing, Trendelenburg
   D. Mechanical ventilation, Trendelenburg

146. Which of the following adverse effects is **NOT** attributable to respiratory or metabolic acidosis?
   A. Increased intracranial pressure
   B. Peripheral vasoconstriction
   C. Increased pulmonary vascular resistance
   D. Increased serum potassium concentration

147. Which of the following maneuvers is **LEAST** likely to raise arterial saturation in a patient in whom the endotracheal tube (ETT) is seated in the right mainstem bronchus? The patient has normal lung function.
   A. Inflating the pulmonary artery catheter balloon (in the left pulmonary artery)
   B. Raising hemoglobin from 8 to 12 mg/dL
   C. Raising F_{IO_2} from 0.8 to 1.0
   D. Increasing cardiac output from 2 to 5 L/min

148. A 100-kg man is 24 hours status post four-vessel coronary artery bypass graft. Which of the following pulmonary parameters would be compatible with successful extubation in this patient?
   A. Vital capacity 2.5 L
   B. Pa_{CO_2} 44 mm Hg
   C. Maximum inspiratory pressure -38 cm H_2O
   D. All of the above

149. Which of the following can cause a rightward shift of the oxyhemoglobin dissociation curve?
   A. Methemoglobinemia
   B. Carboxyhemoglobinemia
   C. Hypothermia
   D. Pregnancy

150. A 24-year-old man is brought to the operating room 1 hour after a motor vehicle accident. He has C7 spinal cord transection and ruptured spleen. Regarding his neurologic injury, anesthetic concerns include
   A. Risk of hyperkalemia with succinylcholine administration
   B. Risk of autonomic hyper-reflexia with urinary catheter insertion
   C. Increased risk of hypothermia
   D. All of the above

151. After sustaining traumatic brain injury, a 37-year-old patient in the ICU develops polyuria and a plasma sodium concentration of 159 mEq/L. What pathologic condition is associated with these clinical findings?
   A. Syndrome of inappropriate antidiuretic hormone (SIADH)
   B. Diabetes mellitus
   C. Diabetes insipidus
   D. Cerebral salt wasting syndrome

152. Which of the following drugs is the best choice for treating hypotension in the setting of severe acidemia?
   A. Norepinephrine
   B. Epinephrine
   C. Phenylephrine
   D. Vasopressin

153. The end-tidal CO_2 measured by an infrared spectrometer is 35 mm Hg. An arterial blood gas sample drawn at exactly the same moment is 45 mm Hg. Which of the following is the **LEAST** plausible explanation for this?
   A. Morbid obesity
   B. Pulmonary embolism
   C. Intrapulmonary shunt
   D. Chronic obstructive pulmonary disease (COPD)

154. A transfusion-related, acute lung injury (TRALI) reaction is suspected in a 48-year-old man in the ICU after a 10-hour operation for scoliosis during which multiple units of blood and factors were administered. Which of the following items is inconsistent with the diagnosis of a TRALI reaction?
   A. Fever
   B. Alveolar-to-arterial (A–a) oxygen gradient of 25 mm Hg
   C. Acute rise in neutrophil count after onset of symptoms
   D. Bilateral pulmonary infiltrates

155. If a central line located in the superior vena cava (SVC) is withdrawn such that the tip of the catheter is just proximal to the SVC, it would be located in which vessel?
   A. Subclavian vein
   B. Brachiocephalic vein
   C. Cephalic vein
   D. Internal jugular vein

156. The time course of anticoagulation therapy is variable after different percutaneous coronary interventions (PCIs). Arrange the interventions in order, starting with the one requiring the shortest course of aspirin and clopidogrel (Plavix) therapy to the one requiring the longest course.
   A. Bare-metal stent, percutaneous transluminal coronary angioplasty (PTCA), drug-eluting stent
   B. Drug-eluting stent, bare-metal stent, PTCA
   C. PTCA, drug-eluting stent, bare-metal stent
   D. PTCA, bare-metal stent, drug-eluting stent

157. A 75-year-old patient in the ICU is intubated and ventilated on AC 12, V_T 500, and "some" PEEP. In a 60-second period, he initiates two spontaneous breaths. The peak airway pressure alarm has not sounded. His minute ventilation would be
   A. Incalculable without knowledge of PEEP value
   B. Incalculable without knowing dead space
   C. Incalculable without knowing magnitude of the two spontaneous breaths
   D. Seven liters

158. Which of the features below is suggestive of weaponized anthrax exposure as opposed to a common flu-like viral illness?
   A. Widened mediastinum
   B. Fever, chills, myalgia
   C. Severe cough
   D. Pharyngitis

159. Which of the following factors could not explain a PaO_2 of 48 mm Hg in a patient breathing a mixture of nitrous oxide and oxygen?

A. Hypoxic gas mixture

B. Eisenmenger syndrome

C. Profound anemia

D. Hypercarbia

160. During a left hepatectomy under general isoflurane anesthesia, arterial blood gases are: O_2 138, CO_2 39, pH 7.38, saturation 99%. At the same time, CO_2 on infrared spectrometer is 26 mm Hg. The most plausible explanation for the difference between CO_2 measured with infrared spectrometer versus arterial blood gas gradient is

A. Mainstem intubation

B. Atelectasis

C. Shunting through thebesian veins

D. Hypovolemia

161. Under which set of circumstances would energy expenditure per day be the greatest?

A. Sepsis with fever

B. 60% burn

C. Multiple fractures

D. 1 hour status post liver transplantation

162. Select the **FALSE** statement regarding amiodarone (Cordarone).

A. It is shown to decrease mortality after myocardial infarction

B. It is indicated for ventricular tachycardia and fibrillation refractory to electrical defibrillation

C. Adverse effects include pulmonary fibrosis and thyroid dysfunction

D. It is useful in treatment of torsades de pointes

163. A 58-year-old woman is awaiting orthotopic liver transplantation for primary biliary cirrhosis in the ICU. An oximetric pulmonary artery catheter is placed, and an SvO_2 of 90% is measured. Which of the following blood pressure interventions is the **LEAST** appropriate for treatment of hypotension in this patient?

A. Milrinone

B. Norepinephrine

C. Vasopressin

D. Phenylephrine

164. A 73-year-old patient is on a ventilator after an MVA. Rate is set at AC 16, V_T 450 with 5 cm H_2O PEEP. The respiratory therapist notes that the measured PEEP is greater than 15 cm H_2O and that the patient is not breathing above the set rate. Which option below is most reasonable for reducing the measured PEEP?

A. Increase the respiratory rate

B. Increase inspiratory flow rate

C. Reverse the I to E ratio

D. Paralyze the patient

165. A 55-year-old man with polycystic liver disease undergoes an 8-hour right hepatectomy. The patient receives 5 units of packed red cells, 1000 mL albumin, and 6 L normal saline. The patient is extubated and taken to a postanesthesia care unit (PACU) where ABGs are: PaO_2 135, $PaCO_2$ 44, pH 7.17, base deficit −11, $[HCO_3^-]$ 12, 97% saturation, $[Cl^-]$ 119, $[Na^+]$ 145, and $[K^+]$ 5.6. The most likely cause for this acidosis is

A. Lactic acid

B. Use of normal saline

C. Diabetic ketoacidosis

D. Polyethylene glycol from bowel prep

166. Which of the following is the **LEAST** appropriate use of noninvasive positive-pressure ventilation (NIPPV)?

A. Acute respiratory distress syndrome (ARDS)

B. COPD exacerbation

C. Obstructive sleep apnea

D. Multiple sclerosis exacerbation

167. A 68-year-old asthmatic drunk driver comes into the ER after being in a motor vehicle accident. After a difficult intubation, you fail to observe end-tidal CO_2 on the monitor. Reasons for this include all of the following **EXCEPT**

A. You intubated the esophagus by mistake

B. You forgot to ventilate the patient

C. The connection between the circuit and monitor has become disconnected

D. The patient also has a pneumothorax, and high airway pressures are needed to adequately ventilate the patient

168. A 30-year-old woman has undergone a 2-hour abdominal surgical procedure and is sent to the ICU intubated for postoperative monitoring, due to suspected sepsis. Three hours later, the ventilator malfunctions and the resident disconnects the patient from the ventilator and hand ventilates the patient with 100% oxygen. The patient has good bilateral breath sounds, the chest rises nicely, and moisture is seen in the ETT. Shortly thereafter, the patient's heart rate slows to 30 beats/min and the blood pressure is 50 mm Hg systolic. The next intervention that should be done, in addition to chest compressions, is

A. Administer atropine

B. Start epinephrine

C. Confirm ETT position

D. Apply external pacemaker

91. (D) A volume-cycled ventilator set to deliver a volume of 750 mL at a rate of 10/min would deliver a minute ventilation of 7.5 L. The measured minute ventilation, however, is only 6 L; therefore, 1.5 L must be absorbed by the breathing circuit. This volume is known as the compression volume. If one divides the volume by 10 (number of breaths/min), then one determines the compression volume/breath. This number (mL) can be further divided by the peak inflation pressure (cm H_2O) to determine the actual compression factor, which in this case is 5 mL/(cm H_2O) *(Miller: Basics of Anesthesia, ed 7, pp 230–231; Ehrenwerth: Anesthesia Equipment Principles and Applications, p 364).*

$$\text{Compression volume} = \frac{(\dot{V}_{delivered} - \dot{V}_{measured}) / \text{Respiratory rate}}{\text{Peak airway pressure (cm } H_2O)} = 5 \text{ mL/(cm } H_2O)$$

92. (B) Endotracheal tubes frequently become partially or completely occluded with secretions. Periodic suctioning of the endotracheal tube in the ICU assures patency of the artificial airway. There are hazards, however, of endotracheal tube suctioning. They include mucosal trauma, cardiac dysrhythmias, hypoxia, increased intracranial pressure, colonization of the distal airway, and psychological trauma to the patient. To reduce the possibility of colonization of the distal airway, it is prudent to keep the suction catheter within the endotracheal tube during suctioning. Pushing the suctioning catheter beyond the distal limits of the endotracheal tube also may produce suctioning trauma to the tracheal tissue *(Tobin: Principles and Practices of Mechanical Ventilation, ed 3, p 1223; Hagberg: Hagberg and Benumof's Airway Management, ed 4, p 796; Goldsmith: Assisted Ventilation of the Neonate, ed 6, p 302).*

93. (D) (Please see diagram and table for explanation with Question 102.) FRC is composed of expiratory reserve volume plus residual volume. It is essential to maximize FRC in the postoperative period to ensure that it will be greater than closing volume. Closing volume is that lung volume at which small-airway closure begins to occur. Maximizing FRC, therefore, reduces atelectasis and lessens the incidence of arterial hypoxemia and pneumonia. Maneuvers aimed at increasing FRC include early ambulation, incentive spirometry, deep breathing, and intermittent positive-pressure breathing *(Barash: Clinical Anesthesia, ed 8, p 376).*

94. (C)

$$PVR = \frac{(PAP_{mean} - PAOP)}{CO} \times 80$$

where PVR is the pulmonary vascular resistance, PAP_{mean} is the mean pulmonary artery pressure, PAOP is the mean pulmonary capillary occlusion pressure, and CO is the cardiac output.

$$PVR = \frac{(20 - 12)}{4} \times 80 = 160 \text{ dyne-sec/cm}^5$$

The normal range for PVR is 50 to 150 dyne-sec/cm^5 *(Miller: Miller's Anesthesia, ed 8, pp 1460–1461; Barash: Clinical Anesthesia, ed 8, p 1708).*

95. (D) For reasons that are not fully understood, patients who have sustained a myocardial infarction and subsequently undergo surgery are most likely to have another infarction 48 to 72 hours postoperatively, so the third postoperative day is the most likely of the choices listed. *(Miller: Basics of Anesthesia, ed 7, p 417).*

96. (B) Calculation of BMI for adults (>20 years of age) can help identify patients who are underweight (BMI <18.5), normal weight (BMI 18.5-24.9), overweight (BMI 25-29.9), class 1 obesity (BMI 30-34.9), class 2 obesity (BMI 35-39.9), class 3 obesity (BMI 40-49.9), and the superobese (BMI >50).

$$BMI = \frac{mass\ (kg)}{(Height)^2\ (meters)} \qquad\qquad BMI = \frac{100}{(2)^2} = 25$$

All major organ systems are affected as a consequence of obesity. The greatest concerns for the anesthesiologist are, however, related to the heart and lungs. Cardiac output must increase about 0.1 L/min for each extra kilogram of adipose tissue. As a consequence, obese patients frequently are hypertensive, and many ultimately develop cardiomegaly and left-sided heart failure. FRC is reduced in obese patients, and management of the airway often can be difficult *(Miller: Miller's Anesthesia, ed 8, pp 2200–2201; Barash: Clinical Anesthesia, ed 8, p 1278).*

97. (B) The forced expiratory volume in 1 second (FEV_1) is the total volume of air that can be exhaled in the first second. Normal healthy adults can exhale approximately 75% to 85% of their forced vital capacity (FVC) in the first second, 94% in 2 seconds, and 97% in 3 seconds. Therefore the normal FEV_1/FVC ratio is 0.75 or higher. In the presence of obstructive airway disease, the FEV_1/FVC ratio less than 70% reflects mild obstruction, less than 60% moderate obstruction, and less than 50% severe obstruction. This ratio can be used to determine the severity of obstructive airway disease and to monitor the efficacy of bronchodilator therapy *(Barash: Clinical Anesthesia, ed 8, p 377).*

98. (C) MAT is a non-reentrant, ectopic atrial rhythm often seen in patients with chronic obstructive pulmonary disease (COPD). It is frequently confused with atrial fibrillation but, in contrast to atrial fibrillation, atrial flutter, and paroxysmal supraventricular tachycardia, DC cardioversion is ineffective in converting it to normal sinus rhythm. Ectopic atrial tachydysrhythmias are not amenable to cardioversion because they lack the re-entrant mechanism, which is necessary for successful termination with electrical counter shock *(Page et al.: 2015 ACC/AHA/HRS Guideline for the Management of Adult Patients With Supraventricular Tachycardia: A Report of the American College of Cardiology/American Heart Association Task Force on Clinical Practice Guidelines and the Hearth Rhythm Society, Circulation 133:e506, 2016).*

99. (C) During apnea, the $PaCO_2$ will increase approximately 6 mm Hg during the first minute and then 3 to 4 mm Hg each minute thereafter *(Miller: Basics of Anesthesia, ed 7, pp 64–65).*

100. (A) TPN therapy is associated with numerous potential complications. Blood sugars need to be carefully monitored because hyperglycemia may develop due to the high glucose load and require treatment with insulin, and hypoglycemia may develop if TPN is abruptly stopped (i.e., infusion turned off or mechanical obstruction in the IV tubing). Other complications include electrolyte disturbances (e.g., hypokalemia, hypophosphatemia, hypomagnesemia, hypocalcemia), volume overload, catheter-related sepsis, renal and hepatic dysfunction, thrombosis of the central veins, and nonketotic hyperosmolar coma. Increased work of breathing is related to increased production of CO_2, most frequently due to overfeeding. Acidosis in these patients is hyperchloremic metabolic acidosis resulting from formation of HCl during metabolism of amino acids. Ketoacidosis is not associated with TPN therapy *(Miller: Basics of Anesthesia, ed 7, p 499).*

101. (B) The O_2 requirement for an adult is 3 to 4 mL/kg/min. The O_2 requirement for a newborn is 7 to 9 mL/kg/min. Alveolar ventilation (V_A) in neonates is double that of adults to help meet their increased O_2 requirements. This increase in V_A is achieved primarily by an increase in respiratory rate as V_T is similar to that of adults (i.e., 7 mL/kg). Although CO_2 production also is increased in neonates, the elevated V_A maintains the $PaCO_2$ near 38 to 40 mm Hg *(Barash: Clinical Anesthesia, ed 8, p 1181).*

102. (A) A comprehensive understanding of respiratory physiology is important for understanding the effects of both regional and general anesthesia on respiratory mechanics and pulmonary gas exchange. The volume of gas remaining in the lungs after a normal expiration is called the functional residual capacity. The volume of gas remaining in the lungs after a maximal expiration is called the residual volume. The difference between these two volumes is called the expiratory reserve volume. Therefore the FRC is composed of the expiratory reserve volume and residual volume *(Barash: Clinical Anesthesia, ed 8, p 376).*

LUNG VOLUMES AND CAPACITIES

Measurement	Abbreviation	Normal Adult Value
Tidal volume	V_T	500 mL (6-8 mL/kg)
Inspiratory reserve volume	IRV	3000 mL
Expiratory reserve volume	ERV	1200 mL
Residual volume	RV	1200 mL
Inspiratory capacity	IC	3500 mL
Functional residual capacity	FRC	2400 mL
Vital capacity	VC	4500 mL (60-70 mL/kg)
Forced exhaled volume in 1 sec	FEV_1	80%
Total lung capacity	TLC	5900 mL

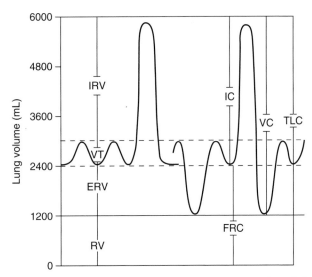

(From Stoelting RK: Pharmacology and Physiology in Anesthetic Practice, ed 3, Philadelphia, Lippincott Williams & Wilkins, 1999.)

---

103. (A) The volume of gas in the conducting airways of the lungs (and not available for gas exchange) is called the anatomic dead space. The volume of gas in ventilated alveoli that is unperfused (and not available for gas exchange) is called the functional dead space. The anatomic dead space together with the functional dead space is called the physiologic dead space. Physiologic dead space ventilation (V_D) can be calculated by the Bohr dead space equation, which is mathematically expressed as follows:

$$V_D/V_T = \frac{(Pa_{CO_2} - PE_{CO_2})}{Pa_{CO_2}}$$

where V_D/V_T is the ratio of V_D to V_T, and a and E represent arterial and mixed expired, respectively. Of the choices given, only the first is correct. A large increase in V_D will result in an increase in Pa_{CO_2} *(West: Respiratory Physiology, ed 9, pp 19–21; Miller: Miller's Anesthesia, ed 8, pp 446–447; Barash: Clinical Anesthesia, ed 8, pp 373–374).*

104. (C) The oxygen content of blood can be calculated with the following formula

$$O_2 \text{ content} = 1.39 \times [Hgb] \times SaO_2 + (0.003 \times PaO_2)$$

$$\text{First oxygen content} = (1.39 \times 15 \times 1.0) + 0.003 \times 120 = 21.2 \text{mL/dL}$$

$$\text{Second oxygen content} = (1.39 \times 15 \times 1.0) + 0.003 \times 150 = 21.30 \text{mL/dL}$$

The difference in the oxygen content is 0.09 mL/dL. This represents a change of 0.42% *(Barash: Clinical Anesthesia, ed 8, p 432)*.

105. (B) The degree of ventilatory depression caused by volatile anesthetics can be assessed by measuring resting Pa_{CO_2}, the ventilatory response to hypercarbia, and the ventilatory response to hypoxemia. Of these techniques, the resting Pa_{CO_2} is the most frequently used index. However, measuring the effects of increased Pa_{CO_2} on ventilation is the most sensitive method of quantifying the effects of drugs on ventilation. In awake unanesthetized humans, inhalation of CO_2 increases minute ventilation ($\dot{V}_E$) by approximately 1 to 1.5 L/min/mm Hg increase in Pa_{CO_2}. Using this technique, halothane, isoflurane, desflurane-N_2O, desflurane-N_2O, and N_2O cause a dose-dependent depression of the ventilation *(Miller: Basics of Anesthesia, ed 7, p 67)*.

106. (A) To create a uniform definition of acute renal insufficiency, the Acute Dialysis Quality Initiative (ADQI) group was convened and, in 2004, proposed the RIFLE (Risk, Injury, Failure, Loss, and End-stage renal disease) criteria. RIF refers to the three levels of renal dysfunction; LE refers to clinical outcomes. The first three criteria have two parts: glomerular filtration rate (GFR) criteria and urine output (UO) criteria.

Risk of renal dysfunction	a. Increased serum creatinine >1.5 × baseline or GFR is decreased >25% b. Urine Output <0.5 mL/kg/hr for 6 hours *(In-hospital mortality Odds Ratio of 2.2)*
Injury to the kidney	a. Increased serum creatinine >2 × baseline or GFR is decreased >50% b. Urine Output <0.5 mL/kg/hr for 12 hours *(In-hospital mortality Odds Ratio of 6.1)*
Failure of kidney function	a. Increased serum creatinine >3 × baseline or GFR is decreased >75% or creatinine >4 mg/dL b. Urine Output <0.3 mL/kg/hr for 24 hours or anuria for 12 hours *(In-hospital mortality Odds Ratio of 8.6)*
Loss of kidney function	- Complete loss of renal function for >4 weeks (need for renal replacement therapy for >4 weeks)
End Stage Renal Disease	- End-stage disease (need for dialysis for >3 months)

(Barash Clinical Anesthesia, 8th ed, p 1529; Miller: Anesthesia, ed 7, p 717; Miller: Anesthesia, ed 8, pp 3047–3048)

107. (C) The presence of hemoglobin species other than oxyhemoglobin can cause erroneous readings by dual-wavelength pulse oximeters. Hemoglobin species such as carboxyhemoglobin and methemoglobin, dyes such as methylene blue and indocyanine green, and some colors of nail polish will cause erroneous readings. Because the absorption spectrum of fetal hemoglobin is similar to that of adult oxyhemoglobin, fetal hemoglobin does not significantly affect the accuracy of these types of pulse oximeters. High levels of bilirubin have no significant effect on the accuracy of dual-wavelength pulse oximeters but may cause falsely low readings by nonpulsatile oximeters *(Miller: Miller's Anesthesia, ed 8, pp 1545–1547; Yao & Artusio: Anesthesiology, ed 8, pp 1097–1098)*.

108. (D) This graph depicts lung volumes as a function of pressure or compliance; one kPa is roughly equal to 10 cm H_2O. Curve A shows an enormous volume with a small pressure (i.e., emphysema). Curve B depicts chronic bronchitis or asthma. The compliance curve is roughly the same as the normal lung, curve C, but volumes have increased. Curve D depicts stiff noncompliant lungs as seen with fibrosis or ARDS *(Miller: Miller's Anesthesia, ed 8, pp 447–448; Barash: Clinical Anesthesia, ed 8, pp 364–365)*.

109. (B) P_{50} is the Pa_{O_2} required to produce 50% saturation of hemoglobin. The P_{50} for adult hemoglobin at a pH of 7.4 and body temperature of 37° C is 26 mm Hg *(Miller: Basics of Anesthesia, ed 7, p 59)*.

110. (B) The work of breathing is defined as the product of transpulmonary pressure and V_T. The work of breathing is related to two factors: the work required to overcome the elastic forces of the lungs, and the work required to overcome airflow or frictional resistances of the airways *(Miller: Miller's Anesthesia, ed 8, p 1563; Barash: Clinical Anesthesia, ed 8, p 365).*

111. (D) Palliative care is an approach provided by a team of physicians, nurses, social workers, and other health care professionals to help patients with life-threatening illnesses improve their quality of life. Palliative care is not limited to patients who are expected to die within 6 months. Goals are directed to help with the patient's pain, anxiety, and depression, as well as to provide family support. Inpatient palliative care teams have been shown to decrease inpatient hospital costs for patients who are discharged from the hospital, as well as for patients who have died in the hospital. In addition, there were fewer deaths in the ICU after palliative care programs were started. Initially, these care teams focused on medical ICUs, but now include surgical ICUs as well as outpatient clinics. Palliative care is appropriate at any stage of a serious illness and can be used in conjunction with "aggressive" care. Hospice care has several similarities to palliative care but usually refers to care for patients on home-based care with a life expectancy <6 months. In the United States 80% of the fees for hospice care are paid by Medicare. Most of the care of patients with hospice care is by a nurse, with physician oversight *(Miller: Anesthesia, ed 8, pp 1919–1924).*

112. (C) The volume of gas exhaled during a maximum expiration is the vital capacity. In a normal healthy adult, the vital capacity is 60 to 70 mL/kg. In a 70-kg patient, the vital capacity is approximately 5 L *(Barash: Clinical Anesthesia, ed 8, p 376).*

113. (C) Carbon monoxide inhalation is the most common immediate cause of death from fire. Carbon monoxide binds to hemoglobin with an affinity 200 times greater than that of oxygen. For this reason, very small concentrations of carbon monoxide can greatly reduce the oxygen-carrying capacity of blood. In spite of this, the arterial PaO_2 often is normal. Because the carotid bodies respond to arterial PaO_2, there would not be an increase in minute ventilation until tissue hypoxia was sufficient to produce lactic acidosis *(Miller: Miller's Anesthesia, ed 8, pp 2679–2680; West: Respiratory Physiology, ed 9, pp 80–82; Barash: Clinical Anesthesia, ed 8, p 368; Miller: Basics of Anesthesia, ed 7, p 742).*

114. (D) Respiratory acidosis is present when the $PaCO_2$ exceeds 44 mm Hg. Respiratory acidosis is caused by decreased elimination of CO_2 by the lungs (i.e., hypoventilation) or increased metabolic production of CO_2. An acute increase in $PaCO_2$ of 10 mm Hg will result in a decrease in pH of approximately 0.08 pH unit. The acidosis of arterial blood will stimulate ventilation via the carotid bodies, and the acidosis of cerebrospinal fluid will stimulate ventilation via the medullary chemoreceptors located in the fourth cerebral ventricle. Volatile anesthetics greatly attenuate the carotid body–mediated and aortic body–mediated ventilatory responses to arterial acidosis, but they have little effect on the medullary chemoreceptor–mediated ventilatory response to cerebrospinal fluid acidosis *(Miller: Basics of Anesthesia, ed 7, p 372).*

115. (C) Paroxetine is a selective serotonin receptor inhibitor (SSRI) and if meperidine is administered, you can induce a serotonin syndrome. Treatment consists of supportive care and since the patient has signs of serotonin syndrome, the best medication treatment listed would be the benzodiazepine lorazepam (Ativan). Cyproheptadine, which binds to serotonin receptors, is a better medication to treat serotonin syndrome but is only available for oral use. Serotonin syndrome is a potentially life-threatening condition associated with increasing serotonergic neurotransmission, commonly associated with two or more serotonergic agents. Signs include altered mentation, tremor, clonus, diaphoresis, and hyperthermia. Severe disease is associated with DIC, rhabdomyolysis, myoglobinuria, renal failure, and ARDS. Treatment includes cessation of all serotonergic agents, treatment with benzodiazepines, and, if necessary, serotonergic antagonists *(Hines: Stoelting's Anesthesia and Co-Existing Disease, 7th ed pp 613–614).*

116. (A) The acid-base disorder described above is a metabolic acidosis with compensatory respiratory alkalosis. If the anion gap were measured, you would also see an increased anion gap (>22 mEq/L). The only item listed above that causes a metabolic acidosis is aspirin toxicity. The other items in the question all cause a metabolic alkalosis *(Hines: Stoelting Anesthesia and Co-Existing Disease, ed 7, pp 422–423).*

117. (D) Mechanical ventilation of the lungs can be accomplished by various modes. These modes are categorized as controlled, assisted, assisted/controlled, controlled with positive end-expiratory pressure (PEEP), and assisted/controlled using intermittent mandatory ventilation (IMV). Assisted/controlled modes of mechanical ventilation are used in patients when the muscles of respiration require rest

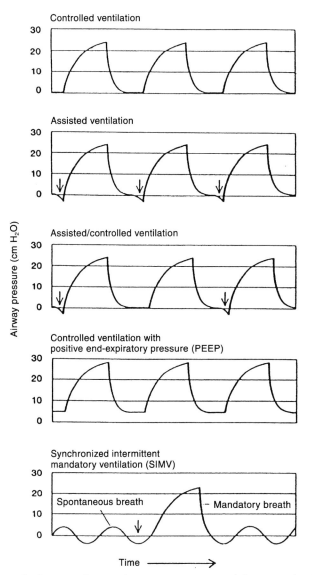

Controlled ventilation

Assisted ventilation

Assisted/controlled ventilation

Controlled ventilation with positive end-expiratory pressure (PEEP)

Synchronized intermittent mandatory ventilation (SIMV)

Spontaneous breath — Mandatory breath

Airway pressure (cm H$_2$O)

Time ⟶

(From Stoelting RK, Dierdorf SF: Anesthesia and Co-Existing Disease, ed 4, New York, Churchill Livingstone, 2001.)

because minimal breathing efforts are required. With the assisted/controlled mode of ventilation, positive-pressure ventilation is triggered by small breathing efforts produced by the patient. The airway pressure tracing shown is typical of that of a patient requiring assisted/controlled ventilation (Miller: Basics of Anesthesia, ed 7, pp 708–709).

118. (D) With a total laryngectomy (TL), a tracheostomy is performed and a wire-reinforced endotracheal tube (ETT) is placed into the trachea early in the procedure. The thyroid gland is usually preserved after dividing the thyroid isthmus, and the entire larynx is then resected, with the pharyngeal connection to the airway completely closed, making the trachea completely independent from the oropharynx. The opening of the trachea is sutured to the anterior skin of the neck, producing a stoma, and often there is no need to keep the ETT placed in the tracheostomy site intraoperatively for postoperative ventilation. However, in cases where there is edema at the stomal site or a free flap is needed, an ETT can remain in place or be replaced with a tracheostomy tube for a period of time postoperatively to maintain an adequate opening to the airway. If the tracheostomy tube becomes occluded and cannot be opened, it needs to be removed and an ETT or another tracheostomy tube placed via the only opening to the airway, the freshly produced stoma. In placing the ETT, be careful not to place it in too far because the distance from the stoma to the carina is short and one can easily pass the ETT past the carina and enter one bronchus *(Jaffe: Anesthesiologist's Manual of Surgical Procedures, ed 5, pp 203–207; Miller: Miller's Anesthesia, ed 8, pp 2542–2543).*

119. (C) A P_{50} less than 26 mm Hg defines a leftward shift of the oxyhemoglobin dissociation curve. This means that at any given PaO_2, hemoglobin has a higher affinity for O_2. A P_{50} greater than 26 mm Hg describes a rightward shift of the oxyhemoglobin dissociation curve. This means that at any given PaO_2, hemoglobin has a lower affinity for O_2. Conditions that cause a rightward shift of the oxyhemoglobin dissociation curve are metabolic and include respiratory acidosis, hyperthermia, increased erythrocyte 2,3-diphosphoglycerate (2,3-DPG) content, pregnancy, and abnormal hemoglobins, such as sickle cell hemoglobin or thalassemia. Alkalosis, hypothermia, fetal hemoglobin, abnormal hemoglobin species, such as carboxyhemoglobin, methemoglobin, and sulfhemoglobin, and decreased erythrocyte 2,3-DPG content will cause a leftward shift of the oxyhemoglobin dissociation curve. Also see explanation to Question 109 *(Miller: Miller's Anesthesia, ed 8, p 1843; West: Respiratory Physiology, ed 9, pp 79–82).*

120. (B) Adult respiratory distress disorder (ARDS) was first reported in adults in 1967 and is associated with decreased lung compliance. Initial therapies for ARDS included mechanical ventilation with tidal volumes of 10 to 15 mL/kg, with rates to achieve a normal pH and $PaCO_2$. In 2000 the National Institutes of Health (NIH) ARDS Network (ARDSNet) trial noted a reduction in mortality for patients with ARDS who were ventilated with low tidal volumes (6 mL/kg predicted body weight [PBW]—mortality rate of 31%) compared with traditional tidal volumes (12 mL/kg PBW—mortality rate of 40%). It was felt that the larger tidal volumes caused overdistention of the alveoli (i.e., produced volume trauma or volutrauma). This increased alveolar volume resulted in mechanical injury and a systemic inflammatory response. It was felt that the stretch and not the pressure (barotrauma) caused the release of the inflammatory cytokinins into the circulation. Because the lower tidal volumes used were associated with an elevation of arterial CO_2 and lower arterial oxygen levels, the term "permissive hypercapnia and hypoxemia" was used. Patients with ARDS also develop atelectasis. Recruitment maneuvers (sustained breaths of increased airway pressures) were used to re-expand atelectatic alveoli to avoid atelectrauma. However, results with the recruitment breaths showed only a transient increase in oxygenation and no change in mortality. Another respiratory technique proposed included the use of inhaled nitric oxide (iNO) that can improve ventilation-perfusion mismatch and improve oxygenation. Randomized controlled studies have shown only limited effectiveness, with no overall improvement in mortality or duration of ventilation. Further studies are looking at iNO for specific conditions (e.g., severe pulmonary hypertension, right ventricular failure, refractory hypoxemia) *(Miller: Miller's Anesthesia, ed 8, pp 3040–3044, 3078–3079; Barash: Clinical Anesthesia, ed 8, pp 1644–1645).*

121. (C) The rate at which a gas diffuses through a lipid membrane is directly proportional to the area of the membrane, the transmembrane partial pressure gradient of the gas, and the diffusion coefficient of the gas, and it is inversely proportional to the thickness of the membrane. The diffusion coefficient of the gas is directly proportional to the square root of gas solubility and is inversely proportional to the square root of the molecular weight of the gas. This is known as Fick's law of diffusion *(Barash: Clinical Anesthesia, ed 8, p 1147).*

122. (A) Aging is associated with reduced ventilatory volumes and capacities, and decreased efficiency of pulmonary gas exchange. These changes are caused by progressive stiffening of cartilage and replacement of elastic tissue in the intercostal and intervertebral areas, which decreases compliance of the thoracic cage. In addition, progressive kyphosis or scoliosis produces upward and anterior rotation of the ribs and sternum, which further restricts chest wall expansion during inspiration. With aging, the FRC, residual volume, and closing volume are increased, whereas the vital capacity, total lung capacity, maximum breathing capacity, FEV_1, and ventilatory response to hypercarbia and hypoxemia are reduced. In addition, age-related changes in lung parenchyma, alveolar surface area, and diminished pulmonary capillary bed density cause ventilation/perfusion mismatch, which decreases resting PaO_2 *(Miller: Basics of Anesthesia, ed 7, pp 612–614).*

123. (C) Physiologic dead space ventilation can be estimated using the Bohr equation (described in the explanation to Question 103):

$$V_D/V_T = \frac{45 \text{ mm Hg} - 30 \text{ mm Hg}}{45 \text{ mm Hg}} = \frac{15 \text{ mm Hg}}{45 \text{ mm Hg}} = 0.33$$

(West: Respiratory Physiology, ed 9, pp 19–21; Miller: Miller's Anesthesia, ed 8, pp 446–447; Barash: Clinical Anesthesia, ed 8, p 374).

124. (A) The ventilation/perfusion ratio is greater at the apex of the lungs than at the base of the lungs. Thus dependent regions of the lungs are hypoxic and hypercarbic compared with the nondependent regions. Also see explanation to Question 132 *(Miller: Miller's Anesthesia, ed 8, pp 451–454; West: Respiratory Physiology, ed 9, pp 21–22, 44–46; Barash: Clinical Anesthesia, ed 8, p 372).*

125. (A) The degree to which a person can hypoventilate to compensate for metabolic alkalosis is limited; hence, this is the least well-compensated acid-base disturbance. Respiratory compensation for metabolic alkalosis is rarely more than 75% complete. Hypoventilation to a $PaCO_2$ greater than 55 mm Hg is the maximum respiratory compensation for metabolic alkalosis. A $PaCO_2$ greater than 55 mm Hg most likely reflects concomitant respiratory acidosis *(Barash: Clinical Anesthesia, ed 8, pp 385–388).*

126. (A) PaO_2 can be estimated using the alveolar gas equation, which is given as follows:

$$PaO_2 = (PB - 47)FIO_2 - \frac{PaCO_2}{R}$$

where PB is the barometric pressure (mm Hg), FIO_2 is the fraction of inspired O_2, $PaCO_2$ is the arterial CO_2 tension (mm Hg), and R is the respiratory quotient *(West: Respiratory Physiology, ed 9, p 59; Barash: Clinical Anesthesia, ed 8, p 375).*

127. (D) When arterial sampling is not possible, "arterialized" venous blood can be used to estimate ABG tensions. Because blood in the veins on the back of the hands has very little O_2 extracted, the O_2 content in this blood best approximates the O_2 content in a sample of blood obtained from an artery *(Miller: Basics of Anesthesia, ed 7, p 367).*

128. (D) Pulmonary function tests can be divided into those that assess ventilatory capacity and those that assess pulmonary gas exchange. The simplest test to assess ventilatory capacity is the FEV_1/FVC ratio. Other tests to assess ventilatory capacity include the maximum midexpiratory flow (FEF 25%-75%), MVV, and flow-volume curves. The most significant disadvantage of these tests is that they are dependent on patient effort. However, because the FEF 25% to 75% is obtained from the midexpiratory portion of the flow-volume loop, it is least dependent on patient effort. Also see explanation to Question 97 *(Barash: Clinical Anesthesia, ed 8, p 377).*

129. (A) Carbon monoxide binds to hemoglobin with an affinity greater than 200 times that of oxygen. This stabilizes the oxygen–hemoglobin complex and hinders release of oxygen to the tissues, leading to a leftward shift of the oxyhemoglobin dissociation curve. The diagnosis is suggested when there is a low oxygen hemoglobin saturation in the face of a normal PaO_2. The two-wave pulse oximeter cannot distinguish oxyhemoglobin from carboxyhemoglobin, so that a normal oxyhemoglobin saturation would be observed in the presence of high concentrations of carboxyhemoglobin. Carbon monoxide poisoning is not associated with cyanosis. See also explanations for Questions 113 and 140 *(Hines: Stoelting's Anesthesia and Co-Existing Disease, ed 7, pp 631–632; Miller: Miller's Anesthesia, ed 8, pp 2679–2680; Barash: Clinical Anesthesia, ed 8, p 1519).*

130. (B) The fraction of total cardiac output that traverses the pulmonary circulation without participating in gas exchange is called the transpulmonary shunt. It can be calculated exactly by the equation:

$$\dot{Q}_S/\dot{Q}_T = \frac{Cc'O_2 - CaO_2}{Cc'O_2 - C\overline{v}O_2}$$

where Cc', Ca, and C_VO_2 stand for the content of oxygen in the alveolar capillary, artery, and mixed venous samples, respectively. This information is not provided in the question; however, the alveolar-to-arterial partial pressure of oxygen difference is using high inspired oxygen concentrations. The alveolar to arterial oxygen difference can be used to estimate venous admixture, most commonly transpulmonary shunt. For every increase in alveolar-arterial O_2 of 20 mm Hg, there is an increase in shunt fraction of 1% of the cardiac output. In the example, 240/20 = 12 and the transpulmonary shunt can be estimated at 12% *(Miller: Miller's Anesthesia, ed 8, p 1557; Miller: Basics of Anesthesia, ed 7, p 374).*

131. (D) Measuring the ventilatory response to increased $PaCO_2$ is a sensitive method for quantifying the effects of drugs on ventilation. In general, all volatile anesthetics (including N_2O), narcotics, benzodiazepines, and barbiturates depress the ventilatory response to increased $Paco_2$ in a dose-dependent manner. The magnitude of ventilatory depression by volatile anesthetics is greater in patients with COPD than in healthy patients. Arterial blood gases (ABGs) may need to be monitored during recovery from general anesthesia in patients with COPD. Ketamine causes minimal respiratory depression. Typically, respiratory rate is decreased only 2 to 3 breaths/min, and the ventilatory response to changes in $Paco_2$ is maintained during ketamine anesthesia. Also see explanation to Question 105 *(Miller: Basics of Anesthesia, ed 6, pp 63–64, 93–94, 110; Miller: Miller's Anesthesia, ed 8, pp 691–693; Barash: Clinical Anesthesia, ed 8, pp 370–371, 493–496).*

132. (D) (See also explanation to Question 124.) The orientation of the lungs relative to gravity has a profound effect on efficiency of pulmonary gas exchange. Because alveoli in dependent regions of the lungs expand more per unit change in transpulmonary pressure (i.e., are more compliant) than alveoli in nondependent regions of the lungs, $\dot{V}_A$ increases from the top to the bottom of the lungs. Because pulmonary blood flow increases more from the top to the bottom of the lungs than does $\dot{V}_A$, the ventilation/perfusion ratio is high in nondependent regions of the lungs and is low in dependent regions of the lungs. Therefore in the upright lungs, the Pao_2 and pH are greater at the apex, whereas the $Paco_2$ is greater at the base *(Miller: Miller's Anesthesia, ed 8, pp 451–454; West: Respiratory Physiology, ed 9, pp 21–22, 44–46; Barash: Clinical Anesthesia, ed 8, p 372).*

133. (A) The work required to overcome the elastic recoil of the lungs and thorax, along with airflow or frictional resistances of the airways, contributes to the work of breathing. When the respiratory rate or airway resistance is high or pulmonary or chest wall compliance is reduced, a large amount of energy is spent overcoming the work of breathing. In the healthy resting adult, only 1% to 3% of total O_2 consumption is used for the work of breathing at rest, but up to 50% may be needed in patients with pulmonary disease. Also see explanation to question 110 *(Miller: Miller's Anesthesia, ed 8, p 1563).*

134. (B) The conducting airways (trachea, right and left mainstem bronchi, and lobar and segmental bronchi) do not contain alveoli and, therefore, do not take part in pulmonary gas exchange. These structures constitute the anatomic dead space. In the adult, the anatomic dead space is approximately 2 mL/kg. The anatomic dead space increases during inspiration because of the traction exerted on the conducting airways by the surrounding lung parenchyma. In addition, the anatomic dead space depends on the size and posture of the subject. Also see explanation to Question 103 *(Stoelting: Pharmacology and Physiology in Anesthetic Practice, ed 4, p 778; Barash: Clinical Anesthesia, ed 7, p 276; Barash: Clinical Anesthesia, ed 8, p 373).*

135. (D) There are three main mechanisms that the body has to prevent changes in pH: the buffer systems (immediate), the ventilatory response (takes minutes), and the renal response (takes hours to days). The buffer systems represent the first line of defense against adverse changes in pH. The $[HCO_3^-]$ buffer system is the most important system and represents greater than 50% of the total buffering capacity of the body. Other important buffer systems include hemoglobin, which is responsible for approximately 35% of the buffering capacity of blood, phosphates, plasma proteins, and bone *(Miller: Basics of Anesthesia, ed 7, p 364).*

136. (C) Cardiac dysrhythmias are a common complication associated with acid-base abnormalities. The etiology of these dysrhythmias is related partly to the effects of pH on myocardial potassium homeostasis. Changes in pH cause potassium to shift in and out of cells. The rise in potassium for a reduction in pH is somewhat variable but will definitely result in an increase; the range spans from 0.2 to 1.7 mEq/L (Mount DB: Potassium Balance In Acid-Base Disorders. UpToDate. Retrieved May 2019, from https://www.uptodate.com/contents/potassium-balance-in-acid-base-disorders)

137. (D) Three main risk factors for death from burns include inhalation injury, burn size (>40%), and age (>60 years). Patients who have sustained major burns from a fire can rapidly deteriorate. Areas of concern include airway management, carbon monoxide (CO) poisoning, pain, edema, fluid management, intravenous access, maintenance of body temperature and prevention of infections.

Airway and lung injury can result from direct tissue injury as well as inflammatory mediators from burned tissues, infection, and fluid resuscitation. Signs of impending airway difficulty include stridor, voice changes, and coughing up carbonaceous material. Explosive injuries involving the head and upper torso are at high risk for airway difficulty. Because upper airway swelling can rapidly lead to airway obstruction and death, securing the airway with an endotracheal tube (0.5-1 mm internal diameter smaller than normal) is advised in patients with major burns. Along with an intravenous anesthetic such as ketamine, the muscle relaxant succinylcholine is safe and often used in the first 24 hours after a burn, but is contraindicated after 48 hours due to the possibility of a hyperkalemia-induced cardiac arrest. In some cases, a sedated fiberoptic intubation may be required. If bronchospasm develops from the aspiration of burned material or gastric contents, then bronchodilators as well as suctioning and fiberoptic evaluation of the airway may be needed.

In addition, prolonged entrapment in a fire area can lead to high carbon monoxide (CO) levels, with resultant tissue hypoxia. Detection of high CO levels may not be obvious because standard pulse oximeters read CO as oxygen. Blood samples analyzed in a blood gas laboratory are required for detection of CO. High-inspired oxygen concentrations are often required to prevent tissue hypoxia, as well as to reduce the half-life of CO in the blood. The half-life of CO is 4 hours when breathing room air, 60 to 90 minutes when breathing 100% oxygen, and 20 to 30 minutes in a hyperbaric chamber breathing 100% oxygen at 2 to 3 atm of pressure. With severe swelling, escharotomies may be needed to treat compartment syndromes *(Barash, Clinical Anesthesia, ed 8, pp 1511–1516; Miller: Basics of Anesthesia, ed 7, pp 740–742).*

138. (D) A patient with a V_D of 150 mL and a V_A of 350 mL (assuming a normal V_T of 500 mL) will have a V_D minute ventilation ($\dot{V}_D$) of 1500 mL and a V_A minute ventilation ($\dot{V}_A$) of 3500 mL ($\dot{V}_E$ of 5000 mL) at a respiratory rate of 10 breaths/min. If the respiratory rate is doubled but $\dot{V}_E$ remains unchanged, then the $\dot{V}_D$ would double to 3000 mL and there would be an increase in $\dot{V}_D$ of 1500 mL and a decrease in $\dot{V}_A$ of 1500 mL. Also see explanation to Questions 103 and 134 *(West: Respiratory Physiology, ed 9, pp 16–17; Barash: Clinical Anesthesia, ed 8, pp 373, 376; Miller: Miller's Anesthesia, ed 8, pp 446–447).*

139. (B) In addition to the items listed in this question, other factors that shift the oxyhemoglobin dissociation curve to the right include pregnancy and all abnormal hemoglobins such as hemoglobin S (sickle cell hemoglobin). For reasons unknown, volatile anesthetics increase the P_{50} of adult hemoglobin by 2 to 3.5 mm Hg. A rightward shift of the oxyhemoglobin dissociation curve will decrease the transfer of O_2 from alveoli to hemoglobin and improve release of O_2 from hemoglobin to peripheral tissues. Also see explanation to Question 109 *(West: Respiratory Physiology, ed 9, pp 79–82; Miller: Basics of Anesthesia, ed 7, p 59).*

140. (B) The most frequent immediate cause of death from fires is carbon monoxide toxicity. Carbon monoxide is a colorless, odorless gas that exerts its adverse effects by decreasing O_2 delivery to peripheral tissues. This is accomplished by two mechanisms. First, because the affinity of carbon monoxide for the O_2 binding sites on hemoglobin is more than 200 times that of O_2, O_2 is readily displaced from hemoglobin. Thus O_2 content is reduced. Second, carbon monoxide causes a leftward shift of the oxyhemoglobin dissociation curve, which increases the affinity of hemoglobin for O_2 at peripheral tissues. Treatment of carbon monoxide toxicity is administration of 100% O_2. Supplemental oxygen decreases the half-time of carboxyhemoglobin from 4 to 6 hours with room air to about 1 hour with 100% oxygen. Breathing 100% oxygen at 3 atm in a hyperbaric chamber reduces the half-time even more to 15 to 30 minutes. See also explanations for Questions 113 and 129 *(Miller: Miller's Anesthesia, ed 8, pp 2679–2680; Barash: Clinical Anesthesia, ed 8, p 1514).*

141. (D) Propofol infusion syndrome is a rare condition associated with prolonged (greater than 48 hour) administration of propofol at a dose of 5 mg/kg/hr (83 μg/kg/min) or higher. This syndrome was first described in children, but later observed in critically ill adults as well. It is manifested by cardiomyopathy with acute cardiac failure, metabolic acidosis, skeletal muscle myopathy, hepatomegaly, hyperkalemia, and lipidemia. It is thought to be related to a failure of free fatty acid transport into the mitochondria and failure of the mitochondrial respiratory chain. Refractory bradycardia can occur with this syndrome and heralds a poor prognosis *(Miller: Miller's Anesthesia, ed 8, p 831; Barash: Clinical Anesthesia, ed 8, pp 487, 492).*

142. (A) Calculating the anion gap (i.e., the unmeasured anions in the plasma) is helpful in determining the cause of a metabolic acidosis. Anion gap = $[Na^+] - ([Cl^-] + [HCO_3^-])$ and is normally 10 to 12 nmol/L. In this case the anion gap = $138 - (115 + 12) = 11$, a normal anion gap. Causes of a high anion gap metabolic acidosis include lactic acidosis, ketoacidosis, acute and chronic renal failure, and toxins (e.g., salicylates, ethylene glycol, methanol). Nonanion gap metabolic acidosis includes renal tubular acidosis, expansion acidosis (e.g., rapid saline infusion), gastrointestinal (GI) bicarbonate loss (e.g., diarrhea, small bowel drainage), drug-induced hyperkalemia, and acid loads (e.g., ammonium chloride, hyperalimentation). Vomiting and nasogastric drainage are some of the many causes of metabolic alkalosis *(Longo: Harrison's Principles of Internal Medicine, ed 18, pp 365–369; Barash: Clinical Anesthesia, ed 8, p 386).*

143. (A) Bloodstream infectious complications with central venous catheters are the most common late complication seen with central catheters (>5%). Current Centers for Disease Control and Prevention (CDC) guidelines do not recommend replacing central venous catheters. All the other statements are true. In addition, evidence is suggesting that the use of ultrasound may decrease the time needed to place catheters and the number of skin punctures needed for central vein access, and may also decrease infections *(Miller: Miller's Anesthesia, ed 8, p 1367; Barash: Clinical Anesthesia, ed 8, pp 1652–1653; O'Grady et al: Guidelines for the prevention of intravascular catheter-related infections, Clin Infect Dis 52(9):e164–e166, 2011).*

144. (C) Sarin (also called GB), like GA (Tabun), GD (Soman), GF, VR, and VX, is a clear liquid organophosphate that vaporizes at room temperatures. These chemical nerve gases mainly bind with acetylcholinesterase and produce clinical signs of excessive parasympathetic activity. The term DUMBELS—Diarrhea, Urination, Miosis, Bronchorrhea and bronchoconstriction, Emesis, Lacrimation, and Salivation—can help you remember several of the signs. Note the eye signs are pupillary constriction (miosis) and not pupillary dilation (mydriasis). Other signs relate to the cardiovascular system and include bradycardia, prolonged QT interval, and ventricular dysrhythmias. These chemicals also affect the GABA and NMDA receptors and may also cause central nervous system (CNS) excitation (i.e., convulsions) *(Miller: Miller's Anesthesia, ed 8, p 2496; Barash: Clinical Anesthesia, ed 8, pp 303–304).*

145. (D) Venous air embolism occurs when air enters the venous system through an incised or cannulated vein. When cannulating or decannulating central veins, it is important to keep a positive venous-to-atmospheric pressure gradient. This is usually accomplished by placing the site below the level of the heart (i.e., Trendelenburg position). In addition, under mechanical ventilation or when the spontaneously breathing patient exhales or performs a Valsalva maneuver, the venous-to-atmospheric pressure is greater than if a spontaneously breathing patient inhales, a time when the venous pressure may be less than atmospheric pressure *(Oropello et al: Critical Care, Chapter 93: Central Venous Access > Positioning > Internal Jugular Vein).*

146. (B) Adverse physiologic effects of respiratory or metabolic acidosis include CNS depression and increased intracranial pressure (ICP), cardiovascular system depression (partially offset by increased secretion of catecholamines and elevated [Ca^{++}]), cardiac dysrhythmias, vasodilation, hypovolemia (which is a result of decreased precapillary and increased postcapillary sphincter tone), pulmonary hypertension, and hyperkalemia *(Barash: Clinical Anesthesia, ed 8, pp 387, 407, 1008).*

147. (C) Withdrawing the tube into the trachea obviously would improve arterial saturation and is the treatment of choice for inadvertent mainstem intubation. Short of pulling the ETT back, all other successful options address ways of improving arterial oxygenation during one-lung ventilation. In essence, any maneuver that improves the saturation of the venous blood will also improve the saturation of arterial blood (in this question). Normal pulmonary circulation is in series with the systemic circulation. Blood exiting the lungs is nearly 100% oxygenated regardless of the saturation of the venous blood when it exits the right ventricle and enters the lungs via the pulmonary artery. In one-lung ventilation, deliberate or accidental, blood exiting the ventilated side of the lungs (the right side in this question) is also essentially fully saturated, but it mixes with nonoxygenated blood. The nonoxygenated blood has effectively bypassed the lungs by passing through an area that is perfused but not ventilated, that is, a shunt. When the blood from the ventilated lung (nearly 100% oxygenated) mixes with the shunted blood, a mixture will be formed that has saturation less than 100%, but higher than the mixed venous O_2 saturation.

$$SvO_2 = SaO_2 - \dot{V}O_2/\dot{Q} \times Hgb$$

where SvO_2 = mixed venous hemoglobin saturation and SaO_2 = arterial oxygen saturation

$$O_2 \text{ content} = 1.39 \times [Hgb] \times SaO_2 + (0.003 \times PaO_2)$$

The exact saturation of the arterial blood in this question depends on the ratio of blood exiting the right lung versus that exiting the left lung. Fortunately, during one-lung ventilation, the nonventilated lung collapses and in so doing raises its resistance to blood flow. This results in preferentially directing blood to the right ventilated lung. A second factor to consider is how well-saturated the shunted blood is. "Red" blood from the right lung mixes with "blue" blood from the left lung to give a mixture of partially saturated blood. The saturation of the shunted "blue" blood depends on the hemoglobin concentration and cardiac output. From the first equation above, you can see that raising either of these would improve the mixed venous oxygen saturation and ultimately the arterial saturation during one-lung ventilation. Inflating the pulmonary artery catheter balloon located in the nonventilated (left) lung would also improve arterial saturation by limiting blood flow to the left lung. Raising the FIO_2 from 80% to 100% will do little if anything to improve arterial saturation, because the blood exiting the "working" lung is already fully saturated. The small rise in PaO_2 that would result from an increase in FIO_2, once multiplied by 0.003 (see the second equation above), would be a very small and insignificant number. In other words, raising FIO_2 does not improve arterial saturation in the presence of a shunt *(Miller: Miller's Anesthesia, ed 8, p 1386; Barash: Clinical Anesthesia, ed 8, pp 374–375, 720).*

148. (D) The decision to stop mechanical support of the lungs is based on a variety of factors that can be measured. Guidelines suggesting that cessation of mechanical inflation of the lungs is likely to be successful include a vital capacity greater than 15 mL/kg, arterial PaO_2 greater than 60 mm Hg (FIO_2 <0.5), alveolar-arterial (A–a) gradient less than 350 mm Hg (FIO_2 = 1.0), arterial pH greater than 7.3, $PaCO_2$ less than 50 mm Hg, dead space/tidal volume ratio less than 0.6, and maximum inspiratory pressure of at least -20 cm H_2O. In addition to these guidelines, the patient should be hemodynamically stable, conscious, oriented, and in good nutritional status *(Barash: Clinical Anesthesia, ed 8, pp 788–790).*

149. (D) A shift to the left in the oxyhemoglobin dissociation curve occurs with fetal hemoglobin, alkalosis, hypothermia, carboxyhemoglobin, methemoglobin, and decreased levels of 2,3-DPG. Storage of blood lowers 2,3-DPG levels in acid-citrate-dextrose stored blood, but minimal changes are seen in 2,3-DPG with citrate-dextrose stored blood. A shift to the right occurs with acidosis, hyperthermia, increased levels of 2,3-DPG, inhaled anesthetics, and pregnancy *(Miller: Basics of Anesthesia, ed 7, pp 59, 341, 556, 742).*

150. (C) With acute spinal cord injuries the major anesthetic concerns are airway management and management of hemodynamic perturbations associated with interruption of the sympathetic nervous system below the level of the transection. Hyperkalemia in response to succinylcholine does not occur until at least 24 hours after the injury. Autonomic hyper-reflexia is not a concern in the acute management of patients with spinal cord injuries. There is no evidence that awake intubation (fiberoptic) is superior to direct laryngoscopy, as long as in-line traction is held in both cases. These patients are more susceptible to hypothermia compared with patients without spinal cord injuries because they lack thermoregulation below the level of the cord injury *(Barash: Clinical Anesthesia, ed 8, pp 1023–1024).*

151. (C) Polyuria of neurogenic (rather than nephrogenic) diabetes insipidus is caused by diminished or absent antidiuretic hormone (ADH) synthesis or release following injury to the hypothalamus, pituitary stalk, or posterior pituitary gland. Hemoconcentration resulting in hypernatremia often results. In contrast, SIADH is associated with excessive amounts of ADH, which in turn causes hyponatremia. Cerebral salt wasting syndrome results from release of brain natriuretic peptide in subarachnoid hemorrhage patients. The resulting natriuresis-mediated electrolyte perturbation is hyponatremia. Diabetes mellitus and spinal shock do not cause hypernatremia *(Longo: Harrison's Principles of Internal Medicine, ed 18, pp 349–351; Barash: Clinical Anesthesia, ed 8, p 403).*

152. (D) Vasopressin, also known as antidiuretic hormone, is a naturally occurring peptide synthesized in the hypothalamus and stored in the posterior pituitary. It is used clinically to treat diabetes insipidus, and in the ICU it is used to treat hypotension. Patients with severe sepsis and septic shock have a relative deficiency of vasopressin, and these patients may be sensitive to vasopressin. Vasopressin interacts with a different receptor and, unlike the catecholamines, it is effective even in the presence of acidemia *(Miller: Basics of Anesthesia, ed 7, p 550).*

153. (C) Confusion may exist between the concepts of shunt versus dead space. Both of these are forms of $\dot{V}/\dot{Q}$ mismatch. With shunts, there is a gradient between the alveolar and the arterial oxygen partial pressures. Alveolar partial pressure (PA) is calculated from the alveolar gas equation. The Pa_{CO_2} with shunt is compensated and is usually normal, even in the presence of a significant $\dot{V}/\dot{Q}$ mismatch. Dead space refers to the portion of a breath that does not reach perfused alveoli. In pathologic conditions, such as COPD, morbid obesity, and pulmonary embolism, dead space is increased because air passes into alveoli that are ventilated but not perfused. This air does not participate in gas exchange and simply exits these unperfused alveoli and "dilutes" the carbon dioxide exiting the lungs from the perfused alveoli. Under these circumstances the mixed expired CO_2 measured with capnometry will be less than the actual arterial CO_2 *(Miller: Basics of Anesthesia, ed 7, pp 62, 64; Barash: Clinical Anesthesia, ed 8, p 1279; Miller: Miller's Anesthesia, ed 8, p 1559).*

154. (C) TRALI reactions are a serious complication of transfusing any product containing plasma, that is, fresh frozen plasma, whole blood, packed red blood cells, platelets, or factor concretes derived from human blood. The clinical diagnosis is made 1 to 2 hours after transfusion (but may occur up to 6 hours later in the ICU). The key features include wide A–a gradient, noncardiogenic pulmonary edema, and leukopenia (not leukocytosis) secondary to sequestration in the lungs. TRALI reactions are one of the leading causes of transfusion-related mortality *(Barash: Clinical Anesthesia, ed 8, p 440).*

155. (B) The right internal jugular vein and the right subclavian vein form the right brachiocephalic vein; similarly, the left internal jugular vein and the left subclavian vein form the left brachiocephalic vein. These two brachiocephalic veins form the SVC *(Netter's Clinical Anatomy, ed 4, Figure 3-28).*

156. (D) Patients who have undergone a PCI are placed on a course of a thienopyridine (ticlopidine or clopidogrel) and aspirin. The thienopyridine is used for at least 2 weeks after PTCA, 1 month after a baremetal stent is placed, and 1 year after a drug-eluting stent is placed. Aspirin is continued for a longer period of time. This is to decrease the chance of thrombosis of the treated coronary artery *(Fleisher et al.: 2014 ACC/AHA Guideline on Perioperative Cardiovascular Evaluation and Management of Patients Undergoing Noncardiac Surgery, J Am Coll Cardiol 64(22):e77–e137, 2014; doi:10.1016/j.jacc.2014.07.944).*

157. (D) Minute ventilation is not the same as alveolar ventilation. The latter does require knowledge of dead space. With the assist control mode, both spontaneous and mandatory breaths are supported to the same degree, 500 mL in the present case. The amount of PEEP does not affect minute ventilation, but could affect alveolar ventilation by decreasing dead space *(Miller: Basics of Anesthesia, ed 7, pp. 708–710).*

158. (A) After an incubation period (commonly within 2 weeks), inhalational anthrax symptoms initially look like viral flu (fever, chills, myalgia, and a nonproductive cough). Although leukocytosis is common with anthrax and rare with viral flu, white blood cell (WBC) counts initially may be normal at the time the patient presents. After a short while, the patient suddenly appears critically ill, and without treatment, death can occur within a few days. Substernal chest pain, hypoxemia, cyanosis, dyspnea, abdominal pain, and sepsis syndrome are common with inhaled anthrax but rare with viral flu. After the anthrax spores are inhaled, macrophages phagocytize the spores and transport them to mediastinal lymph nodes, where the spores germinate, producing enlarged nodes and a widened mediastinum on the chest x-ray film. A widened mediastinum is not seen with viral flu. Pharyngitis is common with viral flu and occasionally is seen with anthrax *(Longo: Harrison's Principles of Internal Medicine, ed 18, pp 1769–1771; Barash: Clinical Anesthesia, ed 8, pp 1697–1698).*

159. (C) To answer this question, it is helpful to review the alveolar gas equation:

$$Pa_{O_2} = F_{IO_2}(P_b - P_{H_2O}) - Pa_{CO_2}/R$$

Pa_{O_2} = partial pressure of oxygen in the alveolar gas; F_{IO_2} = fraction of inhaled oxygen; P_b = barometric pressure; P_{H_2O} = vapor pressure at 100% saturation (47 mm Hg at 37° C); Pa_{CO_2} = partial pressure of CO_2 in the alveolar gas; R = respiratory quotient.

Any factor that lowers Pa_{O_2} (below 100 mm Hg or so) will also lower Pa_{O_2}. Hypoxic gas mixture lowers F_{IO_2}, hence Pa_{O_2}. Hypercarbia makes the term Pa_{CO_2}/R larger and, therefore, reduces Pa_{O_2}. Eisenmenger syndrome results in a larger shunt fraction and lower Pa_{O_2} on that basis (see explanation to Question 147). In normally functioning lungs, anemia has a minimal impact on Pa_{O_2} because physiologic shunt is normally only 2% to 5% of cardiac output *(Barash: Clinical Anesthesia, ed 8, p 375)*.

160. (D) The difference between the Pa_{CO_2} and the CO_2 value measured by the infrared spectrometer is a function of the patient's physiologic dead space. Physiologic dead space is equal to anatomic dead space plus alveolar dead space. Anatomic dead space is roughly 1 mL/lb of body weight. Because anatomic dead space is relatively "fixed," changes in physiologic dead space are mainly attributable to changes in alveolar dead space. Alveoli that are ventilated, but not perfused, add to alveolar dead space. In essence, air goes into these alveoli but does not participate in gas exchanges and merely exits the alveoli upon exhalation. Ventilation of dead space serves no useful purpose but does result in "dilution" of the exhaled CO_2, thus explaining why the CO_2 seen on the infrared spectrometer can be substantially lower than that obtained from arterial blood gas analysis. Several factors increase dead space, including lung diseases such as COPD, cystic fibrosis, and pulmonary emboli. In addition, decreased alveolar perfusion from low cardiac output or hypovolemia may also contribute to increased dead space. Mainstem intubation, atelectasis, shunting through thebesian veins, and ablation of hypoxic pulmonary vasoconstriction by isoflurane are various causes of shunting. Shunting is also a mismatch between ventilation and perfusion, but, in contrast to $\dot{V}/\dot{Q}$ mismatch from dead space ventilation, shunting results in a normal or nearly normal Pa_{CO_2} but a larger-than-expected A–a O_2 gradient. The only choice in this question that would explain an increase in dead space ventilation is hypovolemia *(Barash: Clinical Anesthesia, ed 8, pp 373–374)*.

161. (B) The normal human's resting energy expenditure as well as the postoperative state is about 1800 kcal/24 hr. With starvation (20 days), energy expenditure decreases to about 1080 kcal/day (60% of normal). Patients who have sustained multiple fractures (2160 kcal/day or 120% of normal), major sepsis (2520 kcal/day or 140% of normal), and burns have increased energy expenditures. The energy expenditure in a patient with a major burn also depends on the temperature of the room. The highest energy expenditure is at a room temperature of 25° C (3819 kcal/day or 212% of normal) and is lower at 33° C (3342 kcal/day or 185% of normal) and at 21° C (3600 kcal/day or 200% of normal) *(Miller: Miller's Anesthesia, ed 8, pp 3136–3138)*.

162. (D) Amiodarone is useful in the treatment of a variety of supraventricular and ventricular cardiac arrhythmias. For the treatment of ventricular tachycardia or fibrillation that is refractory to electrical defibrillation, the recommended dose is 300 mg IV. Similar to β-blockers, amiodarone decreases mortality after myocardial infarctions. About 5% to 15% of treated patients develop pulmonary toxicity (especially when doses are >400 mg/day, or underlying lung disease is present), and 2% to 4% develop thyroid dysfunction (amiodarone is a structural analog of thyroid hormone). It has a prolonged elimination half-time of 29 hours and a large volume of distribution. Because it prolongs the QTc interval, it may lead to the production of ventricular tachydysrhythmias and thus is not useful in treating torsades de pointes *(Brunton: Goodman & Gilman's The Pharmacologic Basis of Therapeutics, ed 13, Chapter 30: Antiarrhythmic Drugs > Antiarrhythmic Drugs > Amiodarone)*.

163. (A) Patients with cirrhosis have hyperdynamic circulations, as noted here, with the elevated Sv_{O_2} of 90%. The cardiac output is usually increased, peripheral vascular resistance is low, intravascular volume is increased, and arteriovenous shunts are present. Hypotension is common. Milrinone is a positive inotrope with vasodilating properties, something this patient does not need. If a treatment for hypotension is needed, drugs with α-agonist properties may be helpful. In addition, vasopressin is also a good choice because it increases systemic vascular resistance (SVR) but does not increase the already high cardiac output *(Barash: Clinical Anesthesia, ed 8, pp 311–312, 314, 321–324, 1308–1309)*.

164. (B) The remedy for auto-PEEP is allowing more time for exhalation. Decreasing the respiratory rate allows more time for both exhalation and inspiration and helps with this problem, but increasing the respiratory rate does the exact opposite and is counterproductive. Reversing the I:E ratio is useful with restrictive lung disease, often in conjunction with paralysis, e.g., for ARDs, but is useless, even harmful, in the present scenario. Paralyzing the patient might remedy breath taking with a spontaneously breathing patient, but this too is useless in the present case. Increasing the inspiratory flow rate decreases the inspiratory flow time and, in the face of an unchanged respiratory rate, would allow for more time to exhale and thus reduce the problem with auto-PEEP *(Miller: Basics of Anesthesia, ed 7, p 709)*.

165. (B) This patient has a metabolic acidosis. Recall that anion gap = $[Na^+] - ([Cl^-] + [HCO_3^-])$ and is normally 10 to 12 nmol/L. In this case the anion gap = $145 - (119 + 12) = 14$, which is slightly above the normal anion gap range. In looking at this case, the acidosis is quite profound and would most likely be related to the rapid infusion of normal saline. Lactic acid, ketoacidosis, and ethylene glycol produce a high anion gap metabolic acidosis. Narcotics may produce respiratory but not metabolic acidosis. See also Question 142 *(Longo: Harrison's Principles of Internal Medicine, ed 18, pp 365–369; Barash: Clinical Anesthesia, ed 8, pp 385–390).*

166. (A) Noninvasive positive-pressure ventilation (NIPPV) refers to delivering positive-pressure ventilation to patients by way of a nasal mask, or full face mask, without the placement of an endotracheal or tracheostomy tube. This mode of therapy requires conscious and cooperative patients and does not protect the airway. NIPPV has been very useful in COPD patients and in immunosuppressed patients in acute respiratory failure. It most likely will fail (i.e., intubation would be needed) in patients with pneumonia and ARDS *(Miller: Miller's Anesthesia, ed 8, p 3068; Barash: Clinical Anesthesia, ed 8, pp 1643–1645).*

167. (D) Capnography has been a valuable monitor for the cardiac and pulmonary systems, as well as for checking the anesthetic equipment. Forgetting to ventilate the patient, intubating the esophagus, and having the sensing tube become disconnected from the monitor quickly will show no CO_2 detected. Any significant reduction in lung perfusion (i.e., air embolism, decreased cardiac output, or decreased blood pressure) increases alveolar dead space and leads to a lowering of the detected CO_2. A cardiac arrest where there is no blood flow to the lungs and hence no carbon dioxide going to the lungs would also result in no detectable CO_2. As CPR is started, detectable CO_2 would be a sign of lung perfusion and ventilation. A patient with a pneumothorax and high airway pressures would still give you CO_2 readings *(Barash: Clinical Anesthesia, ed 8, pp 711–712).*

168. (C) Always confirm an adequate Airway and Breathing before treating a Cardiac rhythm (A, B before C). Having the ETT in proper position for several hours does not ensure that it remains in proper position. In this case the ETT slipped out of the trachea and went into the esophagus. The only way you know the ETT is in the trachea is to see the tube passing between the vocal cords directly with a conventional laryngoscope or by putting a fiberoptic bronchoscope through the tube and seeing carina. Other forms of confirmation such as bilateral breath sounds, adequate chest rise, and moisture in the tube are helpful but could also be seen with an esophageal intubation. Getting a consistent and adequate end tidal CO_2 on a monitor confirms some gas exchange, but in cases where blood does not get to the lungs, as in a cardiac arrest, CO_2 cannot be removed from the lungs. The first part in the treatment of bradycardia is adequate ventilation with oxygen. After that the other choices may be indicated *(Miller: Miller's Anesthesia, ed 8, p 1654; Barash: Clinical Anesthesia, ed 8, p 1247).*

CHAPTER 3

Pharmacology and Pharmacokinetics of Intravenous Drugs

DIRECTIONS (Questions 169 through 282): Each of the questions or incomplete statements in this section is followed by answers or by completions of the statement, respectively. Select the ONE BEST answer or completion for each item.

169. Which of the following muscle relaxants is eliminated the most by renal excretion?
  A. Pancuronium
  B. Vecuronium
  C. Atracurium
  D. Rocuronium

170. All of the following conditions may develop when using propofol for prolonged sedation in the intensive care unit (ICU) **EXCEPT**
  A. Pancreatitis
  B. Hyperlipidemia
  C. Metabolic acidosis
  D. Adrenal suppression

171. Under which scenario should dantrolene be withheld in a patient in whom malignant hyperthermia (MH) is suspected?
  A. Concomitant treatment with a calcium channel blocker
  B. History of previous uneventful anesthetic with volatile anesthetic
  C. History of negative genetic test for ryanodine mutation
  D. Never

172. A 78-year-old patient with Parkinson disease undergoes a cataract operation under general anesthesia. In the recovery room, the patient has two episodes of emesis and complains of severe nausea. Which of the following antiemetics would be the best choice for treatment of nausea in this patient?
  A. Droperidol
  B. Promethazine
  C. Ondansetron
  D. Metoclopramide

173. Which of the following diseases is associated with increased resistance to neuromuscular blockade with succinylcholine?
  A. Myasthenia gravis
  B. Myasthenic syndrome
  C. Huntington chorea
  D. Polymyositis

174. Sedation with which of the following drugs is most likely to resemble normal sleep?
  A. Propofol
  B. Midazolam
  C. Dexmedetomidine
  D. Ketamine

175. Which of the following intravenous anesthetics is converted from a water-soluble to a lipid-soluble drug after exposure to the bloodstream?
  A. Propofol
  B. Midazolam
  C. Ketamine
  D. None of the above

176. A 33-year-old, 70-kg patient is brought to the operating room for resection of an anterior pituitary prolactin-secreting tumor. Anesthesia is induced with sevoflurane, nitrous oxide, and oxygen. The patient is intubated, and nitrous oxide is discontinued. Anesthesia is maintained with 1.2 minimum alveolar concentration (MAC) sevoflurane in oxygen. The surgeon plans to inject epinephrine into the nasal mucosa to minimize bleeding. What is the maximum volume of a 1:100,000 epinephrine solution that can be administered safely to this patient without producing ventricular arrhythmias?
  A. 55 mL
  B. 45 mL
  C. 35 mL
  D. 25 mL

177. Patients receiving antihypertensive therapy with propranolol are at increased risk for each of the following **EXCEPT**
  A. Blunted response to hypoglycemia
  B. Bronchoconstriction
  C. Rebound tachycardia after discontinuation
  D. Orthostatic hypotension

178. Atropine causes each of the following **EXCEPT**
  A. Decreased gastric acid secretion
  B. Inhibition of salivary secretion
  C. Increased lower esophageal sphincter tone
  D. Mydriasis

179. Which of the following drugs is capable of crossing the blood-brain barrier?
   A. Neostigmine
   B. Pyridostigmine
   C. Edrophonium
   D. Physostigmine

180. Which drug exerts its main central nervous system (CNS) action by inhibiting the *N*-methyl-D-aspartate (NMDA) receptors?
   A. Propofol
   B. Midazolam
   C. Etomidate
   D. Ketamine

181. Which of the following opioid-receptor agonists has anticholinergic properties?
   A. Morphine
   B. Hydromorphone
   C. Sufentanil
   D. Meperidine

182. Which of the following statements about ketamine is **FALSE?**
   A. In the United States it is a racemic mixture of two isomers
   B. It is a potent cerebral vasodilator and can increase intracranial pressure (ICP)
   C. Respiratory depression rarely occurs with induction doses
   D. Its metabolite norketamine is more potent than the parent compound

183. Which of the following vasopressor agents increases systemic blood pressure (BP) indirectly by stimulating the release of norepinephrine from sympathetic nerve fibers and directly by binding to adrenergic receptors?
   A. Vasopressin
   B. Ephedrine
   C. Epinephrine
   D. Phenylephrine

184. Methadone-induced constipation could be reversed without loss of analgesic effect with which of the following opioid antagonists?
   A. Naloxone
   B. Nalmefene
   C. Naltrexone
   D. Methylnaltrexone

185. The treatment of patients with human immunodeficiency virus (HIV) may include indinavir, nelfinavir, or ritonavir. What anesthetic consideration is significant with these drugs?
   A. Decreased platelet function
   B. Increased sensitivity to midazolam
   C. Hypoglycemia
   D. Hyperkalemia

186. Neurokinin-1 (NK1) antagonists such as aprepitant have all the following properties **EXCEPT**
   A. Anxiolytic
   B. Antidepressant
   C. Analgesic
   D. Antiemetic

187. Which of the following drugs should be administered with caution to patients receiving echothiophate for the treatment of glaucoma?
   A. Atropine
   B. Succinylcholine
   C. Ketamine
   D. Remifentanil

188. When one of four thumb twitches in the train-of-four (TOF) stimulation of the ulnar nerve can be elicited, how much suppression would there be if you were measuring a single twitch?
   A. 20 to 25
   B. 45 to 55
   C. 75 to 80
   D. 90 to 95

189. Which of the following muscle relaxants causes slight histamine release at two to three times the ED_{95} (effective dose in 95% of subjects) dose?
   A. Rocuronium
   B. Pancuronium
   C. Atracurium
   D. Cisatracurium

190. Termination of action of the neurotransmitter norepinephrine is achieved predominately by which mechanism?
   A. Reuptake into postganglionic sympathetic nerve endings (uptake 1)
   B. Dilution by diffusion away from receptors
   C. Metabolism by catechol-*O*-methyltransferase (COMT)
   D. Metabolism by monoamine oxidase (MAO)

191. The incidence of unpleasant dreams associated with emergence from ketamine anesthesia can be reduced by the administration of
   A. Caffeine
   B. Droperidol
   C. Physostigmine
   D. Midazolam

192. The principal advantage of Ryanodex over conventional formulations of dantrolene is
    A. Cost
    B. Speed of reconstitution and administration
    C. Absence of large amounts of mannitol
    D. Need for lower dose

193. Eplerenone (Inspra) inhibits the renin-angiotensin-aldosterone system by which mechanism?
    A. Blocks aldosterone receptor
    B. Blocks conversion angiotensinogen to angiotensin I
    C. Blocks angiotensin receptor
    D. Prevents formation of renin

194. Each of the following drugs can enhance the neuromuscular blockade produced by nondepolarizing muscle relaxants **EXCEPT**
    A. Calcium
    B. Aminoglycoside antibiotics
    C. Magnesium
    D. Intravenous lidocaine

195. The primary site of action of lisinopril is
    A. Heart
    B. Lungs
    C. Kidney
    D. Metarterioles

196. Circulating BNP (B-type natriuretic peptide) is a powerful biomarker predicting outcomes of which of the following?
    A. Heart
    B. CNS
    C. Kidneys
    D. Organ rejection

197. Hyperkalemia is **NOT** a risk for patients receiving succinylcholine with which of the following?
    A. Multiple sclerosis (MS)
    B. Myasthenia gravis
    C. Guillain-Barré syndrome
    D. Becker muscular dystrophy

198. Which of the antibiotics below does **NOT** augment neuromuscular blockade?
    A. Clindamycin
    B. Neomycin
    C. Streptomycin
    D. Erythromycin

199. A 43-year-old woman with ascites, hepatopulmonary syndrome, and bleeding esophageal varices is admitted to the ICU. Which of the therapies below is **LEAST** likely to improve symptoms associated with hepatic encephalopathy (HE)?
    A. Amino acid–rich total parenteral nutrition (TPN)
    B. Neomycin
    C. Lactulose
    D. Flumazenil

200. 100 mg succinylcholine is administered to a 70-kg anesthetized man before intubation. The patient remains paralyzed for 20 minutes. Which of the parameters below is **NOT** consistent with this finding?
    A. Dibucaine number 70
    B. Heterozygous for atypical cholinesterase
    C. Incidence of 1/480
    D. Presence of fasciculations with this dose

201. In which of the following situations is succinylcholine most likely to cause severe hyperkalemia?
    A. 24 hours after a right hemisphere stroke
    B. 14 days after a severe burn injury
    C. 24 hours after a midthoracic spinal cord transection
    D. 2 days with a severe abdominal infection

202. The most common minor side effect reported after flumazenil administration in anesthesia is
    A. Nausea and/or vomiting
    B. Dizziness
    C. Tremors
    D. Hypertension

203. Ketorolac
    A. Is a selective cyclooxygenase-2 (COX-2) inhibitor
    B. Does not inhibit thromboxane A_2 (TXA_2)
    C. Does not inhibit prostaglandin I_2
    D. Exhibits a dose ceiling effect with regard to analgesia

204. A 37-year-old patient with a history of acute intermittent porphyria is scheduled for knee arthroscopy under general anesthesia. Which of the following drugs is contraindicated in this patient?
    A. Fentanyl
    B. Isoflurane
    C. Propofol
    D. Etomidate

205. A 57-year-old male is discharged after tooth extraction of two molars. His only medication is paroxetine (Paxil), which he takes for depression. Codeine is a poor analgesic choice for this patient because
    A. It is likely to be ineffective
    B. It is likely to cause extreme sedation
    C. He is at increased risk for nausea
    D. He is at increased risk for serotonin syndrome

206. If etomidate were accidentally injected into a left-sided radial arterial line, the most appropriate step to take would be
    A. Left stellate ganglion block
    B. Administer intra-arterial clonidine
    C. Slowly inject dilute (0.1 mEq/L) [HCO_3^-]
    D. Observe

207. The most important reason for the more rapid onset and shorter duration of action of fentanyl with single dose compared with morphine is the difference in
  A. Volume of distribution
  B. Hepatic clearance
  C. Protein binding
  D. Lipid solubility

208. A narcotic infusion is initiated in a patient without a bolus (loading dose). Of the following drugs, which would reach steady state after 2 hours or less of continuous infusion (fentanyl, remifentanil, alfentanil, and morphine)?
  A. All of these
  B. Remifentanil and alfentanil
  C. Alfentanil only
  D. Remifentanil only

209. The period of vulnerability after three courses of bleomycin for testicular cancer is
  A. 1 month
  B. 1 year
  C. Lifelong
  D. No vulnerability with just three courses

210. The unique advantage of rocuronium over other muscle relaxants is its
  A. Short duration of action
  B. Metabolism by pseudocholinesterase
  C. Onset of action
  D. Lack of need for reversal

211. Which of the following statements regarding the efficacy of neuromuscular blockade in the setting of acute hypokalemia is correct?
  A. There is no effect with depolarizing or nondepolarizing muscle relaxants
  B. There is resistance to effects of both depolarizing and nondepolarizing muscle relaxants
  C. There is increased sensitivity to effects of both depolarizing and nondepolarizing muscle relaxants
  D. There is resistance to depolarizing muscle relaxants and increased sensitivity to nondepolarizing muscle relaxants

212. A patient undergoing which of the following operations would be at highest risk for operative recall?
  A. Laparoscopic cholecystectomy with total intravenous anesthesia (TIVA) (no volatile)
  B. Cervical spine fusion with MEP (motor evoked potentials) monitoring
  C. Pneumonectomy with one-lung ventilation
  D. Emergency splenectomy after falling from a ladder

213. A 58-year-old patient is brought to the emergency room with the following symptoms: miosis, abdominal cramping, salivation, loss of bowel and bladder control, bradycardia, ataxia, and skeletal muscle weakness. The most likely diagnosis is
  A. Central anticholinergic syndrome
  B. Malignant neuroleptic syndrome
  C. Anticholinesterase poisoning
  D. Serotonin syndrome

214. Flumazenil
  A. Is contraindicated in narcotic addicts
  B. Can be given orally as well as intravenously
  C. Can produce seizures in chronic benzodiazepine users
  D. Has a longer elimination half-life compared with midazolam

215. What percentage of neuromuscular receptors could be blocked and still allow patients to carry out a 5-second head lift?
  A. 5%
  B. 15%
  C. 25%
  D. 50%

216. A 25-year-old woman undergoes thyroidectomy under general anesthesia. Ondansetron 4 mg IV is administered as nausea prophylaxis. She complains of nausea in the recovery room. Which of the following agents is **LEAST** likely to be of benefit to her for treatment (rescue) of postoperative nausea and vomiting (PONV)?
  A. Aprepitant
  B. Granisetron
  C. Promethazine
  D. Droperidol

217. Which of the following drugs can prevent tachyarrhythmias in patients with Wolff-Parkinson-White (WPW) syndrome?
  A. Droperidol
  B. Pancuronium
  C. Ketamine
  D. Verapamil

218. The half-life of pseudocholinesterase is
  A. 1 hour
  B. 12 hours
  C. 1 week
  D. 2 weeks

219. A patient with CYP2D6 polymorphism is tested and shown to be an ultrarapid metabolizer. Which of the following statements regarding PONV prophylaxis with serotonin receptor antagonists is true?
  A. Neither granisetron nor ondansetron would likely be efficacious
  B. Granisetron would likely be more efficacious than ondansetron
  C. Ondansetron would likely be more efficacious than granisetron
  D. Both would likely be efficacious

220. Which of the following equals the anti-inflammatory activity of 50 mg of prednisone (Deltasone)?
  A. 100 mg cortisol (Solu-Cortef)
  B. 80 mg methylprednisolone (Solu-Medrol)
  C. 7.5 mg dexamethasone (Decadron)
  D. 4 mg betamethasone (Celestone)

221. The recovery index (RI) of which of the following nondepolarizing muscle relaxants is **NOT** altered by aging?
  A. Atracurium
  B. Vecuronium
  C. Rocuronium
  D. Pancuronium

222. Side effects associated with cyclosporine therapy include each of the following **EXCEPT**
  A. Nephrotoxicity
  B. Pulmonary toxicity
  C. Seizures
  D. Limb paresthesias

223. What is the predominant mechanism for succinylcholine-induced tachycardia in adults?
  A. Direct sympathomimetic effect at postjunctional muscarinic receptors
  B. Stimulation of nicotinic receptors at autonomic ganglia
  C. Blockade of nicotinic receptors at autonomic ganglia
  D. Direct vagolytic effect at postjunctional muscarinic receptors

224. A 72-year-old patient with a history of type 2 diabetes and hypertension is brought to the ICU after aortobifemoral bypass grafting. The patient is up 3 kilograms since surgery, and diuretic therapy is initiated to enhance urine output. Which of the choices below is **LEAST** likely to cause hypokalemic, hypochloremic metabolic acidosis?
  A. Triamterene
  B. Furosemide
  C. Bumetanide
  D. Oral thiazide

225. Which of the commonly used drugs below is **NOT** metabolized by nonspecific esterases?
  A. Propofol
  B. Esmolol
  C. Atracurium
  D. Remifentanil

226. Succinylcholine is contraindicated for routine tracheal intubation in children because of an increased incidence of which of the following side effects?
  A. Hyperkalemia
  B. Malignant hyperthermia
  C. Masseter spasm
  D. Sinus bradycardia

227. From **MOST** to **LEAST** rapid, select the correct temporal sequence of neuromuscular blockade in the adductor of the thumb, the orbicularis oculi, and the diaphragm after administration of an intubating dose of vecuronium to an otherwise healthy patient.
  A. Diaphragm, orbicularis oculi, thumb
  B. Orbicularis oculi, diaphragm, thumb
  C. Orbicularis oculi, thumb, diaphragm
  D. Orbicularis oculi same as diaphragm, thumb

228. Select the **TRUE** statement regarding interaction of nondepolarizing neuromuscular blocking drugs when durations of action are dissimilar.
  A. If a long-acting drug is administered after an intermediate-acting drug, the duration of the long-acting drug will be longer than normal
  B. If a long-acting drug is administered after an intermediate-acting drug, the duration of the long-acting drug will be about the same as expected
  C. If an intermediate-acting drug is administered after a long-acting drug, the duration of the intermediate-acting drug will be about the same as expected
  D. If an intermediate-acting drug is administered after a long-acting drug, the duration of action of the intermediate-acting drug will be longer than expected

229. Select the correct statement regarding the effects of volatile anesthetics on nondepolarizing neuromuscular blocking drugs and the reversal agents.
  A. Volatile anesthetics potentiate neuromuscular blockade but retard reversal agents
  B. Volatile anesthetics potentiate both neuromuscular blocking drugs and reversal agents
  C. Volatile anesthetics retard both neuromuscular blocking drugs and reversal agents
  D. Volatile anesthetics retard neuromuscular blocking drugs but potentiate reversal agents

230. Meperidine is contraindicated in patients taking which of the following drugs for Parkinson disease?
  A. Bromocriptine
  B. Trihexyphenidyl (Artane)
  C. Selegiline (Eldepryl)
  D. Amantadine (Symmetrel)

231. Emergence delirium (ED) occurs most often with
  A. Sevoflurane
  B. Desflurane
  C. Ketamine
  D. Propofol

232. The most common reason for patients to rate anesthesia with etomidate as unsatisfactory is
  A. PONV
  B. Pain on injection
  C. Recall of intubation
  D. Postoperative hiccups

233. Which of the following muscle relaxants inhibits the reuptake of norepinephrine by the adrenergic nerves?
  A. Pancuronium
  B. Vecuronium
  C. Rocuronium
  D. Atracurium

234. The most common side effect of oral dantrolene used to prevent MH is
  A. Nausea and vomiting
  B. Muscle weakness
  C. Blurred vision
  D. Tachycardia

235. A 65-year-old patient is admitted for right upper quadrant pain. Acute cholecystitis is diagnosed, and laparoscopic cholecystectomy planned. The patient has no major medical problems other than type 2 diabetes, for which she takes metformin, and depression, for which she takes paroxetine (selective serotonin reuptake inhibitor [SSRI]). Which of the following best describes the rationale for discontinuation of metformin 48 hours before surgery?
  A. Risk of metabolic acidosis
  B. Risk of hypoglycemia
  C. Risk of serotonin syndrome
  D. None of the above

236. A 37-year-old man is brought to the operating room for repair of a broken mandible sustained in a motor vehicle accident. No other injuries are significant. The patient has been in treatment for alcohol abuse and takes disulfiram and naltrexone. Which of the following would be the best technique for management of this patient's postoperative pain?
  A. Continue naltrexone with round-the-clock low-dose methadone
  B. Continue naltrexone with small doses of morphine every 4 hours as needed
  C. Continue naltrexone with small doses of nalbuphine every 4 hours as needed
  D. Discontinue naltrexone and treat pain with morphine as needed

237. Context sensitive half-time for a pharmacologic agent is most closely related its
  A. Lipid solubility
  B. Duration of administration
  C. Concentration
  D. Route of administration

238. The neuromuscular effects of an intubation dose of vecuronium are terminated by
  A. Diffusion from the neuromuscular junction back into the plasma
  B. Nonspecific plasma cholinesterases
  C. The kidneys
  D. The liver

239. Respiratory depression produced by which of the following analgesics is not readily reversed by administration of naloxone?
  A. Meperidine
  B. Methadone
  C. Hydromorphone
  D. Buprenorphine

240. Which of the following intravenous anesthetic agents is associated with the highest incidence of nausea and vomiting?
  A. Midazolam
  B. Etomidate
  C. Ketamine
  D. Propofol

241. If naloxone were administered to a patient who is receiving ketorolac for postoperative pain, the most likely result would be
  A. Bradycardia
  B. Hypotension
  C. Pain
  D. None of the above

242. Which drug produces strong pulmonary arterial dilation with the least amount of systemic artery dilation?
A. Nitroprusside
B. Prostaglandin E_1
C. Phentolamine
D. Nitric oxide

243. The action of succinylcholine at the neuromuscular junction is terminated by which mechanism?
A. Hydrolysis by pseudocholinesterase
B. Diffusion into extracellular fluid
C. Reuptake into nerve tissue
D. Reuptake into muscle tissue

244. The **LEAST** likely side effect of dexmedetomidine in a healthy patient is
A. Respiratory arrest
B. Bradycardia
C. Sinus arrest
D. Hypotension

245. Which of the following signs is **NOT** seen in patients suffering from thyrotoxicosis in whom thyroid storm is suspected
A. Tachycardia
B. Altered consciousness
C. Hypothermia
D. Weakness

246. Which of the following features of chronic morphine therapy is **NOT** subject to tolerance?
A. Analgesia
B. Respiratory depression
C. Constipation
D. All are subject to tolerance

247. A 78-year-old woman with a history of reactive airway disease takes cimetidine (Tagamet) 400 mg at night. An additional dose is given IV 30 minutes before induction of anesthesia for an exploratory laparotomy. Possible side effects associated with this drug include all of the following **EXCEPT**
A. Bradycardia
B. Delayed awakening
C. Confusion
D. Increased metabolism of diazepam

248. Intraoperative allergic reactions are **LEAST** common after patient exposure to
A. Ketamine
B. Latex
C. Muscle relaxants
D. Hydroxyethyl starch

249. Which of the following medications would be useful in the definitive treatment of sarin nerve gas poisoning?
A. Sodium nitroprusside
B. Methylene blue
C. Atropine
D. All the above are useful

250. Alfentanil
A. Has a more rapid onset of action compared with fentanyl
B. Has a longer duration of action compared with fentanyl
C. Is 250 times more potent than fentanyl
D. Is excreted unchanged in the urine

251. Which of the following medications is **NOT** useful in the immediate management of status asthmaticus?
A. Terbutaline
B. Subcutaneous (SQ) epinephrine
C. Magnesium sulfate
D. Cromolyn

252. Clonidine
A. Is an α_2 blocker
B. Increases CNS sympathetic response to painful stimuli
C. Can be given orally as well as intravenously, but not epidurally or intrathecally
D. Decreases postanesthetic shivering

253. The plasma half-time of which of the following drugs is prolonged in patients with end-stage cirrhotic liver disease?
A. Diazepam
B. Pancuronium
C. Alfentanil
D. All are prolonged

254. A 24-year-old, 100-kg patient is brought to the emergency room by the fire department after suffering smoke inhalation and third-degree burns on the abdomen, chest, and thighs 30 minutes earlier. The best muscle relaxant choice for the most rapid intubation would be
A. 2 mg vecuronium followed by succinylcholine
B. 1 mg of vecuronium, then 2 to 4 minutes later, 9 mg vecuronium
C. Rocuronium
D. Succinylcholine

255. Clonidine is useful in each of the following applications **EXCEPT**
  A. Reducing BP with pheochromocytoma
  B. Treatment of postoperative shivering
  C. Protection against perioperative myocardial ischemia
  D. As an agent for prolonging a bupivacaine spinal

256. A 79-year-old man is brought to the operating room for elective repair of bilateral inguinal hernias. The patient has a history of awareness during general anesthesia and refuses regional anesthesia. The patient is preoxygenated before induction of general anesthesia; 5 mg of midazolam and 250 mg of fentanyl are administered. One minute later the patient loses consciousness, and chest wall stiffness develops to the extent that positive-pressure ventilation is very difficult. The most appropriate therapy for reversal of chest wall stiffness at this point could include
  A. Flumazenil
  B. Naloxone
  C. Succinylcholine
  D. Albuterol

257. Respiratory depression is **LEAST** after the induction dose of which of the following drugs?
  A. Etomidate
  B. Ketamine
  C. Fentanyl
  D. Propofol

258. A 64-year-old man with colon cancer is anesthetized for hepatic resection of liver metastases. Medical history is significant for ileal conduit surgery for bladder cancer, diabetes treated with glyburide, 50-pack-per-year smoking history, and family history of Malignant hyperthermia. Anesthesia is provided with morphine, midazolam, oxygen, and a propofol infusion. After a 3-unit packed red blood cell (RBC) transfusion and 8 hours of surgery, the following blood gas values are recorded: pH 7.2, CO_2 34, $[HCO_3^-]$ 14, base deficit -13, $[Na^+]$ 135, $[K^+]$ 5, $[Cl^-]$ 95, glucose 240 mg/dL. The most likely cause of this patient's acidosis is
  A. Excessive infusion of normal saline
  B. Renal tubular acidosis
  C. Propofol infusion syndrome
  D. Diabetic ketoacidosis (DKA)

259. Treatment of neuroleptic malignant syndrome (NMS) may be carried out with administration of the following drugs **EXCEPT**
  A. Amantadine
  B. Dantrolene
  C. Bromocriptine
  D. Physostigmine

260. A patient with a normal quantity of pseudocholinesterase (plasma cholinesterase) has a dibucaine number of 57. A 1 mg/kg dose of intravenous succinylcholine would likely result in
  A. Hyperkalemic cardiac arrest
  B. Paralysis lasting 5 to 10 minutes
  C. Paralysis lasting 20 to 30 minutes
  D. Paralysis lasting more than 1 to 3 hours

261. Aprepitant exerts its pharmacologic effect by interaction with which receptor?
  A. Neurokinin-1 (NK_1)
  B. 5-HT_3
  C. Histamine (H_1)
  D. Dopamine (D_2)

262. A prolonged neuromuscular block with succinylcholine can be seen in all of the following patients **EXCEPT** those
  A. Chronically exposed to malathion
  B. Treated with echothiophate for glaucoma
  C. Treated with cyclophosphamide for metastatic cancer
  D. Having a C_5 isoenzyme variant

263. Which of the following statements concerning midazolam is **FALSE**?
  A. Midazolam has greater amnestic than sedative properties
  B. Its breakdown is inhibited by cimetidine
  C. It produces retrograde amnesia
  D. It facilitates the actions of the inhibitory neurotransmitter γ-aminobutyric acid (GABA) in the CNS

264. After a 2-hour vertical gastric banding procedure under desflurane, oxygen, and remifentanil anesthesia, the trocar is removed and the wound is closed. Upon emergence, the most likely scenario is
  A. Adequate analgesia for 2 hours
  B. Delayed emergence from narcotic
  C. Pain
  D. Respiratory depression in postanesthesia care unit (PACU)

265. An oral surgeon is about to perform a full mouth extraction on a 70-kg, 63-year-old man under conscious sedation. What is the maximum dose of lidocaine with epinephrine that he can safely infiltrate?
  A. 200 mg
  B. 300 mg
  C. 400 mg
  D. 500 mg

266. Postanesthetic shivering can be treated with all of the following **EXCEPT**
   A. Naloxone
   B. Physostigmine
   C. Magnesium sulfate
   D. Dexmedetomidine

267. The main disadvantage of Sugammadex compared with neostigmine is
   A. Recurarization
   B. Contraindicated with renal failure
   C. Not effective with benzylisoquinolinium relaxants
   D. High incidence of allergic reactions

268. Which of the biologic substances listed below is by itself the greatest determinant of serum osmolality?
   A. AVP (arginine vasopressin)
   B. Angiotensin I
   C. Aldosterone
   D. Renal prostaglandins (PGE_2)

269. Remimazolam
   A. Is less potent than its main metabolite
   B. Is suitable for patients with liver disease
   C. Is metabolized rapidly by amine precursor uptake and decarboxylation (APUD) cells in the gastrointestinal (GI) tract
   D. Is a commercially available mixture of remifentanil plus midazolam

270. Important interactions involving chlorpromazine include all of the following **EXCEPT**
   A. Potentiation of the depressant effects of narcotics
   B. Lowering of the seizure threshold
   C. Prolongation of the QT interval
   D. Potentiation of neuromuscular blockade

271. Amrinone
   A. Is a positive inotropic drug
   B. Is antagonized by esmolol
   C. Is a vasoconstrictor
   D. All the above

272. Which statement concerning tricyclic antidepressants in patients receiving general anesthesia is **TRUE**?
   A. They should be discontinued 2 weeks before elective operations
   B. They may decrease the requirement for volatile anesthetics (decrease MAC)
   C. Meperidine may produce hyperpyrexia in patients taking tricyclic antidepressants
   D. They may exaggerate the response to ephedrine

273. Which of the following types of insulin preparations has the fastest onset of action if administered subcutaneously?
   A. Glargine (Lantus)
   B. Lispro (Humalog)
   C. Regular (Humulin-R)
   D. NPH (Humulin-N)

274. Which of the following mechanisms best explains the anticoagulative properties of tirofiban?
   A. Cyclooxygenase (COX) inhibition
   B. Interaction with von Willebrand factor (vWF)
   C. Interaction with antithrombin III
   D. Enhanced anti-Xa activity

275. The duration of action of remifentanil is attributable to which mode of metabolism?
   A. Spontaneous degradation in blood (Hofmann elimination)
   B. Hydrolysis by nonspecific plasma esterases
   C. Hydrolysis by pseudocholinesterase
   D. Rapid metabolism in the large intestine

276. Pain at the intravenous site is **LEAST** with which IV drug?
   A. Diazepam
   B. Etomidate
   C. Ketamine
   D. Propofol

277. A 35-year-old patient with a history of grand mal seizures is anesthetized for thyroid biopsy under general anesthesia consisting of 4 mg midazolam with infusion of propofol (150 μg/kg/min) and remifentanil (1 μg/kg/min). The patient takes phenytoin for control of seizures. After 30 minutes, the infusion is stopped and the patient is transported intubated to the recovery room, where he is arousable but not breathing. The most reasonable course of action would be
   A. Administer naloxone
   B. Administer flumazenil
   C. Administer naloxone and flumazenil
   D. Ventilate by hand

278. Which of the following α-antagonists produces an irreversible blockade?
   A. Phentolamine
   B. Prazosin
   C. Phenoxybenzamine
   D. Labetalol

279. Which of the following drugs should **NOT** be used in the treatment of severe bradycardia induced by an excess of the beta-adrenergic receptor blockade as a result from a propranolol overdose?
  A. Atropine
  B. Isoproterenol
  C. Dopamine
  D. Glucagon

280. A dose of 150 mg of IV dantrolene is administered to a 24-year-old, 75-kg man in whom incipient MH is suspected. An expected consequence of this therapy would be
  A. Muscle spasticity in the postoperative period
  B. Hypothermia
  C. Cardiac dysrhythmias
  D. Diuresis

281. Atracurium differs from cisatracurium in which way?
  A. Molecular weight
  B. Formation of laudanosine
  C. Histamine release
  D. No renal metabolism

282. Signs and symptoms of opioid withdrawal include all of the following **EXCEPT**
  A. Increased BP and heart rate
  B. Seizures
  C. Abdominal cramps
  D. Jerking of the legs

DIRECTIONS (Questions 283 through 320): Each group of questions consists of several numbered statements followed by lettered headings. For each numbered statement, select the ONE lettered heading that is most closely associated with it. Each lettered heading may be selected once, more than once, or not at all.

Group 283-287

283. Adrenal suppression

284. Thrombosis, phlebitis, specific antagonist available

285. Pain on injection, severe hypotension in elderly

286. Increases ICP

287. Lactic acidosis may develop with prolonged use
  A. Ketamine
  B. Diazepam
  C. Etomidate
  D. Propofol

Group 288-292

288. Reduces MAC

289. Blockade of angiotensin receptor

290. With high doses may cause a systemic lupus erythematosus–like syndrome

291. Produces α-adrenergic receptor and β-adrenergic receptor blockade

292. May result in severe rebound hypertension when abruptly discontinued
  A. Clonidine
  B. Hydralazine
  C. Losartan
  D. Labetalol

Group 293-297

293. Alternative to heparin for cardiopulmonary bypass

294. Glycoprotein (GP)IIb/IIIa inhibition

295. Direct thrombin inhibition

296. Used after angioplasty often for a year or more to prevent restenosis

297. Anti-Xa activity mechanism of action
  A. Argatroban
  B. Clopidogrel
  C. Abciximab
  D. Fondaparinux

Group 298-301

298. Of the list, most likely to be associated with opioid-induced hyperalgesia (OIH)

299. Demonstrates ceiling effect with regard to respiratory depression

300. Antagonism of NMDA receptors

301. Norepinephrine reuptake inhibitor (NRI)
  A. Methadone
  B. Remifentanil
  C. Tapentadol (Nucynta)
  D. Butorphanol

Group 302-305

302. Block is antagonized with anticholinesterase drugs

303. Block is enhanced with anticholinesterase drugs

304. Post-tetanic facilitation occurs

305. Sustained response to tetanic stimulus is seen
   A. True of nondepolarizing blockade only
   B. True of phase I depolarizing blockade only
   C. True of phase II depolarizing blockade only
   D. True of nondepolarizing and phase II depolarizing blockade

Group 306-315

306. Amphetamines

307. α_2 Agonists (clonidine, dexmedetomidine)

308. Hyperthyroidism

309. Acute ethanol ingestion

310. Lidocaine

311. Lithium

312. Opioids

313. Duration of anesthesia

314. Pregnancy

315. Pao_2 35 mm Hg
   A. No change in MAC
   B. Increases MAC
   C. Decreases MAC
   D. Acute administration increases MAC; chronic administration decreases MAC

Group 316-320

316. Least effective antisialagogue

317. Produces best sedation

318. Causes greatest increase in heart rate

319. Does not produce central anticholinergic syndrome

320. May produce mydriasis and cycloplegia when placed topically in the eye
   A. Atropine
   B. Glycopyrrolate
   C. Scopolamine
   D. Atropine and scopolamine

Pharmacology and Pharmacokinetics of Intravenous Drugs
Answers, References, and Explanations

169. (A) The duration of action of neuromuscular blocking drugs is related to the dose administered, as well as to how the drug is metabolized or handled in the body. Succinylcholine normally is rapidly metabolized by plasma cholinesterase and has an ultrashort duration of action. The intermediate-duration neuromuscular blockers atracurium and cisatracurium undergo chemical breakdown in the plasma (Hofmann elimination), as well as ester hydrolysis. Vecuronium and rocuronium also have intermediate duration of actions and undergo primarily hepatic metabolism and biliary excretion with limited renal excretion (10%-25%). Only the long-duration neuromuscular blocker pancuronium is primarily excreted in the urine (80%). In patients with renal failure, the duration of action of neuromuscular blockers is not prolonged with atracurium or cisatracurium; is slightly prolonged with vecuronium and rocuronium; and is markedly prolonged with D-tubocurarine, pancuronium, doxacurium, and pipecuronium. Of the long-duration drugs, 80% of pancuronium, 70% of doxacurium, and 70% of pipecuronium are renally excreted unchanged in the urine. D-tubocurarine has a little more liver excretion and a little less renal elimination compared with pancuronium. *(Miller: Basics of Anesthesia, ed 7, pp 164–165).*

COMPARATIVE PHARMACOLOGY OF NONDEPOLARIZING NEUROMUSCULAR BLOCKING DRUGS

Drug	ED$_{95}$ (mg/kg)	Onset to Maximum Twitch Depression (min)	Duration to Return to ≥25%*	Intubating Dose (mg/kg)	Continuous Infusion (mg/kg/min)	Renal Excretion (% Unchanged)	Hepatic Degradation (%)	Biliary Excretion (% Unchanged)	Hydrolysis in Plasma
Pancuronium	0.07	3-5	60-90	0.1		80	10	5-10	No
Vecuronium	0.05	3-5	20-35	0.08-0.1	1	15-25	20-30	40-75	No
Rocuronium	0.3	1-2	20-35	0.6-1.2		10-25	10-20	50-70	No
Atracurium	0.2	3-5	20-35	0.4-0.5	6-8	NS	NS	NA	Enzymatic, spontaneous
Cisatracurium	0.05	3-5	20-35	0.1	1-1.5	NS	NS	NS	Spontaneous
Mivacurium	0.08	2-3	12-20	0.25	5-6	NS	NS	NS	Enzymatic

NA, not applicable; NS, not significant.
*Control twitch height (minutes).
From Miller: Basics of Anesthesia, ed 7, Philadelphia, Elsevier, 2017, p 165, Table 11.4.

170. (D) Pancreatitis has been reported in patients on long-term propofol infusions. Because of the high fat content of propofol solutions (propofol is insoluble in aqueous solutions and is marketed as an emulsion containing 10% soybean oil, 2.25% glycerol, and 1.2% purified egg phosphatide), patients on long-term infusion should be checked for hyperlipidemia, and patients receiving TPN should have the Intralipid portion of the TPN reduced. Propofol infusion syndrome is commonly defined as an acute onset of metabolic acidosis associated with cardiac dysfunction (e.g., bradycardia or right bundle branch block) and one of the following: rhabdomyolysis, hypertriglyceridemia, enlarged liver, or renal failure. Propofol decreases myocardial contractility and reduces systemic vascular resistance but does not cause adrenal suppression. The latter is a feature of etomidate administration *(Brunton: Goodman & Gilman's The Pharmacological Basis of Therapeutics, ed 13, pp 389–392; Miller: Basics of Anesthesia, ed 7, pp 718–719).*

171. (D) Patients who develop the inherited MH disorder have an abnormality of the type 1 ryanodine receptor (RyR1) in skeletal muscle. The ryanodine receptor is involved with proper intracellular calcium function. When the RyR1 receptor is abnormal and the cell is exposed to triggering drugs (e.g., all volatile anesthetics and/or depolarizing muscle relaxants such as succinylcholine), a loss of control of intracellular calcium may develop, leading to excessive release of calcium from the sarcoplasmic reticulum (SR), which stimulates a marked increase in metabolic function and CO_2 production. Other signs include an increase in oxygen consumption, tachycardia, tachypnea, hyperkalemia, rhabdomyolysis, fever, and multiorgan failure. Dantrolene, the only medication that can reverse MH by reducing calcium release from the SR, appears to rapidly restore normal calcium function in the cell and reverses the metabolic stimulation over the course of several minutes.

Although calcium channel blockers decrease the influx of calcium into the cell, they are inadequate to treat MH. In addition, calcium channel blockers interact with dantrolene to produce hyperkalemia and myocardial depression. However, if MH develops in a patient on calcium channel blockers, dantrolene should be administered cautiously.

In a patient who is MH susceptible, the likelihood of developing MH is unpredictable. In one study, 50% of patients who developed MH had previously received two or more uneventful general anesthetics before the anesthetic triggered an MH response.

Between 50% and 80% of patients who have had clinical MH and a positive muscle biopsy have one of the >210 RyR1 abnormal receptors. Thus a negative genetic test for the ryanodine mutation does not eliminate the possibility of developing clinical MH.

Before the introduction of IV dantrolene (approved by the U.S. Food and Drug Administration [FDA] in 1979), the mortality rate for MH was about 70%. Since IV dantrolene was approved and advances in anesthetic monitoring have allowed earlier detection of MH, during the course of an anesthetic (e.g., with use of end tidal CO_2 monitoring), the mortality rate has been reduced considerably and is currently <5%.

Treatment consists of stopping administration of the triggering agent, suspending surgery as soon as possible, administering dantrolene, hyperventilating with 100% oxygen at high fresh gas flows, inserting fresh activated charcoal filters into the breathing circuit, managing the metabolic acidosis, cooling the patient as needed, and administering diuretics to help prevent kidney injury from myoglobinuria by maintaining a urine output >1 mL/kg/hr *(Cote: A Practice of Anesthesia for Infants and Children, ed 5, pp 817–834; Hines: Stoelting's Anesthesia and Co-Existing Disease, ed 7, pp 666–669; Malignant Hyperthermia Association of the United States – MHAUS website http://www.mhaus.org; Miller: Miller's Anesthesia, ed 8, pp 1287–1300).*

172. (C) Parkinson disease (paralysis agitans or shaking palsy) is a degenerative CNS disease. It is caused by greater than 80% destruction of dopaminergic neurons in the substantia nigra of the basal ganglia. Dopamine acts as a neurotransmitter to inhibit the rate of firing of neurons that control the extrapyramidal motor system. The imbalance of neurotransmitters that results leads to the extrapyramidal symptoms of this disease. Symptoms include bradykinesia (slowness of movement), muscular rigidity, resting tremor (that lessens with voluntary movement), and impaired balance. Drugs that can produce extrapyramidal effects, such as the dopamine antagonists droperidol, promethazine, and thiethylperazine, as well as the dopamine and serotonin antagonist metoclopramide, are contraindicated. Ondansetron, a 5-hydroxytryptamine type 3 (5-HT$_3$) receptor antagonist, is the preferred drug to treat nausea and vomiting for this patient *(Barash: Clinical Anesthesia, ed 8, p 621; Hines: Stoelting's Anesthesia and Co-Existing Disease, ed 7, pp 293–295).*

173. (A) In order for depolarizing muscle relaxants such as succinylcholine to work, the drug must interact with the receptor at the myoneural junction. Patients with myasthenia gravis have fewer acetylcholine receptors on the muscle and are more resistant to succinylcholine but are much more sensitive to nondepolarizing muscle relaxants. Patients with myasthenic syndrome (Eaton-Lambert syndrome) have a decreased release of acetylcholine at the myoneural junction; however, the number of receptors is normal. Patients with myasthenic syndrome are more sensitive to both depolarizing and nondepolarizing muscle relaxants. Huntington chorea is a degenerative CNS disease that is associated with decreased plasma cholinesterase activity, and prolonged responses to succinylcholine use have been seen. The response to depolarizing and nondepolarizing muscle relaxants appears to be unchanged in patients with polymyositis. Succinylcholine is contraindicated in patients with Duchenne muscular dystrophy because of the risks of rhabdomyolysis, hyperkalemia, and cardiac arrest. Nondepolarizing muscle relaxants have a normal response in patients with Duchenne muscular dystrophy, although some patients have prominent coexisting skeletal muscle weakness *(Hines: Stoelting's Anesthesia and Co-Existing Disease, ed 7, pp 295, 516–524).*

174. (C) Sedation is commonly used in the ICU to prevent patient injury, decrease anxiety, reduce pain, reduce sympathetic stimulation, and help with ventilator dyssynchrony. Many different drugs have been used, including barbiturates, narcotics (e.g., fentanyl, morphine), benzodiazepines (e.g., midazolam, loraze-pam), etomidate, ketamine, antipsychotics (e.g., haloperidol), propofol, and α_2-adrenergic agonists (e.g., dexmedetomidine). Although deep sedation was commonly used, more recent evidence has suggested that patients tend to have fewer complications with light sedation and daily awakening (e.g., shorter duration of mechanical ventilation, less cardiovascular depression, and shorter ICU stays). The choice of drugs depends on the particular indications. Dexmedetomidine has several desirable effects, especially in the neurosurgical ICU, including sedation, analgesia, and little effect on respiratory drive. Its sedative properties resemble normal sleep in that the sedated patient can be easily aroused with stimulation and then rapidly fall back to sleep after stimulation ends. Dexmedetomidine does have some disadvantages, such as cost and FDA-approved use for only 24 hours *(Barash: Clinical Anesthesia, ed 8, pp 498–497; Miller: Basics of Anesthesia, ed 7, pp 118–119).*

175. (B) Diazepam (Valium) and lorazepam are water-insoluble benzodiazepines and are usually mixed with pro-pylene glycol to become soluble solutions. These propylene glycol solutions are painful when injected. Midazolam has an imidazole ring that allows the drug to be water soluble in an acid pH (pH 3.5). When injected into the bloodstream, midazolam is exposed to the higher physiologic pH, the ring changes shape, and the drug becomes lipid soluble. The lipid-soluble form readily crosses the blood-brain barrier to exert its pharmacologic effects. None of the other drugs change form with different pH *(Hemmings: Pharmacology and Physiology for Anesthesia, pp 144–145; Brunton: Goodman & Gilman's The Pharmacological Basis of Therapeutics, ed 13, p 396).*

176. (C) The amount of submucosally injected epinephrine required to produce ventricular cardiac dysrhyth-mias (i.e., three or more premature ventricular contractions during or after injection) varies with the volatile anesthetic administered. Patients under halothane anesthesia are particularly sensitive to ven-tricular arrhythmias, whereas patients with isoflurane, desflurane, and sevoflurane are less sensitive to epinephrine. Fifty percent of patients have ventricular arrhythmias when a dose of 2.1 µg/kg of epi-nephrine is administered submucosally into patients under halothane anesthesia. Ventricular arrhyth-mias do not seem to occur when a dose of up to 5 µg/kg of epinephrine is injected submucosally into patients under 1.2 MAC of sevoflurane or isoflurane in oxygen anesthesia. However, when the dose of epinephrine is increased to between 5 and 15 µg/kg, then about one third of patients will exhibit ven-tricular ectopy under sevoflurane or isoflurane anesthesia. Thus using the 5 µg/kg maximum dose, a 70-kg patient could receive up to 350 µg of epinephrine (70 kg × 5 µg/kg) or 35 mL of this 1:100,000 solution (10 µg/mL) without ventricular arrhythmias *(Johnston: A comparative interaction of epinephrine with enflurane, isoflurane and halothane in man. Anesth Analg 55:709–712, 1976; Navarro: Humans anesthetized with sevoflurane or isoflurane have similar arrhythmic response to epinephrine. Anesthesiology 80:545–549, 1994; Miller: Miller's Anesthesia, ed 8, p 713).*

177. (D) β-Adrenergic receptor antagonists are effective in the treatment of essential hypertension and angina pectoris. They can be used to decrease mortality in patients suffering myocardial infarctions; to treat hyperthyroidism or hypertrophic obstructive cardiomyopathy; and to prevent migraine headaches. Although they are useful drugs, their use is limited by many side effects, which include bronchocon-striction, suppression of insulin secretion, blunting of the catecholamine response to hypoglycemia, excessive myocardial depression, atrioventricular heart block, accentuated increases in plasma concen-trations of potassium with intravenous infusion of potassium chloride, fatigue, and rebound tachycardia associated with abrupt drug discontinuation. An important advantage of β-adrenergic receptor antag-onists used in treating hypertension is the lack of orthostatic hypotension *(Brunton: Goodman & Gil-man's The Pharmacological Basis of Therapeutics, ed 13, pp 214–216, 513).*

178. (C) Anticholinergics are rarely given with premedication today unless a specific effect is needed (e.g., drying of the mouth before fiberoptic intubation, prevention of bradycardia, and, rarely, as a mild sedative). Side effects are many and include relaxation or a decrease of the lower esophageal sphincter tone that may make patients more likely to regurgitate gastric contents. Although these drugs can decrease gastric acid secretion and increase gastric pH, the pH effects are small and the dose needed to accomplish this is much higher than clinically used. The following table compares the effects of various anticholinergics *(Brunton: Goodman & Gilman's The Pharmacological Basis of Therapeutics, ed 13, pp 153–158; Miller: Basics of Anesthesia, ed 7, pp 80–81).*

COMPARATIVE EFFECTS OF ANTICHOLINERGICS ADMINISTERED INTRAMUSCULARLY AS PHARMACOLOGIC PREMEDICATION

Effect	Atropine	Scopolamine	Glycopyrrolate
Antisialagogue effect	+	+++	++
Sedative and amnesic effects	+	+++	0
Increased gastric fluid pH	0	0	0/+
Central nervous system toxicity	+	++	0
Relaxation of lower esophageal sphincter	++	++	++
Mydriasis and cycloplegia	+	+++	0
Heart rate	++	0/+	+

From Miller: Basics of Anesthesia, *ed 7, Philadelphia, Elsevier, 2017, p 81, Table 6.3.*

179. (D) Neostigmine, pyridostigmine, edrophonium, and physostigmine are anticholinesterase drugs. Neostigmine, pyridostigmine, and edrophonium are quaternary ammonium compounds and do not pass the blood-brain barrier. However, physostigmine is a tertiary amine and does cross the blood-brain barrier. This property makes physostigmine useful in the treatment for central anticholinergic syndrome (also called postoperative delirium or atropine toxicity) *(Barash: Clinical Anesthesia, ed 8, pp 550–551).*

180. (D) Whereas propofol, barbiturates, etomidate, and benzodiazepines exert much, if not all, of their pharmacologic effects via the GABA receptors, ketamine has only weak activity on the GABA receptors. Ketamine's mechanism of action is complex, with most of the effects due to interaction with NMDA receptors. Ketamine also interacts with monoaminergic, muscarinic, and opioid receptors, as well as voltage-sensitive calcium ion channels *(Miller: Basics of Anesthesia, ed 7, pp 115–117).*

181. (D) All of the drugs listed are opioids. Meperidine is structurally similar to atropine and possesses mild anticholinergic properties. In contrast to other opioid-receptor agonists, meperidine rarely causes bradycardia but can increase heart rate. Normeperidine, a metabolite of meperidine with some CNS-stimulating properties, may cause delirium and seizures if the level is high enough. This is more likely in patients who have renal impairment and are receiving meperidine over several days *(Brunton: Goodman & Gilman's The Pharmacological Basis of Therapeutics, ed 13, pp 372–373).*

182. (D) In the United States, ketamine is prepared as a mixture of the two isomers S(+) and R(−). In some countries, the S(+) isomer, which is more potent and has fewer side effects, is available. All of the statements are true except for answer D. Norketamine (ketamine's primary active metabolite) is one fifth to one third as potent as ketamine and can contribute to prolonged effects *(Barash: Clinical Anesthesia, ed 8, pp 493–496; Miller: Basics of Anesthesia, ed 7, pp 115–117).*

183. (B) Direct-acting sympathomimetic drugs work directly on the receptors. Indirect-acting sympathomimetic drugs have their effects primarily by entering the neurons and then displacing norepinephrine and causing the release of norepinephrine from the postganglionic sympathetic nerve fibers. Ephedrine, mephentermine, and metaraminol are primarily indirect-acting sympathomimetic agents that also may have some direct-acting properties. The following table summarizes the sympathomimetic agents and their effects on the adrenergic receptors *(Miller: Basics of Anesthesia, ed 7, p 77).*

CLASSIFICATION AND COMPARATIVE PHARMACOLOGY OF SYMPATHOMIMETICS

Sympathomimetic	α	β₁	β₂	Mechanism of Action
Amphetamine	++	+	+	Indirect
Dobutamine	0	+++	0	Direct
Dopamine	++	++	+	Direct
Ephedrine	++	+	+	Indirect and some direct
Epinephrine	+	++	++	Direct
Isoproterenol	0	+++	+++	Direct
Mephentermine	++	+	+	Indirect
Metaraminol	++	+	+	Indirect and some direct
Methoxamine	+++	0	0	Direct
Norepinephrine	+++	++	0	Direct
Phenylephrine	+++	0	0	Direct

From Stoelting RK: Pharmacology and Physiology in Anesthetic Practice, *ed 4, Philadelphia, Lippincott Williams & Wilkins, 2006, p 293.*

184. (D) Naloxone, naltrexone, and nalmefene are opioid receptor antagonists that can reverse the central and peripheral effects of opioids (e.g., methadone). Methylnaltrexone is a quaternary ammonium opioid receptor antagonist that does not penetrate the CNS (i.e., does not reverse analgesia) but does antagonize peripheral opioid receptors (i.e., blocks the GI tract's opioid receptors and can treat opioid-induced constipation). Because of its structure, it is not absorbed after oral administration, so it is administered by injection *(Brunton: Goodman & Gilman's The Pharmacological Basis of Therapeutics, ed 13, pp 370, 930).*

185. (B) Patients with HIV take at least three drugs simultaneously during their treatment. A variety of antiretroviral drugs such as nucleoside reverse transcriptase inhibitors (NRTIs), non-nucleoside reverse transcriptase inhibitors (NNRTIs), entry inhibitors, integrase inhibitors, and/or protease inhibitors are used. Indinavir, nelfinavir, and ritonavir are three of many protease inhibitors currently available. All protease enzyme inhibitors have metabolic drug interactions. Most (especially ritonavir in clinical doses) irreversibly inhibit CYP3A4, and this inhibition could last for 2 to 3 days after the drug is stopped.

CYP3A4 is involved in the metabolism of benzodiazepines (e.g., midazolam) and many opioids (e.g., fentanyl), and these drugs will have higher concentrations and prolonged elimination times when protease inhibitors are used. Protease inhibitors can also induce the production of the CYP enzymes, allowing some drugs (e.g., estrogens) to be metabolized more quickly. In addition, protease inhibitors may cause glucose intolerance, disorders in lipid metabolism, premature atherosclerosis, and diastolic dysfunction leading to heart failure, as well as acute tubular necrosis and nephrolithiasis *(Brunton: Goodman & Gilman's The Pharmacological Basis of Therapeutics, ed 13, pp 1139–1154; Hines: Stoelting's Anesthesia and Co-Existing Disease, ed 7, pp 561–562).*

186. (C) Aprepitant is an NK1 antagonist (substance P antagonist) with a long half-life of 9 to 13 hours. It is orally administered for the prevention and treatment of PONV, although it seems better in preventing vomiting. NK1 antagonists may act synergistically with 5-HT₃ antagonists and/or dexamethasone. Aprepitant is not associated with QTc prolongation. Although marketed for its antiemetic effects, it has some anxiolytic and mild antidepressant effects as well *(Brunton: Goodman & Gilman's The Pharmacological Basis of Therapeutics, ed 13, p 937; Miller: Miller's Anesthesia, ed 8, pp 2637, 2967–2968).*

187. (B) Echothiophate is an organophosphate that inhibits acetylcholinesterase as well as pseudocholinesterase, which is responsible for the metabolism of succinylcholine and ester-type local anesthetics. It does this by forming a phosphorylated complex with acetylcholinesterase. The topical solution is instilled in the eye for treatment of refractory open-angle glaucoma. The amount of drug absorbed may be sufficient to inhibit acetylcholinesterase and cause prolongation in the duration of action of succinylcholine or mivacurium. Because of this, it is "recommended" to wait at least 3 weeks after the stoppage of echothiophate before the administration of these two muscle relaxants. One must wonder about these "recommendations" because clinical cases have shown that when cholinesterase activity is decreased (from echothiophate) to no activity, the increase in duration of neuromuscular block from succinylcholine was less than 25 minutes *(Miller: Basics of Anesthesia, ed 7, p 525)*.

188. (D) Monitoring neuromuscular blockade for nondepolarizing muscle relaxants can be done in a variety of ways. The simplest way is to measure the reduction or suppression of a single twitch height. This is commonly performed by observing the twitch response of the thumb's adductor pollicis muscle, after ulnar nerve stimulation. At 90% to 95% reduction of twitch height (i.e., ED_{90} to ED_{95}), there is good muscle relaxation for intubation and intra-abdominal surgery. However, measuring the reduction of twitch height is not practical. Because there is good correlation between reduction of twitch height and the number of thumb twitches that can be elicited by TOF stimulation, TOF stimulation is more commonly used where four twitches are administered over 2 seconds. If only one twitch of a TOF is demonstrated, single twitch height is depressed at least 85%; with two to four thumb twitches, 70% to 85% depression is seen. Note that the presence of four twitches does not mean that neuromuscular function has completely recovered; in fact, a significant number of receptors may still be occupied by the muscle relaxant *(Barash: Clinical Anesthesia, ed 8, pp 542–544)*.

189. (C) There are two major chemical classes of nondepolarizing muscle relaxants: the aminosteroids (-onium drugs) and the benzylisoquinolinium (-urium) drugs. In general, the aminosteroids cause no significant histamine release (at the clinical doses of 2-3 × ED_{95}), whereas some of the benzylisoquinolinium drugs can. The histamine release primarily occurs with rapid administration of atracurium but does not occur with cisatracurium or doxacurium. The amount of histamine released is rarely of clinical significance. The cardiovascular effects of neuromuscular blocking drugs occur by three main mechanisms: (1) drug-induced histamine release; (2) effects at cardiac muscarinic receptors; or (3) effects on nicotinic receptors at autonomic ganglia. The following table summarizes the mechanisms for the cardiovascular effects of muscle relaxants *(Barash: Clinical Anesthesia, ed 8, pp 537–538)*.

CLINICAL AUTONOMIC EFFECTS OF NEUROMUSCULAR BLOCKING DRUGS

Drug	Autonomic Ganglia	Cardiac Muscarinic Receptors	Histamine Release
Depolarizing Substance			
Succinylcholine	Stimulates	Stimulates	Slight
Benzylisoquinolinium Compounds			
Mivacurium	None	None	Slight
Atracurium	None	None	Slight
Cisatracurium	None	None	None
D-tubocurarine	Blocks	None	Moderate
Steroidal Compounds			
Vecuronium	None	None	None
Rocuronium	None	Blocks weakly	None
Pancuronium	None	Blocks moderately	None

From Miller RD: Miller's Anesthesia, ed 7, Philadelphia, Saunders, 2011, p 882, Table 29-11.

190. (A) Postganglionic sympathetic nerve fibers release norepinephrine from the synaptic vesicles in the nerve terminals. Eighty percent of the released norepinephrine rapidly undergoes reuptake into the sympathetic nerve terminals (uptake 1) and reenters storage vesicles for future release. Only a small amount of the norepinephrine that is reabsorbed is metabolized in the cytoplasm by MAO. Twenty percent of the norepinephrine is diluted by diffusion away from the receptors and can gain access to the circulation. COMT, which is located primarily in the liver, metabolizes this norepinephrine *(Barash: Clinical Anesthesia, ed 8, pp 341–342)*.

191. (D) Administration of ketamine may be associated with visual, auditory, and proprioceptive hallucinations. These unpleasant side effects of ketamine occur on emergence and may progress to delirium. The incidence of emergence delirium from ketamine is dose dependent and occurs in approximately 5% to 30% of patients. Emergence delirium is less frequent after repeated administrations of ketamine. The most effective prevention for emergence delirium is administration of a benzodiazepine (midazolam being more effective than diazepam) about 5 minutes before induction of anesthesia with ketamine. Atropine and droperidol given perioperatively may increase the incidence of emergence delirium *(Miller: Basics of Anesthesia, ed 7, p 116)*.

192. (B) The original formulations of dantrolene (Dantrium, Revonto) required the contents of each 20-mg vial to be reconstituted with 60 mL of sterile water for injection; then the contents are shaken until the solution is clear. Thus large volumes of fluid are administered. These formulations also contain 3000 mg of mannitol/20-mg vial.

Ryanodex (FDA approval in 2014) is at least twice as expensive as other formulations of IV dantrolene, but its main advantage is fast reconstitution and administration. Each 250-mg vial is reconstituted with only 5 mL of sterile water for injection and shaken to ensure a uniformly opaque orange-colored suspension. A 250-mg dose of Ryanodex can be reconstituted and administered in less than 1 minute. If you reconstituted the same 250-mg of IV dantrolene using the original preparations (12.5 20-mg vials), the same dose would take >15 minutes to administer. Ryanodex has a low amount of mannitol (125 mg/vial), which is insufficient to maintain a brisk diuresis.

Dosage of dantrolene is the same between products. Starting dose of dantrolene is 2.5 mg/kg and repeated as needed every 5 to 10 minutes up to a maximum of 10 mg/kg (product labeling). MHAUS does not have an upper limit of the dantrolene dose, but you should seriously consider other etiologies if a total dose of 10mg/kg of dantrolene does not give you the desired response. *(Cote: A Practice of Anesthesia for Infants and Children, ed 5, pp 817–834; Hines: Stoelting's Anesthesia and Co-Existing Disease, ed 7, pp 666–669; Malignant Hyperthermia Association of the United States – MHAUS website http://www.mhaus.org; Ryanodex.com)*.

193. (A) Mineralocorticoids are produced in the adrenal cortex and are involved in Na^+ reabsorption, as well as K^+ and H^+ excretion by the kidney. The main mineralocorticoid produced is aldosterone. Spironolactone (Aldactone) and eplerenone (Inspra) are competitive inhibitors of aldosterone's binding to the mineralocorticoid receptors. As with all inhibitors, their actions depend on the amount of aldosterone circulating. They are especially useful in advanced stages of heart failure associated with high levels of aldosterone. Eplerenone is a more selective inhibitor of aldosterone compared with spironolactone, and the side effect of gynecomastia (a progesterone-related side effect of spironolactone) is less. *(Brunton: Goodman and Gilman's The Pharmacological Basis of Therapeutics, ed 12, pp 692–695; Hines: Stoelting's Anesthesia and Co-Existing Disease, ed 7, p 208)*.

194. (A) Many drugs can enhance the neuromuscular block produced by nondepolarizing muscle relaxants. These include volatile anesthetics, aminoglycoside antibiotics, magnesium, intravenous local anesthetics, furosemide, dantrolene, calcium channel blockers, and lithium. Calcium does not enhance neuromuscular blockade and, in fact, actually antagonizes the effects of magnesium. In patients with hyperparathyroidism and hypercalcemia, there is a decreased sensitivity to nondepolarizing muscle relaxants and shorter durations of action *(Miller: Basics of Anesthesia, ed 7, p 165)*.

195. (B) Lisinopril (Prinivil/Zestril) is a lysine analog of enalapril (Vasotec), and both drugs are angiotensin-converting enzyme (ACE) inhibitors. Angiotensin I is converted in the lungs to the potent vasoconstrictor angiotensin II by ACE. Angiotensin II also stimulates the release of aldosterone from the adrenal cortex of the kidneys. The half-life of lisinopril is 12 hours, and it is primarily excreted unchanged in the urine. ACE inhibitors are commonly used to treat hypertension (especially those related to increased renin secretion) and congestive heart failure and to help reduce the risk of death in patients who have had myocardial infarctions *(Flood: Stoelting's Pharmacology and Physiology in Anesthetic Practice, ed 5, pp 505–507; Miller: Basics of Anesthesia, ed 7, p 484)*.

196. (A) About 40 years ago it was noted that kidney response varies with the type of shock. In canines, hypovolemic shock reduced renal blood flow to 10% of controls, whereas cardiogenic shock reduced renal blood flow to only 75% of controls. The main difference seemed to be related to the atrial pressures (decreased in hypovolemic shock but increased in cardiogenic shock). About 10 years later, a peptide was isolated from the atrium of rats, named atrial or A-type natriuretic peptide (ANP). Later a natriuretic peptide was isolated from porcine brains and was named brain or BNP. In humans, BNP is mainly produced in the cardiac ventricles. Natriuretic peptides are primarily released from the atria (ANP) and ventricles (BNP) when the chambers are overdistended. Thus in the failing heart, BNP is released. Natriuretic peptides have a main effect on the kidneys to excrete sodium and water. They have vasodilating properties and inhibit the release of renin. Blood levels of BNP are used as a marker for the severity of cardiovascular disease and may have a role in preoperative cardiac risk assessment. Nesiritide is a recombinant BNP and is being studied for the treatment of acute heart failure *(Barash: Clinical Anesthesia, ed 8, pp 591–592; Hines: Stoelting's Anesthesia and Co-Existing Disease, ed 7, pp 203–205).*

197. (B) MS is an acquired inflammatory autoimmune disease in which there is demyelination of nerve fibers within the CNS. In patients with MS and profound neurologic deficits, succinylcholine may cause hyperkalemia and should be avoided, and nondepolarizing muscle relaxants appear safe.

Guillain-Barré syndrome is an inflammatory polyneuritis affecting the peripheral nervous system and associated with muscle weakness. In patients with Guillain-Barré, succinylcholine may cause hyperkalemia and should be avoided, whereas nondepolarizing muscle relaxants are not contraindicated but are avoided because of increased sensitivity and possible prolonged muscle weakness in the postoperative period.

Duchenne muscular dystrophy and the less common Becker muscular dystrophy are both X-linked recessive diseases. They are characterized by progressive muscle weakness. In 1992 the FDA issued a warning with regard to the use of succinylcholine in children and adolescents because succinylcholine has been associated with several deaths when administered to patients with unsuspected muscular dystrophy (many developed hyperkalemia and were later diagnosed as having muscular dystrophy). Nondepolarizing muscle relaxants appear safe, but a slower onset may exist.

Myasthenia gravis patients have fewer postsynaptic receptors at the myoneural junction, and, if succinylcholine is administered, they appear to be resistant. Larger doses appear needed (1.5-2 mg/kg) for intubation, and there is no associated hyperkalemic response. The duration of action of succinylcholine, on the other hand, will be prolonged because these patients receive anticholinesterase therapy (pyridostigmine). They are, however, very sensitive to nondepolarizing muscle relaxants, and a greatly reduced dose of a nondepolarizer should be administered, if at all *(Hines: Stoelting's Anesthesia and Co-Existing Disease, ed 7, pp 296–298, 321–322, 516–517, 521–524).*

198. (D) Several antibiotics potentiate neuromuscular blockade. The aminoglycosides (neomycin, streptomycin, gentamicin, and tobramycin) and the lincosamides (clindamycin and lincomycin) can augment neuromuscular blockade. The only drug in question that does not affect neuromuscular blockade is erythromycin (of the macrolide antibiotic group). In addition, tetracyclines, penicillins, and cephalosporins do not affect neuromuscular blockade *(Barash: Clinical Anesthesia, ed 8, p 538; Brunton: Goodman & Gilman's The Pharmacological Basis of Therapeutics, ed 13, p 183).*

199. (D) With liver failure, the liver cannot adequately detoxify noxious chemicals. Among patients with end-stage liver disease, 50% to 70% develop HE. Symptoms vary from mild confusion, drowsiness, and stupor to coma. The etiology of HE is complex. Because an elevation in blood ammonia levels (easily measured) is strongly associated with HE, treatment is aimed at lowering the ammonia level. Other toxins also contribute to HE. To lower the ammonia level, lactulose (which decreases the absorption of ammonia) and neomycin (which reduces the production of ammonia by reducing the ammonia-producing intestinal flora) are commonly administered. Protein restriction is commonly done to decrease ammonia production, so amino acid–rich TPN is not helpful. Flumazenil (a GABA receptor antagonist) has been shown to produce short-duration reversal of the symptoms of HE in some patients and thus suggests that GABA receptors are somehow activated during HE. GABA receptors are responsible for inhibitory neurotransmission in the CNS *(Hines: Stoelting's Anesthesia and Co-Existing Disease, ed 7, pp 354–355).*

200. (A) In most patients, an intravenous intubating dose of succinylcholine (1 mg/kg = 2 × the ED_{95}) will show neuromuscular blockade that lasts 5 to 10 minutes. The reason for the short duration of action relates to succinylcholine's very rapid metabolism by typical plasma cholinesterase (also called pseudocholinesterase or butyrylcholinesterase). Some patients, however, have a prolonged effect, which could be due to either a decrease in the quantity or a genetic qualitative change in the enzyme. Quantitative decreases can be seen in patients with malnutrition, liver disease, pregnancy, burns, or advanced age.

Cholinesterase activity can also be decreased by the coadministration of various medications, including anticholinesterase drugs (e.g., neostigmine), metoclopramide, and esmolol. A marked quantitative reduction (e.g., severe liver disease) can prolong succinylcholine activity about three times the normal duration of block. A marked prolongation of effect is due to the genetic production of atypical pseudocholinesterase (an inactive form). To investigate the genetic or qualitative change, a dibucaine inhibition test is done. The local anesthetic dibucaine can inhibit a normal enzyme more so than an abnormal enzyme. People with a normal dibucaine number of 70 to 80 are homozygous for the normal typical plasma cholinesterase and have the normal 5- to 10-minute neuromuscular blockade. People who are heterozygous (incidence of 1/480) for the atypical plasma cholinesterase have a dibucaine number of 50 to 60 and a block duration of 20 minutes. Patients who are homozygous for the atypical plasma cholinesterase (incidence 1/3200) have a dibucaine number of 20 to 30 and a block duration from 1 to 3 hours. This genetic variation of plasma cholinesterase is the most common abnormality; however, there are also other, less frequent genetic changes in the plasma cholinesterase. See also Question 260 *(Miller: Basics of Anesthesia, ed 7, pp 162–163).*

201. (B) In normal patients, potassium levels increase about 0.5 mEq/L after the administration of succinylcholine. However, in some acquired conditions the potassium level may increase 5 to 7 mEq/L above the baseline potassium level after administration of succinylcholine. This marked elevation of potassium may lead to cardiac arrest. These acquired conditions include the following: (1) denervation injury as caused by spinal cord injury leading to skeletal muscle atrophy; (2) skeletal muscle injury resulting from third-degree burns (until scarring occurs); (3) acute upper motor neuron injury such as stroke; (4) severe skeletal muscle trauma; and (5) severe abdominal infections. In these acquired conditions the potential to increase potassium levels after succinylcholine usually takes a few days to develop, peaks 10 to 50 days after the initial injury, and may persist for 6 months or more. All factors considered, it might be prudent to avoid administration of succinylcholine to any patient more than 24 hours after the conditions listed here. This vulnerability to hyperkalemia may reflect a proliferation of extrajunctional cholinergic receptors, which provide more sites for potassium to leak outward across the cell membrane during depolarization. Some have suggested that the number of receptors is unchanged but that the receptors themselves have altered affinity to acetylcholine or drugs. Similar marked elevations of potassium may develop in cases of undiagnosed myopathy *(Miller: Basics of Anesthesia, ed 7, p 163).*

202. (A) Although flumazenil (a specific benzodiazepine antagonist) inhibits the activity at the GABA receptor, it works only at the benzodiazepine recognition site and has no effect in reversing other drugs that work on the GABA site (e.g., barbiturates, etomidate, propofol). It has a fast onset (within minutes), with peak brain levels occurring within 6 to 10 minutes, and a relatively short duration of action. Flumazenil can reverse all benzodiazepine CNS effects, including sedative, amnestic, muscle relaxant, and anticonvulsant effects. Side effects are rare, the most common being nausea, vomiting, or both (about 10%). Nausea occurs more commonly when flumazenil is given to patients after general anesthesia than after conscious sedation. Due to its short clinical duration of action, patients receiving flumazenil should be monitored for possible resedation and respiratory depression *(Brunton: Goodman & Gilman's The Pharmacological Basis of Therapeutics, ed 13, p 346).*

203. (D) Nonsteroidal anti-inflammatory drugs (NSAIDs) (e.g., aspirin, acetaminophen, indomethacin, ibuprofen, diclofenac, and ketorolac) inhibit COX enzymes that are involved in the conversion of arachidonic acid to prostaglandin, thromboxane, and prostacyclin. COX-1 is involved with platelet aggregation and gastric mucosal protection; COX-2 is involved with pain, inflammation, and fever. TXA_2 has prothrombotic and vasoconstricting properties. Prostacyclin I_2 has antithrombotic and vasodilating properties. Ketorolac is a nonselective inhibitor of both COX-1 and COX-2 enzymes. Selective COX-2 drugs (e.g., only celecoxib, currently available in the United States) can be used, but in general these have been shown to cause a small increase in thrombotic issues (but fewer effects on gastric mucosa and platelet activity). Because of a ceiling effect with regard to analgesia, ketorolac has only mild-to-moderate analgesic effects *(Barash: Clinical Anesthesia, ed 8, p 1232; Brunton: Goodman & Gilman's The Pharmacological Basis of Therapeutics, ed 13, p 698).*

204. (D) Acute intermittent porphyria is the most serious form of porphyria. This disease affects both the central and peripheral nervous systems. An acute intermittent porphyria attack can be triggered by a variety of conditions, including starvation, dehydration, stress, sepsis, and some drugs, such as etomidate and barbiturates. Drugs that are safe or *probably safe* include local anesthetics, inhaled anesthetics, neuromuscular blocking drugs, some intravenous anesthetics (propofol and ketamine), some analgesics (acetaminophen, aspirin, morphine, fentanyl, sufentanil), antiemetics (droperidol, H_2 blockers, metoclopramide, ondansetron), and neostigmine and naloxone. Drugs that are contraindicated include some intravenous anesthetics (barbiturates), some analgesics (ketorolac, pentazocine), and hydantoin anticonvulsants *(Barash: Clinical Anesthesia, ed 8, pp 623–625; Hines: Stoelting's Anesthesia and Co-Existing Disease, ed 7, pp 380–382).*

205. (A) Cytochrome P450 (CYP) enzymes are involved in the metabolism of many medications. There are many such isoforms, and these are further characterized into families with an Arabic number and further characterized into subfamilies (capital letter). The clinical activity of these enzymes can be increased (induced) or decreased (inhibited) by age, genetics, medications, and some foods. CYP2D6 is needed to convert the inactive codeine to the active morphine. Similarly, CYP2D6 also metabolizes oxycodone into active oxymorphone, and inactive hydrocodone into active hydromorphone. CYP2D6 is inhibited by selective serotonin reuptake inhibitors, as well as with quinidine. SSRIs include fluoxetine (Prozac), sertraline (Zoloft), paroxetine (Paxil), fluvoxamine (Luvox), citalopram (Celexa), and escitalopram (Lexapro). Thus patients taking SSRIs or quinidine will get a poor analgesic effect with codeine, oxycodone, and hydrocodone *(Brunton: Goodman & Gilman's The Pharmacological Basis of Therapeutics, ed 13, pp 90–91, 269–274, 381).*

206. (D) Although etomidate causes pain on intravenous injection in up to 80% of patients, the unintentional administration of etomidate into an artery does not result in detrimental effects to the artery *(Barash: Clinical Anesthesia, ed 8, pp 492–493).*

207. (D) Fentanyl is more lipid soluble than morphine, so it passes through the blood-brain barrier more easily and has a faster onset of action. Fentanyl also has a larger volume of distribution, slower plasma clearance, and longer elimination half-life than morphine. However, the duration of action of fentanyl (when given in small doses) is much shorter than that of morphine because fentanyl is rapidly redistributed from the brain to inactive tissue sites (e.g., lipid sites). In larger doses, these tissue sites can become saturated, and the pharmacologic action of fentanyl becomes considerably prolonged *(Brunton: Goodman & Gilman's The Pharmacological Basis of Therapeutics, ed 13, pp 369–370, 372; Miller: Basics of Anesthesia, ed 7, pp 125–127).*

208. (D) This question illustrates the concept of infusion front-end kinetics. This concept is useful for comparing the kinetics of various intravenous agents used in anesthesia. Remifentanil reaches the steady state in less than 1 hour of continuous infusion. Approximately 8 hours are required to reach the steady state with alfentanil and sufentanil, whereas fentanyl and morphine have not achieved the steady state concentration even after 10 hours of continuous infusion.

Another important concept is the time after bolus to reach peak effect: bolus front-end kinetics. This concept is more intuitive to most anesthesia providers. Comparing the same narcotics used in this question, alfentanil and remifentanil reach peak concentration at nearly the same time and fentanyl only slightly later *(Miller: Basics of Anesthesia, ed 7, p 127).*

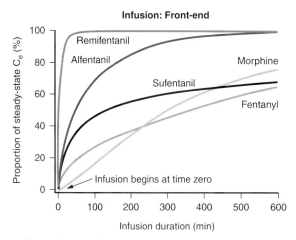

From Miller RD: Basics of Anesthesia, *ed 7, Figure 9.3 p 127.*

209. (C) Bleomycin is used primarily in the treatment of Hodgkin lymphoma and testicular tumors. Bleomycin causes oxidative damage to nucleotides, which leads to breaks in DNA. Although the more common side effects of bleomycin use are mucocutaneous, dose-related pulmonary toxicity is the most serious side effect. Early signs and symptoms of pulmonary toxicity include dry cough, fine rales, and diffuse infiltrates on x-ray. Approximately 5% to 10% of patients will develop pulmonary toxicity, and about 1% will die of this complication. Most believe that the risk of pulmonary toxicity increases with dose (especially total dose >250 mg), in patients older than 40 years of age, in patients with a creatinine clearance (CrCl) of less than 80 mL/min, and in patients with prior chest radiation or preexisting pulmonary disease. Although a relationship appears to exist between the use of bleomycin and the use of high concentrations of oxygen, the details are unclear. Currently, it has been suggested to use the lowest concentration of oxygen consistent with patient safety, with a careful evaluation of oxygen saturation with pulse oximetry in any patient who has received bleomycin *(Barash: Clinical Anesthesia, ed 8, pp 589, 595; Brunton: Goodman & Gilman's The Pharmacological Basis of Therapeutics, ed 13, p 1193).*

210. (C) The first two letters of the word "rocuronium" stand for "rapid onset." Of the nondepolarizing muscle relaxants currently available, rocuronium has the most rapid onset of action at clinically useful dosages. Rocuronium is a nondepolarizing neuromuscular relaxant with an intermediate duration of action similar to that of vecuronium, atracurium, and cisatracurium. At an ED_{95} dose (0.3 mg/kg), the onset time is 1.5 to 3 minutes, whereas with the other intermediate nondepolarizing muscle relaxants, the onset time is 3 to 7 minutes. At larger doses (i.e., $2 \times ED_{95}$ or 0.6 mg/kg), onset time can be reduced to 1 to 1.5 minutes *(Miller: Basics of Anesthesia, ed 7, p 167).*

211. (D) An acute decrease in serum potassium causes hyperpolarization of cell membranes. This causes resistance to depolarizing neuromuscular blockers and an increased sensitivity to nondepolarizing neuromuscular blockers *(Stoelting: Pharmacology and Physiology in Anesthetic Practice, ed 4, pp 226–227).*

212. (D) Awareness during general anesthesia is the postoperative recall of events that happened during the anesthetic. Overall incidence has decreased from about 1% 50 years ago to about 0.1% today (with some variations from study to study). Patients at increased risk include patients undergoing cardiac surgery, endoscopic airway surgery, cesarean sections, and trauma surgery *(Miller: Basics of Anesthesia, ed 7, p 816).*

213. (C) The symptoms described in this patient are consistent with cholinergic stimulation or increased levels of acetylcholine that occur with anticholinesterase poisoning. Stimulation of the parasympathetic nervous system produces miosis, abdominal cramping, excess salivation, loss of bowel and bladder control, bradycardia, and bronchoconstriction. These symptoms are treated with atropine. The acetylcholinesterase reactivator pralidoxime sometimes is added to treat the nicotinic effects of elevation of acetylcholine at the neuromuscular junction of skeletal muscle (i.e., skeletal muscle weakness, apnea). CNS effects of elevated acetylcholine levels can include confusion, ataxia, and coma. In addition, supportive therapy (the ABCs of resuscitation [Airway, Breathing, Circulation, etc.]) is provided as needed *(Miller: Basics of Anesthesia, ed 7, p 764).*

214. (C) Flumazenil is a benzodiazepine antagonist used to antagonize the benzodiazepine effects on the CNS. It does not reverse the effects of barbiturates, opiates, or alcohol. Seizures can be precipitated in patients who have been on benzodiazepines for long-term sedation or in patients showing signs of serious cyclic antidepressant overdosage (e.g., twitching, rigidity, widened QRS complex, hypotension). Flumazenil has a shorter elimination half-life (0.7-1.3 hours) compared with midazolam (2-2.5 hours). Flumazenil is poorly absorbed orally *(Brunton: Goodman & Gilman's The Pharmacological Basis of Therapeutics, ed 13, p 346).*

215. (D) Adequate recovery from neuromuscular blockade is believed to occur when 50% or less of receptors are occupied with muscle relaxants. This can be measured with sustained tetanus at 100 Hz, but this test is very painful. Another method requires patient cooperation and consists of a sustained head lift for 5 seconds in the supine position. The "head lift" test is the standard test to determine adequate muscular function *(Miller: Basics of Anesthesia, ed 7, p 171).*

216. (B) PONV is the second-most common complaint reported in the perioperative period (pain is the number one complaint). Many drugs have been used to both prevent (prophylaxis) and to treat (rescue) PONV. Antiemetics were often administered alone, but now combination therapy of two or more drugs such as dopamine antagonists (e.g., droperidol, metoclopramide), histamine antagonists (e.g., diphenhydramine, promazine), anticholinergics (e.g., scopolamine), steroids (e.g., dexamethasone), neurokinin antagonists (e.g., aprepitant), and serotonin antagonists (e.g., ondansetron, dolasetron, granisetron, and palonosetron) are commonly used. Once a serotonin antagonist is given for prophylaxis, adding more of a serotonin antagonist in the PACU does not seem to help. It is better to use an antiemetic from another class of drugs *(Miller: Basics of Anesthesia, ed 7, pp 687–689).*

217. (A) Patients with WPW syndrome are predisposed to develop supraventricular arrhythmias. Sympathetic stimulation (e.g., anxiety, hypovolemia), as well as many drugs (e.g., pancuronium, meperidine, ketamine, ephedrine, digoxin, verapamil), can induce tachyarrhythmias, often by enhancing conduction through accessory atrial pathways. Although verapamil is used to treat supraventricular tachyarrhythmias because of its depressant effects on alveolar nodal conduction, it actually may increase the heart rate in patients with WPW syndrome because it can increase conduction of the accessory pathways. Droperidol, in addition to its antidopaminergic properties, has antidysrhythmic properties that protect against epinephrine-induced dysrhythmias. Proposed mechanisms include α-adrenergic receptor blockade and mild local anesthetic effects. Large doses of droperidol (0.2-0.6 mg/kg) can reduce impulse transmission via the accessory pathways responsible for the tachyarrhythmias that occur in patients with WPW syndrome *(Stoelting: Pharmacology and Physiology in Anesthetic Practice, ed 4, pp 413–415, 766; Hines: Stoelting's Anesthesia and Co-Existing Disease, ed 7, p 160).*

218. (B) Pseudocholinesterase (also called plasma cholinesterase) is an enzyme found in plasma and most other tissues (except erythrocytes). Pseudocholinesterase metabolizes the acetylcholine released at the neuromuscular junction, as well as certain drugs such as succinylcholine, mivacurium, and ester-type local anesthetics. It is produced in the liver and has a half-life of approximately 8 to 16 hours. Pseudocholinesterase levels may be reduced in patients with advanced liver disease. The decrease must be greater than 75% before significant prolongation of neuromuscular blockade occurs with succinylcholine *(Stoelting: Pharmacology and Physiology in Anesthetic Practice, ed 4, p 218; Barash: Clinical Anesthesia, ed 8, pp 1229–1230).*

219. (B) CYP2D6 (also called cytochrome P450 2D6) is a member of the cytochrome P450 mixed-function oxidase system and is involved in metabolism and elimination of approximately 25% of clinically used medications. In addition, it is involved in the metabolism of dopamine and serotonin. CYP2D6 isoenzymes are highly polymorphic, with large variations between individuals as to the number of gene copies. Patients are often classified as being in one of four groups (poor or slow metabolizers, intermediate metabolizers, normal or extensive metabolizers, and ultrarapid or fast metabolizers). Ondansetron is extensively metabolized by CYP1A2, CYP2D6, and CYP3A4. In patients who are ultrarapid metabolizers, such as this patient, ondansetron will be metabolized faster and will have fewer clinical effects. Granisetron is not metabolized by CYP2D6 but is metabolized by CYP3A, so its activity is not affected in this patient, who is an ultra-rapid metabolizer of CYP2D6. CYP2D6 inactivates many medications, including β-blockers, antidepressants, and antipsychotic medications, as well as tamoxifen. CYP2D6 also converts prodrugs such as codeine to its active form, morphine *(Barash: Clinical Anesthesia, ed 8, p 517; Brunton: Goodman and Gilman's The Pharmacological Basis of Therapeutics, ed 12, pp 156–159, 1341–1342).*

220. (C) The adrenal cortex secretes two classes of steroids: the corticosteroids (glucocorticoids and mineralocorticoids) and the androgens. The main glucocorticoid is hydrocortisone, also called cortisol. The glucocorticoids are used primarily for their anti-inflammatory and immunosuppressive effects, but they also have mineralocorticoid activity (i.e., sodium-retaining effects). These drugs differ in potency, amount of mineralocorticoid effect, and duration of action. The normal amount of cortisol produced daily is about 10 mg, but under stress, the level can increase tenfold. The main mineralocorticoid is aldosterone. The normal amount of aldosterone produced daily is about 0.125 mg. Because fludrocortisone has such significant mineralocorticoid activity, it is used only for this. The following table compares several corticosteroids. In this case 50 mg of prednisone is equivalent in glucocorticoid activity to 7.5 mg of dexamethasone and 200 mg of hydrocortisone *(Miller: Basics of Anesthesia, ed 7, p 506).*

COMPARATIVE PHARMACOLOGY OF CORTICOSTEROIDS

Agent	Anti-inflammatory Potency	Equivalent Glucocorticoid Dose (mg)	Sodium-Retaining Potency	Duration of Action (hr)
Hydrocortisone or cortisol (Cortef)	1	20	1	8-12
Cortisone (Cortone)	0.8	25	0.8	8-36
Prednisolone (Hydeltrasol)	4	5	0.8	12-36
Prednisone (Deltasone)	4	5	0.8	18-36
Methylprednisolone (Solu-Medrol)	5	4	0.5	12-36
Triamcinolone (Kenalog)	5	4	0	12-36
Betamethasone (Celestone)	25	0.75	0	36-54
Dexamethasone (Decadron)	25	0.75	0	36-54
Fludrocortisone (Florinef)	10	2	250	24
Aldosterone	0	NA	3000	

NA, not applicable.

From Stoelting RK: Pharmacology and Physiology in Anesthetic Practice, *ed 4, Philadelphia, Lippincott Williams & Wilkins, 2006, p 462.*

221. (A) The RI of neuromuscular blocking drugs is the time needed for spontaneous recovery of a twitch height from 25% to 75% of the baseline height. The elderly, who tend to have reduced renal and hepatic function, have a prolonged RI for nondepolarizing muscle relaxants that are dependent on renal or hepatic elimination (e.g., vecuronium, D-tubocurarine, pancuronium, rocuronium). The RI for atracurium and cisatracurium, which are broken down in the plasma, are not prolonged in the elderly *(Barash: Clinical Anesthesia, ed 8, p 537).*

222. (B) Cyclosporine is a drug that selectively inhibits helper T-lymphocyte–mediated but not B-lymphocyte–mediated immune responses. It is mainly used alone or in combination with corticosteroids to prevent or treat organ rejection. Other uses include the treatment of Crohn disease, uveitis, psoriasis, and rheumatoid arthritis. Side effects that may accompany the administration of cyclosporine include nephrotoxicity (25%-38%), hypertension, limb paresthesias (50%), headaches, confusion, somnolence, seizures, elevation of liver enzymes, allergic reactions, gum hyperplasia, hirsutism, and hyperglycemia. There appears to be no pulmonary toxicity associated with cyclosporine therapy *(Brunton: Goodman & Gilman's The Pharmacological Basis of Therapeutics, ed 13, p 642).*

223. (B) Succinylcholine is basically two acetylcholine molecules hooked together. Succinylcholine may exert cardiovascular effects by: (1) inducing histamine release from mast cells; (2) stimulating autonomic ganglia, which increases neurotransmission at both the sympathetic and parasympathetic nervous systems; and (3) directly stimulating postjunctional cardiac muscarinic receptors. The effect of succinylcholine on heart rate is variable, with both bradycardia and tachycardia possible. The final heart rate depends on many factors, including the amount of nicotinic stimulation of the sympathetic and parasympathetic ganglia, which is greater for the nondominant autonomic nervous system. For example, when sympathetic nervous system tone is high (as in children), bradycardia is more likely to develop when succinylcholine is administered. When parasympathetic nervous system tone is high (as in many adults), tachycardia, although not common, is more likely to occur when succinylcholine is administered. Bradycardia is more likely to occur when a second intravenous dose of succinylcholine is administered 4 to 5 minutes after the first dose, especially when difficult laryngoscopy (e.g., intense vagal stimulation) is being performed *(Barash: Clinical Anesthesia, ed 8, pp 529–532).*

224. (A) Triamterene is a potassium-sparing, distal tubule diuretic.

The mechanism is to directly interfere with Na^+ entry through the Na^+ channels in the apical membrane of the collecting tubule. Because K^+ secretion is coupled with Na^+ entry in this segment, these agents are also effective K^+-sparing diuretics (*Hemmings: Pharmacology and Physiology for Anesthesia pp 609–610*).

225. (A) Propofol's chemical structure is 2,6-diisopropylphenol (i.e., is not an ester) and thus is not metabolized by esterases. Propofol is rapidly metabolized by the liver to more water-soluble compounds that are then renally excreted. Esmolol is an ester compound and is rapidly metabolized by RBC esterases (short half-life of 9-10 minutes). Atracurium and cisatracurium primarily undergo Hofmann elimination, which is a chemical reaction. Atracurium has a second metabolic route: metabolism by nonspecific plasma esterases. Interestingly, cisatracurium, which is an isolated form of atracurium (1 of the 10 stereoisomers), does not undergo metabolism by nonspecific plasma esterases.

The short duration of action of remifentanil is due to its ester structure, which is metabolized by blood and tissue nonspecific esterases. Because of the nonspecific metabolism, its duration of action is not prolonged in patients with pseudocholinesterase deficiency (*Miller: Basics of Anesthesia, ed 7, pp 80, 105–106, 133–134, 167*).

226. (A) Hyperkalemia, MH, masseter spasm, sinus bradycardia, nodal rhythms, and myalgias are side effects that can be seen after the administration of succinylcholine. In recent years, there have been several case reports of intractable cardiac arrest in apparently healthy children after the administration of succinylcholine. In these cases, hyperkalemia, rhabdomyolysis, and acidosis were documented. Later, muscle biopsy samples demonstrated that many of these cases were subclinical cases of Duchenne muscular dystrophy. For this reason of occasional severe hyperkalemia, succinylcholine is contraindicated for routine tracheal intubation in children (*Barash: Clinical Anesthesia, ed 8, p 532*).

227. (D) To make intubation easier, it is important to know when the muscles of the airway are maximally relaxed after administration of a neuromuscular relaxant. This often is done with neuromuscular monitoring. However, which muscles one monitors is important because neuromuscular blockade develops faster, lasts a shorter time, and recovers more quickly in the central muscles of the airway (i.e., the larynx, jaw, and diaphragm) than in the more peripheral abductor muscles of the thumb (e.g., ulnar nerve monitoring). Also important is the observation that the pattern of blockade in the orbicularis oculi (e.g., facial nerve monitoring) is similar to that of the laryngeal muscles and the diaphragm. Therefore, when the orbicular oculi muscles are maximally relaxed, intubation would be optimal. When adductor function of the thumb returns to normal, the diaphragm and laryngeal muscles will have recovered (*Barash: Clinical Anesthesia, ed 8, p 548*).

228. (D) Rarely, it is necessary to change from one nondepolarizing drug to another. A general rule to determine the duration of action of a drug given after another drug of different duration is a matter of simple kinetics. Three half-lives will be required for a clinical changeover so that 95% of the first drug will have cleared for the block duration to begin to take on the characteristics of the second drug. For example, if an intermediate-acting muscle relaxant such as vecuronium is given after a long-acting agent such as pancuronium, the duration of action of vecuronium is prolonged after the first two maintenance doses of vecuronium. After the third maintenance dose the duration of vecuronium is not prolonged (*Barash: Clinical Anesthesia, ed 8, pp 537–538*).

229. (A) Volatile anesthetics enhance neuromuscular blockade in a dose-dependent fashion. Recent studies have suggested that antagonism of neuromuscular block is slowed by volatile anesthetics; thus, volatile anesthetic vapor concentrations should be reduced as much as possible at the end of the case to help ensure that reversal will take place as promptly as possible (*Barash: Clinical Anesthesia, ed 8, pp 552–553*).

230. (C) Selegiline is an MAO inhibitor (MAOI) that is sometimes used in the treatment of Parkinson disease. Meperidine is the original phenylpiperidine from which a number of other congeners are derived (e.g., fentanyl, sufentanil, alfentanil, remifentanil). Meperidine is rarely used as an analgesic but rather as an anti-shivering drug. Meperidine (as well as methadone and tramadol) is contraindicated in patients taking MAOIs because of the possibility of serotonin syndrome (e.g., agitation, skeletal muscle rigidity, hyperpyrexia) or depression (e.g., hypotension, depressed ventilation, coma) that may result (*Hines: Stoelting's Anesthesia and Co-Existing Disease, ed 7, p 294*).

231. (A) Some children awaken from general anesthesia and appear restless and inconsolable during the early recovery period from general anesthesia. This is called emergence "excitement" delirium (ED), and more intensive nursing will be needed to prevent such children from hurting themselves, as well as prevent them from pulling out intravenous lines or surgical drains. This usually resolves quickly when the child awakens more fully. Although untreated pain is often considered an instigating factor, many children can be pain free and still develop ED. Risk factors include age younger than 5 years (peak incidence, 2-4 years of age), the use of volatile anesthetics (sevoflurane has the highest frequency of ED), otolaryngologic and ophthalmologic surgeries, and anxious parents. Prophylactic treatment with a single IV dose of fentanyl (2.5 µg/kg), clonidine (2 µg/kg), ketamine (0.25 mg/kg), nalbuphine (0.1 mg/kg), or dexmedetomidine (0.15 µg/kg) can decrease the incidence. Some have used IV propofol (1 mg/kg) after turning off sevoflurane at the conclusion of surgery to decrease the incidence of ED. Intranasal fentanyl (1 µg/kg) may be useful when the IV route is unavailable *(Barash: Clinical Anesthesia, ed 8, p 1253).*

232. (A) Etomidate, an imidazole derivative, is used most often for induction of general anesthesia, but it also can be used for maintenance of general anesthesia. Etomidate has a relatively short duration of action and provides very stable hemodynamics, even in patients with limited cardiovascular reserve. However, it is associated with several adverse effects. These adverse effects include a high incidence of nausea and vomiting (greater than after thiopental), pain on injection, thrombophlebitis, myoclonic movements, and, sometimes, hiccups. Nausea and vomiting constitute the most common reason patients rate anesthesia with etomidate as unsatisfactory. The addition of fentanyl to etomidate to decrease the pain of injection also increases the incidence of nausea and vomiting *(Miller: Miller's Anesthesia, ed 8, p 852).*

233. (A) Pancuronium tends to increase the heart rate, mean arterial BP, and cardiac output. This may be related to several mechanisms, including a moderate vagolytic effect, norepinephrine release, and decreased reuptake of norepinephrine by adrenergic nerves. The other listed drugs rarely cause direct adrenergic stimulation and do not inhibit the uptake of norepinephrine by adrenergic nerves *(Barash: Clinical Anesthesia, ed 8, pp 535–536).*

234. (B) Dantrolene is a muscle relaxant used orally to help control skeletal muscle spasticity in patients with upper motor neuron lesions, and it can be used acutely in the prevention of MH in patients undergoing anesthesia. It is given intravenously in the treatment of MH. Dantrolene has little or no effect on smooth or cardiac muscle at clinical doses. Dantrolene works directly on skeletal muscle by decreasing the amount of calcium released from the SR. This decreases the excitation–contraction coupling needed for the muscle to contract. The most common side effect of dantrolene administration is skeletal muscle weakness. Other acute side effects include nausea, diarrhea, and blurred vision. When the drug is given intravenously, a brisk diuresis occurs and is related to the mannitol added to make the intravenous solution isotonic. With chronic oral use, patients may rarely develop hepatitis and pleural effusions *(Hines: Stoelting's Anesthesia and Co-Existing Disease, ed 7, p 667).*

235. (D) (Please also see explanation to Question 435.) Diabetes mellitus is a disease characterized by altered metabolism of carbohydrates (usually manifested by hyperglycemia), lipids, and proteins. Ninety percent of diabetic patients in the United States have non–insulin-dependent diabetes mellitus (NIDDM) or type 2 diabetes and a relative deficiency in circulating insulin. Diabetic patients also can have a decreased tissue response to circulating insulin (insulin resistance). Oral hypoglycemic agents, most commonly of the sulfonylurea chemical class, can be used in patients with NIDDM. These sulfonylurea drugs have many metabolic effects, including the initial stimulation of the pancreas to release insulin (chronically, insulin secretion is not increased, but the hypoglycemic effects are maintained). Tolbutamide (Orinase) and chlorpropamide (Diabinese) are first-generation analogs.

The biguanides metformin (Glucophage) and phenformin work by increasing the action of circulating insulin on peripheral tissues and are called antihyperglycemic, not hypoglycemic, agents. There is no risk of hypoglycemia with metformin, even with overnight fasting.

Phenformin was withdrawn from the market because of an association with lactic acidosis. Metformin, long thought to cause metabolic acidosis, is now understood to do so only in patients who have abnormal kidney or liver function.

SSRIs are drugs commonly used for depression. SSRIs have serious side effects, including hyperpyrexia. There have been reports of serotonin syndrome with SSRI and methylene blue, but not with metformin *(Hines: Stoelting's Anesthesia and Co-Existing Disease, ed 7, pp 451–452).*

236. (D) Disulfiram and naltrexone occasionally are administered orally in alcoholic rehabilitation programs. Disulfiram alters the metabolism of alcohol by irreversibly inactivating the enzyme aldehyde dehydrogenase. If the patient drinks alcohol, there is a buildup of acetaldehyde in the blood. This produces the unpleasant effects of flushing, headache, nausea, vomiting, chest pain, tachycardia, hypotension, and confusion. The alcohol sensitivity with disulfiram use may last up to 2 weeks after the drug is stopped. Naltrexone is used with disulfiram in the treatment of alcohol addiction. It appears to block some of the reinforcing properties of alcohol. Patients taking naltrexone with disulfiram have a lower rate of relapse for alcohol. Naltrexone is a pure opioid antagonist. Patients taking naltrexone at the time of surgery will have markedly elevated opioid requirements if opioids are chosen for pain relief. The duration of action of naltrexone is 24 hours, and the drug should be stopped during the hospitalization to allow better pain control with narcotics, as would be desirable in this major surgical procedure *(Brunton: Goodman & Gilman's The Pharmacological Basis of Therapeutics, ed 13, pp 376–377; Hines: Stoelting's Anesthesia and Co-Existing Disease, ed 7, p 625).*

237. (A) Context sensitive half-time (or context sensitive half-life) is used to describe the time needed to decrease the blood or plasma concentration of a drug by 50% after an intravenous infusion is discontinued. The actual context sensitive half-time depends on the duration of the infusion. With time, drugs will distribute to various tissues. When the intravenous infusion is stopped, the blood level will decrease as a result of drug clearance (e.g., metabolism or renal excretion). However, drugs that are highly lipid soluble will be stored in adipose tissue and, when the infusion is discontinued, will slowly be released from the less-perfused adipose tissue back into the bloodstream over time. Therefore with longer duration of an infusion, the drugs with high lipid solubility will have a longer context sensitive half-time. If the drug is rapidly metabolized (e.g., remifentanil), the context sensitive half-time is not significantly affected by the duration of the infusion because the drug going back to the bloodstream is rapidly cleared. A drug with slower clearance (e.g., fentanyl) will have a much longer context sensitive half-time with increasing drug infusion times *(Barash: Clinical Anesthesia, ed 8, pp 264–266, 511–512, 828–831; Miller: Basics of Anesthesia, ed 7, p 106).*

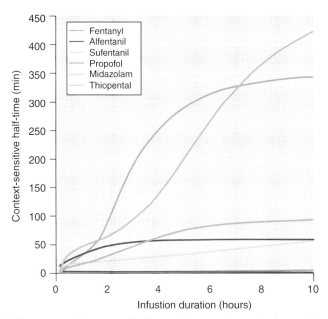

Context-sensitive half-times as a function of infusion duration (context) derived from pharmacokinetic models of fentanyl, sufentanil, alfentanil, remifentanil, Propofol, midazolam, and thiopental.(Adapted from Hughes MA, Glass PSA, Jacobs JR: Context-senstive half-time in multicompartment pharmacokinetic models for intravenous anesthetic drugs. Anesthesiology 76:334-341, 1992).

238. (A) The effects of nondepolarizing neuromuscular drugs are based on the drug being at the receptor. After intravenous injection of a muscle relaxant, plasma drug concentration immediately starts to decrease. To produce paralysis, the drug must diffuse from the plasma to the neuromuscular junction after injection and bind to the receptors. The drug effect is later terminated by diffusion of drug back into the plasma. Recovery of neuromuscular function occurs when the muscle relaxant diffuses from the neuromuscular junction back into the plasma to be metabolized and/or eliminated from the body *(Barash: Clinical Anesthesia, ed 8, pp 533–536)*.

239. (D) Buprenorphine (Buprenex) is a mixed agonist-antagonist opioid with a very strong affinity for μ receptors. Because of its strong affinity (33 times greater than morphine) and slow dissociation from the receptors, it has a prolonged duration of effect (>8 hours) and shows resistance to reversal from naloxone. In rare cases of respiratory depression, reversal may not be achieved with high doses of naloxone *(Brunton: Goodman & Gilman's The Pharmacological Basis of Therapeutics, ed 13, pp 375–376)*.

240. (B) Nausea and vomiting may be associated with any of the drugs listed. Propofol, and perhaps midazolam, may actually be protective in some patients. Of the listed drugs in this question, etomidate has the highest incidence of nausea and vomiting, with some reporting an incidence as high as 40% *(Miller: Basics of Anesthesia, ed 7, p 118)*.

241. (D) Naloxone is a pure opioid antagonist (affinity but no intrinsic activity) at all opioid receptors. It mainly is used to reverse narcotic-induced toxicity. In large doses, naloxone may reverse the effects of endogenous opioids that are elevated in conditions of stress (e.g., shock or stroke). Naloxone has no effect on NSAIDs (e.g., ketorolac) *(Brunton: Goodman & Gilman's The Pharmacological Basis of Therapeutics, ed 13, p 376)*.

242. (D) Nitric oxide, nitroglycerin, nitroprusside, phentolamine, amrinone, milrinone, and prostaglandin E all have a vasodilatory effect on the pulmonary arterial tree. However, only nitric oxide has basically no effect on the systemic circulation. The following table compares the relative efficacy of various intravenous vasodilators *(Miller: Miller's Anesthesia, ed 8, pp 3084–3088)*.

RELATIVE EFFICACY OF INTRAVENOUS VASODILATORS ON HEMODYNAMIC VARIABLES

	Dilation			
	Venous	**Pulmonary Arterial**	**Systemic Arterial**	**Cardiac Output**
Nitric oxide	0	+++	0	±
Nitroglycerin IV	+++	+	+	I, D*
Nitroprusside	+++	+++	+++	I, D*
Phentolamine	+	+	+++	I
Hydralazine	0	?	+++	I
Nicardipine	0	?	+++	I
Amrinone[†]	+	+	+	I
Milrinone[†]	+	+	+	I
Prostaglandin E₁[‡]	+	+++	+++	I, D*

0, none; ±, small and variable; +, mild; +++, strongest effect of that particular drug; D, decrease; I, increase.
*Effect on cardiac output depends on net balance of effects on preload, afterload, and myocardial oxygenation.
[†]Amrinone and milrinone are inodilators (they have inotropic plus vasodilating effects).
[‡]Prostaglandin E₁ almost always requires left atrial infusion of norepinephrine to sustain adequate systemic blood pressure.
From Stoelting RK, Miller RD: Basics of Anesthesia, ed 5, Philadelphia, Churchill Livingstone, 2006, p 1794.

243. (B) Succinylcholine is rapidly metabolized in the blood by pseudocholinesterase (plasma cholinesterase). This accounts for the large dose required to facilitate intubation. Because pseudocholinesterase is not present at the neuromuscular junction, succinylcholine's action is terminated after it diffuses into the extracellular fluid *(Miller: Basics of Anesthesia, ed 7, p 162)*.

244. (A) Dexmedetomidine is a highly selective α_2-adrenergic agonist that is mainly used for sedation. It has a rapid onset of action (<5 minutes) and a peak effect in about 15 minutes. In normovolemic healthy patients, the cardiovascular effects include a decrease in heart rate and cardiac output. The heart-rate changes can be profound, and occasionally sinus arrest may develop. After an IV injection, the BP initially increases (due to peripheral α stimulation), then within 15 minutes returns to normal and is followed by an approximately 15% decrease in BP within an hour. This is related to its CNS α-adrenergic stimulation overriding the peripheral effects. Respiratory changes are minimal, provided that excessive sedation does not produce obstructive apnea. At clinical doses of 1 to 2 µg/kg/min only a mild decrease in tidal volume (V_T) is seen, with no change in respiratory rate. With high doses, the $Paco_2$ may increase about 20% due to a decrease in V_T as the respiratory rate increases *(Miller: Basics of Anesthesia, ed 7, pp 118–119)*.

245. (C) Thyroid storm is a severe hyperthyroid condition due to an overproduction of thyroid hormone and can be precipitated in a thyrotoxic patient by trauma (especially to the thyroid gland), infection, diabetic ketoacidosis, drugs (e.g., pseudoephedrine), and surgery (thyroid as well as nonthyroid). It presents abruptly as a hypermetabolic syndrome (very similar to MH) with tachycardia (sinus rhythm >140 bpm, atrial fibrillation), extreme anxiety, cardiovascular instability, fever (>41° C), sweating, weakness, and altered consciousness. In spite of treatment, thyroid storm has a mortality rate of about 30%. Treatment consists of cooling blankets, ice packs, IV fluids to treat dehydration, steroids to decrease hormonal release and conversion of T4 to the more potent T3 (e.g., dexamethasone 2 mg q 6 hours or cortisol 100-200 mg q 8 hours), antithyroid drugs (propylthiouracil 200-400 mg every 8 hours), and β-blockers to decrease the heart rate (aim is <90 beats per minute) and also decrease the conversion of T4 to T3 (this takes 1-2 weeks). Propranolol is the most frequently used β-adrenergic blocker, but other β-blockers (e.g., atenolol, metoprolol, and esmolol) can be used. Propranolol blocks both β_1- and β_2- adrenergic receptors, whereas atenolol, metoprolol, and esmolol are β_1-adrenergic blockers. Urinary excretion of propranolol is <0.5%, for metoprolol is 10%, for atenolol is 94%. Esmolol undergoes ester hydrolysis in the RBCs. Metoprolol is less lipid soluble and undergoes about 10% renal excretion. Propranolol is the oldest, most studied β-adrenergic blocker for the treatment of thyroid storm and the least expensive IV β-blocker *(Barash: Clinical Anesthesia, ed 8, pp 1329–1330; Brunton: Goodman and Gilman's The Pharmacologic Basis of Therapeutics, ed 12, pp 1905, 1953, 1968; Hines: Stoelting's Anesthesia and Co-Existing Disease, ed 7, pp 458–461; Pardo Jr: Miller: Basics of Anesthesia, ed 7, pp 80, 502–503)*.

246. (C) In addition to analgesia, respiratory depression, nausea, and euphoria, tolerance to sedation with chronic analgesic therapy with morphine will develop after 2 to 3 weeks of treatment. Miosis and constipation occur with narcotic administration, regardless of length of therapy. The concept of tolerance is not applicable to these two side effects *(Brunton: Goodman & Gilman's The Pharmacological Basis of Therapeutics, ed 13, pp 362–363)*.

247. (D) H_2-receptor antagonists (e.g., cimetidine, ranitidine, famotidine, nizatidine) can be used preoperatively to increase gastric fluid pH before induction of anesthesia. Elevation of gastric fluid pH (above 2.5) is desirable to decrease the incidence and severity of lung damage if aspiration of gastric contents occurs. H_2-receptor antagonists are not uncommonly used as a premedication for parturients, patients with symptomatic gastroesophageal reflux, and obese patients (who tend to have very acidic gastric fluid compared with nonobese patients). H_2-receptor antagonists, in contrast to metoclopramide, have no effect on lower esophageal sphincter tone, intestinal motility, or gastric emptying. Although the incidence of side effects is low, side effects occasionally may develop in patients, especially when the drug is administered intravenously and when the drugs are administered to the elderly or to patients with hepatic or renal dysfunction. Bradycardia may develop and may be related to the effects on cardiac H_2 receptors. Reversible elevation of plasma aminotransaminase enzymes may occur. H_2-receptor antagonists cross the blood-brain barrier and may lead to mental confusion or delayed awakening. Cimetidine impairs the metabolism of drugs such as lidocaine, propranolol, and diazepam. This impairment may be related to the binding of cimetidine to the cytochrome P-450 enzymes *(Brunton: Goodman & Gilman's The Pharmacological Basis of Therapeutics, ed 13, pp 912–913)*.

248. (A) Drug sensitivity has been reported in about 3% to 4% of anesthetic-related deaths. Allergic drug reactions have been reported to occur with most drugs administered during anesthesia, with the exception of ketamine and the benzodiazepines. Although most drug-induced allergic reactions occur within 5 to 10 minutes of exposure, reactions to latex products may take longer than 30 minutes to develop *(Hines: Stoelting's Anesthesia and Co-Existing Disease, ed 7, pp 576–580)*.

249. (C) Atropine is administered in doses of 2 to 6 mg and is repeated every 5 to 10 minutes until secretions begin to decrease. In most cases, 2 mg every 8 hours is needed. However, doses of 15 to 20 mg are not uncommon, and occasionally doses over 1000 mg have been needed. Pralidoxime 600 mg removes the organophosphate compounds from acetylcholinesterase and is often used in conjunction with atropine. Benzodiazepines are often administered to counter the effects of the nerve gases on the GABA system *(Hines: Stoelting's Anesthesia and Co-Existing Disease, ed 7, pp 630–631)*.

250. (A) Alfentanil (a fentanyl analog) is less potent (1/5-1/10), has a more rapid onset (within 1.5 minutes), and has a shorter duration of action than fentanyl. The brief duration of action of alfentanil is a result of redistribution to inactive tissue sites and to its rapid hepatic metabolism (96% cleared within 1 hour). Renal failure does not alter the clearance of alfentanil *(Barash: Clinical Anesthesia, ed 8, pp 1574–1575)*.

251. (D) Asthma is an inflammatory illness associated with bronchial hyper-reactivity and bronchospasm. Medications effective in the management of acute exacerbations of bronchial asthma include the rapid-onset inhaled β_2-adrenergic receptor agonists (e.g., albuterol, pirbuterol, terbutaline), anticholinergic drugs (e.g., inhaled ipratropium), and IV corticosteroids. In an acute attack, ipratropium (slower in onset than β_2-adrenergic receptor agonists) can be effective when used in combination with the rapid-onset β_2 agonists. When unresolving bronchospasm occurs and is considered life-threatening, the diagnosis of status asthmaticus is made. Although treatment often starts with β_2 agonists (two to four puffs every 15-20 minutes), when alveolar ventilation is reduced, inhaled agents may not be successful. In this case SQ epinephrine (adult dose of 0.2-1 mg or 0.2-1 mL of 1:1000 solution) can be given. Corticosteroids enhance and prolong the response to β_2 agonists, and, in status asthmaticus, IV corticosteroids such as cortisol (Solu-Cortef) 2 mg/kg IV bolus followed by 0.5 mg/kg/hr, or methylprednisolone (Solu-Medrol) 60 to 125 mg every 6 hours, are administered early in the treatment (but may take several hours to work). Supplemental oxygen is given to keep the oxygen saturation greater than 90%. Because Heliox (70% helium and 30% oxygen) is one third the density of oxygen, it can be tried. IV terbutaline starting at a rate of 0.1 μg/kg/min and increased until improvement is seen or significant tachycardia develops may be useful. Magnesium sulfate at a dose of 25 to 40 mg/kg (maximum of 2 g) administered over 20 minutes has been used. Broad-spectrum antibiotics are also started. In severe cases where fatigue sets in and the $Paco_2$ is rising (e.g., >70-80 mm Hg), general anesthesia with mechanical ventilation may be needed. The volatile anesthetics such as isoflurane, halothane, or sevoflurane can be used not only to sedate but also to relax the smooth muscle in the constricted airways. Cromolyn, however, does not relieve bronchospasm. Cromolyn is used prophylactically because it inhibits antigen-induced release of histamine and other autacoids, such as leukotrienes, from mast cells. Aminophylline once was widely used to treat acute asthma but is rarely used today because it adds little to β_2-agonist activity and has significant side effects *(Hines: Stoelting's Anesthesia and Co-Existing Disease, ed 7, pp 19–20)*.

252. (D) Clonidine is an α_2-adrenergic agonist. Unlike many peripherally acting antihypertensive drugs (e.g., guanethidine, propranolol, captopril), clonidine primarily stimulates central adrenergic receptors and decreases the sympathetic response. As with other drugs that affect the central release of catecholamines, clonidine not only reduces anesthetic requirements (as represented by a decrease in MAC) but also decreases extremes in arterial BP during anesthesia. Clonidine has analgesic properties and reduces the requirements for opioids. Clonidine has been given orally, intravenously, epidurally, intrathecally, and in peripheral nerve blocks and potentiates the analgesic effect of local anesthetics. α_2-Adrenergic agonists can reduce the muscle rigidity seen with the administration of narcotics and can be used to decrease postanesthetic shivering. Patients chronically taking clonidine should not have it discontinued before surgery and should keep taking clonidine to prevent clonidine withdrawal and hypertensive crisis *(Barash: Clinical Anesthesia, ed 8, pp 315–316, 854, 1243, 1600)*.

253. (D) Chronic liver disease may interfere with the metabolism of drugs because of the decreased number of enzyme-containing hepatocytes, decreased hepatic blood flow, or both. Prolonged elimination half-times for morphine, alfentanil, diazepam, lidocaine, pancuronium, and, to a lesser extent, vecuronium have been demonstrated in patients with cirrhosis of the liver. In addition, severe liver disease may decrease the production of cholinesterase (pseudocholinesterase) enzyme, which is necessary for the hydrolysis of ester linkages in drugs such as succinylcholine, and the ester local anesthetics such as procaine *(Miller: Basics of Anesthesia, ed 7, p 491)*.

254. (D) Succinylcholine is the drug of choice (unless contraindicated) when rapid-sequence tracheal intubation is needed. Although hyperkalemic cardiac arrest is a complication of succinylcholine administrations to patients who have sustained burns (as well as crush injuries, spinal cord trauma, or other denervation injuries, chronic illness polyneuropathy, and chronic illness myopathy), the susceptibility for hyperkalemia after a burn injury peaks at 7 to 10 days but may begin as early as 2 days after sustaining a thermal injury. The first 24 hours after the injury are considered safe. Adding a defasciculating dose of a nondepolarizing neuromuscular blocking drug before succinylcholine use to the regimen would slow down achievement of paralysis. Although the "priming" technique of giving 10% of the intubating dose followed 2 to 4 minutes later by the rest of the intubating dose has been used to speed conditions for intubation, it is still slower than succinylcholine, and this technique is rarely used because rocuronium (which provides the most rapid intubating conditions among the nondepolarizing neuromuscular blocking drugs and is a close second behind succinylcholine) is available. An intubating dose of D-tubocurarine should never be given as a bolus because of its moderate histamine release *(Miller: Basics of Anesthesia, ed 7, p 163)*.

255. (A) Clonidine, a centrally acting α-agonist, decreases sympathetic nervous system outflow and decreases plasma catecholamine concentrations in normal patients, but it has no effect in patients with pheochromocytomas. It is used as an antihypertensive agent for treating essential hypertension, an analgesic when injected epidurally or into the subarachnoid space alone, a drug that prolongs the effect of regional local anesthetics, a drug that can be used to stop shivering (75 µg IV), a drug that can help protect against perioperative myocardial ischemia (when given preoperatively and typically for 4 days after surgery), and a drug that can help decrease the symptoms of narcotic and alcohol withdrawal *(Barash: Clinical Anesthesia, ed 8, pp 315–316, 854, 1243, 1600; Hines: Stoelting's Anesthesia and Co-Existing Disease, ed 7, pp 464–467)*.

256. (C) Skeletal muscle spasm, particularly of the thoracoabdominal muscles ("stiff chest" syndrome), may occur when large doses of opioids are given rapidly. This may be significant enough to prevent adequate ventilation. Although the administration of a muscle relaxant or an opioid antagonist such as naloxone will terminate the skeletal muscle rigidity, reversing the narcotic effect may not be desirable if surgery is needed *(Miller: Basics of Anesthesia, ed 7, p 129)*.

257. (B) One of the advantages of ketamine is the minimal effect on respirations. After the intravenous induction dose of 2 mg/kg, general anesthesia is induced within 30 to 60 seconds with, at most, a transient decrease in respirations (Pa_{CO_2} rarely increases more than 3 mm Hg). With unusually high doses, or if opioids are also administered, apnea can occur *(Miller: Basics of Anesthesia, ed 7, pp 107, 114–116)*.

258. (C) This patient has a partially compensated metabolic acidosis. Metabolic acidosis is commonly divided into those with a normal ion gap, also called hyperchloremic metabolic acidosis (bicarbonate loss is counterbalanced by an increase in chloride levels), and those with a high anion gap. The anion gap can be calculated by determining the difference between the sodium concentration and the sum of the chloride and bicarbonate concentrations (i.e., $[Na^+] - [Cl^-] + [HCO_3^-]$) and is normally 8 to 14 mEq/L. In this case the anion gap is $135 - [95 + 14] = 26$. This patient, therefore, has a high anion gap acidosis. This question has two forms of acidosis that have a high anion gap: DKA and propofol infusion syndrome, which causes a lactic acidosis. Because this patient is a type 2 (non–insulin-dependent) diabetic, DKA does not occur, and the cause must be propofol infusion syndrome *(Barash: Clinical Anesthesia, ed 8, pp 386–387)*.

259. (D) NMS can be seen in up to 1% of patients treated with antipsychotic drugs. The syndrome has many features that resemble the condition malignant hyperthermia, including increased metabolism, tachycardia, muscle rigidity, rhabdomyolysis, fever, and acidosis. The mortality rate may be 20% to 30%. There are many differences between NMS and malignant hyperthermia. NMS is not inherited and usually takes 24 to 72 hours to develop after the use of neuroleptic drugs (e.g., phenothiazines, haloperidol), whereas malignant hyperthermia presents more acutely. Stopping the antipsychotic medication is obviously necessary. Because dopamine depletion appears to play a role in causing NMS, the dopamine agonists bromocriptine and amantadine appear useful in the treatment. Abrupt withdrawal of levodopa may also cause this syndrome. Succinylcholine and volatile anesthetics, which are known triggers for malignant hyperthermia, are not triggers for NMS. Dantrolene has been used to treat this condition (*Hines: Stoelting's Anesthesia and Co-Existing Disease, ed 7, pp 614, 618–619*).

260. (C) Normal pseudocholinesterase is inhibited 80% by dibucaine (dibucaine number of 80), whereas patients with atypical cholinesterase show only 20% inhibition (dibucaine number of 20). Patients who are heterozygous for atypical pseudocholinesterase (as in this case) have intermediate dibucaine numbers ranging from 50% to 60%. Succinylcholine paralysis after an intubating dose of 1 mg/kg lasts up to 10 minutes with normal pseudocholinesterase, up to 30 minutes in patients with the atypical heterozygous pseudocholinesterase, and may persist for 3 hours or longer in patients who have atypical cholinesterase paralysis. See also Question 200 (*Miller: Basics of Anesthesia, ed 7, pp 162–163*).

261. (A) Several different receptors may be involved in producing nausea and vomiting, and more than one antiemetic is often needed. Antiemetic drugs used to prevent and treat nausea and vomiting include serotonin 5-HT$_3$ receptor antagonists (e.g., ondansetron, granisetron, dolasetron, palonosetron), histamine (H$_1$) antagonists (e.g., dimenhydrinate, diphenhydramine, promethazine), dopamine (D$_2$) receptor antagonists (e.g., droperidol, haloperidol, metoclopramide), muscarinic cholinergic receptor antagonists (e.g., scopolamine), opioid receptor antagonists (e.g., alvimopan), corticosteroids (e.g., dexamethasone), GABA$_A$ agonists (e.g., midazolam, lorazepam, diazepam, propofol) and, more recently, the NK$_1$ receptor antagonists (e.g., aprepitant, fosaprepitant). Aprepitant is administered orally with other premedications, has a half-life of 9 to 13 hours, and does not prolong the QTc interval. It is often administered along with other antiemetics, such as dexamethasone and 5-HT$_3$ receptor antagonists (*Hemmings: Pharmacology and Physiology for Anesthesia, pp 503–519; Miller: Miller's Anesthesia, ed 8, pp 2635–2637*).

262. (D) The duration of neuromuscular block by succinylcholine can be markedly prolonged when the total amount of plasma cholinesterase is very low, the amount is normal but of an abnormal type (i.e., atypical plasma cholinesterase), or an anticholinesterase drug (e.g., neostigmine, echothiophate, or the organophosphate insecticide malathion) is administered. To evaluate a prolonged response to succinylcholine, one needs to evaluate both the total amount of cholinesterase (i.e., quantitative test) and the type of cholinesterase (i.e., qualitative test). Atypical plasma cholinesterase is an inherited disorder that occurs in approximately 1 of every 480 patients with heterozygous genome and in approximately 1 of 3200 patients with homozygous genome. The local anesthetic dibucaine can inhibit normal plasma cholinesterase enzyme better than an abnormal enzyme. In patients with normal plasma cholinesterase, the dibucaine inhibition test reports a number around 80 or produces 80% inhibition. Heterozygotes have a dibucaine number of around 50, and patients who are homozygous for the atypical plasma cholinesterase have a number around 20. Total plasma cholinesterase levels can be reduced with decreased production, as occurs with severe chronic liver disease or with the use of some chemotherapeutic drugs (e.g., cyclophosphamide). The dibucaine number is normal when the total plasma cholinesterase levels are reduced, as well as after the use of anticholinesterase drugs. Patients with a C$_5$ isoenzyme variant have increased plasma cholinesterase activity, a more rapid breakdown of succinylcholine, and a shorter duration of action (*Miller: Basics of Anesthesia, ed 7, pp 162, 525; Brunton: Goodman & Gilman's The Pharmacological Basis of Therapeutics, ed 13, pp 167–169*).

263. (C) Benzodiazepines are drugs that have the chemical structure of a benzene ring attached to a seven-member diazepine ring. Midazolam, lorazepam, oxazepam, and diazepam are benzodiazepine agonists, and flumazenil is an antagonist. Benzodiazepine agonists are all sedatives and possess a number of favorable pharmacologic characteristics, including production of sedation, anxiolysis, anterograde amnesia (acquisition of new information), and anticonvulsant activity. The amnestic properties are greater than the sedative properties, which is why patients sometimes forget what you tell them after the benzodiazepine is given, despite their having what appears to be a lucid discussion with you. They do not produce retrograde amnesia (stored information). They rarely cause significant respiratory or cardiovascular depression and rarely are associated with the development of significant tolerance or physical dependence. The agonist actions of benzodiazepines most likely reflect the ability of these drugs to facilitate the inhibitory neurotransmitter GABA actions in the CNS. Midazolam and diazepam undergo oxidative metabolism, and their metabolites are conjugated with glucuronide before renal excretion.

Cimetidine inhibits oxidative metabolism and may prolong the duration of these drugs. Lorazepam and oxazepam primarily undergo conjugation with glucuronic acid, which is not influenced by cimetidine usage or alterations in hepatic function *(Miller: Basics of Anesthesia, ed 7, pp 111–114)*.

264. (C) Remifentanil is an ultrashort-acting opioid most commonly administered by an IV infusion. Its short duration of action is due to its ester linkage, which allows for rapid breakdown by nonspecific plasma and tissue esterases (primarily within erythrocytes). Its metabolism is not significantly influenced by renal failure, hepatic failure, or pseudocholinesterase levels (because it is not metabolized to any significant extent by plasma pseudocholinesterase). The clinical elimination half-time is less than 6 minutes. For monitored anesthesia care sedation after 2 mg of midazolam, an infusion rate of 0.05 to 0.1 µg/kg/min is used in healthy adults. For analgesia during general anesthesia with controlled respirations, a rate of 0.1 to 1.0 µg/kg/min is commonly used. A loading dose of 1 µg/kg of remifentanil (or 0.5 µg/kg, if a benzodiazepine was also given) can be given IV over 60 to 90 seconds before starting the infusion. Although it effectively suppresses autonomic and hemodynamic responses to painful stimuli and decreases respirations as well, its rapid dissipation of opioid effect produces rapid onset of postoperative pain (in painful surgical operations), unless other analgesics are administered for postoperative pain before stopping the infusion *(Barash: Clinical Anesthesia, ed 8, pp 516–517)*.

265. (D) The maximum recommended single dose of lidocaine given by infiltration is 300 mg of lidocaine without epinephrine and 500 mg of lidocaine with epinephrine. Careful injection in the mouth is recommended due to the vascular nature of that area *(Barash: Clinical Anesthesia, ed 8, p 575)*.

266. (A) Postoperative shivering can be caused by many factors, including hypothermia, transfusion reactions, and pain, as well as anesthetics. It is uncomfortable for patients and can make monitoring more difficult, but it also can lead to significant increases in oxygen consumption (up to 200%). The exact etiology in many cases is unclear, but, after routine skin surface warming, pharmacologic treatment may be needed. Clonidine, dexmedetomidine, propofol, ketanserin, tramadol, physostigmine, magnesium sulfate, and narcotics (especially meperidine) have been used. Naloxone use may increase pain and does not help decrease shivering *(Barash: Clinical Anesthesia, ed 8, pp 1555–1556)*.

267. (C) Sugammadex is a cyclodextrin (cyclic oligosaccharide) compound that encapsulates nondepolarizing steroidal muscle relaxants (rocuronium > vecuronium >> pancuronium) and produces rapid reversal of profound block (e.g., reversal of 0.6 mg/kg rocuronium in 3 minutes). Because it has no effect on acetylcholinesterase, there is no need to combine it with the anticholinergics atropine or glycopyrrolate. It works only with steroidal muscle relaxants and has no effect on reversing the benzylisoquinolinium relaxants (e.g., atracurium, cisatracurium, doxacurium, D-tubocurarine). Severe bradycardia requiring CPR and atropine is extremely rare but can occur with sugammadex administration. *(Miller: Basics of Anesthesia, ed 7, p 173)*.

268. (A) Arginine vasopressin (AVP), also called antidiuretic hormone (ADH), has many actions, but its primary role involves controlling serum osmolality by regulating diuresis. AVP is released by the hypothalamus and directly causes the collecting tubules in the kidney to increase water permeability and reabsorption. This increases blood volume and lowers serum osmolality. Below a serum osmolality of 280 mOsm/kg, AVP is barely detectable; however, when the osmolality is greater than 290 mOsm/kg, AVP is maximally secreted. AVP is also secreted when the intravascular volume is detected to be low (e.g., hemorrhage, heart failure, hepatic cirrhosis, and adrenal insufficiency). Angiotensin I is converted to angiotensin II, which is a potent vasoconstrictor and increases aldosterone secretion from the adrenal cortex. Aldosterone is a mineralocorticoid and is involved in sodium reabsorption and potassium excretion in the renal tubules. Aldosterone secretion is stimulated by hypovolemic states. Renal prostaglandins are released from the kidney by sympathetic stimulation or by angiotensin II and help modulate the effects of AVP *(Barash: Clinical Anesthesia, ed 8, pp 350, 390–391, 396, 400)*.

269. (B) Remimazolam is an ultrashort-acting intravenous benzodiazepine with a rapid onset and offset. Like midazolam, it acts as an agonist on GABA receptors and has hypnotic and amnestic properties. Unlike most benzodiazepines, which primarily undergo hepatic metabolism, remimazolam is rapidly metabolized by plasma and tissue esterases to an inactive metabolite, making it useful in patients with liver disease. Like other benzodiazepines, it can be reversed by flumazenil. APUD cells are widely distributed, especially in the GI tract. These APUD cells are peptide-secreting endocrine cells that concentrate amino acid precursors of certain amines and decarboxylate them to form several amines that function as neurotransmitters (e.g., epinephrine, norepinephrine, dopamine, serotonin, encephalin) *(Barash: Clinical Anesthesia, ed 8, pp 501–502; Miller: Basics of Anesthesia, ed 7, p 112; https://medical-dictionary.thefreedictionary.com).*

270. (D) Phenothiazines, such as chlorpromazine (Thorazine), are effective antipsychotic (neuroleptic) drugs that block D_2 dopaminergic receptors in the brain. Extrapyramidal effects are not uncommon with these drugs. They also possess antiemetic effects. Phenothiazines with low potency, such as chlorpromazine, have prominent sedative effects, which gradually decrease with treatment. The effects of CNS depressants (e.g., narcotics and barbiturates) are enhanced by concomitant administration of phenothiazines. Lowering the seizure threshold is more common with aliphatic phenothiazines with low potency (e.g., chlorpromazine) compared with piperazine phenothiazines. These drugs are associated with cholestatic jaundice, impotence, dystonia, and photosensitivity. Electrocardiographic abnormalities, such as prolongation of the QT or PR intervals, blunting of T waves, depression of the ST segment, and, on rare occasions, premature ventricular contractions and torsades de pointes, are seen. The antihypertensive effects of guanethidine and guanadrel are blocked by phenothiazines. These drugs have no effect on neuromuscular *(Miller: Miller's Anesthesia, ed 8, p 1219; Hemmings: Pharmacology and Physiology for Anesthesia, pp 189–192).*

271. (A) Amrinone is a noncatecholamine, nonglycoside cardiac inotropic drug that works as a selective phosphodiesterase III (PDE III) inhibitor. Amrinone increases cyclic adenosine monophosphate (cAMP) levels by decreasing cAMP breakdown in the myocardium and vascular smooth muscle. Because the actions of PDE III inhibitors work by a different mechanism than catecholamines (cAMP levels are increased by β-adrenergic receptor stimulation), amrinone can work in the presence of β-blockade and in cases where patients become refractory to catecholamine use. The catecholamine actions can be enhanced with PDE III inhibitors. Amrinone produces both positive inotropic and vasodilatory effects but has no antidysrhythmic effects *(Kaplan: Essentials of Cardiac Anesthesia, ed 2, pp 733–734; Miller: Basics of Anesthesia, ed 7, p 436).*

272. (D) Tricyclic antidepressants often are administered as the initial treatment of mental depression; however, the more recently developed SSRIs are more frequently used because of fewer side effects. Tricyclic antidepressants work by inhibiting the reuptake of released norepinephrine (and serotonin) into the nerve endings. Although at one time it was recommended to stop tricyclic antidepressants before elective surgery, this has not been shown to be necessary. However, alterations in patient responses to some drugs should be anticipated. The increased availability of neurotransmitters in the CNS can result in increased anesthetic requirements (i.e., increased MAC). In addition, the increased availability of norepinephrine at postsynaptic receptors in the peripheral sympathetic nervous system can be responsible for an exaggerated BP response after administration of an indirect-acting vasopressor such as ephedrine. If a vasopressor is required, a direct-acting drug such as phenylephrine may be preferred. If hypertension occurs and requires treatment, deepening the anesthetic or adding a peripheral vasodilator such as nitroprusside may be needed. The potential for an exaggerated BP response (i.e., hypertensive crisis) is greatest during the acute treatment phase (the first 14-21 days). Chronic treatment is associated with downregulation receptors and a decreased likelihood of an exaggerated BP response after administration of a sympathomimetic. Tricyclics have significant anticholinergic side effects (e.g., dry mouth, blurred vision, increased heart rate, urinary retention), and caution is especially important in elderly patients, who may develop anticholinergic delirium despite the therapeutic doses administered. Caution is advised with the use of meperidine in patients taking MAOIs (not tricyclic antidepressants) because of the possibility of inducing seizure, hyperpyrexia, or coma *(Hines: Stoelting's Anesthesia and Co-Existing Disease, ed 7, pp 613–614).*

273. (B) In normal, nondiabetic patients, about 40 units of insulin are secreted every day. There are many SQ insulin preparations available. After SQ administration the onset of action is very rapid with Lispro and Aspart (15 minutes); rapid with Regular (30 minutes); intermediate with NPH or Lente (1-2 hours); and slow with Glargine (1.5 hours) and Ultralente (4-6 hours) *(Hines: Stoelting's Anesthesia and Co-Existing Disease, ed 7, pp 452–455).*

INSULIN PREPARATIONS

Insulin Preparation		Hours after Subcutaneous Administration		
		Onset	**Peak**	**Duration**
Very rapid acting	Lispro (Humalog)	0.25	1-2	3-6
	Aspart (NovoLog)	0.25	1-2	3-6
Rapid acting	Regular (Humulin-R, Novolin-R)	0.5	2-4	5-8
Intermediate acting	NPH (Humulin-N)	1-2	6-10	10-20
	Lente	1-2	6-10	10-20
Long acting	Glargine (Lantus)	1-2	Peakless	About 24
	Ultralente	4-6	8-20	24-48

From Hines RL: Stoelting's Anesthesia and Co-Existing Disease, *ed 5, Philadelphia, Saunders, 2008, p 371.*

274. (B) The GPIIb/IIIa receptor is specific for platelets. Platelet activation changes the shape of the receptor and increases its affinity for fibrinogen and vWF. GPIIb/IIIa receptor antagonists (e.g., tirofiban, abciximab, and eptifibatide) reversibly bind to the platelet GPIIb/IIIa receptor and block the binding of fibrinogen to platelets. They do not prolong the prothrombin time or the activated partial thromboplastin time. These drugs are administered intravenously as a bolus and then as a continuous infusion. The plasma half-life after a bolus intravenous injection is 2 hours for tirofiban, 2.5 hours for eptifibatide, and only 30 minutes for abciximab. The biologic half-life of these drugs is 4 to 8 hours for tirofiban, 4 to 6 hours for eptifibatide, and 12 to 24 hours for abciximab. The longer duration of action for abciximab is primarily due to clearance by the reticuloendothelial system (tirofiban and eptifibatide are cleared by the kidney) and its stronger affinity to the receptor *(Brunton: Goodman & Gilman's The Pharmacological Basis of Therapeutics, ed 13, pp 598–599).*

275. (B) Remifentanil is rapidly hydrolyzed by nonspecific plasma and tissue esterases, making it ideal for an infusion where precise control is sought. The onset and offset of remifentanil is rapid (clinical half-time of <6 minutes). Because the activity of these nonspecific esterases is not usually affected by liver and renal failure, remifentanil is well suited for such patients *(Miller: Basics of Anesthesia, ed 7, pp 133–134).*

276. (C) Pain with the intravenous injection is common with diazepam, etomidate, methohexital, and propofol. It is very rare after thiopental and ketamine *(Miller: Basics of Anesthesia, ed 7, pp 108, 113–114, 118).*

277. (D) Patients anesthetized with total intravenous anesthesia (TIVA), in this case consisting of midazolam, remifentanil, and propofol, sometimes require a few minutes to resume breathing after the infusions are stopped. Although it may seem appropriate to reverse this patient and avoid the need for hand ventilation, reversing benzodiazepines (midazolam) with flumazenil may precipitate seizures in epileptic patients, and, because remifentanil has such a short elimination half-life (<6 minutes), reversal with naloxone is not necessary. The patient needs a brief period to allow the propofol to wear off, during which hand or mechanical ventilation will be necessary (until the patient breathes spontaneously). Also, muscle weakness must be ruled out if a muscle relaxant has been used, and normocapnia should be assured, given that hyperventilation may reduce the arterial CO_2 below the apneic threshold *(Barash: Clinical Anesthesia, ed 8, pp 1544–1545; Hines: Stoelting's Anesthesia and Co-Existing Disease, ed 7, pp 298–300).*

278. (C) Phentolamine, prazosin, yohimbine, tolazoline, and terazosin are competitive and reversible α-adrenergic antagonists. Phenoxybenzamine produces an irreversible α-adrenergic blockade. Once phenoxybenzamine's α blockade develops, even massive doses of sympathomimetics are ineffective until phenoxybenzamine's action is terminated by metabolism. Phentolamine and phenoxybenzamine are nonselective α_1 and α_2 antagonists, prazosin is a selective α_1 antagonist, and yohimbine is a selective α_2 antagonist *(Brunton: Goodman & Gilman's The Pharmacological Basis of Therapeutics, ed 13, pp 208–211).*

279. (C) Symptomatic bradycardia as a result of excessive β-adrenergic receptor blockade can be treated with a variety of drugs, as well as with a pacemaker. Treatment depends on severity of symptoms. Atropine can block any parasympathetic nervous system contribution to the bradycardia. If atropine is not effective, then a pure β-adrenergic receptor agonist can be tried. For excessive cardioselective β_1 blockade, dobutamine can be used; for a noncardiac selective β_1 and β_2 blockade, isoproterenol can be chosen. Dopamine is not recommended because the high doses needed to overcome β-adrenergic receptor blockade will cause significant α-adrenergic receptor–induced vasoconstriction. Glucagon at an initial dose of 1 to 10 mg intravenously followed by an infusion of 5 mg/hr often is believed to be the drug of choice for β-adrenergic blockade overdosage. Glucagon increases myocardial contractility and heart rate, primarily by increasing cAMP formation (not via β-adrenergic receptor stimulation) and, to a lesser extent, by stimulating the release of catecholamines. Other drugs that have been used include aminophylline and calcium chloride. Aminophylline inhibits phosphodiesterase, resulting in an increase in cAMP. Thus like glucagon, aminophylline increases cardiac output and heart rate via a non–β-adrenergic receptor–mediated mechanism. Calcium chloride may prove useful to counteract any decrease in myocardial contractility induced by the β blockade; however, this effect may be transient *(Stoelting: Pharmacology and Physiology in Anesthetic Practice, ed 4, pp 331–332).*

280. **(D)** Dantrolene is a skeletal muscle relaxant that is effective in the treatment of malignant hyperthermia. Dantrolene is formulated with mannitol (300 mg mannitol/20 mg dantrolene) so that diuresis is promoted during dantrolene therapy. Myoglobinuria from malignant hyperthermia–associated muscle breakdown accumulates in the renal tubules and can cause kidney failure if urine output is not maintained. Dantrolene works within the muscle cell to reduce intracellular levels of calcium. In the usual clinical doses, dantrolene has little effect on cardiac muscle contractility. In fulminant malignant hyperthermia, cardiac dysrhythmias may occur, but this is related to perturbations in pH and electrolytes. (Verapamil should not be used, because it interacts with dantrolene and may produce hyperkalemia and myocardial depression. Lidocaine appears safe.) Some side effects of short-term administration include muscle weakness (which may persist for 24 hours after dantrolene therapy is discontinued), nausea and vomiting, diarrhea, blurred vision, and phlebitis. Hypothermia may also occur with malignant hyperthermia treatment but is related to ice packing, not to dantrolene administration per se. When decreasing the fever, cooling should be stopped when core temperature reaches 38° C to avoid hypothermia. Hepatotoxicity has been demonstrated only with long-term use of oral dantrolene *(Hines: Stoelting's Anesthesia and Co-Existing Disease, ed 7, pp 667–668).*

281. **(C)** Cisatracurium is a stereoisomer of atracurium and as such has the same molecular weight. Both drugs undergo Hofmann elimination and form laudanosine. Atracurium is also estimated to undergo two thirds of its metabolism via ester hydrolysis catalyzed by nonspecific plasma esterases (not pseudocholinesterase). Neither drug requires renal or hepatic input for its degradation; hence, both can be used with renal or hepatic failure. Atracurium causes histamine release, whereas cisatracurium does not *(Miller: Basics of Anesthesia, ed 7, p 167).*

282. **(B)** Withdrawal from opioids is rarely life-threatening but may complicate postoperative care. Opioid withdrawal may spontaneously start within 6 to 12 hours after the last dose of a short-acting opioid and as long as 72 to 84 hours after a long-acting opioid in addicted patients. The duration of withdrawal symptoms also depends on the opioid; for heroin, withdrawal symptoms last 5 to 10 days, and for methadone, even longer. Opioid withdrawal can be precipitated within seconds if naloxone is administered intravenously to an addict. (Naloxone is contraindicated in opioid addicts for this reason.) Signs and symptoms of withdrawal include craving for opioids, restlessness, anxiety, irritability, nausea, vomiting, abdominal cramps, muscle aches, insomnia, and sympathetic stimulation (increased heart rate, increased BP, mydriasis, diaphoresis) as well as tremors, jerking of the legs (origin of the term "kicking the habit"), and hyperthermia. Seizures, however, are very rare, and if seizures occur, one should consider that withdrawal from other drugs may also be occurring (e.g., from barbiturates) or that an underlying seizure disorder may also exist. Recently, naloxone can be given *nasally* by first responders (e.g., police, emergency medical technicians, fire personnel and others) to help treat *acute* narcotic overdosage in patients with severely depressed respirations to help save the patient's life. Nasal naloxone is available over the counter in pharmacies. *(Hines: Stoelting's Anesthesia and Co-Existing Disease, ed 7, pp 624–625).*

For Questions 283-287: Side effects of each of the intravenous induction agents (thiopental, diazepam, etomidate, propofol, and ketamine) occur. Some are unique for each drug.

283. **(C)** Etomidate is unique among the intravenous induction agents because it can cause adrenocortical suppression by inhibiting the conversion of cholesterol to cortisol. This can occur after a single induction

dose and may persist for 4 to 8 hours. The clinical significance of this temporary adrenocortical suppression is unclear. However, in the ICU with prolonged sedation, clinical adrenal insufficiency may develop (i.e., hypotension, hyponatremia, and hyperkalemia). Here corticosteroids should be administered in stress doses (e.g., cortisol 100 mg/day) *(Miller: Basics of Anesthesia, ed 7, pp 117–118).*

284. (B) Diazepam is a benzodiazepine drug and was widely used intravenously for anesthesia until midazolam was developed. Although it is an effective sedative and amnestic drug, diazepam causes significant pain on injection and, at times, venous irritation and thrombophlebitis. This does not seem to occur with midazolam. Benzodiazepines do not suppress the adrenal gland. The most significant problem with benzodiazepines is respiratory depression. Benzodiazepines are unique among the intravenous sedatives because a specific benzodiazepine receptor antagonist is available (flumazenil). One problem with flumazenil is its relatively short duration of action (half-life about 1 hour), which is shorter than that of diazepam (21-37 hours) and midazolam (1-4 hours) *(Miller: Basics of Anesthesia, ed 7, pp 112–113).*

285. (D) Pain on injection is common with diazepam, etomidate, and propofol but rare with thiopental and ketamine. However, hemodynamic stability is common with etomidate and diazepam, whereas hypotension is common after propofol and thiopental, especially in patients who are volume-depleted or elderly. Hypertension may develop with ketamine use due to its sympathetic nervous system stimulation *(Miller: Basics of Anesthesia, ed 7, p 107).*

286. (A) ICP tends to fall after the administration of thiopental, etomidate, and propofol and can either fall or remain unchanged with benzodiazepines. Ketamine, however, can increase ICP and should be avoided in patients with intracranial mass lesions and elevated ICP because it can further increase the ICP *(Miller: Basics of Anesthesia, ed 7, p 116).*

287. (D) Propofol infusion syndrome (lactic acidosis) may develop when high-dose infusions (i.e., >75 µg/kg/min) are infused for longer than 24 hours. Early signs include tachycardia; later on, severe metabolic acidosis, bradyarrhythmias, and myocardial failure may develop. The cause appears to be related to impaired fatty acid oxidation in the mitochondria *(Miller: Basics of Anesthesia, ed 7, p 107).*

For Questions 288-292: Antihypertensive agents are used primarily in the treatment of essential hypertension to reduce BP toward normal. These agents include direct-acting smooth muscle relaxants or vasodilators (e.g., hydralazine), centrally acting α_2-sympathetic receptor agonists (e.g., clonidine), peripheral adrenergic receptor antagonists (e.g., labetalol), calcium channel blockers, diuretics, ACE inhibitors (e.g., captopril, lisinopril), and angiotensin receptor blockers (ARBs) (Barash: Clinical Anesthesia, ed 8, pp 315–316, 320, 325, 329).

288. (A) Central-acting sympathomimetic agents such as clonidine produce some sedative effects and can reduce the anesthetic requirement or MAC *(Barash: Clinical Anesthesia, ed 8, pp 315–316, 320, 325, 329).*

289. (C) Losartan (Cozaar) blocks the hormone angiotensin at the receptor. It is pharmacologically similar to ACE inhibitors, but with fewer side effects. It is useful for treatment of diabetic patients and those with cardiovascular disease. Hyperkalemia is a potential side effect of therapy with this drug *(Barash: Clinical Anesthesia, ed 8, pp 315–316, 320, 325, 329).*

290. (B) Approximately 10% to 20% of patients who are chronically taking hydralazine (i.e., >6 months) develop a systemic lupus erythematosus–like syndrome, especially if the daily dose is high (e.g., >200 mg). The systemic lupus erythematosus–like syndrome will resolve once hydralazine therapy is discontinued *(Barash: Clinical Anesthesia, ed 8, pp 315–316, 320, 325, 329).*

291. (D) Labetalol is an α_1-adrenergic receptor and nonselective β-adrenergic receptor antagonist *(Barash: Clinical Anesthesia, ed 8, pp 315–316, 320, 325, 329).*

292. (A) Abrupt discontinuation of chronically administered clonidine (especially if the dose is >1.2 mg/day) may result in severe rebound hypertension within 8 to 36 hours after the last dose *(Barash: Clinical Anesthesia, ed 8, pp 315–316, 320, 325, 329).*

For Question 293: Some drugs inhibit coagulation and do so through a myriad of different pathways. An understanding of these drugs and their mechanisms is helpful to the anesthesia provider.

293. (A) Patients susceptible to HIT-2 (heparin-induced thrombocytopenia) should wait 3 months for a clinically significant decrease in the antibody titer before receiving heparin. If waiting is not possible and surgery involving cardiopulmonary bypass cannot be delayed, direct thrombin inhibitors like hirudin, bivalirudin, or argatroban can be used as anticoagulants for bypass surgery *(Miller: Basics of Anesthesia, ed 7, p 389)*.

294. (C) Abciximab (ReoPro, plasma half-life 30 minutes), tirofiban (Aggrastat, plasma half-life 2 hours), and eptifibatide (Integrilin, plasma half-life 2.5 hours) are potent inhibitors of platelet activity. They block the binding of vWF and fibrinogen to the GPIIb/IIIa receptors on platelets. These drugs are used in the treatment of acute coronary syndrome. If surgery is required, therapy with eptifibatide and tirofiban should be stopped for 24 hours. Abciximab should be stopped for 72 hours before an operation. All three of these drugs produce thrombocytopenia and are metabolized by the kidney, but dialysis as reversal is only effective with tirofiban *(Brunton: Goodman & Gilman's The Pharmacological Basis of Therapeutics, ed 13, pp 598–599)*.

295. (A) Argatroban is a direct thrombin inhibitor. Please see explanation and reference for Question 293 *(Miller: Basics of Anesthesia, ed 7, pp 389–390)*.

296. (B) The thienopyridine compounds, ticlopidine and clopidogrel, are P2Y12 adenosine diphosphate (ADP) receptor antagonists. Binding to this ADP receptor suppresses expression of GPIIb/IIIa and prevents fibrinogen from binding to platelets. Although platelet function studies, per se, are not a reliable way to test the effects of clopidogrel, there is a test to measure the inhibition of the GPIIb/IIIa receptor. Clopidogrel is an inactive prodrug that must be metabolized into the active form by liver oxidases. A genetic polymorphism exists whereby patients are unable to oxidize clopidogrel into the active compound, thus making it therapeutically ineffective *(Brunton: Goodman & Gilman's The Pharmacological Basis of Therapeutics, ed 13, p 597)*.

297. (D) Fondaparinux is an antagonist of factor Xa. It also binds with antithrombin III. Its principal use is deep vein thrombosis prophylaxis, and there is no antidote for it other than stopping therapy and letting it wear off. Because it is renally eliminated, dose must be reduced in patients with renal failure. It is not approved for patients with history of heparin-induced thrombocytopenia *(Miller: Basics of Anesthesia, ed 7, p 389)*.

298. (B) Both acute tolerance to opioids and OIH require more analgesics to treat pain. With tolerance the pharmacologic response is less over time; thus, more opioids are needed to relieve the same amount of pain (e.g., chronic back pain). With OIH there is an exaggerated response to painful stimuli. This can occur under certain situations such as an exaggerated response to pain when a remifentanil infusion is stopped (rapid offset of analgesia). To prevent this when using remifentanil-based anesthesia, it is wise to add a longer duration opioid (e.g., morphine) and/or to add nonopioid analgesics before stopping a remifentanil infusion (if pain is expected in the postoperative period). Although the etiology of OIH is unknown, it may involve both central and peripheral nervous system adaptations involving the NMDA receptor *(Barash: Clinical Anesthesia, ed 8, p 516)*.

299. (D) Mixed agonist-antagonist drugs, such as butorphanol, nalbuphine, and pentazocine, are partial agonists at the κ receptor and complete competitive antagonists at the μ receptor. Both the analgesia and respiratory depressant effects of these drugs approach a ceiling effect. They are used as analgesics for mild-to-moderate pain. They are also used to reverse excessive opioid-induced respiratory depression due to their μ antagonism, while maintaining some analgesia at the κ receptor *(Miller: Basics of Anesthesia, ed 7, p 134)*.

300. (A) Although opioids are mainly thought to work on opioid receptors, methadone is also a most potent NMDA receptor antagonist (6-18 times that of morphine). This property appears to be useful in reducing the effects of opioid tolerance and withdrawal syndrome *(Barash: Clinical Anesthesia, ed 8, pp 1575–1576)*.

301. (C) Tapentadol (Nucynta) is a new opioid marketed for fewer GI and CNS side effects. It has a dual mechanism of action: as an agonist for the μ receptor site and as an NRI. It should not be used in patients taking MAOIs, because an adrenergic crisis may develop. It is also contraindicated with SSRIs, because it may lead to serotonin syndrome. It is only available orally *(Brunton: Goodman & Gilman's The Pharmacological Basis of Therapeutics, ed 13, p 375).*

For Questions 302-305: Depolarizing neuromuscular blockade usually is described as having two phases. Phase I blockade occurs with depolarization of the postjunctional membrane. Phase II blockade occurs when the postjunctional membrane has become repolarized but does not respond normally to acetylcholine (i.e., often termed desensitized, but other factors are involved). This can occur when the dose of succinylcholine is greater than 2 to 4 mg/kg. The response of a muscle to electrical nerve stimulation for a phase II block is similar to that for a nondepolarizing block. Nondepolarizing neuromuscular blockade is only of one type (Miller: Basics of Anesthesia, ed 7, pp 161–162).

302. (D) Although the mechanisms of a nondepolarizing and a phase II depolarizing block likely are different, they both can be antagonized with anticholinesterase drugs.

303. (B) Only a phase I depolarizing block is enhanced with the use of anticholinesterase drugs.

304. (D) Post-tetanic facilitation occurs when a single twitch that is induced a short period of time after tetanic stimulation is larger than the amplitude of the tetanus. This occurs with a phase II depolarizing blockade as well as with a nondepolarizing blockade.

305. (B) The amplitude of the muscle response to sustained tetanic stimulation remains the same with phase I depolarizing blockade, but it shows a marked fade with a phase II depolarizing blockade or a nondepolarizing blockade.

SUMMARY OF MUSCULAR RESPONSES TO NERVE STIMULATION WITH DIFFERENT TYPES OF BLOCKADE

Stimulation	Phase I Depolarizing	Phase II Depolarizing	Nondepolarizing
Single twitch	Decreased	Decreased	Decreased
Tetanic stimulation	Decreased height but no fade	Fade	Fade
Post-tetanic facilitation	None	Yes	Yes
Train of four	All twitches same, decrease in height	Marked fade	Marked fade
Train-of-four ratio	>0.7	<0.4	<0.7
Anticholinesterase	Enhances	Antagonizes	Antagonizes

For Questions 306-315: A simple way to measure the potency of inhaled drugs is to measure their MAC values. MAC is the minimum alveolar concentration of an inhaled drug at 1 atmosphere (atm) (1 atm = 760 mm Hg) where 50% of patients do not move in response to a painful stimulus. It is commonly measured as the end-expired drug concentration. Various physiologic or pharmacologic factors can increase or decrease MAC. In general, factors that increase metabolic function of the brain (e.g., hyperthermia) or elevate brain catecholamines (e.g., MAOIs, tricyclic antidepressants, cocaine, acute amphetamine use) increase MAC, and factors that depress function (e.g., intravenous anesthetics, acute ethanol use, narcotics, hypothermia) decrease MAC. Recently it has been suggested that there might be a genetic component to MAC, because redheaded females have about a 20% increase in MAC compared with dark-haired females. (Barash: Clinical Anesthesia, ed 8, pp 469–471).

306. (D) Acute amphetamine use increases MAC, whereas chronic amphetamine use decreases MAC.

307. (C) α_2 Agonists decrease MAC.

308. (A) Changes in thyroid function (e.g., hyperthyroidism, hypothyroidism) do not seem to affect MAC. However, the cardiovascular response to volatile drugs is altered with thyroid function.

309. (C) With acute administration, ethanol is a CNS depressant and decreases MAC. Chronic ethanol administration increases MAC.

310. (C) Lidocaine use decreases MAC.

311. (C) Patients on lithium therapy have lower MAC values. This may be related to the lower catecholamine levels in the brain.

312. (C) Opioids produce a dose-dependent decrease in MAC (up to about 50%).

313. (A) The duration of anesthesia, as well as the gender of the patient, does not affect MAC.

314. (C) Pregnancy lowers MAC. This may be related to the sedative effects of progesterone. Pregnant patients also are very sensitive to local anesthetics.

315. (C) Severe hypoxia (PaO_2 of 38 mm Hg), as well as severe anemia (<4.3 mL/oxygen/dL of blood), decreases MAC.

For Questions 316-320: The goals of pharmacologic premedication must be individualized to meet each patient's requirements. Some of these goals include amnesia, relief of anxiety, sedation, analgesia, reduction of gastric fluid volume, elevation of gastric fluid pH, prophylaxis against allergic reactions, and reduction of oral and respiratory secretions. The drugs most commonly used to achieve these goals include benzodiazepines, barbiturates, opioids, H_2-receptor antagonists, nonparticulate antacids, antihistamines, and anticholinergic agents. The anticholinergics atropine, scopolamine, and glycopyrrolate are rarely given with premedication today unless a specific effect is needed (e.g., drying of the mouth before fiberoptic intubation, prevention of bradycardia, and, rarely, as a mild sedative). Atropine and scopolamine are tertiary compounds that can readily cross lipid membranes such as the blood-brain barrier. These tertiary amines can produce sedation, amnesia, CNS toxicity (central anticholinergic syndrome manifested as delirium or prolonged somnolence after anesthesia), mydriasis, and cycloplegia (whereas glycopyrrolate, a quaternary compound, does not cross lipid membranes well). All three anticholinergics can cause drying of airway secretions by inhibiting salivation, can cause tachycardia (although bradycardia can be seen in some patients), can decrease the lower esophageal sphincter tone, and can increase body temperature by inhibiting sweating. The main differences are listed in the table following the explanation to Question 178 (Miller: Basics of Anesthesia, ed 7, pp 80–81).

316. (A) All three anticholinergics can cause drying of airway secretions by inhibiting salivation, but atropine is the least effective of these drugs.

317. (C) To produce sedation, the drug must pass the blood-brain barrier. This is much more prominent with scopolamine and much less so with atropine. Glycopyrrolate does not cause any sedation.

318. (A) Atropine has the best blocking effect on muscarinic receptors of the heart.

319. (B) The toxic state known as central anticholinergic syndrome requires passage of the drug across the blood-brain barrier and, therefore, precludes glycopyrrolate from causation.

320. (D) Both atropine and scopolamine can cause ocular effects (scopolamine more so than atropine), including mydriasis and cycloplegia when applied topically to the eye. Caution is suggested when scopolamine is given intramuscularly to patients with glaucoma. IV administration of atropine to prevent or treat bradycardia appears to have little effect on the eye. If a scopolamine patch is placed to help prevent PONV, one needs to carefully wash one's hands after application, because rubbing an eye with any scopolamine on the fingers may lead to unilateral mydriasis.

CHAPTER 4

Pharmacology and Pharmacokinetics of Volatile Anesthetics

DIRECTIONS (Questions 321 through 377): Each question or incomplete statement in this section is followed by answers or by completions of the statement, respectively. Select the ONE BEST answer or completion for each item.

321. The minimum alveolar concentration (MAC) is highest in neonates (0-30 days old) versus other age groups with which of the following?
    A. Isoflurane
    B. Sevoflurane
    C. Desflurane
    D. N_2O

322. The rate of increase in the alveolar concentration of a volatile anesthetic relative to the inspired concentration (FA/FI) plotted against time is steep during the first moments of inhalation, with all volatile anesthetics. The reason for this observation is that
    A. Volatile anesthetics reduce alveolar ventilation (V_A)
    B. There is minimal anesthetic uptake from the alveoli into pulmonary venous blood
    C. Volatile anesthetics increase cardiac output initially
    D. The volume of the anesthetic breathing circuit is small

323. During spontaneous breathing, volatile anesthetics
    A. Increase tidal volume (V_T) and decrease respiratory rate
    B. Increase V_T and increase respiratory rate
    C. Decrease V_T and decrease respiratory rate
    D. Decrease V_T and increase respiratory rate

324. Which of the following can **NOT** be considered an advantage of low-flow anesthesia?
    A. Conservation of fossil fuel
    B. Less ozone depletion
    C. Reduced room pollution
    D. Conservation of absorbent

325. The main reason desflurane is not used for inhalation induction in clinical practice is because of
    A. Its low blood/gas partition coefficient
    B. Its propensity to produce hypertension in high concentrations
    C. Its propensity to produce airway irritability
    D. Its propensity to produce tachyarrhythmias

326. A 24-year-old is undergoing open reduction of an ankle fracture under general anesthesia with sevoflurane, N_2O, and O_2 through a laryngeal mask airway (LMA). Just after the vaporizer dial is turned up to 2%, the patient begins spontaneously breathing, but the inspiratory valve is not fully closing. The likely result of this (malfunctioning valve) is an increase in the inspired concentration of
    A. N_2O
    B. CO_2
    C. O_2
    D. All of the above

327. Select the **TRUE** statement regarding blood pressure when 1.5 MAC N_2O-isoflurane is substituted for 1.5 MAC isoflurane-oxygen.
    A. Blood pressure is less than awake value but greater than that seen with isoflurane-O_2
    B. Blood pressure is equal to awake value
    C. Blood pressure is greater than awake value
    D. Blood pressure is less than isoflurane-O_2 pressure

328. Which of the following volatile anesthetics decreases systemic vascular resistance?
    A. Sevoflurane
    B. Isoflurane
    C. Desflurane
    D. All of the above

329. With which of the following inhalational agents is cardiac output moderately increased?
    A. N_2O
    B. Sevoflurane
    C. Desflurane
    D. Isoflurane

330. Select the **FALSE** statement about isoflurane (≤ 1 MAC).
    A. May attenuate bronchospasm
    B. Increases right atrial pressure
    C. Decreases mean arterial pressure
    D. Decreases cardiac output

331. Abrupt and large increases in the delivered concentration of which of the following inhalational anesthetics may produce transient increases in systemic blood pressure and heart rate?
  A. Desflurane
  B. Isoflurane
  C. Sevoflurane
  D. N_2O

332. Discontinuation of 1 MAC of which volatile anesthetic followed by immediate introduction of 1 MAC of which second volatile anesthetic would temporarily result in the greatest combined anesthetic potency?
  A. Isoflurane followed by desflurane
  B. Sevoflurane followed by desflurane
  C. Desflurane followed by isoflurane
  D. Desflurane followed by sevoflurane

333. Cardiogenic shock has the greatest impact on the rate of increase in F_A/F_I for which of the following volatile anesthetics?
  A. Isoflurane
  B. Desflurane
  C. Sevoflurane
  D. N_2O

334. The vessel-rich group receives what percent of the cardiac output?
  A. 45%
  B. 60%
  C. 75%
  D. 90%

335. What percent desflurane is present in the vaporizing chamber of a desflurane vaporizer (pressurized to 1500 mm Hg and heated to 23° C)?
  A. Nearly 100%
  B. 85%
  C. 65%
  D. 45%

336. A 25-year-old man is undergoing lymph node dissection for testicular cancer under general anesthesia. He has received four courses of bleomycin. The sevoflurane vaporizer is set at 1.8%, the oxygen at 100 mL/min, and air at 900/mL/min. The F_{IO_2} of the fresh gas flow is
  A. 26%
  B. 29%
  C. 34%
  D. 41%

337. How would a right mainstem intubation affect the rate of increase in arterial partial pressure of volatile anesthetics?
  A. It would be reduced to the same degree for all volatile anesthetics
  B. It would be accelerated to the same degree for all volatile anesthetics
  C. It would be reduced the most for highly soluble agents
  D. It would be reduced the most for poorly soluble agents

338. During a breast biopsy with the patient under general anesthesia, the end-tidal carbon dioxide ($ETCO_2$) is 25 mm Hg on infrared spectrometer. Which of the following could **NOT** account for these findings?
  A. Mainstem intubation
  B. Enormous dead space
  C. Incipient cardiac arrest
  D. Overventilation

339. Isoflurane, when administered to healthy patients in concentrations less than 1.0 MAC, will decrease all of the following **EXCEPT**
  A. Cardiac output
  B. Myocardial contractility
  C. Stroke volume
  D. Systemic vascular resistance

340. Increased V_A will accelerate the rate of rise of the F_A/F_I ratio the **MOST** for
  A. Desflurane
  B. Sevoflurane
  C. Isoflurane
  D. N_2O

341. Select the correct order from greatest to least for anesthetic requirement.
  A. Adults > infants > neonates
  B. Adults > neonates > infants
  C. Infants > neonates > adults
  D. Neonates > adults > infants

342. Which of the following **MOST** closely determines anesthetic effect?
  A. Volume percent administered to patient
  B. Partial pressure at the level of the central nervous system (CNS)
  C. Solubility in blood
  D. End-tidal concentration

343. A 31-year-old moderately obese woman is receiving a general anesthetic for cervical spinal fusion. After induction and intubation, the patient is mechanically ventilated with isoflurane at a vaporizer setting of 2.4%. The N_2O flow is set at 500 mL/min, and the oxygen flowmeter is set at 250 mL/min. The infrared spectrometer displays an inspired isoflurane concentration of 1.7% and an expired isoflurane concentration of 0.6%. Approximately how many MAC of anesthesia would be represented by the alveolar concentration of anesthetic gases?
A. 0.85 MAC
B. 1.1 MAC
C. 1.8 MAC
D. 2.1 MAC

344. The graph in the figure depicts

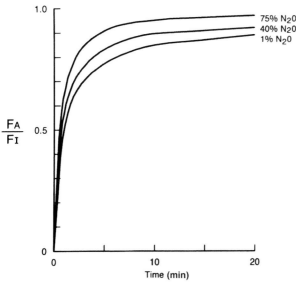

A. The second gas effect
B. The concentration effect
C. The concentrating effect
D. The effect of solubility on the rate of rise of F_A/F_I

345. The rate of induction of anesthesia with isoflurane would be slower than expected in patients
A. With anemia
B. With chronic renal failure
C. In shock
D. With a right-to-left intracardiac shunt

346. Which of the antihypertensives below reduces MAC?
A. Lisinopril (Zestril)
B. Losartan (Cozaar)
C. Triamterene (Dyrenium)
D. Verapamil (Calan SR)

347. A left-to-right tissue shunt, such as arteriovenous fistula, physiologically most resembles which of the following?
A. A left-to-right intracardiac shunt
B. A right-to-left intracardiac shunt
C. Ventilation of unperfused alveoli
D. A pulmonary embolism

348. A fresh gas flow rate of 2 L/min or greater is recommended for administration of sevoflurane because
A. The vaporizer cannot accurately deliver the volatile at lesser flow rates
B. It prevents the formation of fluoride ions
C. It prevents the formation of compound A
D. It diminishes rebreathing

349. Select the true statement regarding the arrangement of the reservoir (sump) and bypass chamber in the Datex-Ohmeda Anesthesia Delivery Unit.
A. All volatiles share a common sump and separate bypass chambers
B. Sevoflurane and isoflurane share a common sump and bypass chamber, and desflurane has its own
C. Sevoflurane and desflurane share a common sump and bypass chamber, and isoflurane has its own
D. All volatiles have independent sumps but share a common bypass chamber

350. Smokers are **MOST** likely to show a mild but transient increase in airway resistance after intubation and general anesthesia with which of the following?
A. Isoflurane
B. Sevoflurane
C. Halothane
D. Desflurane

351. If a patient is anesthetized with 6% desflurane in a hyperbaric chamber at 1 atm and the pressure is increased to 2 atm, the desflurane dial should be set to which setting if the anesthesia provider wishes to maintain the anesthetic at the same level?
A. 3%
B. 6%
C. 12%
D. Cannot be determined without knowledge of F_{IO_2}

352.

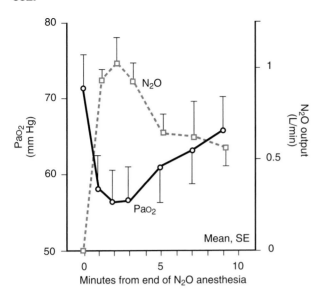

The graph above depicts which of the following?
A. Diffusion hypoxia
B. Second gas effect
C. Context sensitive half-time of desflurane
D. Concentration effect

353. Which of the following organs is **NOT** considered a member of the vessel-rich group?
A. Lungs
B. Brain
C. Heart
D. Kidney

354. In isovolumic normal human subjects, 1 MAC of isoflurane anesthesia depresses mean arterial pressure by approximately 25%. The single **BEST** explanation for this is
A. Reduction in heart rate
B. Venous pooling
C. Myocardial depression
D. Decreased systemic vascular resistance

355. If cardiac output and V_A are doubled, the effect on the rate of rise of F_A/F_I for isoflurane compared with that which existed immediately before these interventions will be
A. Doubled
B. Somewhat increased
C. Unchanged
D. Somewhat decreased

356. Which of the following characteristics of inhaled anesthetics most closely correlates with recovery from inhaled anesthesia?
A. Blood/gas partition coefficient
B. Brain/blood partition coefficient
C. Fat/blood partition coefficient
D. MAC

357. After a 12-hour 60% N_2O-desflurane anesthetic, evidence of N_2O can be best detected by histologic examination of
A. Bone marrow
B. Renal tubules
C. Hepatocytes
D. None of the above

358. An unconscious, spontaneously breathing patient is brought to the operating room (OR) from the intensive care unit for wound débridement. Which of the following maneuvers would serve to slow induction of inhalational anesthesia through the tracheostomy?
A. Using isoflurane instead of sevoflurane (using MAC-equivalent inspired concentrations)
B. Increasing fresh gas flow from 2 to 6 L/min
C. Esmolol 30 mg intravenously
D. None of the above

359. Which of the settings below would give the highest arterial oxygen concentration during inhalation induction of general anesthesia with sevoflurane?

		Oxygen	Air	N_2O
A.	L/min	1	2	0
B.	L/min	2	0	2
C.	L/min	2	2	2
D.	L/min	2	3.5	0

360. If a patient were anesthetized 90 minutes with 1.25 MAC isoflurane followed by 30 minutes of 1.25 MAC sevoflurane anesthesia, wake-up would be
A. The same as 2 hours of isoflurane anesthesia
B. The same as 2 hours of sevoflurane anesthesia
C. Less than 2 hours of isoflurane anesthesia, but greater than 2 hours of sevoflurane
D. Greater than 2 hours of isoflurane anesthesia

361. An anesthesia circuit is primed in preparation for an inhalation induction (with open adjustable pressure-limiting valve). The anesthesia hose is occluded with a flow of 6 L/min. The anesthesia circuit (canisters, hoses, mask, anesthesia bag) contains 6 L. A machine malfunction allows administration of 100% N_2O. Approximately how much N_2O would there be in the circuit when the malfunction is discovered at the 1-minute mark?
   A. 32%
   B. 48%
   C. 63%
   D. 86%

362. Which of the following factors lowers MAC for volatile anesthetics?
   A. Serum sodium 151 mEq/L
   B. Red hair
   C. Body temperature 38° C
   D. Acute ethanol ingestion

363. Each of the following factors can influence the partial pressure gradient necessary for the achievement of anesthesia **EXCEPT**
   A. Inspired anesthetic concentration
   B. Cardiac output
   C. V_A
   D. Ventilation of nonperfused alveoli (dead space)

364. Which of the following volatile anesthetics is unique in containing preservative?
   A. Sevoflurane
   B. Desflurane
   C. Isoflurane
   D. None of the above

365. If the alveolar-to-venous partial pressure difference of a volatile anesthetic (PA − Pv) is positive (i.e., PA > Pv) and the arterial-to-venous partial pressure difference (Pa − Pv) is negative (i.e., Pv > Pa), which of the following scenarios is **MOST** likely to be true?
   A. The vaporizer has been shut off at the end of the case
   B. Induction has just started
   C. Steady state has been achieved
   D. The vaporizer was shut off during emergence, then turned back on

366. Anesthetic loss to the plastic and rubber components of the anesthetic circuit, hindering achievement of an adequate inspired concentration, is a factor with which of the following anesthetics?
   A. Desflurane
   B. Isoflurane
   C. Sevoflurane
   D. N_2O

367. Factors predisposing to formation and/or rebreathing of compound A include each of the following **EXCEPT**
   A. Low fresh gas flow
   B. Use of calcium hydroxide lime versus soda lime
   C. High absorbent temperatures
   D. Fresh absorbent

368. The purpose of the check valve in the desflurane vaporizer in the Datex-Ohmeda Aladin Cassette Vaporizer is to prevent
   A. Gas flow from vaporizing chamber to bypass chamber
   B. Gas flow from bypass chamber to vaporizing chamber
   C. Hypoxic gas delivery
   D. Rebreathing

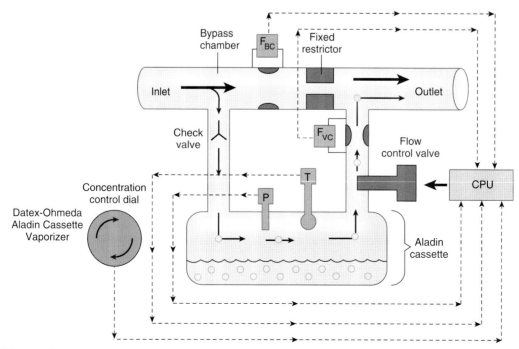

(Modified from Andrews JJ: Operating principles of the Datex-Ohmeda Aladin Cassette Vaporizer: a collection of color illustrations, *Washington, D.C., 2000, Library of Congress.)*

369. The following volatile agents are correctly matched with their degree of metabolism (determined by metabolite recovery):
A. Sevoflurane 2%
B. Isoflurane 0.2%
C. Desflurane 0.02%
D. All are correctly matched

370. Which of the components below is **NOT** considered in the process of "washin" of the anesthesia circuit at the onset of administration?
A. Infrared spectrometer tubing and reservoir
B. Expiratory limb
C. Anesthesia bag
D. CO_2 absorber

371. Which of the following maneuvers would **NOT** increase the rate of an inhalation induction?
A. Giving the patient an inotropic infusion
B. Substituting sevoflurane for isoflurane
C. Overpressurizing
D. Carrying out the induction in San Diego instead of Denver

372. Which of the following anesthetics would undergo 90% elimination the most rapidly after a 6-hour Whipple procedure under 1 MAC for the duration of the operation?
A. Isoflurane
B. Sevoflurane
C. Desflurane
D. Sevoflurane and desflurane are tied

373. After induction and intubation of a healthy patient and institution of a ventilator, the sevoflurane vaporizer is set at 2%, and fresh gas flow is 1 L/min (50% N_2O and 50% O_2). The inspired concentration on the infrared spectrometer 1 minute later is 1.4%. The **MAIN** reason for the difference between the dial setting and the concentration shown on the infrared spectrometer is
A. Rapid uptake of sevoflurane
B. Insufficient fresh gas flow for correct vaporizer function
C. Second gas effect
D. Dilution

374. After cessation of general anesthesia that consisted of air, oxygen, and a volatile agent only, the patient is given 100% oxygen. Each of the following serves as a reservoir for volatile anesthesia and may delay emergence **EXCEPT**
A. Rebreathed exhaled gases
B. The absorbent
C. The patient
D. Gases emerging from the common gas outlet

375. Which of the following characteristics of volatile anesthetics is necessary for calculation of the time constant?
A. Blood/gas partition coefficient
B. Brain/blood partition coefficient
C. Oil/gas partition coefficient
D. All of the above

376. The concept of "context sensitive half-time" emphasizes the importance of the relationship between half-time and
A. V_A
B. Blood solubility
C. Concentration
D. Duration

377. Select the **FALSE** statement regarding pharmacokinetics for volatile anesthetics. After three time constants
A. 6 to 12 minutes have elapsed for "modern anesthetics"
B. The arterial-to-venous partial pressure difference (for the volatile) for the brain is very small
C. The expired volatile concentration will rise much less slowly than in the preceding 12 minutes
D. The venous blood will contain 95% of volatile content of arterial blood

DIRECTIONS (Questions 378 through 381): Match the inhalational agents with the characteristics to which they most closely correspond. Each lettered heading (A through D) may be selected once, more than once, or not at all.

378. Halothane (1 MAC)

379. Isoflurane (1 MAC)

380. Desflurane (1 MAC)

381. Sevoflurane (1 MAC)

	Heart Rate	Systemic Vascular Resistance	Cardiac Index
A	No change	No change	Decreased
B	Decreased	Decreased	Decreased
C	Increased	Decreased	No change or slight increase
D	Increased	Decreased	Decreased

321. (B) The MAC for inhalation agents varies with age. For most volatile anesthetics, the highest MAC values are for infants 1 to 6 months old. In infants younger than 1 month or older than 6 months, the MAC is lower for isoflurane, halothane, and desflurane. Sevoflurane is different. For sevoflurane, the MAC for neonates 0 to 30 days old is 3.3%, for infants 1 to 6 months old it is 3.2%, and for infants 6 to 12 months old it is 2.5% *(Miller: Miller's Anesthesia, ed 8, p 2764)*.

322. (B) The alveolar partial pressure of a volatile anesthetic, which ultimately determines the depth of general anesthesia, is determined by the relative rates of input to removal of the anesthetic gases to and from the alveoli. Removal of anesthetic gases from the alveoli is accomplished by uptake into the pulmonary venous blood, which is most dependent on an alveolar partial pressure difference. During the initial moments of inhalation of an anesthetic gas, there is no volatile anesthetic in the alveoli to create this partial pressure gradient. Therefore the uptake for all volatile anesthetic gases will be minimal until the resultant rapid increase in alveolar partial pressure establishes a sufficient alveolar-to-venous partial pressure gradient to promote uptake of the anesthetic gas into the pulmonary venous blood. This will occur in spite of other factors, which are discussed in the explanation to Question 333 *(Miller: Miller's Anesthesia, ed 8, pp 648–649)*.

323. (D) At concentrations of 1 MAC or less, volatile anesthetics, as well as the inhaled anesthetic N_2O, will produce dose-dependent increases in the respiratory rate in spontaneously breathing patients. This trend continues at concentrations greater than 1 MAC for all of the inhaled anesthetics except isoflurane. With the exception of N_2O, the evidence suggests that this effect is caused by direct activation of the respiratory center in the CNS rather than by stimulation of pulmonary stretch receptors. Additionally, volatile anesthetics decrease V_T and significantly alter the breathing pattern from the normal awake pattern of intermittent deep breaths separated by varying time intervals to one of rapid, shallow, regular, and rhythmic breathing *(Miller: Miller's Anesthesia, ed 8, pp 691–692)*.

324. (D) Barium-containing absorbents that interact with volatile anesthetics and produce carbon monoxide and compound A are no longer used in clinical practice. They have been replaced with calcium-containing products such as Amsorb Plus. Consequently, absorbent granules are "consumed" by CO_2 produced by the patient, not by the total flow of anesthetic gases. On the contrary, with low flow techniques, recirculation (rebreathing) of expired gases results in more rapid depletion of the CO_2 absorbent.

Volatile anesthetics are organic compounds, specifically alkanes (halothane) and substituted methyl-ethyl ethers (desflurane, isoflurane) or substituted isopropyl methyl ether (sevoflurane). They are ultimately derived from petroleum sources and are then halogenated to become substituted organic compounds. They join a myriad of other organic halides such as hairspray, propellants, refrigerants, and solvents that collectively contribute to the depletion of the ozone layer in the earth's atmosphere.

The main greenhouse gases are CO_2, methane, and N_2O. N_2O constitutes roughly 5% of the greenhouse gases. Another rationale for the use of low-flow anesthesia is the introduction of less waste into the OR.

The disadvantage of low-flow anesthesia is that the FIO_2 will continually drop during the administration of anesthesia (unless 100% oxygen is administered), and vigilance is required because this drop may approach or even reach the level of a hypoxic mixture *(Miller: Miller's Anesthesia, ed 8, pp 664–665)*.

325. (C) Although desflurane has a low blood/gas partition coefficient (0.42) and should produce rapid induction of anesthesia, its marked pungency and airway irritation make inhalation inductions very difficult. Not only do patients dislike the scent, but the airway irritation often leads to coughing, increased salivation, breath holding, and sometimes laryngospasm (especially if the concentration is rapidly increased). In addition, with abrupt increases in concentration, patients often experience tachycardia and hypertension, thought to be due to increased sympathetic discharge *(Miller: Basics of Anesthesia, ed 7, p 100)*.

326. (B) If the inspiratory valve becomes stuck in the open position, it will "malfunction" only during exhalation because during inhalation it is supposed to be open. During the exhalation phase of breathing, exhaled gases will exit through the expiratory valve into the expiratory limb of the circuit and beyond (proper path), as well as through the inspiratory valve into the inspiratory limb of the circuit (errant path). Gases traveling into the inspiratory limb (old gas) will be returned to the patient with the next breath. The volume of recently exhaled gas is now drawn back into the patient's lungs along with the "new" gas that would be inspired in a fully functional breathing circuit. The net effect is that oxygen, sevoflurane, and N_2O will all be diluted, but the patient rebreathes CO_2; thus, it will be the only gas with an increased inspired concentration (normal inspired CO_2 is zero) as a result of the stuck inspiratory valve *(Miller: Basics of Anesthesia, ed 7, p 229).*

327. (A) When N_2O is substituted for an equal MAC value of isoflurane, the resulting blood pressure is greater than that seen with the same MAC value achieved with isoflurane as the sole anesthetic agent. When administered alone, N_2O does not alter arterial blood pressure, stroke volume, systemic vascular resistance, or baroreceptor reflexes. The administration of N_2O increases heart rate slightly, which may result in a mild increase in cardiac output. In vitro, N_2O has a dose-dependent direct depressant effect on myocardial contractility, which is probably overcome in vivo by sympathetic activation *(Miller: Basics of Anesthesia, ed 7, p 98).*

328. (D) All of the present-day volatile anesthetics reduce blood pressure in a dose-dependent fashion. Desflurane, sevoflurane, and isoflurane cause this primarily through reductions in systemic vascular resistance. The obsolete agents, halothane and enflurane, produce hypotension via direct myocardial depression *(Miller: Basics of Anesthesia, ed 7, p 95).*

329. (A) The older agent halothane tended to decrease the cardiac output, whereas sevoflurane, desflurane, and isoflurane tend to maintain cardiac output. N_2O tends to increase cardiac output primarily because of the mild increase in sympathetic tone *(Stoelting: Pharmacology and Physiology in Anesthetic Practice, ed 5, pp 123–124).*

330. (D) At concentrations of 1 MAC, isoflurane may attenuate antigen-induced bronchospasm, presumably by decreasing vagal tone. At similar concentrations, isoflurane will not reduce cardiac output in patients with normal left ventricular function. Additionally, isoflurane will decrease stroke volume, mean arterial pressure, and systemic vascular resistance in a dose-dependent manner. Cardiac output remains unchanged because decreases in systemic vascular resistance result in a reflex increase in heart rate that is sufficient to offset the decrease in stroke volume. However, dose-dependent decreases in both stroke volume and cardiac index can be seen when isoflurane is administered in concentrations greater than 1 MAC *(Miller: Basics of Anesthesia, ed 7, pp 95–100).*

331. (A) Desflurane can (but does not always) produce increased blood pressure and heart rate when the concentrations are rapidly increased. This may be related to airway irritation and a sympathetic response. This has also occurred with isoflurane, but to a much less frequent and usually lower extent. The other agents listed do not cause this sympathetic response with a rapid increase in concentration. If desflurane is increased slowly or a prior dose of narcotic is given, this increase in blood pressure and heart rate may not occur *(Miller: Basics of Anesthesia, ed 7, pp 97–98).*

332. (A) Of all the options listed, desflurane has the lowest solubility constant, which results in a very rapid rise in FA/FI. The rate of rise is very similar to that seen with N_2O and results in the most rapid attainment of 1 MAC concentration once the new volatile anesthetic has been initiated. Isoflurane has the highest blood/gas solubility coefficient of all the options, reflecting the largest quantity of gas stored in the blood. This reservoir will result in the slowest decline in the alveolar concentration of this volatile agent upon discontinuation. The combination of these different solubilities will ultimately result in the highest combined MAC when 1 MAC of isoflurane is discontinued and 1 MAC of desflurane is introduced *(Miller: Basics of Anesthesia, ed 7, pp 91, 93–94; Butterworth: Morgan & Mikhail's Clinical Anesthesiology, ed 5, pp 154–159).*

333. (A) The alveolar partial pressure of an anesthetic is determined by the rate of input relative to removal of the anesthetic from the alveoli, as explained in Question 322. During induction, the anesthetic gas is removed from the alveoli by uptake into the pulmonary venous blood. The rate of uptake is influenced by cardiac output, the blood/gas solubility coefficient, and the alveolar-to-venous partial pressure difference of the anesthetic. At a lower cardiac output, a slower rate of uptake of volatile anesthetic from the alveoli into the pulmonary venous blood results in a faster rate of increase in the alveolar concentration. This will result in an increased FA/FI. Uptake of poorly soluble anesthetic gases from the alveoli is minimal, and the rate of rise of FA/FI is rapid and virtually independent of cardiac output. Uptake of the more soluble anesthetics, such as isoflurane, from the alveoli into the pulmonary venous blood can be considerable and will be reflected by a slower rate of rise of the FA/FI ratio. Cardiogenic shock will have the smallest impact on the most insoluble agents, such as desflurane, sevoflurane, and N_2O, whereas the impact on the rate of rise of FA/FI of the relatively soluble anesthetic gases, such as isoflurane, will be more profound *(Miller: Miller's Anesthesia, ed 8, pp 645–646).*

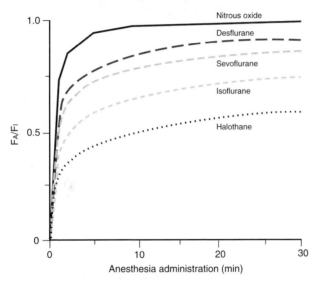

(From Miller RD: Miller's Anesthesia, ed 6, Philadelphia, Saunders, 2005, Figure 5-2. Data from Yasuda N et al: Kinetics of desflurane, isoflurane, and halothane in humans, Anesthesiology 74: 489-498, 1991; and Yasuda N et al: Comparison of kinetics of sevoflurane and isoflurane in humans, Anesth Analg 73:316–324, 1991.)

334. (C) The vessel-rich group that receives approximately 75% of the cardiac output is composed of the brain, heart, spleen, liver, splenic bed, kidneys, and endocrine glands. This group, however, constitutes only 10% of the total body weight. Because of this large blood flow relative to tissue mass, these organs take up a large volume of volatile anesthetic and equilibrate with the partial pressure of the volatile anesthetic in the blood and alveoli during the earliest moments of induction *(Miller: Basics of Anesthesia, ed 7, p 93; Miller: Miller's Anesthesia, ed 8, pp 647–648).*

335. (D) Desflurane is unique among the current commonly used volatile anesthetics because of its high vapor pressure of 664 mm Hg. Because of this, the vaporizer is pressurized to 1500 mm Hg and is electrically heated to 23° C to give more predicable concentrations: 664/1500 = about 44%. If the desflurane is used at 1 atm, the concentration will be about 88% *(Barash: Clinical Anesthesia, ed 8, pp 668–672; Miller: Basics of Anesthesia, ed 7, pp 88, 224).*

336. (B) Fresh gas flow = 1 L per minute (1000 mL/min).

$$FIO_2 = [(100\,mL/min) + (900 \times 0.21\,mL/min)]/1000\,mL/min = (100 + 180)/1000 = 289/1000$$
$$= 29\%$$

Anesthetic flow meters are designed to deliver gases very accurately *(Miller: Miller's Anesthesia, ed 8, pp 760–761).*

337. (D) The situation described here is a transpulmonary shunt. In patients with transpulmonary shunting, blood emerging from unventilated alveoli contains no anesthetic gas. This anesthetic-deficient blood mixes with blood from adequately ventilated, anesthetic-containing alveoli, producing an arterial anesthetic partial pressure considerably less than expected. Because uptake of anesthetic gas from the alveoli into pulmonary venous blood will be less than normal, transpulmonary shunting accelerates the rate of rise in the FA/FI ratio but reduces the rate of increase in the arterial partial pressure of all volatile anesthetics. The degree to which these changes occur depends on the solubility of the given volatile anesthetic. For poorly soluble anesthetics, such as N_2O, transpulmonary shunting only slightly accelerates the rate of rise in the FA/FI ratio, but it significantly reduces the rate of increase in arterial anesthetic partial pressure. The opposite occurs with highly soluble volatile anesthetics, such as halothane and isoflurane *(Miller: Miller's Anesthesia, ed 8, pp 646–647)*.

338. (A) CO_2 is a very soluble gas, making the $ETCO_2$ at the level of the alveoli virtually identical to arterial CO_2 ($Paco_2$). Because we measure $ETCO_2$ on the total exhaled gas, the alveolar CO_2 is diluted with the gas in the dead space (e.g., alveoli are ventilated but are not perfused as well as the respiratory passageways). A gradient of 2 to 5 mm Hg between $Paco_2$ and $ETCO_2$ is seen in normal healthy patients. Any condition that increases dead space or reduces lung perfusion (i.e., increases V/Q) such as pulmonary embolism, severe hypotension, low cardiac output, and cardiac arrest will decrease $ETCO_2$. $ETCO_2$ can also decrease with an increase in minute ventilation (increased removal of CO_2) and can decrease with hypothermia (decreased production of CO_2). Of course, $ETCO_2$ can rapidly decrease to zero with any failure to ventilate (e.g., esophageal intubation, circuit disconnection, failure to turn the ventilator on after manual ventilation is stopped) as well as with disruption of the sampling lines. Because CO_2 rapidly equilibrates between the bloodstream and the alveolar gas, an endotracheal tube that slips into a mainstem gives the same minute ventilation as an endotracheal tube in the trachea (airway pressure, however, would increase). Increased $ETCO_2$ can have many causes, including hypoventilation, rebreathing of exhaled gas, increased absorption of CO_2 from the abdomen distended with CO_2 during laparoscopy, malignant hyperthermia, sepsis, and administration of bicarbonate used to treat metabolic acidosis *(Barash: Clinical Anesthesia, ed 8, pp 711–712; Miller: Basics of Anesthesia, ed 7, pp 342–345; Butterworth: Morgan & Mikhail's Clinical Anesthesiology, ed 5, pp 123–127)*.

339. (A) Isoflurane is unique among the volatile agents in that it does not reduce cardiac output (cardiac index) at concentrations of 1 MAC or less in healthy volunteers *(Miller: Basics of Anesthesia, ed 7, pp 96–97)*.

340. (C) The rate of input of volatile anesthetics from the anesthesia machine to the alveoli is influenced by three factors: VA, the inspired anesthetic partial pressure, and the characteristics of the anesthetic breathing system. Increased VA will accelerate the rate of increase in FA/FI for all volatile anesthetics. However, the magnitude of this effect is dependent on the solubility of the inhaled anesthetic. The rate of increase in FA/FI depends very little on VA for poorly soluble anesthetics because the uptake of these is minimal. In contrast, the rate of increase in FA/FI for highly soluble anesthetics depends significantly on VA. Isoflurane is the most soluble inhaled anesthetic listed in this question (blood/gas solubility coefficient 1.46). Therefore an increase in VA will accelerate the rate of increase in FA/FI the most for isoflurane. Blood/gas solubility coefficients for the other volatile anesthetics are as follows: halothane 2.54, enflurane 1.90, sevoflurane 0.69, desflurane 0.42, and N_2O 0.46 *(Miller: Miller's Anesthesia, ed 8, pp 647–650)*.

341. (C) Anesthetic requirement increases from birth until approximately age 3 to 6 months. Then, with the exception of a slight increase at puberty, anesthetic requirement progressively declines with aging. For example, the MAC for halothane in neonates is approximately 0.87%, in infants it is approximately 1.2%, and in young adults it is approximately 0.75%. A notable exception to this pattern is seen with sevoflurane, for which MAC is the highest with neonates. If the question pertained only to sevoflurane, the correct response would have been C. Please review the answer to Question 321 *(Miller: Miller's Anesthesia, ed 8, p 2764)*.

342. (B) The exact mechanism in which volatile anesthetics exert their effects is not fully understood and remains a topic of considerable research. The most obvious effect of general anesthesia, unconsciousness (hypnosis), is produced at the level of the brain. The end-tidal concentration of the volatile in question reflects the level of anesthesia "seen" by the brain, but only once equilibrium has been reached. At equilibrium, $P_{alveolar} = P_{arterial} = P_{CNS}$. After three (95% equilibrium) to four (99% equilibrium) time constants, the end-tidal concentration and the partial pressure of the anesthetic at the brain (and blood for that matter) would be the same, provided delivery has remained constant. A time constant is defined as capacity (of the brain) divided by flow (of anesthetic-laden blood) and is expressed by the following equation:

$$\tau = V\lambda \div Q$$

The time constant, τ, is about 3 to 4 minutes for modern volatile anesthetics. Accordingly, 10 to 15 minutes must elapse before assuming that the partial pressure of the anesthetic has reached equilibrium in the brain. For this reason, choice D is an incorrect response for this question, because no mention is made of time *(Barash: Clinical Anesthesia, ed 8, pp 461–462; Miller: Basics of Anesthesia, ed 7, pp 91–92; Hemmings: Pharmacology and Physiology for Anesthesia, ed 1, pp 50–51).*

343. (B) Two principles of MAC must be considered in this situation. First, MAC is additive, so the fraction of MAC of each individual gas must be added to arrive at total MAC. The second is that alveolar concentrations of soluble agents are reflected more accurately by end-expiratory concentrations rather than by either inspiratory concentrations or gradients between inspiratory and expiratory concentrations. Because N_2O is very insoluble, it is reasonable to assume that equilibrium will be established early. The inspiratory concentration of N_2O, approximately 0.6 MAC, should approximate the alveolar concentration. However, the expiratory concentrations of the more soluble volatile anesthetics should be used to estimate the alveolar concentration. The end-expiratory isoflurane concentration of 0.6 reflects approximately 0.5 MAC, which in addition to the 0.6 MAC of N_2O would be closest to answer B: 1.1 MAC *(Miller: Basics of Anesthesia, ed 7, p 89).*

344. (B) The figure shown in this question depicts the concentration effect. Note that the inspired anesthetic concentration influences not only the maximum attainable alveolar concentration but also the rate at which the maximum alveolar concentration can be attained. The greater the inhaled anesthetic concentration, the faster the increase in FA/FI *(Miller: Basics of Anesthesia, ed 7, pp 89–90).*

345. (D) The depth of general anesthesia is directly proportional to the alveolar anesthetic partial pressure. The faster the rate of increase in FA/FI, the faster the induction of anesthesia. With the exception of a right-to-left intracardiac shunt (see explanation to Question 337 on effect of shunt on the rate of increase in FA/FI), all of the conditions listed in this question will accelerate the rate of increase in FA/FI and thus the rate of induction of anesthesia *(Stoelting: Pharmacology and Physiology in Anesthetic Practice, ed 5, p 109).*

346. (D) The Minimal Alveolar Concentration (MAC) of an inhaled anesthetic is defined as the concentration of the vapor at 1 atm that is needed to prevent movement in 50% of patients after a painful stimuli (e.g., surgical incision). The MAC values are usually based on 40-year-old patients. Factors that increase MAC include drugs that increase neurotransmitter levels (monoamine oxidase inhibitors, ephedrine, levodopa, cocaine, acute amphetamine use), hyperthermia, hypernatremia, chronic ethanol abuse, age <40 (especially infants), lower atmospheric pressure, and red hair (19% increase over dark hair). Factors that decrease MAC include drugs that decrease neurotransmitter levels (e.g., reserpine, alpha-methyldopa, chronic amphetamine use), hypothermia, hyponatremia, hypoxia, severe anemia (e.g., <5 g/dL), acute ethanol ingestion, acute tetrahydrocannabinol use, age >40 (22% decrease in MAC between 40 and 80 years of age), higher atmospheric pressure (e.g., hyperbaric chamber), IV sedatives and anesthetics (e.g., barbiturates, benzodiazepines, chlorpromazine, dexmedetomidine, etomidate, ketamine, propofol), other medications (e.g., lidocaine, lithium, opioids, verapamil), and pregnancy. Factors that do not affect MAC include gender, type of surgical stimulation, and thyroid function *(Barash: Clinical Anesthesia, ed 8, pp 469–471; Miller: Basics of Anesthesia, ed 7, pp 86–87).*

347. (A) Both a left-to-right intracardiac shunt and a left-to-right tissue shunt, such as an arteriovenous fistula, will result in a higher partial pressure of anesthetic gas in the blood returning to the lungs, ultimately resulting in a more rapid rise in FA/FI. However, this effect is minimal and in most cases is clinically insignificant *(Stoelting: Pharmacology and Physiology in Anesthetic Practice, ed 5, p 109).*

348. (D) Sevoflurane is a highly insoluble volatile anesthetic that combines with CO_2 absorbents to form a vinyl ether known as compound A. The blood/gas partition coefficient for sevoflurane is 0.69. The vaporizer manufactured by Ohmeda is capable of delivering concentrations ranging from 0.2% to 8% at fresh gas flow rates of 0.2 to 15 L/min. Its vapor pressure is 160 mm Hg at 20° C, which is similar to the vapor pressure for the other volatile anesthetics except desflurane (664 mm Hg at 20° C). Gas flows greater than 2 L/min prevent the rebreathing of compound A (not the formation of it), thus reducing the possibility of renal toxicity associated with it *(Miller: Miller's Anesthesia, ed 8, p 662)*.

349. (D) Modern vaporizers have two components, just as their measured flow predecessors, the Copper Kettle and Vernitrol, had. The vast majority of gas (oxygen, nitrogen, and N_2O) passes through the bypass chamber, and a small portion passes through the reservoir (sump). This fraction is determined by the splitting ratio.

The Datex-Ohmeda Aladin Cassette is freely movable and is engaged into the Anesthesia Delivery Unit (or removed) when the choice of agent is made for a given episode of care. These cassettes contain the reservoir for the various volatiles, and each is unique and independent. Any common sump space would result in the delivery of a mixture of volatiles known as an azeotrope, which is highly undesirable. In the Datex-Ohmeda Anesthesia Delivery Unit, however, in contrast to older vaporizers, the bypass chamber is located inside the machine (not in the cassette) and is common for all volatiles *(Miller: Basics of Anesthesia, ed 7, p 87)*.

350. (D) Volatile anesthetics produce minimal bronchodilation unless airway resistance is increased (bronchospasm). This is explained by the fact that airway smooth muscle tone is ordinarily low, and additional bronchodilation is difficult to demonstrate. The irritating effects of desflurane can be reduced by prior administration of fentanyl or morphine *(Miller: Basics of Anesthesia, ed 7, p 100)*.

351. (A) Please see also Question 342 and its answer. The determinant of anesthetic effect is partial pressure, ultimately at the CNS. If a patient is in a hyperbaric chamber under 2 atm (1520 torr), the effective partial pressure from a desflurane vaporizer would be doubled for any given dial setting in comparison with sea level. A 6% setting at sea level would be 760×0.06, or 45.6 mm Hg desflurane. The desflurane vaporizer is unique in that it is more akin to a dual gas blender. To achieve a partial pressure of 45.6 mm Hg (at 2 atm), the dial should be set at 3% *(Miller: Miller's Anesthesia, ed 8, pp 771–772)*.

352. (A) This classic graph depicts the effect of switching from 21% oxygen and 79% N_2O to 21% oxygen and 79% nitrogen—that is, air. When this occurs, large volumes of N_2O are released into the lungs and dilute all gases, including oxygen and CO_2. The reduction in O_2 results in hypoxia, and the resulting fall in CO_2 reduces the drive to breathe. This combination occurs at a time when most patients have narcotics and other respiratory depressants in the body. For this reason, it is wise to administer 100% oxygen to patients for several minutes after they emerge from general anesthesia *(Miller: Miller's Anesthesia, ed 8, pp 656–657; Modified from Sheffer L, Steffenson JL, Birch AA: Nitrous oxide-induced diffusion hypoxia in patients breathing spontaneously, Anesthesiology 37:436–439, 1972.)*.

353. (A) The vessel-rich group receives 75% of the cardiac output (CO) and represents 10% of the weight of a lean adult. In a sense, the lungs receive virtually 100% of the cardiac output, but this is the right-sided CO (the supply side for oxygen) and therefore does not "count" in the classic definition. Lung parenchyma, ironically, uses a very small quantity of oxygen compared with the brain, liver, kidney, and myocardium *(Miller: Miller's Anesthesia, ed 8, p 648)*.

354. (D) At 1 MAC concentrations, isoflurane depresses mean arterial pressures primarily by decreasing systemic vascular resistance. The decrease in mean arterial pressure may be greater than that seen with the administration of halothane. However, heart rate will be increased, and stroke volume will decrease to a lesser extent than is seen with the administration of 1 MAC halothane *(Miller: Miller's Anesthesia, ed 8, p 712)*.

355. (B) Changes in both cardiac output and V_A will affect the rates of rise of F_A/F_I, but in opposite directions. An increase in cardiac output will decrease the rate of F_A/F_I, whereas an increase in V_A will increase the rate of F_A/F_I. However, these two opposing options do not completely offset each other because the increased cardiac output also accelerates the equilibrium of the anesthetic between the blood and the tissues. This equilibrium results in a narrowing of the alveolar-to-venous partial pressure difference and attenuates the impact of the increased cardiac output on uptake. The net result will be a slight increase in the rate of rise of F_A/F_I *(Miller: Miller's Anesthesia, ed 8, p 646)*.

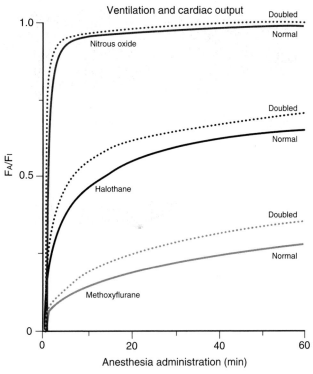

Ventilation and cardiac output

(Modified from Eger EI II, Bahlman SH, Munson ES: Effect of age on the rate of increase of alveolar anesthetic concentration, Anesthesiology 35:365–372, 1971.)

356. (A) Blood/gas partition coefficient is the option listed that most closely correlates with recovery from inhaled anesthesia. A higher blood/gas partition coefficient reflects a larger quantity of gas dissolved in the blood for a given alveolar concentration. Other factors that affect emergence from anesthesia include V_A, cardiac output, tissue concentrations, and metabolism *(Miller: Miller's Anesthesia, ed 8, p 654).*

357. (A) N_2O interferes with the enzyme methionine synthetase, which catalyzes the conversion of homocysteine to methionine. Chronic exposure to N_2O leads to a disease state similar to vitamin B_{12} deficiency, but with one important difference: It is not alleviated with vitamin B_{12} supplementation.

In healthy patients, megaloblastic changes can be seen in the bone marrow after just 12 hours of exposure to 50% N_2O (or higher). In patients who are seriously ill, these changes can be seen even earlier. The other disease caused by vitamin B_{12} deficiency, subacute combined degeneration of the spinal cord, appears only after months of exposure, as is seen in long-term N_2O abusers *(Miller: Miller's Anesthesia, ed 8, p 664).*

358. (A) Four main factors affect the total or rate of rise of the alveolar concentration of anesthetic (F_A) and hence the inhalation induction of anesthetics. These factors are the inspired concentration of anesthetic (F_I), the solubility of the anesthetic, the V_A, and the cardiac output. The rate of rise in F_A/F_I is faster with the less soluble anesthetics, as noted by the blood/gas partition coefficients. The blood/gas partition coefficient measured at 37° C is the least with desflurane (0.45), followed closely by N_2O (0.47), then sevoflurane (0.65), isoflurane (1.4), enflurane (1.8), and halothane (2.5); it is the highest with ether (12). Thus replacing sevoflurane with isoflurane would slow down induction. Increasing the minute ventilation as well as increasing the fresh gas flow rate allows more of the anesthetic to get into the lungs and offset the uptake of anesthetic by the blood, thus speeding the induction of inhalational anesthesia. Decreasing the cardiac output also accelerates the rise of F_A/F_I, resulting in faster inhalation induction (decreases the amount of blood exposed to the lung and decreases the uptake of anesthesia) *(Miller: Miller's Anesthesia, ed 8, pp 647–650; Miller: Basics of Anesthesia, ed 7, pp 89–92).*

359. (B) The table below contains a fifth column, F_{IO_2}. Choices B and D appear to be tied at 50%. The question asks for arterial oxygen concentration (not F_{IO_2}). During induction of general anesthesia, N_2O is rapidly taken up into the blood, resulting in the so-called second gas effect and a concentrating effect.

Concentration of oxygen in this manner is termed "alveolar hyperoxygenation" and results in a transient increase in PaO_2 of approximately 10% *(Miller: Basics of Anesthesia, ed 7, p 90)*.

		Oxygen	Air	N_2O	FIO_2
A.	L/min	1	2	0	0.47
B.	L/min	2	0	2	0.50
C.	L/min	2	2	2	0.40
D.	L/min	2	3.5	0	0.50

360. (A) The insoluble volatile agent desflurane has the advantage of rapid washout and therefore rapid recovery. The downside is the higher cost of desflurane compared with isoflurane. A study was devised to test wake-up after volunteers were anesthetized with isoflurane for the first 75% of the anesthetic and switched to sevoflurane for the last 25%. The results showed that the "hybrid" lasted as long as an anesthetic that consisted of isoflurane alone and proved the futility of this strategy *(Miller: Miller's Anesthesia, ed 8, pp 656–657)*.

361. (C) Calculation of the washin of N_2O requires use of the concept of time constant. Given a volume of 6 L for the circle system, the time constant is 6 L/(6 L/min) or 1 minute. The numbers to remember for time constants are 63%, 84%, and 95% for 1, 2, and 3 time constants, respectively. A properly functioning anesthesia machine would never allow the administration of 100% N_2O, but this nightmare scenario is given purely for illustrative purposes *(Barash: Clinical Anesthesia, ed 8, p 463)*.

362. (D) Acute ethanol ingestion is the only factor listed that will reduce MAC. Acute amphetamine ingestion raises MAC, as do hypernatremia, hyperthermia, and naturally occurring red hair. Gender, thyroid function, and $PaCO_2$ between 15 and 95 mm Hg and PaO_2 greater than 38 mm Hg have no effect on MAC *(Miller: Basics of Anesthesia, ed 7, p 86)*.

363. (D) This table summarizes the factors that influence the partial pressure gradients. A right-to-left intrapulmonary shunt affects the delivery of inhaled anesthetics, but lung dead space does not, because the latter does not produce a dilutional effect on the arterial partial pressure of the anesthetic in question *(Miller: Basics of Anesthesia, ed 7, pp 89–93)*.

FACTORS DETERMINING PARTIAL PRESSURE GRADIENTS NECESSARY FOR ESTABLISHMENT OF ANESTHESIA

Input from Anesthesia Machine to Alveoli	Uptake from Alveoli to Pulmonary Blood	Uptake from Arterial Blood to Brain
Inspired anesthetic concentration	Blood gas partition coefficient	Brain/blood partition coefficient
Alveolar ventilation	Cardiac output	Cerebral blood flow
Characteristics of the anesthesia breathing system	Alveolar-to-venous partial pressure difference	Arterial-to-venous partial pressure difference

From Stoelting RK, Miller RD: Basics of Anesthesia, ed 4, New York, Churchill Livingstone, 2000, p 26.

364. (D) Halothane was the only "modern" volatile anesthetic (methoxyflurane also contained a preservative) that contains a preservative, thymol. Because halothane was at risk for degradation into chloride, hydrochloric acid, bromide, hydrobromic acid, and phosgene, it was stored in amber-colored bottles, and thymol was added to prevent spontaneous oxidation. None of the currently used volatile agents contains a preservative *(Stoelting: Pharmacology and Physiology in Anesthetic Practice, ed 5, pp 100–102)*.

365. (D) The delivery of anesthetic gases to a patient is a complex series of events that starts with the anesthesia machine and culminates with achievement of an anesthetic partial pressure in the brain (PBr). The partial pressure measured in the blood for any volatile agent is either rising (at first rapidly, then more slowly) or falling (rapidly at first, then more slowly). The vessel-rich group reaches steady state in about 12 minutes (for any dialed level of volatile agent). The rest of the body, however, approaches, but virtually never reaches, equilibrium (e.g., the equilibrium half-time for the fat group is 30 hours for sevoflurane). Hence, a true zero gradient is never achieved in the steady state. When the anesthetic is discontinued or reduced, there is a fall in the arterial partial pressure such that it is less than the venous partial pressure. In fact, when the venous partial pressure exceeds the arterial partial pressure, it means that the volatile agent has been reduced (or shut off) because the lungs are "cleansing" the blood as the volatile-filled blood passes through them. The newly "cleansed" blood then finds its way to the left ventricle with a very low PA for the volatile agent in question *(Barash: Clinical Anesthesia, ed 8, pp 462–465)*.

366. (B) Anesthetic agents are soluble in the rubber and plastic components found in the anesthesia machine. This fact can impede the development of anesthetic concentrations of these drugs. The worst offender is the obsolete volatile agent methoxyflurane. However, both isoflurane and halothane are soluble in rubber and plastic, but to a lesser degree. Sevoflurane, desflurane, and N_2O have little or no solubility in rubber or plastic. A different but important issue should be borne in mind regarding the loss of sevoflurane. This agent can be destroyed in appreciable quantities by Baralyme (no longer available) and soda lime, but not calcium hydroxide lime (Amsorb) *(Miller: Miller's Anesthesia, ed 8, pp 660–661)*.

367. (B) Compound A is an ether that forms when sevoflurane interacts with absorbent granules. In rats, compound A is a nephrotoxin that causes damage to the proximal renal tubule. It is believed that compound A is not nephrotoxic in humans, at least not at the concentrations that are achieved clinically (even with fresh gas flows as low as 1 L/min). The factors that lead to increased concentrations of compound A are use of fresh absorbent, use of soda lime or Baralyme instead of calcium hydroxide lime, high absorbent temperatures, higher concentrations of sevoflurane in the anesthesia system, and closed-circuit or low-flow anesthesia. Calcium hydroxide lime (Amsorb plus) does not contain KOH or NaOH and does not interact with sevoflurane to produce compound A or other volatile agents to produce carbon monoxide *(Miller: Miller's Anesthesia, ed 8, p 790)*.

368. (A) The Aladin Cassette Vaporizer is a variable-bypass vaporizer in which concentration of volatile is tightly regulated by a flow control valve that is controlled by a central processing unit (CPU). Most of the gas from the flowmeters bypasses the sump, and the portion that does pass through the sump (vaporing chamber) must be carefully metered. Desflurane is unique among the volatiles, with its low boiling point of 73° F. If room temperature exceeds 73°, the volatile will boil and lead to retrograde flow between the sump chamber and the bypass chamber (in the absence of a properly working check valve). This would lead to an overdose of agent. The check valve effectively eliminates the "alternate" pathway for desflurane vapor *(Miller: Miller's Anesthesia, ed 8, pp 778–779)*.

369. (D) Each of the volatile agents is correctly paired with its percentage of recovered metabolites. Sevoflurane is metabolized 2% to 5% through oxidative pathways using the cytochrome P-450 enzyme pathway. Likewise, the other volatile agents are all oxidatively metabolized in varying degrees. The obsolete anesthetic methoxyflurane underwent 50% metabolism, resulting in high concentrations of fluoride ions and resultant renal failure in some patients. Halothane is unique among the volatile agents in that it can undergo reductive metabolism in the face of low oxygen availability in the liver *(Stoelting: Pharmacology and Physiology in Anesthetic Practice, ed 5, pp 146–149)*.

370. (A) By definition, the washin of the anesthesia circuit refers to the filling of the components of the circuit with anesthetic gases. The total washin volumes are around 7 L and break down as follows: anesthesia bag 3 L, anesthesia hoses 2 L, and anesthesia absorbent compartment 2 L. All of the components listed are part of the anesthesia circuit except the infrared spectrometer tubing. The infrared spectrometer and mass spectrometer take away (sample) from incoming gases through aspiration but do not dilute them *(Miller: Miller's Anesthesia, ed 8, pp 660–661)*.

371. (A) Increasing minute ventilation is one of two methods for manipulating ventilation to increase the rate of establishing anesthesia. Another method is increasing inspired concentration, which can be achieved by turning up the dial above the desired steady-state concentration (overpressurizing) to reach steady state more quickly, or increasing fresh gas flow to reduce or eliminate rebreathing (dilution). Substituting a less soluble anesthetic, such as sevoflurane for isoflurane, also establishes anesthesia more rapidly. Carrying out the induction in San Diego instead of Denver constitutes administering the anesthetic at higher atmospheric (barometric) pressure, which decreases the uptake and hence increases the rate of rise of F_A/F_I—that is, accelerates the establishment of anesthesia. The administration of an inotropic agent increases cardiac output, which also increases uptake and slows the rate of induction *(Barash: Clinical Anesthesia, ed 8, pp 463–465; Miller: Basics of Anesthesia, ed 7, pp 90–93)*.

372. (C) In a comparison of the pharmacokinetics of elimination for volatile anesthetics, desflurane is the fastest. The time for a 50% reduction (decrement) in the alveolar partial pressure of the "modern" anesthetics is roughly the same: about 5 minutes, regardless of anesthetic duration. For longer anesthetics, however, the 80% and 90% decrement times become markedly different. In the present example, the 90% decrement time for desflurane after a 6-hour anesthetic is 14 minutes. This is in stark contrast to sevoflurane (65 minutes) and isoflurane (86 minutes). Please see Question 376 and its explanation *(Miller: Basics of Anesthesia, ed 7, pp 93–95; Miller: Miller's Anesthesia, ed 8, pp 654–655)*.

373. (D) A properly functioning vaporizer will produce the concentration set on the dial (plus or minus a small tolerance) provided the fresh gas flow rate is greater than 250 mL/min and less than 15 L/min. The 1 L/min rate in this question is well within the limits of the vaporizer. The fact that rebreathing occurs with a circular anesthesia system causes a significant dilutional effect. It is true that uptake would enhance dilution, but it (uptake), per se, is not the main reason for this discrepancy. Uptake is considered in the discussion of the F_A/F_I ratio. This question addresses the characteristics of the anesthesia machine and the relationship between dial setting and delivered concentration. To achieve a desired concentration (e.g., 2%), you must either raise the fresh gas flow to convert the system to a nonrebreathing system or set the vaporizer to a higher level than is actually desired: the concept of overpressurization. In this era of cost containment, the latter is more economical *(Miller: Basics of Anesthesia, ed 7, p 228)*.

374. (D) The anesthesia circuit can delay emergence significantly if the patient is not disconnected (functionally) from it. Anesthetic gases become dissolved in the rubber and plastic components of the breathing circuit. Likewise, the soda lime can serve as a depository for anesthetics, as well as the patient's own exhaled gases. To reduce these effects to nearly zero, the fresh gas flow should be raised to at least 5 L/min. Fresh gases emerge via the common gas outlet and do not contain volatile agents or N_2O because they (volatile agents and N_2O) are shut off during emergence *(Miller: Miller's Anesthesia, ed 8, pp 660–661)*.

375. (B) The time constant is defined as capacity divided by flow. The time constant for a volatile anesthetic is determined by the capacity of a tissue to hold the anesthetic relative to the tissue blood flow. The capacity of a tissue to hold a volatile anesthetic depends both on the size of the tissue and on the affinity of the tissue for the anesthetic. The brain time constant of a volatile anesthetic can be estimated by doubling the brain/blood partition coefficient for the volatile anesthetic. For example, the time constant of halothane (brain/blood partition coefficient of 2.6) for the brain (mass of approximately 1500 g, blood flow of 750 mL/min) is approximately 5.2 minutes *(Eger: Anesthetic Uptake and Action, ed 1, pp 85–87; Miller: Basics of Anesthesia, ed 7, pp 91–92)*.

376. (D) This concept highlights the fact that the difference in half-time values among the volatile anesthetics is similar for all volatiles, if the anesthetic duration is very brief. With the administration of volatile anesthetics for longer times, the differences in recovery time become more profound. For example, after a 1-hour anesthetic with desflurane (blood/gas tissue coefficient 0.45), a 95% reduction in the alveolar concentration can be reached in 5 minutes. With an hour-long sevoflurane anesthetic (blood/gas tissue coefficient 0.65), a 95% reduction requires 18 minutes, and an hour-long isoflurane anesthetic (blood/gas tissue coefficient 1.4) requires more than 30 minutes to reach a 95% reduction in the alveolar concentration *(Miller: Basics of Anesthesia, ed 7, pp 94–95; Miller: Miller's Anesthesia, ed 8, pp 654–655)*.

377. (D) After a period of time equal to three time constants, the venous blood exiting the vessel-rich group will be at the 95% level, but the blood as a whole will have a level of less than 95%. The venous blood contains a mixture of blood from the vessel-rich group, the muscle group, the fat group, and the vessel-poor group, and at the three time constant mark will be less than 95% *(Miller: Basics of Anesthesia, ed 7, pp 91–93)*.

378. (A) *Miller: Basics of Anesthesia, ed 7, pp 95–98*

379. (C) *Miller: Basics of Anesthesia, ed 7, pp 95–98*

380. (D) *Miller: Basics of Anesthesia, ed 7, pp 95–98*

381. (B) The information for these questions is summarized in the graphs below. Halothane is unique among the volatile agents listed in that it does not affect the heart rate or systemic vascular resistance in the MAC ranges studied. Sevoflurane reduces heart rate until about 1 MAC, at which time it produces a dose-dependent increase in heart rate *(Miller: Basics of Anesthesia, ed 7, pp 95–98)*.

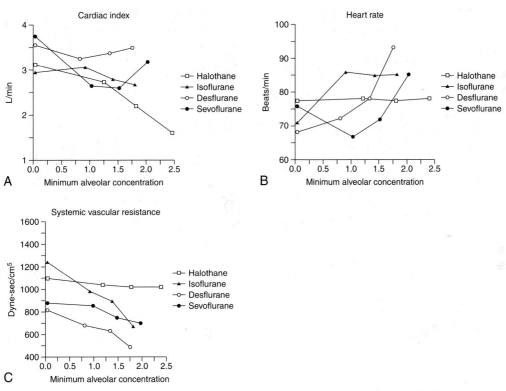

(From Cahalan MK: Hemodynamic Effects of Inhaled Anesthetics. Review Courses, Cleveland, International Anesthesia Research Society, 1996, pp 14–18.)

CHAPTER 5

Blood Products, Transfusion, and Fluid Therapy

DIRECTIONS (Questions 382 through 415): Each question or incomplete statement in this section is followed by answers or by completions of the statement, respectively. Select the ONE BEST answer or completion for each item.

382. Each of the following treatments might be useful in decreasing a prolonged prothrombin time (PT) **EXCEPT**
    A. Recombinant factor VIII
    B. Vitamin K
    C. Fresh frozen plasma (FFP)
    D. Cryoprecipitate

383. Which of the following practices for releasing platelets is most beneficial in avoiding future hemolytic reactions (from alloantibodies) in the recipient?
    A. Serologic crossmatch
    B. Extended phenotype matching
    C. RhD matching
    D. ABO matching

384. Which of the fluids below has the greatest osmolality?
    A. Normal saline
    B. Lactated Ringer solution
    C. D5 ½NS normal saline
    D. 5% Albumin

385. In a 70-kg patient, 1 dose of platelets (1 apheresis platelet or six pooled units of whole blood–derived platelets) should increase the platelet count by
    A. 12,000 to 30,000/mm^3
    B. 30,000 to 60,000/mm^3
    C. 90,000 to 120,000/mm^3
    D. 120,000 to 150,000/mm^3

386. A 68-year-old patient receives a 1-unit transfusion of packed red blood cells (RBCs) in the recovery room after a laparoscopic prostatectomy. As the blood is slowly dripping into his peripheral intravenous line, the patient complains of itching on his chest and arms, but his vital signs remain stable. The antibody most likely responsible for this is directed against
    A. Rh
    B. ABO
    C. MN, P, and Lewis
    D. None of the above

387. The likelihood of a clinically significant hemolytic transfusion reaction resulting from administration of type-specific blood is less than
    A. 1 in 250
    B. 1 in 500
    C. 1 in 1000
    D. 1 in 10,000

388. Which of the following is **NOT** tested in the first or immediate phase of blood crossmatching?
    A. ABO
    B. Rh
    C. MN
    D. Lewis

389. Which of the following clotting factors has the shortest half-life?
    A. Factor II
    B. Factor V
    C. Factor VII
    D. Factor IX

390. Which of the measures below does **NOT** reduce the incidence of transfusion-related acute lung injury (TRALI)?
  A. Exclusion of female donors
  B. Use of autologous blood
  C. Leukocyte reduction
  D. Use of blood less than 14 days old

391. A 42-year-old woman is anesthetized for resection of a large (22-kg), highly vascular sarcoma in the abdomen. During the resection, 20 units of RBCs, 6 units of platelets, 10 units of cryoprecipitate, 5 units of FFP, and 1 L of albumin are administered. At the conclusion of the operation, the patient's vital signs are stable, and she is transported to the intensive care unit. Three and a half hours later, a diagnosis of sepsis is made, and antibiotic therapy is started. Which of the items below would be the most likely cause of sepsis in this patient?
  A. Packed RBCs
  B. Cryoprecipitate
  C. Platelets
  D. FFP

392. Blood is routinely tested for
  A. Hepatitis A
  B. Severe acute respiratory syndrome (SARS)
  C. West Nile virus
  D. Bovine spongiform encephalitis (BSE, or mad cow disease)

393. The blood volume of a 10-kg, 1-year-old infant is
  A. 600 mL
  B. 800 mL
  C. 1000 mL
  D. 1300 mL

394. Which of the infections below has the highest risk of causing a transfusion-transmitted infection?
  A. Human T-cell lymphotropic virus (HTLV)-II
  B. Hepatitis B
  C. Hepatitis C
  D. Human immunodeficiency virus (HIV)

395. A 40-year-old, 78-kg patient with hemophilia A is scheduled for a right total knee arthroplasty. His laboratory test results show a hematocrit of 40, a factor VIII level of 0%, and no inhibitors to factor VIII. How much factor VIII concentrate do you need to give him to bring his factor VIII level to 100%?
  A. 3000 units
  B. 2500 units
  C. 2000 units
  D. 1500 units

396. A 38-year-old man is undergoing a total colectomy under general anesthesia. Urine output has been 20 mL/hr for the last 2 hours. Volume replacement has been adequate. The rationale for administering 5 to 10 mg of furosemide to this patient is to
  A. Offset the effects of increased antidiuretic hormone (ADH)
  B. Improve renal blood flow
  C. Convert oliguric renal failure to nonoliguric renal failure
  D. Offset the effects of increased renin

397. A 65-year-old man involved in a motor vehicle accident (MVA) is brought to the emergency room with a blood pressure of 60 mm Hg systolic. He is transfused with 4 units of type O, Rh-negative whole blood and 4 L of normal saline solution. After the patient is brought to the operating room, his blood type is determined to be A positive. Which of the following is the most appropriate blood type for further intraoperative transfusions?
  A. Type A, Rh-positive whole blood
  B. Type O, Rh-negative RBCs
  C. Type A, Rh-positive RBCs
  D. Type O, Rh-negative whole blood

398. The criterion used to determine how long blood can be stored before transfusion is
  A. 90% of transfused erythrocytes must remain in circulation for 24 hours
  B. 70% of transfused erythrocytes must remain in circulation for 24 hours
  C. 70% of transfused erythrocytes must remain in circulation for 72 hours
  D. 75% of transfused erythrocytes must remain in circulation for 7 days

399. The rationale for storage of platelets at room temperature (22° C) is
  A. There is less splenic sequestration
  B. It preserves platelet survival
  C. It reduces the chance for infection
  D. It decreases the incidence of allergic reactions

400. An 18-year-old woman involved in an MVA is brought to the emergency room in shock. She is transfused with 10 units of type O, Rh-negative whole blood over 30 minutes. After infusion of the first 5 units, bleeding is controlled, and her blood pressure rises to 85/51 mm Hg. During the next 15 minutes, as the remaining 5 units are infused, her blood pressure slowly falls to 60 mm Hg systolic. The patient remains in sinus tachycardia at 120 beats/min, but the QT interval is noted to increase from 310 to 470 msec, and the central venous pressure increases from 9 to 20 mm Hg. Her breathing is rapid and shallow. The most likely cause of this scenario is
  A. Citrate toxicity
  B. Hyperkalemia
  C. Hemolytic transfusion reaction
  D. Tension pneumothorax

401. A 20-kg, 5-year-old child with a hematocrit of 40% could lose how much blood and still maintain a hematocrit of 30%?
- **A.** 140 mL
- **B.** 250 mL
- **C.** 350 mL
- **D.** 450 mL

402. A 68-year-old man with recent cardiac stent placement is taking 75 mg clopidogrel (Plavix) daily. He is scheduled for retinal surgery, and a thromboelastogram (TEG) is ordered before surgery. The likely result of the TEG will show
- **A.** Increased R + K
- **B.** Increased alpha
- **C.** Increased MA 30
- **D.** Normal TEG

403. Paramedics respond to an MVA site and immediately stabilize the neck, secure the airway, and place an intravenous line into a 19-year-old, 70-kg man lying in a pool of blood. Before the infusion is started, 3 mL of blood are withdrawn for hemoglobin and drug screening. The first responders estimate that the patient has lost one half of his entire blood volume. Given a starting value of 18 g/dL, the new value would likely be
- **A.** 9 g/dL
- **B.** 11 g/dL
- **C.** 14 g/dL
- **D.** 17 g/dL

404. A 23-year-old woman who has been receiving total parenteral nutrition (TPN) (15% dextrose, 5% amino acids, and intralipids) for 3 weeks is scheduled for surgery for severe Crohn disease. Induction of anesthesia and tracheal intubation are uneventful. After peripheral intravenous access is established, the old central line is removed and a new central line is placed at a different site. At the end of the operation, a large volume of fluid is discovered in the chest cavity on chest x-ray film. Arterial blood pressure is 105/70 mm Hg, heart rate is 150 beats/min, and SaO_2 is 96% (pulse oximeter). The most appropriate initial step is to
- **A.** Place a chest tube
- **B.** Change the single-lumen to a double-lumen endotracheal tube
- **C.** Start a dopamine infusion
- **D.** Check the blood glucose level

405. In an emergency when there is a limited supply of type O-negative RBCs, type O-positive RBCs are preferable for transfusion for each of the following patients **EXCEPT**
- **A.** A 60-year-old woman with diabetes who was involved in an MVA
- **B.** A 23-year-old man who sustained a gunshot wound to the upper abdomen
- **C.** An 84-year-old man with a ruptured abdominal aortic aneurysm
- **D.** A 21-year-old, gravida 2, para 1 woman with placenta previa who is bleeding profusely

406. Hetastarch exerts an anticoagulative effect through interference with the function of
- **A.** Antithrombin III
- **B.** Factor VIII
- **C.** Fibrinogen
- **D.** Prostacyclin

407. All of the following characterize packed RBCs that have been stored for 35 days at 4° C in citrate phosphate dextrose adenine-1 (CPDA-1) anticoagulant preservative **EXCEPT**
- **A.** Serum potassium greater than 70 mEq/L
- **B.** pH less than 7.0
- **C.** Blood glucose less than 100 mg/dL
- **D.** P_{50} of 28

408. Which of the following statements about coagulation factor Xa (FXa) (recombinant) inactivated-zhzo is **FALSE**?
- **A.** It is used only to reverse the FXa inhibitors (apixaban and rivaroxaban)
- **B.** It is used only if the patient has life-threatening or uncontrolled bleeding
- **C.** Urinary tract infections and pneumonia occur in >5% of patients
- **D.** Thromboembolic risks are rare (<2%) and usually occur within 24 hours

409. In the adult, the liver is the primary organ for
- **A.** Hemoglobin synthesis
- **B.** Hemoglobin degradation
- **C.** Factor VIII synthesis
- **D.** Antithrombin III synthesis

410. Anticoagulation with low-molecular-weight heparin (LMWH) can be best monitored through which of the following laboratory tests?
- **A.** Activated partial thromboplastin time (aPTT)
- **B.** Anti-Xa assay
- **C.** Thrombin time
- **D.** Reptilase test

411. Heparin resistance is likely in patients with which of the following heritable conditions?
   A. Factor V Leiden mutation
   B. Prothrombin *G20210A* gene mutation
   C. Protein S deficiency
   D. Antithrombin or antithrombin III (AT3) deficiency

412. Type 1 von Willebrand disease (vWD) could be treated by any of the following **EXCEPT**
   A. Cryoprecipitate
   B. Desmopressin (DDAVP)
   C. FFP
   D. Recombinant factor VIII

413. The significance of immunoglobulin A (IgA) antibodies in transfusion medicine is related to
   A. Allergic reaction
   B. Febrile reaction
   C. Delayed hemolytic reaction (immune extravascular reaction)
   D. Diagnosis of TRALI reaction

414. The most common cause of mortality associated with administration of blood is
   A. TRALI
   B. Non-ABO hemolytic transfusion reaction
   C. Microbial infection
   D. Anaphylactic reaction

415. Fluid resuscitation during major abdominal surgery with which of the following agents is associated with the **BEST** survival data?
   A. 5% Albumin
   B. 6% Hydroxyethyl starch
   C. Dextran 70
   D. None of the above

DIRECTIONS (Questions 416 and 417): Choose the correct response below for the following questions:

A. Washing erythrocytes
B. Reduction of leukocytes
C. Irradiation
D. Storage in Adsol

416. Which of the following processes reduces the possibility of transmission of cytomegalovirus (CMV) to a susceptible recipient via transfusion of RBCs?

417. What is the process aimed at reducing graft-versus-host disease (GVHD) in transfusion recipients?

Blood Products, Transfusion, and Fluid Therapy
Answers, References, and Explanations

382. (A) PT and aPTT are common tests used to evaluate coagulation factors. The PT primarily tests for factor VII in the extrinsic pathway, as well as factors I, II, V, and X of the common pathway. The aPTT primarily tests for factors VIII and IX of the intrinsic pathway, as well as factors I, II, V, and X of the common pathway. Although not thought of as important for in vivo hemostasis, factor XII, high-molecular kininogen, and prekallikrein also influence aPTT results. Although the PT is prolonged with deficient function of factors I, II, V, VII, or X, it is more sensitive to deficiencies of factor VII but less so with deficiencies of factor I or II. In fact, the PT is not prolonged until the level of fibrinogen (factor I) is less than 100 mg/dL and may be prolonged for only 2 seconds when the level of factor II (prothrombin) is 10% of normal. Factors II, VII, IX, and X are vitamin K–dependent factors, and their formation is blocked with Coumadin therapy. Administering factor VIII will not help a prolonged PT *(Miller: Miller's Anesthesia, ed 8, pp 1872–1874; Basics of Anesthesia, ed 7, p 407; Kandice Kottke-Marchant, MD, PhD, FCAP: An Algorithmic Approach to Hemostasis Testing, pp 7–8).*

383. (C) Platelets are complicated cell fragments that have several different antigens on them that can cause problems in the future. In addition to human platelet antigens (HPAs) and human leukocyte antigens (HLAs), they also express ABO antigens. Antibodies to any of these can result in lower than expected yields from platelet transfusions, as they are removed from circulation once "tagged" with antibody. Interestingly, platelets do not express Rh antigens. Modern practices now result in platelet products that have very low volumes of contaminating RBCs (less than 2 mL per standards), and an apheresis platelet may have as low as about 0.5 mL of RBCs. Due to this very low volume of red cells, platelets do not require serologic crossmatching (compared with a unit of RBCs). Extended phenotype matching may be performed to prevent alloimmunization to red cell antigens in the chronically transfused (such as sickle cell patients). Because ABO antibodies are naturally occurring, ABO matching platelets will not prevent the formation of antibodies and therefore prevent future hemolytic reactions. The best answer here is to RhD-match platelets. Even though there is a very small number of red cells in a unit of platelets, the RhD antigen is highly immunogenic and may cause alloimmunization if given to RhD-negative patients, where a new anti-D antibody may lead to future hemolysis. Common practice is to reserve RhD-negative platelets for children or women of childbearing age. If RhD-positive units must be given to these groups due to inventory concerns, RhIG may be offered within 72 hours of the transfusion *(AABB Technical Manual, ed 19, p 514).*

384. (C) Osmotic pressure is proportional to the number of particles in solution. Osmolality measures the amount of dissolved particles in a fluid. For calculations keep in mind that mEq/L = mOsmol/L for Na^+, K^+, Cl^-, and lactate. Normal saline solution (0.9% NaCl) contains 154 mEq/L of sodium + 154 mEq/L chloride = 308 mOsm/L. Lactated Ringer solution contains 130 mEq/L of sodium + 4 mEq/L of potassium + 2.7 mEq/L of calcium + 109 mEq/L of chloride + 28 mEq/L of lactate = 273.7 mOsmol/L. Because dextrose solutions are not listed as mEq/L, you need to calculate the mOsmol/L from the weight of dextrose. To do this you need to know the molecular weight of the dextrose and when preparing the solution the monohydrate is used. The gram molecular weight of dextrose is 180 g/mole and the gram molecular weight of water is 18 g/mole = 198.

D5 (5% dextrose solution) contains 50 g (50,000 mg) of dextrose per liter of fluid. The dextrose in solution is the monohydrate form, so 50,000 mg/198 mg = 252 mOmol/L. D5 − 0.45% solution (5% dextrose with ½ normal saline) contains 252 mOsm/L of dextrose + 77 mEq/L of sodium + 77 mEq/L of chloride = 406 mOsm/L.

The NaCl concentration of albumin solutions varies depending on the manufacturer. 5% albumin osmolality is approximately 330 mOsm/L *(Miller: Basics of Anesthesia, ed 7, p 397; Miller: Miller's Anesthesia, ed 8, pp 1779–1783).*

385. (B) Each transfusion dose will increase the platelet count by 30,000 to 60,000/mm^3 in the typical 70-kg patient. Each whole blood unit contains greater than 5.5×10^{10} platelets and is classically pooled with six individual donations and transfused as a "six pack" with about 3×10^{11} platelets to make a dose. An alternative approach to this is with apheresis platelets, where 3×10^{11} platelets are collected from one donor, and this constitutes an apheresis platelet dose *(AABB Technical Manual, ed 19, p 514).*

386. (D) This is an example of a typical allergic reaction. All of the other choices in this question may be involved in hemolytic reactions. Allergic reactions are a form of nonhemolytic transfusion reactions, which are thought to be caused by foreign proteins in the transfused blood. The reactions occur in about 3% of all transfusions, and they present with urticaria, erythema, pruritus, fever, and sometimes respiratory symptoms. When such a reaction occurs, the transfusion is stopped and supportive therapy, including antihistamines, is administered. If the symptoms resolve and there are no signs of a hemolytic reaction (no free hemoglobin in the plasma or urine) or a severe anaphylactic reaction, the transfusion can be resumed after consultation with the transfusion service *(Miller: Miller's Anesthesia, ed 8, p 1853; Basics of Anesthesia, ed 7, p 410).*

387. (C) Hemolytic transfusion reactions are often the result of clerical error. Three main blood compatibility tests can be performed to reduce the chance of a hemolytic reaction: ABO Rh typing, antibody screening, and crossmatching. With correct ABO and Rh typing, the possibility of an incompatible transfusion is less than 1 per 1000. If you add a type and screen, the possibility of an incompatible transfusion is less than 1 per 10,000. Optimal safety occurs when crossmatching is performed *(Miller: Miller's Anesthesia, ed 8, p 1840; Basics of Anesthesia, ed 7, p 403).*

388. (B) A blood crossmatch is performed to determine whether donor blood is compatible with the recipient and takes about 45 minutes to an hour to perform. There are three phases to complete crossmatching of blood: the immediate phase, the incubation phase, and the antiglobulin phase. Phase 1, or the immediate phase, takes 1 to 5 minutes to complete and is used to detect ABO incompatibilities, as well as the naturally occurring antibodies in the MN, P, and Lewis systems. Phase 2, incubation phase, involves the incubation of first-phase reactions at 37° C in albumin (30-45 minutes) or in low-ionic-strength salt solution (10-20 minutes) and primarily detects antibodies of the Rh system. Phase 3, antiglobulin phase, involves adding antiglobulin sera to the incubated test tubes and is used to detect most of the incomplete antibodies including the Rh, Kell, Kidd, and Duffy systems *(Miller: Miller's Anesthesia, ed 8, p 1838).*

389. (C) Factor VII is one of the four vitamin K–dependent clotting factors (factors II, VII, IX, and X). It also has the shortest half-life of all the clotting factors (4-6 hours) and is the first factor to become deficient in patients with severe hepatic failure, warfarin (Coumadin) anticoagulation therapy, and vitamin K deficiency. The PT is most sensitive to decreases in factor VII *(Basics of Anesthesia, ed 7, pp 388–389).*

390. (C) TRALI occurs within 6 hours of blood component administration. Patients experience noncardiogenic pulmonary edema with acute bilateral pulmonary infiltrates and hypoxemia ($PaO_2/FIO_2 \leq 300$ mm Hg or oxygen saturation $\leq 90\%$ on room air with no evidence of left atrial hypertension). The pathologic changes associated with TRALI are complex and may involve low-pressure pulmonary edema secondary to neutrophil activation and sequestration in the lungs. Older transfusion products (>14 days), female donors (especially multiparous patients), and pooled platelets compared with apheresis platelets are associated with a higher frequency of this condition. Interestingly, because donor antibodies are the usual cause, leukocyte reduction does not seem to significantly decrease the incidence of TRALI but does decrease the incidence of febrile reactions and the risk of CMV, and it may decrease leukocyte-induced immunomodulation. Treatment for TRALI reactions is supportive *(Miller: Miller's Anesthesia, ed 8, p 1859; Basics of Anesthesia, ed 7, p 408; Transfusion Reactions, ed 4, pp 199–209).*

391. (C) Of the five blood products listed in this question, platelets are the most likely to cause bacterial sepsis. Platelet-related sepsis is estimated to occur in 1 case per 12,000. The source of bacteria can be donor blood or contamination during the collection, processing, and storage of the blood. If platelets are cooled, then rewarmed, the platelets tend not to function very effectively. Because platelets are stored at room temperature of 20° to 24° C, bacteria may survive and multiply. New pathogen reduction technologies are used by some blood banks that may alleviate some of this risk by inactivating many pathogens; however, this is not yet widespread. All other listed blood products are cooled. Whole blood and packed RBCs are cooled to 4° C (unless they are frozen, which would be colder). FFP and cryoprecipitate are frozen to below −70° C. Albumin is heat sterilized, making it a sterile preparation that then can be safely stored at room temperatures *(Miller: Miller's Anesthesia, ed 8, pp 1859–1860; Basics of Anesthesia, ed 7, pp 406–407; AABB Technical Manual, ed 19, pp 193–195).*

392. (C) Hepatitis A transmission is very rare and is screened for by history alone (not serologically) because there is no carrier state for the virus and the disease is relatively mild. A decrease in the transmission for various other infectious agents has been attributed to the recent addition of nucleic acid testing (see table). At present, there are no screening tests available for malaria, SARS, variant Creutzfeldt-Jakob disease, or BSE *(Miller: Miller's Anesthesia, ed 8, pp 1856–1858; Basics of Anesthesia, ed 7, pp 407–408).*

TESTS USED FOR DETECTING INFECTIOUS AGENTS IN ALL UNITS OF BLOOD, 2017

Infectious Agent	NA Minipool	Antibody To
Human immunodeficiency virus 1/2 (HIV)	Nucleic acid technology	HIV-1, HIV-2
Hepatitis C virus (HCV)	Nucleic acid technology	HCV
Hepatitis B virus (HBV)	Nucleic acid technology	HBV surface and core
Human T-cell lymphotropic virus I/II (HTLV)		HTLV-1, HTLV-2
West Nile virus	Nucleic acid technology	
Trypanosoma cruzi (Chagas)		Chagas (may perform only once per donor life)
Syphilis		Treponemal or nontreponemal antigens

Table modified from Table 7-3, AABB Technical Manual, ed 19, pp 166–167.

393. (B) Blood volume decreases with age. A preterm newborn has a blood volume of 100 to 120 mL/kg, a term newborn has a blood volume of about 90 mL/kg, an infant (3-12 months) has a blood volume of 80 mL/kg, a child older than 1 year has a blood volume of 70 mL/kg, and an adult has a blood volume of 65 mL/kg. This 10-kg, 1-year-old infant would have an estimated blood volume (EBV) of 800 *(Basics of Anesthesia, ed 7, p 743).*

394. (B) The risk of transfusion-transmitted infection with a unit of screened blood in the United States varies from study to study, but it is very infrequent with CMV because of leukocyte-reduced blood: 1 in 843,000 to 1,208,000 for hepatitis B, 1 in 1,149,000 for hepatitis C, 1 in 1,467,000 for HIV, 1 in 2,993,000 for HTLV-II, and 1 in more than 1,100,000 for West Nile virus. Thus the highest-risk transfusion-transmitted viral infection in the United States is now hepatitis B. The infective agent for syphilis does not survive at 4° C, making transmission unlikely for whole blood, packed RBCs, FFP, or cryoprecipitate. It is possible for platelets (stored at room temperature) to transmit syphilis *(Miller: Miller's Anesthesia, ed 8, pp 1856–1858; AABB Technical Manual, ed 19, p 179).*

395. (A) The most common type of hemophilia is hemophilia A, an X-linked recessive disease causing a reduction in factor VIII activity. The disease occurs with a frequency of 1 in 5000 male individuals. This disease can be severe (<1% factor VIII), moderate (1%-4% factor VIII), or mild (5%-30% factor VIII). Patients with mild hemophilia rarely have spontaneous bleeding. Laboratory studies show a normal platelet count and normal PT, but a prolonged aPTT. The primary goal of preoperative preparation of patients with hemophilia A is to increase plasma factor VIII activity to a level that will ensure adequate hemostasis (i.e., 50%-100%), then maintain a level (>40% factor VIII levels) for 7 to 10 days. One unit of factor VIII is equal to 1 mL of 100% activity of normal plasma. Thus to calculate the initial dose, first calculate the patient's blood and then the plasma volume. Then calculate the amount of activity needed to increase the factor VIII level. In this case the blood volume is 78 kg × 65 mL/kg, or about 5000 mL. Knowing that the RBC volume is 40% (i.e., hematocrit is 40) makes the plasma volume 60%. Thus the plasma volume is 5000 mL × 0.6, or about 3000 mL. Because the patient is starting at 0% activity and you wish to raise it to 100% activity, you will need 3000 units. (If you wish to raise the activity by 40%, then 3000 mL of plasma × 0.4 for 40% activity = 1200 units.) In addition, because the half-life of factor VIII is about 12 hours, about 1500 units will remain after 12 hours. An infusion of 1500 units in 12 hours, or 125 units per hour, will be a good starting maintenance infusion rate. Factor VIII can be administered as factor VIII concentrate or cryoprecipitate (about 10 units/mL). Patients with factor VIII inhibitors (10%-20% of patients with hemophilia) require more factor VIII. Hematology consultation should be considered for all patients with hemophilia, and routine checking of factor VIII levels should be performed *(Marx: Rosen's Emergency Medicine, ed 8, p 1614; Miller: Miller's Anesthesia, ed 8, p 1215).*

396. (A) Serum ADH levels increase during painful stimulation associated with surgery, as well as during positive-pressure mechanical ventilation. Small doses of furosemide (i.e., 0.1 mg/kg) will counteract this effect during surgery *(Miller: Miller's Anesthesia, ed 8, p 1773).*

397. (B) In an emergency transfusion of a patient with unknown blood type, type O RhD negative is the classic "universal donor" product. After a recent standards change, rare hospitals will also utilize group O whole blood with a low titer of anti-A and anti-B as a resuscitation product because it is a "balanced" product with the usual ratios of RBCs, plasma, and platelets. Importantly, although low titer, O whole blood does still contain some O plasma and therefore anti-A and anti-B. If a patient were to receive a significant volume of O whole blood, there could be a risk of intravascular hemolysis if they are transfused with red cells containing A or B antigens. This question is highlighting the difference between universal red cells (O) and universal plasma (AB). In reality, there may be very good reasons to switch a patient to type-specific blood in this situation; however, the best answer to the question as written is to transfuse O-positive red cells to prevent immediate hemolysis. Also, once it is known that the patient is RhD positive, there is no need to continue to transfuse a scarce resource (O RhD negative), and you would surely transfuse RhD-positive units instead *(AABB Standards for Blood Banks and Transfusion Services, ed 31, p 44).*

398. (B) The requirement for blood storage states that at least 70% of the erythrocytes must remain in circulation for 24 hours after a transfusion for the transfusion to be successful. Erythrocytes that survive longer than 24 hours after transfusion appear to have a normal life span *(Miller: Miller's Anesthesia, ed 8, p 1841; Basics of Anesthesia, ed 7, p 404).*

399. (B) At a pH below 6.0 or in cold temperatures such as 4° C (the temperature used for red cell storage), platelets undergo irreversible shape changes, and they are promptly removed from circulation. To maximize post-transfusion platelet count yields, the optimal temperature for platelet storage is 22° C ± 2° C, or room temperature. There are two major problems with platelet storage at this recommended temperature. First, the pH falls because of platelet metabolism. Second, bacterial growth is possible, which could potentially lead to sepsis and death. Recent evidence suggests that cold-stored platelets are "pre-activated," and although they don't last as long in circulation, they may be MORE hemostatic. Nonetheless, the standard is still room temperature storage (22° C), with maximum duration set at 5 days *(Miller: Miller's Anesthesia, ed 8, pp 1859–1861; AABB Technical Manual, ed 19, pp 142–143).*

400. (A) Whole blood is rarely used today except in emergency cases, when the rapid infusion of blood and volume is needed. Stored blood contains citrate, an anticoagulant that binds ionized calcium. When whole blood is rapidly transfused (i.e., >50 mL/70 kg/min), the citrate binds with calcium, producing transient decreases in ionized calcium. The abrupt decrease in ionized calcium can lead to prolonged QT intervals, an increase in left ventricular end-diastolic pressure, and arterial hypotension. Within 5 minutes of stopping the transfusion, ionized calcium levels return to normal. The volume of an average unit of whole blood is 500 mL. This patient received 10 units of whole blood, or 5000 mL, over 30 minutes, then another 5 units in 15 minutes. This averages to a rate greater than 160 mL/min *(Miller: Miller's Anesthesia, ed 8, pp 1840–1841; Basics of Anesthesia, ed 7, p 409).*

401. (C) A 20-kg, 5-year-old child has an EBV of 70 mL/kg = 1400 mL. The acceptable blood loss can be determined by use of the following formula: maximum allowable blood loss (in mL) = EBV × (Hcts − Hct1)/Hcts where EBV is the estimated blood volume (in mL), Hcts is the starting hematocrit, and

Hct1 is the lowest acceptable hematocrit. For this patient, the maximal allowable blood loss = 1400 × (40 - 30/40) = 1400 × (10/40) = 350 mL. This assumes that the patient is getting volume expansion with crystalloid (3 mL per mL of blood loss). Also see explanation to Question 393 *(Basics of Anesthesia, ed 7, p 594)*.

402. (D) Classically, in vivo hemostasis occurs when platelets activate and form an initial platelet plug (primary hemostasis), which is followed by coagulation factor activation on platelet surfaces and subsequent fibrin deposition at the site of injury (secondary hemostasis). Although whole blood viscoelastic tests are commonly thought to provide the answers to all hemostatic abnormalities, they unfortunately do not. Classic TEG activates whole blood via the intrinsic pathway (adding kaolin, for example), which then generates large amounts of thrombin and forms an in vitro clot, including activating and incorporating platelets into the evolving clot. Note that compared with in vivo hemostasis, where platelet plug precedes coagulation, this is the inverse; this produces an interesting artifact of the test. See in the figure that platelets can be activated by a whole host of agonists (e.g., ADP, epinephrine, collagen, thromboxane A2 etc.) that all have a relatively conserved intracellular mechanism of increasing intracellular Ca, which activates the platelet. If one of these pathways is blocked, such as when clopidogrel prevents ADP activation of platelets, this produces an in vivo antiplatelet effect, but the TEG will be normal because thrombin is generated in huge amounts and the platelet thrombin receptors are unaffected. Overall, the platelet doesn't care where it gets its Ca from, and thrombin is stellar at doing it.

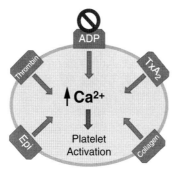

(Kandice Kottke-Marchant, MD, PhD, FCAP: An Algorithmic Approach to Hemostasis Testing, ed 2)

403. (D) Hemoglobin is usually measured in grams per volume of blood. During the initial phase of rapid blood loss, whole blood is lost, meaning both the numerator and denominator are lost in equal proportions. Although the circulating red cell mass is decreasing rapidly during the bleed, the *concentration* doesn't start to drop until extravascular fluid redistributes to the intravascular space or fluid resuscitation is initiated, both of which take some time to occur. For this reason, initial reliance on labs during a bleed can lead to false reassurance as they may not highlight the severity of the situation until later. In this case though, the blood sample is drawn before the fluid infusion is started, so the hemoglobin drawn should be similar to his hemoglobin concentration immediately before the MVA *(Butterworth: Morgan & Mikhail's Clinical Anesthesiology, ed 5, pp 1161–1164; Basics of Anesthesia, ed 7, pp 397–400)*.

404. (D) Abrupt discontinuation of TPN that contains 10% to 20% dextrose may result in profound rebound hypoglycemia. Tachycardia in this patient may signify hypoglycemia. Prompt diagnosis and treatment of severe hypoglycemia are essential if neurologic damage is to be avoided. Whenever a central line is placed for TPN, it should be properly checked before the hypertonic infusion is started *(Miller: Miller's Anesthesia, ed 8, p 1782)*.

405. (D) In an emergency when massive amounts of blood are immediately required and the supply of O-negative RBCs in the blood bank is low, it is acceptable to transfuse O-positive RBCs into male patients or into female patients past the age of childbirth before the patient's blood type is known. This is because delaying blood transfusion for blood typing may be more hazardous to the patient than the risk of a significant transfusion reaction based on Rh type for these patients. However, for the female patient who has the potential for pregnancy, administration of Rh-positive RBCs is not recommended (unless no Rh-negative RBCs are available). This is because an Rh-negative patient who receives

Rh-positive RBCs would experience isoimmunization. For these women, future pregnancies with Rh-positive fetuses could be associated with erythroblastosis fetalis *(Turgeon: Clinical Hematology, ed 1, pp 50–51; Basics of Anesthesia, ed 7, p 403).*

406. (B) Hetastarch (hydroxyethyl starch) and dextran 70 (glucose polymers with mean molecular weights of 70,000) are colloid solutions that are used for intravascular fluid volume expansion. Both hetastarch and dextran have been associated with allergic reactions, can interfere with coagulation, and can cause hypervolemia. Hetastarch, unlike dextran, does not interfere with crossmatching of blood at the recommended maximal daily dose of 20 mL/kg. Neither compound needs to be administered through a filter.

Hetastarch also reduces levels of vWF significantly, as well as availability of glycoprotein IIb/IIIa, and it can become directly incorporated into the fibrin clot. Because of these potential issues, these products have mostly fallen out of favor *(Miller: Miller's Anesthesia, ed 8, p 1783; Basics of Anesthesia, ed 7, p 398).*

407. (D) RBCs are cooled to about 4° C to decrease cellular metabolism. CPDA-1 is a preservative anticoagulant solution often added to blood. It contains citrate, phosphate, dextrose, and adenine. The citrate is used to bind calcium and acts as an anticoagulant. Phosphate acts as a buffer. Dextrose is added as an energy source for cellular metabolism on the day of donation to raise the blood sugar to greater than 400 mg/dL. At 35 days, the glucose level drops below 100 mg/dL. Adenine is added as a substrate source so that the cells can produce adenosine triphosphate. Other biochemical changes include a fall in pH to about 6.7 and a rise in plasma potassium from around 4 mEq/L on the day of donation to 76 mEq/L at 35 days. Concentrations of 2,3-diphosphoglycerate fall below 1 μM/mL, which causes a leftward shift in the oxyhemoglobin dissociation curve that allows for an increased oxygen affinity for the hemoglobin. This leftward shift produces a P50 value less (not greater) than the normal 26 mm Hg *(Miller: Miller's Anesthesia, ed 8, pp 1841–1842).*

408. (D) In May 2018, the FDA approved the use of FXa (recombinant) inactivated-zhzo (Andexxa) to reverse the anticoagulation effects of the FXa inhibitors apixaban and rivaroxaban when there is life-threatening or uncontrolled bleeding. The mechanism of action consists of binding and sequestering the FXa inhibitors. Common adverse reactions (>5%) include urinary tract infections and pneumonia. Serious and life-threatening adverse effects include arterial and venous thromboembolic events, ischemic events (e.g., myocardial infarction, ischemic stroke), cardiac arrest, and sudden death or other possible thromboembolic events. Thromboembolic events have been reported in >15% of patients, with a mean time of occurrence equal to 6 days. Because of the significant risk for thromboembolic events, a black box warning for thromboembolic risks, ischemic risks, cardiac arrest, and sudden deaths has been made. Patients who take FXa inhibitors for the anticoagulation effects are prone to thromboembolism, and reversing FXa inhibitors may lead to thrombosis, which is why it is recommended to restart anticoagulation as soon as possible *(Portola Pharmaceuticals, Inc., Package insert for Andexxa, www.andexxa.com; Miller: Miller's Anesthesia, ed 8, p 1873).*

409. (D) The liver produces most of the coagulation factors except for factor III (tissue thromboplastin), factor IV (calcium), and factor VIII (von Willebrand factor [vWF]). The liver also produces the coagulation regulatory protein C, protein S, and antithrombin III. Fetal RBCs are produced exclusively by the liver; in the adult, 80% of RBCs are produced by the bone marrow and only 20% are produced in the liver. The degradation of blood is primarily by the reticuloendothelial system *(Basics of Anesthesia, ed 7, p 381).*

410. (B) LMWH is produced by the fractionation or cleaving of "unfractionated heparin" (UFH) into shorter fragments. The anticoagulant properties of UFH and LMWH are complex and somewhat different; however, both require antithrombin to be effective. UFH binds to and activates antithrombin (more effectively than LMWH) to antagonize thrombin and can be monitored easily with the aPTT. At the usual clinical doses of LMWH, aPTT is not prolonged. When bound to antithrombin, LMWH is more effective in inactivating factor Xa and can be monitored by anti-Xa levels (although commonly this is not performed because of the more predictable action of prophylactic dosing of LMWH). At high doses of LMWH, antifactor Xa values are more commonly measured. Thrombin time is a measure of the ability of thrombin to convert fibrinogen to fibrin. It is prolonged with low amounts of fibrinogen, heparin, and fibrin degradation products (FDPs). A reptilase test is done by adding reptilase to plasma and waiting for a clot to form and is prolonged in the presence of FDPs, fibrinogen deficiency, or abnormal fibrinogen. It is not prolonged in the presence of heparin *(Miller: Miller's Anesthesia, ed 8, pp 1872–1874; Basics of Anesthesia, ed 7, p 389).*

411. (D) The four selections to this question are four of the five major hereditary conditions associated with hypercoagulation. They cause an increased likelihood of clot formation by either increasing prothrombotic proteins (e.g., factor V Leiden mutation, prothrombin G20210A gene mutation) or decreasing endogenous antithrombotic proteins (e.g., antithrombin deficiency, protein C deficiency, protein S deficiency). Clot may also develop if heparin resistance occurs (usual doses produce less than the expected prolongation of the partial thromboplastin time or the activated clotting time) and is not recognized, as during cardiopulmonary bypass. It may occur as a result of excessive binding of heparin to plasma proteins or an insufficient amount of antithrombin. Because heparin binds to and potentiates antithrombin's activity, conditions with low amounts of antithrombin show resistance. Treatment of ATIII deficiency is replacement of ATIII with either specific AT III concentrate (Thrombate III) or FFP. Replacement of antithrombin to 100% activity is recommended before cardiac surgery in patients with congenital ATIII deficiency *(Miller: Miller's Anesthesia, ed 8, pp 1871–1872, 1876–1877; Young: Clinical Hematology, ed 1, pp 1116–1118).*

412. (D) vWD is the most common inherited abnormality affecting platelet function and is caused by a quantitative or qualitative deficiency of a protein called vWF. vWF is produced by endothelial cells and platelets and appears to have two main functions: It acts as an adhesion protein that diverts platelets to sites of vascular injury, and it helps protect factor VIII from inactivation and clearance. Patients with vWD have prolonged bleeding times and a reduced amount of factor VIII. Patients with hemophilia A also have a decrease in factor VIII, but normal bleeding times. Type 1 vWD is the most common type (60%-80%) and is associated with a quantitative decrease in circulating plasma vWF caused by a decrease in release of available vWF. Type 2 vWD (20%-30%) has several subtypes and is associated with qualitative deficiency of vWF. Type 3 vWD is the least frequent (1%-5%) and the most severe form, wherein there is almost no vWF and very low factor VIII levels (3%-10% of normal). Treatment of vWD may include DDAVP, which increases the release of available vWF, or blood products that contain vWF and factor VIII (e.g., cryoprecipitate, FFP, or factor VIII concentrates). Of note, not all types of vWD use the same treatment approach (DDAVP is not recommended in Type 2B), so expert consultation is often recommended. Recombinant factor VIII is not used because it does not contain vWF *(Miller: Miller's Anesthesia, ed 8, pp 1123, 1872; Basics of Anesthesia, ed 7, p 381; Practical Hemostasis and Thrombosis, ed 3, pp 105–109).*

413. (A) Although allergic reactions after blood transfusions are common (up to 3%), true nonhemolytic anaphylactic reactions are rare. When anaphylactic reactions develop (often with only a few milliliters of blood or plasma transfused), the signs and symptoms may include dyspnea, bronchospasm, laryngeal edema, chest pain, hypotension, and shock. Classically, these reactions are caused by the transfusion of "foreign" IgA protein to patients who have hereditary IgA deficiency and have formed anti-IgA antibody. Importantly, simply being IgA deficient (about 1 in 700 Caucasians) is not sufficient, as you must also form the anti-IgA antibody. Although this is listed as the most common cause of anaphylaxis to blood transfusion, it only explains the cause in about 40% of cases, and in the remainder, no cause is determined. Treatment includes stopping the transfusion and administering epinephrine and steroids. If further transfusion is needed, one should discuss the special needs for washed cellular components (RBCs and platelets) or components from IgA-deficient donors with the transfusion service. Notably, it may take days to obtain IgA-deficient blood products *(Miller: Miller's Anesthesia, ed 8, p 1853; Transfusion Reactions, ed 4, pp 108–125).*

414. (A) For the years 2012 to 2016, 186 confirmed transfusion-related fatalities were listed by the U.S. Food and Drug Administration (FDA) in the United States. The most common cause was TRALI (34%). Considering that about 17 million components are transfused each year (2015 calendar year) in the United States, the reported incidence of death is quite small *(www.fda.gov/cber/blood/fatal/0506.htm; Miller: Miller's Anesthesia, ed 8, pp 1855–1860; Basics of Anesthesia, ed 7, pp 407–408; https://www.fda.gov/downloads/BiologicsBloodVaccines/SafetyAvailability/ReportaProblem/TransfusionDonationFatalities/UCM598243.pdf).*

TRANSFUSION-RELATED FATALITIES IN THE UNITED STATES, 2004 TO 2006

Complication	Total Number	Total %
Transfusion-associated acute lung injury	64	34%
Transfusion-associated circulatory overload	56	30%
Hemolytic transfusion reactions (non-ABO)	19	10%
Contamination	19	10%
Hemolytic transfusion reaction (ABO)	14	8%
Anaphylaxis	11	6%
Hypotensive reaction	3	2%

From Fatalities reported to FDA following blood collection and transfusion annual summary for FY2016, Table 3 Transfusion Associated Fatalities by Complication, FY2012-2016. (https://www.fda.gov/downloads/BiologicsBloodVaccines/SafetyAvailability/ReportaProblem/TransfusionDonationFatalities/UCM598243.pdf).

415. (D) There is controversy not only as to which intravenous fluid is the best but also how much to give. Most would suggest that isotonic crystalloids should be the initial resuscitative fluids to any trauma patients, and they are certainly less expensive than 5% albumin, 6% hydroxyethyl starch, and dextran 70. Clear advantages of one fluid over another are hard to find *(Miller: Miller's Anesthesia, ed 8, p 1800; Basics of Anesthesia, ed 7, pp 396–401).*

416. (B) Transmission of CMV to patients who have normal immune mechanisms is benign and self-limiting, but in patients who are immunocompromised (e.g., premature newborns, solid organ and bone marrow transplant patients, acquired immunodeficiency syndrome patients), CMV infection can be serious and life-threatening. Leukocyte reduction can reduce CMV transmission, but restriction of blood products from seronegative donors is preferred *(Miller: Miller's Anesthesia, ed 8, pp 1857–1858).*

417. (C) GVHD is an often fatal condition that occurs in patients who are immunocompromised. It occurs when donor lymphocytes (graft) establish an immune response against the recipient (host). Blood products that have a significant amount of lymphocytes include RBCs and platelets. FFP and cryoprecipitate appear to be safe. Although directed donor units from first-degree relatives and leukoreduction may reduce the incidence of GVHD, only irradiated products (which inactivate donor lymphocytes) or their equivalent (such as with pathogen reduction technologies) can prevent GVHD *(Miller: Miller's Anesthesia, ed 8, p 1858; Basics of Anesthesia, ed 7, p 594; AABB Technical Manual, ed 19, p 194).*

CHAPTER 6

General Anesthesia

DIRECTIONS (Questions 418 through 546): Each of the questions or incomplete statements in this section is followed by answers or by completions of the statement, respectively. Select the ONE BEST answer or completion for each item.

418. A 78-year-old patient with a history of hypertension and adult-onset diabetes for which she takes chlorpropamide (Diabinese) is admitted for elective cholecystectomy. On the day of admission, blood glucose is noted to be 270 mg/dL, and the patient is treated with 15 units of regular insulin subcutaneously (SQ) in addition to her regular dose of chlorpropamide. Twenty-four hours later after overnight fasting, the patient is brought to the operating room (OR) without her daily dose of chlorpropamide and is anesthetized. A serum glucose is measured and found to be 35 mg/dL. The **MOST** likely explanation for this is
    A. Insulin
    B. Chlorpropamide
    C. Hypovolemia
    D. Effect of general anesthesia

419. Select the **TRUE** statement.
    A. Dibucaine is an ester-type local anesthetic
    B. A dibucaine number of 20 is normal
    C. The dibucaine number represents the quantity of normal pseudocholinesterase
    D. None of the above

420. A 56-year-old patient with a history of liver disease and osteomyelitis is anesthetized for tibial débridement. After induction and intubation, the wound is inspected and débrided with a total blood loss of 300 mL. The patient is transported intubated to the recovery room, at which time the systolic blood pressure falls to 50 mm Hg. Heart rate is 120 beats/min, arterial blood gases (ABGs) are PaO_2 103, $PaCO_2$ 45, pH 7.3, with 97% O_2 saturation with 100% FIO_2. Mixed venous blood gases are PVO_2 60 mm Hg, $PVCO_2$ 50, and pH 7.25. Which of the following diagnoses is **MOST** consistent with this clinical picture?
    A. Hypovolemia
    B. Congestive heart failure (CHF)
    C. Cardiac tamponade
    D. Sepsis with acute respiratory distress syndrome (ARDS)

421. Normal tracheal capillary pressure is
    A. 10 to 15 mm Hg
    B. 15 to 20 mm Hg
    C. 25 to 30 mm Hg
    D. 35 to 40 mm Hg

422. How many hours should elapse before performing a single-shot spinal anesthetic in a patient who is receiving 1 mg/kg enoxaparin (Lovenox) twice a day for the treatment of a deep vein thrombosis?
    A. 6 hours
    B. 12 hours
    C. 24 hours
    D. 48 hours

423. A 46-year-old female with low back pain and left-sided L4 radiculopathy presents for an L4/L5 lumbar discectomy. Her past medical history includes hypothyroidism, insulin-dependent diabetes type 1, and chronic low back pain, for which she is maintained on sublingual buprenorphine/naloxone, with the last dose having been received the morning of surgery.

     Compared with a patient who has **NOT** received buprenorphine/naloxone, which **ONE** of the following **BEST** describes her anticipated response to perioperative administration of opioids?
    A. DECREASED response due to upregulation of the cytochrome P450 system
    B. DECREASED response secondary to opioid receptor antagonism by naloxone
    C. DECREASED response due to high-affinity binding of buprenorphine to the opioid receptor
    D. No DIFFERENCE in response IF an opioid agonist with a high binding affinity is administered

424. Which of the following is the most plausible explanation for the lack of analgesia with codeine administration?
    A. Lack of CYP2D6 enzyme
    B. VKORC1 polymorphism
    C. CYP3A4 polymorphism
    D. Lack of μ receptors

425. A 62-year-old patient with a bare-metal stent in the mid portion of the left anterior descending artery is scheduled for rotator cuff repair under general anesthesia. The stent was placed 6 weeks before surgery, and the patient is on dual therapy (aspirin and clopidogrel). Which of the paradigms below would be best for managing his anticoagulation before surgery?
    A. Continue both up to the day of surgery
    B. Stop both 7 to 10 days before surgery
    C. Stop aspirin and continue clopidogrel
    D. Stop clopidogrel and continue aspirin

426. A patient with which of the following eye diseases would be at greatest risk for retinal damage from hypotension during surgery?
  A. Strabismus
  B. Open eye injury
  C. Glaucoma
  D. Severe myopia

427. Naltrexone is
  A. A narcotic with local anesthetic properties
  B. An opioid agonist-antagonist similar to nalbuphine
  C. A pure opioid antagonist with a shorter duration of action than naloxone
  D. An opioid antagonist used for treatment of previously detoxified heroin addicts

428. Which of the following mechanisms is most frequently responsible for hypoxia in the recovery room?
  A. Ventilation/perfusion mismatch
  B. Hypoventilation
  C. Hypoxic gas mixture
  D. Intracardiac shunt

429. Hypoparathyroidism secondary to the inadvertent surgical resection of the parathyroid glands during total thyroidectomy typically results in airway symptoms of hypocalcemia how many hours postoperatively?
  A. 1 to 2 hours
  B. 3 to 12 hours
  C. 12 to 24 hours
  D. 24 to 72 hours

430. Damage to which nerve may lead to wrist drop?
  A. Radial
  B. Axillary
  C. Median
  D. Ulnar

431. A 25-year-old woman with a body mass index (BMI) 42 kg/m^2 is to be anesthetized for laparoscopic bariatric surgery. She has a history of knee pain while walking. She has no medication allergies and takes multivitamins and an oral contraceptive. Her American Society of Anesthesiologists (ASA) designation should be
  A. ASA I
  B. ASA II
  C. ASA III
  D. ASA IV

432. A 6-year-old child is transported to the recovery room after a tonsillectomy. The patient was anesthetized with isoflurane, fentanyl, and N_2O. Twenty minutes before emergence and tracheal extubation, droperidol was administered. The anesthesiologist is called to the recovery room because the patient is "making strange eye movements." The patient's eyes are rolled back into his head, and his neck is twisted and rigid. The most appropriate drug for treatment of these symptoms is
  A. Dantrolene
  B. Diazepam
  C. Glycopyrrolate
  D. Diphenhydramine

433. A 22-year-old with multiple medical problems lists 5-HT$_3$ antagonists on her allergy band. With which of the medications listed below was this allergy most likely discovered?
  A. Granisetron (Kytril)
  B. Paroxetine (Paxil)
  C. Milrinone
  D. Cyproheptadine (Periactin)

434. Pheochromocytoma would be **MOST** likely to coexist with which of the following?
  A. Insulinoma
  B. Pituitary adenoma
  C. Primary hyperaldosteronism (Conn syndrome)
  D. Medullary carcinoma of the thyroid

435. Which of the following oral antidiabetic drugs is unique in that it does **NOT** produce hypoglycemia when administered to a fasting patient?
  A. Glyburide (Micronase)
  B. Glipizide (Glucotrol)
  C. Tolbutamide (Orinase)
  D. Metformin (Glucophage)

436. The onset of delirium tremens (DTs) after abstinence from alcohol usually occurs in
  A. 8 to 24 hours
  B. 24 to 48 hours
  C. 2 to 4 days
  D. 4 to 7 days

437. A 78-year-old retired coal miner with an intraluminal tracheal tumor is scheduled for tracheal resection. Which of the following is a relative contraindication for tracheal resection?
A. Need for postoperative mechanical ventilation for underlying lung disease
B. Tumor located at the carina
C. Documented liver metastases
D. Ischemic heart disease with a history of CHF

438. A 78-year-old patient with multiple myeloma is admitted to the intensive care unit (ICU) for treatment of hypercalcemia. The primary risk associated with anesthetizing patients with hypercalcemia (levels of 14-16 mg/dL) is
A. Coagulopathy
B. Cardiac dysrhythmias
C. Hypotension
D. Laryngospasm

439. Just before induction of general anesthesia for an 85-year-old demented man with an ischemic bowel, he mentions to you that he forgot to take his green-capped eye drops. He states that not taking it daily will result in blindness. The green-capped eye drops are
A. NaCl drops used to prevent his eye from drying out
B. Antibiotic drops
C. Steroids
D. Used to produce miosis

440. A normal, healthy 3-year-old child was involved in a motor vehicle accident (MVA). He is coming emergently to the OR. Drug doses need to be calculated, but his weight is not known. What value should be used to estimate the 3-year-old child's weight?
A. 8 kg
B. 10 kg
C. 12 kg
D. 14 kg

441. A 16-year-old patient presents for extraction of multiple teeth. In her history, it is noted that she is on a ketogenic diet. The likely reason for this is history of
A. Phenylketonuria (PKU)
B. Mitochondrial myopathies
C. Intractable seizures
D. Glycogen storage disease

442. A 28-year-old obese patient has diminished breath sounds bilaterally at the lung bases 18 hours after an emergency appendectomy under general anesthesia. Which of the following maneuvers would be **LEAST** effective in preventing postoperative pulmonary complications in this patient?
A. Coughing
B. Voluntary deep breathing
C. Performing a forced vital capacity (FVC)
D. Use of incentive spirometry

443. Easily discernable improvement in patient outcomes can be observed through which measure of quality improvement?
A. Process measure (e.g., timing of antibiotics with incision)
B. Structural measures (e.g., electronic medical record)
C. Outcome measures (e.g., incidence of wound infection)
D. None of the above

444. A 67-year-old patient is mechanically ventilated in the ICU 2 days after repair of a ruptured abdominal aortic aneurysm. To maintain PaO_2 in the 60 to 65 range, 10 cm H_2O positive end-expiratory pressure (PEEP) is added to the ventilator cycle. The patient's blood pressure has averaged 110/65 before addition of PEEP. After addition of PEEP, the blood pressure is noted to slowly fall to an average of approximately 95/50. The best explanation for this decrease in blood pressure is
A. Tension pneumothorax
B. Decreased venous return to the heart
C. Increased afterload on the right side of the heart
D. Increased afterload on the left side of the heart

445. The mechanism of action of clopidogrel is
A. Adenosine diphosphate (ADP) receptor blockade ($P2Y_{12}$)
B. Platelet glycoprotein IIB/IIIa antagonism
C. Cyclooxygenase COX-1 and COX-2 inhibition
D. Direct thrombin inhibition

446. Which of the following is most closely associated with minimum alveolar concentration (MAC)?
A. Blood/gas partition coefficient
B. Oil/gas partition coefficient
C. Vapor pressure
D. Brain/blood partition coefficient

447. By federal law, any breach in protected health information (PHI) must be disclosed to
A. Department of Health and Human Services (HHS)
B. Department of Justice (DOJ)
C. Joint Commission on Accreditation of Healthcare Organizations (JCAHO)
D. American Accreditation HealthCare Commission/ Utilization Review Accreditation Commission (AAHC/URAC)

448. Scopolamine should not be given as a premedication in patients with which of the following neurologic diseases?
A. Parkinson disease
B. Alzheimer disease
C. Multiple sclerosis
D. Narcolepsy

449. A 45-year-old female patient with a history of depression and previous intraoperative awareness is anesthetized for gastric bypass. A 2-mg dose of midazolam is administered 1 hour preoperatively to alleviate anxiety. The anesthetic consists of a low-dose propofol infusion (50 μg/kg/min), fentanyl, and sevoflurane. The next day she reports awareness during the procedure itself, which she describes as "painful." The provider reviews the anesthetic records and notes no episode of end-tidal sevoflurane below 1.5%. The proper next step would be
  A. Sympathetic listening, apology, offer counseling
  B. Avoid contact with patient until legal advice has been sought
  C. Immediate psychiatric evaluation
  D. Sympathetic listening with nondefensive explanation that recall would be essentially impossible under these circumstances

450. A 53-year-old woman with endometrial cancer is undergoing an abdominal hysterectomy under general anesthesia with desflurane. During the first hour of anesthesia, urine output is 100 mL. Blood loss is minimal. When the patient is placed in the Trendelenburg position, the urine output declines to virtually zero. The most likely explanation for this sudden decrease in urine output in this patient is
  A. Pooling of urine in the dome of the bladder
  B. Increased central venous pressure
  C. Increased antidiuretic hormone (ADH) production from surgical stimulation
  D. Hypovolemia

451. Which of the following diseases is **NOT** associated with a decrease in DLCO?
  A. Emphysema
  B. Obesity
  C. Pulmonary emboli
  D. Anemia

452. Each of the following postoperative complications of thyroid surgery can result in upper airway obstruction **EXCEPT**
  A. Cervical hematoma
  B. Tetany
  C. Bilateral superior laryngeal nerve injury
  D. Bilateral recurrent laryngeal nerve injury

453. The **MOST** sensitive early sign of malignant hyperthermia (MH) during general anesthesia is
  A. Tachycardia
  B. Hypertension
  C. Fever
  D. Increased end-expiratory CO_2 tension ($PECO_2$)

454. A 78-year-old woman is anesthetized for a right hemicolectomy for 3 hours. At the end of the operation the patient's blood pressure is 130/85 mm Hg, heart rate is 84 beats/min, core body temperature is 35.4° C, and $PECO_2$ on infrared spectrometer is 38 mm Hg. Which of the following would be the **LEAST** plausible reason for prolonged apnea in this patient?
  A. Residual neuromuscular blockade
  B. Narcotic overdose
  C. Unrecognized obstructive pulmonary disease and high baseline $PaCO_2$
  D. Persistent intraoperative hyperventilation

455. A 68-year-old woman with severe rheumatoid arthritis undergoes pulmonary function evaluation before an elective abdominal surgery. Forced expiratory volume in 1 second (FEV_1) and FVC are within normal limits; however, the maximum voluntary ventilation (MVV) is only 40% of predicted. The next step in the pulmonary function evaluation of this patient should be to
  A. Obtain ABGs on room air
  B. Obtain a flow-volume loop
  C. Obtain a measurement of peak flow
  D. Obtain a ventilation/perfusion scan

456. Which of the following is **NOT** a component of the postanesthetic discharge scoring system (PADSS) used to evaluate the suitability of a patient to be discharged from an ambulatory surgical facility?
  A. Drinking
  B. Ambulation
  C. Absence of nausea and vomiting
  D. Pain control

457. During emergency repair of a mandibular jaw fracture in an otherwise healthy 19-year-old man, the patient's temperature is noted to rise from 37° C on induction to 38° C after 2 hours of surgery. Which of the following informational items would be **LEAST** useful in ruling out MH in this patient?
  A. Normal heart rate and blood pressure
  B. History of negative caffeine-halothane contracture test carried out 6 months earlier
  C. History of an uncomplicated general anesthetic at age 16 years with halothane and succinylcholine
  D. Normal ABGs drawn when the patient's temperature reached 38° C

458. Which of the following drugs is useful in the treatment of asthma by specifically interfering with the leukotriene pathway?
  A. Fluticasone (Flovent)
  B. Ipratropium bromide (Atrovent)
  C. Triamcinolone (Azmacort)
  D. Montelukast (Singulair)

459. A 68-year-old, 100-kg patient is undergoing a transurethral resection of the prostate gland under general anesthesia. Upon arrival in the recovery room, the patient appears restless and confused. Serum sodium is checked and found to be 110 mEq/L. How many mEq of sodium are needed to raise the serum $[Na^+]$ to 120 mEq/L?
A. 300 mEq
B. 400 mEq
C. 500 mEq
D. 600 mEq

460. Which of the intravenous (IV) anesthetics below is **LEAST** useful in the treatment of status epilepticus?
A. Phenobarbital
B. Dexmedetomidine
C. Propofol
D. Midazolam

461. A 45-year-old man is brought to the OR emergently for repair of a ruptured abdominal aortic aneurysm. Anesthesia is induced with ketamine 2 mg/kg IV, and tracheal intubation is facilitated with succinylcholine 1.5 mg/kg IV. Immediately after tracheal intubation, the patient's blood pressure falls from 110/80 to 50/20 mm Hg. What is the **MOST** likely cause of the sudden severe hypotension in this patient?
A. Hypovolemia
B. Direct myocardial depression from ketamine
C. Vasovagal response to direct laryngoscopy
D. Arteriolar vasodilation from succinylcholine-mediated histamine release

462. MH is believed to involve a generalized disorder of membrane permeability to
A. Sodium
B. Potassium
C. Calcium
D. Magnesium

463. A 25-year-old man with a history of testicular cancer is scheduled to undergo an exploratory laparotomy under general anesthesia. He has received bleomycin for metastatic disease. Which of the following is an important consideration concerning the pulmonary toxicity of bleomycin?
A. N_2O should not be used
B. Preoperative pulmonary function tests should be obtained
C. The patient should be ventilated at a slow rate and inspiratory-to-expiratory (I:E) ratio of 1:3
D. FIO_2 should be less than 0.3

464. A 39-year-old obese woman undergoes an abdominal hysterectomy under general anesthesia. Induction of anesthesia is uneventful. SaO_2 is 98% during the first 15 minutes of the operation, with 50% oxygen and 50% N_2O. Then, at the request of the surgeon, N_2O is discontinued (now 50% oxygen, 50% N_2), the head is flexed, and the patient is placed in the Trendelenburg position to improve surgical exposure, and SaO_2 falls to 90%. The **MOST** likely explanation for this desaturation is
A. Diffusion hypoxia
B. Decreased functional residual capacity (FRC)
C. Mainstem intubation
D. Decreased cardiac output

465. How long after intravitreal injection of sulfur hexafluoride and air can N_2O be used without risk of increasing intraocular pressure?
A. 1 hour
B. 24 hours
C. 10 days
D. 1 month

466. A 54-year-old woman is undergoing a total thyroidectomy under general anesthesia. The patient is awakened in the OR, the mouth and pharynx are suctioned, and after intact laryngeal reflexes are demonstrated, the endotracheal tube is removed. Two days later, the anesthesiologist is consulted because the patient has severe stridor and upper airway obstruction. The most likely cause of airway obstruction in this patient is
A. Damage to the recurrent laryngeal nerve
B. Hematoma
C. Tracheomalacia
D. Hypocalcemia

467. A 27-year-old obese woman is scheduled to undergo foot surgery under general anesthesia. She underwent a subtotal thyroidectomy 3 years ago and takes levothyroxine (Synthroid). Which of the following laboratory tests would be the **MOST** useful in evaluating whether this patient is euthyroid?
A. Total plasma thyroxine (T_4)
B. Total plasma triiodothyronine (T_3)
C. Thyroid-stimulating hormone (TSH)
D. Resin triiodothyronine uptake

468. An 85-year-old man with no previous medical history except for cataracts is undergoing a transurethral resection of the prostate gland under spinal anesthesia. Twenty minutes into the procedure the patient becomes restless. Over the next 20 minutes, his blood pressure increases from 110/70 to 140/90 mm Hg and his heart rate slows from 90 to 50 beats/min. The patient is noted to have some difficulty breathing. The most likely cause of these symptoms in this patient is
  A. Volume overload
  B. Hyponatremia
  C. High spinal
  D. Bladder perforation

469. A 17-year-old patient with third-degree burns over 30% of his body is scheduled for débridement and skin grafting 12 days after sustaining a thermal injury. Select the **TRUE** statement regarding the use of depolarizing and nondepolarizing muscle relaxants in this patient, compared with normal patients.
  A. Sensitivity to both depolarizing and nondepolarizing muscle relaxants is increased
  B. Sensitivity to both depolarizing and nondepolarizing muscle relaxants is decreased
  C. Sensitivity to depolarizing muscle relaxants is increased while sensitivity to nondepolarizing muscle relaxants is decreased
  D. Sensitivity to depolarizing muscle relaxants is decreased while sensitivity to nondepolarizing muscle relaxants is increased

470. A patient undergoes parotid gland removal under general anesthesia. Each of the following assesses facial nerve function **EXCEPT**
  A. Clenching teeth
  B. Closing eyes
  C. Pursing lips
  D. Eyebrow lift

471. A 65-year-old patient with a history of chronic obstructive pulmonary disease (COPD) and coronary artery disease (CAD) undergoes a laparoscopic nephrectomy uneventfully under general desflurane anesthesia. In the recovery room, ABGs are as follows: PaO_2 60 mm Hg, $PaCO_2$ 50 mm Hg, pH 7.35, and hemoglobin 8.1 g/dL. Which of the following steps would produce the greatest increase in O_2 delivery to the myocardium?
  A. Administration of 100% O_2 with a close-fitting mask
  B. Administration of 35% O_2 with a Venturi mask
  C. Administer 1 ampule of HCO_3
  D. Transfuse with 2 units of packed red blood cells (RBCs)

472. Allergic reactions occurring during the immediate perioperative period are **MOST** commonly attributable to administration of
  A. Muscle relaxants
  B. Local anesthetics
  C. Antibiotics
  D. Opioids

473. Caution is advised when using succinylcholine in patients with Huntington chorea because
  A. They are at increased risk for MH
  B. Potassium release may be excessive
  C. They may have a decreased concentration of pseudocholinesterase
  D. There may be adverse interactions between succinylcholine and phenothiazine

474. Which of the following would **NOT** result in an increase in intraocular pressure?
  A. Increase in $PaCO_2$ from 35 to 40 mm Hg
  B. 100 mg intramuscular (IM) succinylcholine
  C. Acute rise in venous pressure from coughing
  D. 100 mg IV succinylcholine in a patient in whom eye muscles have been detached from the globe

475. An apnea-hypopnea index (AHI) of 30 means
  A. Episodes of hypopnea are 30 times more common than apnea
  B. Apnea/hypopnea episodes occur at a rate of 30 per sleep cycle
  C. Episodes of apnea and hypopnea occur at a rate of 30 per hour
  D. Apnea/hypopnea episodes last 30 seconds

476. The reversal agent Andexxa is indicated for life threatening or uncontrollable hemorrhage in patients receiving
  Enoxaparin (Lovenox)
  Apixaban (Eliquis)
  Pradaxa (Dabigatran)
  Clopidogrel (Plavex)

477. A 26-year-old man is undergoing an emergency exploratory laparotomy under general anesthesia with isoflurane. SaO_2 is 89% on the pulse oximeter. PaO_2 on ABGs is 77 mm Hg. The patient's core body temperature is 35° C. What is the corrected PaO_2?
  A. 68 mm Hg
  B. 72 mm Hg
  C. 77 mm Hg
  D. 86 mm Hg

478. A 27-year-old patient with a 10-year history of Crohn disease is scheduled to undergo drainage of a rectal abscess under general anesthesia. His preoperative medications include prednisone, sulfasalazine, and cyanocobalamin. He has no known allergies and is otherwise healthy. Before induction of anesthesia, the patient is noted to have central cyanosis, and the pulse oximeter shows an SaO_2 of 89%, which does not increase after the administration of 100% O_2 for 2 minutes. ABGs are as follows: PaO_2 490 mm Hg, $PaCO_2$ 32 mm Hg, pH 7.43, SaO_2 89%. The **MOST** likely cause of these findings is
A. Presence of sulfhemoglobin
B. Presence of methemoglobin
C. Presence of cyanhemoglobin
D. Presence of carboxyhemoglobin

479. Low-molecular-weight heparin (LMWH)
A. Is as likely to cause heparin-induced thrombocytopenia (HIT) as unfractionated heparin
B. Should be monitored with partial thromboplastin time (PTT) for clinical effect
C. Can be fully reversed with protamine
D. LMWH has a longer plasma half-life than unfractionated heparin

480. In a given patient, if a creatinine of 1.0 corresponds to a glomerular filtration rate (GFR) of 120 mL/min, a creatinine of 4.0 would correspond to
A. 20 mL/min
B. 30 mL/min
C. 40 mL/min
D. 50 mL/min

481. The incidence of each of the following is increased in patients with Down syndrome (trisomy 21) **EXCEPT**
A. MH
B. Congenital heart disease
C. Smaller trachea
D. Occipito-atlantoaxial instability

482. A 55-year-old man is to undergo a laparoscopic cholecystectomy under general anesthesia. The patient has a 40-pack-per-year smoking history and a history of CHF. The patient receives metoclopramide and scopolamine preoperatively. General anesthesia is induced with ketamine, and the patient undergoes the procedure uneventfully. However, in the recovery room the patient complains of not being able to see objects "up close." Which of the following would be the **MOST** likely cause of this complaint?
A. Emergence delirium from ketamine anesthesia
B. Effect of scopolamine
C. Effect of Trendelenburg position
D. Corneal abrasion

483. MH and neuroleptic malignant syndrome share each of the following characteristics **EXCEPT**
A. Generalized muscular rigidity
B. Hyperthermia
C. Effectively treated with dantrolene
D. Flaccid paralysis after administration of vecuronium

484. What of the following statements about vasopressin is true?
A. It has a potent vasopressor effect at high doses in normal subjects
B. Plasma levels are inappropriately high in patients immediately after cardiopulmonary bypass
C. Plasma levels are inappropriately low in the setting of septic shock
D. It causes pulmonary vasoconstriction secondary to inhibition of endothelial nitric oxide release

485. Remifentanil is metabolized primarily by
A. Kidneys
B. Liver
C. Nonspecific esterases
D. Pseudocholinesterase

486. A term infant with good muscle tone and strong cry has an 83% saturation on room air 5 minutes after delivery. The **MOST** appropriate action at this point would be
A. Bag and mask ventilation with 100% oxygen
B. Intubate and ventilate with 100% oxygen
C. Spontaneous breathing with 100% oxygen
D. Observe

487. Patients who undergo extracorporeal shock wave lithotripsy are at increased risk for
A. Venous air embolism
B. Pneumothorax
C. Hypotension with regional anesthesia at the end of the procedure
D. Postdural puncture headache with spinal anesthesia

488. The most common reason for admitting outpatients to the hospital following general anesthesia is
A. Nausea and vomiting
B. Inability to void
C. Inability to ambulate
D. Surgical pain

489. A 37-year-old man with myasthenia gravis arrives in the emergency room confused and agitated after a 2-day history of weakness and increased difficulty breathing. ABGs on room air are PaO_2 60 mm Hg, $PaCO_2$ 51 mm Hg, HCO_3^- 25 mEq/L, pH 7.3, SaO_2 of 90%. His respiratory rate is 30 breaths/min, and tidal volume (VT) is 4 mL/kg. After administration of edrophonium 2 mg IV, his VT declines to 2 mL/kg. What should be the most appropriate step in the management of this patient at this time?

A. Tracheal intubation and mechanical ventilation

B. Repeat the test dose of edrophonium

C. Administer neostigmine

D. Administer atropine for cholinergic crisis

490. Select the **FALSE** statement regarding tramadol (Ultram).

A. Ondansetron may interfere with part of tramadol's analgesia

B. Tramadol is associated with seizures in patients taking selective serotonin reuptake inhibitors (SSRIs)

C. It is relatively safe in patients whose pain makes them suicidal

D. Its analgesic effects are partially antagonized by naloxone

491. In statistical hypothesis testing, if the P value is less than the predetermined α value, which of the following is most likely?

A. The observed result is unlikely under the null hypothesis

B. The observed result is unlikely under an alternative hypothesis

C. The sample size is too small

D. The predetermined power is too low

492. A 72-year-old man undergoes emergency repair of an abdominal aortic aneurysm. In the first hour after release of the suprarenal cross-clamp, urine output is only 10 mL. After administration of furosemide 20 mg IV, urine output increases to 100 mL/hr. Urine [Na^+] is 43 mEq/L, and urine osmolality is 210 mOsm/L. The **MOST** likely cause of the initial oliguria is

A. Increased ADH

B. Renal hypoperfusion

C. Acute tubular necrosis

D. Impossible to differentiate

493. Brice Questionnaire is used to estimate

A. Risk of sleep apnea

B. Intraoperative awareness

C. Postoperative nausea and vomiting (PONV)

D. Suitability for postanesthesia care unit (PACU) discharge

494. A 40-year-old man is undergoing a left inguinal hernia repair under general anesthesia in San Diego, California. N_2O is administered at 3 L/min, O_2 at 1 L/min, and isoflurane at 0.85%. What MAC is this patient receiving?

A. 0.8

B. 1.25

C. 1.50

D. 1.75

495. An otherwise healthy 140-kg, 24-year-old man is scheduled for vocal cord surgery under general anesthesia. Which of the following statements concerning his cardiac output at 140 kg compared with his cardiac output at his ideal body weight (70 kg) is **CORRECT**?

A. Cardiac output is the same

B. Cardiac output is increased by 10%

C. Cardiac output is increased by 50%

D. Cardiac output is doubled

496. After a single 150-mg dose of propofol to a 75-kg healthy patient, which of the following statements is **FALSE**?

A. The peak plasma concentration is reached in <1 minute

B. The peak plasma concentration of propofol is 7 to 8 µg/mL

C. The therapeutic plasma concentration range for propofol is 1.5-5 µg/mL

D. It takes about 15 to 20 minutes for the drug level to fall to a subtherapeutic level

497. A 58-year-old hemophiliac is scheduled for total knee arthroplasty. His factor VIII levels are 35% of normal. Which of the following would be the most appropriate therapy before surgery?

A. Administer sufficient cryoprecipitate to raise factor VIII levels to 50% normal

B. Administer factor VIII concentrates to achieve levels of 100% normal

C. Transfuse fresh frozen plasma until factor VIII levels are 100% normal

D. None of the above

498. A 16-year-old boy whose maternal uncle has hemophilia A is scheduled for wisdom tooth extraction. Which test below would be the best screening test for hemophilia A?

A. PTT

B. Prothrombin time (PT)

C. Thrombin time

D. Bleeding time

499. Five minutes after a single 150-mg dose of propofol to a 75-kg patient, which of the following is most likely regarding the cytosol (intracellular) concentration of propofol in the various tissues?
  A. The concentration in the brain would be rising
  B. The concentration in the spinal cord would be rising
  C. The concentration in the leg muscles would be falling
  D. The concentration in fat would be rising

500. A 57-year-old man is undergoing a right eye enucleation under general anesthesia. The patient has no history of cardiac disease. During the operation, 5-mm ST-segment elevation is noted on lead II, and the patient develops complete heart block. The coronary artery most likely affected is
  A. Circumflex coronary artery
  B. Right coronary artery
  C. Left main coronary artery
  D. Left anterior descending coronary artery

501. Each of the following may increase MAC for volatile anesthetics **EXCEPT**
  A. Cocaine
  B. Hyperthyroidism
  C. Hypernatremia
  D. Tricyclic antidepressants

502. A 37-year-old patient with a history of manic-depressive illness is scheduled to undergo surgery for removal of an intramedullary rod in the left tibia. Which of the following statements regarding potential untoward effects of lithium therapy is **NOT** true?
  A. Long-term administration may be associated with nephrogenic diabetes insipidus
  B. Administration of succinylcholine to patients treated with lithium may result in hyperkalemia
  C. Long-term therapy may be associated with hypothyroidism
  D. Duration of action of vecuronium may be prolonged

503. Treatment of hypotension in a patient anesthetized for resection of metastatic carcinoid would be best accomplished with
  A. Epinephrine
  B. Ephedrine
  C. Vasopressin (DDAVP)
  D. Octreotide

504. You are asked to evaluate a patient in the recovery room after having undergone an exploratory laparotomy for a colonic perforation. Which of the following factors in the quick Sequential Organ Failure Assessment (qSOFA) would be associated with an in-hospital mortality of 10%?
  A. Respiratory rate of 24/min; confusion; blood pressure of 110/60
  B. Lactate of 3.0 mmol/L; confusion; blood pressure of 110/60
  C. Lactate of 5.0 mmol/L; confusion; blood pressure of 110/60
  D. Respiratory rate of 24/min; awake, in pain; blood pressure of 110/60

505. A 31-year-old patient has been in the ICU on a ventilator for 24 hours after an MVA. The patient does not open his eyes to any stimulus and has no verbal or motor response. The Glasgow Coma Scale corresponding to this patient would be
  A. 0
  B. 1
  C. 2
  D. 3

506. Hypoglycemia is more likely to occur in the diabetic surgical patient with which of the following diseases?
  A. Renal disease
  B. Rheumatoid arthritis requiring high-dosage prednisone
  C. Chronic obstructive lung disease treated with a terbutaline inhaler and aminophylline
  D. Manic-depressive disorder treated with lithium

507. Which of the following is most likely to be associated with a falsely elevated SaO_2 as measured by pulse oximetry (dual wave)?
  A. Hemoglobin F
  B. Carboxyhemoglobin
  C. Methylene blue dye
  D. Fluorescein dye

508. Select the **FALSE** statement regarding clinical performance and sleep deprivation
  A. A period of vulnerability has been identified between 2 AM and 7 AM
  B. There is an increased incidence of MVAs in post-call house staff
  C. When patient simulation was used to study sleep deprivation in anesthesia residents, no reduction in clinical performance was demonstrable
  D. After inception of restriction of resident work hours in July 2003, a reduction in patient death rates was shown to be less in hospitals with large numbers of resident physicians versus those with fewer

509. Gabapentin (Neurontin) as used in the treatment of chronic pain belongs to the same broad class of drugs as
A. Carbamazepine
B. Imipramine
C. Clonidine
D. Fluoxetine (Prozac)

510. A 72-year-old man with a history of smoking, hypertension, and CHF undergoes a colonoscopy under sedation. The night before the procedure, he took his bowel prep but omitted his metoprolol and lisinopril. At the end of the procedure, his oxygen saturation is 83% and blood pressure is 175/85 mm Hg, and the electrocardiogram (ECG) shows sinus rhythm with a heart rate of 120. Rales are easily heard in both lung fields. The patient is intubated. Echocardiogram shows 80% ejection fraction (EF). Which of the items below would be **LEAST** helpful in management?
A. PEEP
B. Furosemide
C. Increase FIO_2
D. Esmolol

511. A 47-year-old morbidly obese patient develops bilateral blindness (only able to perceive light) after a 6-hour, three-segment laminectomy and fusion. The patient received 6 units of blood and 5 L of lactated Ringer solution. A mean arterial blood pressure was maintained at 50 to 60 mm Hg. The **MOST** likely structure involved in this visual loss is
A. Central retinal artery
B. Optic nerve
C. Retina
D. Cerebral cortex

512. Each of the following statements regarding postoperative shivering is true **EXCEPT**
A. It may increase metabolism and oxygen consumption significantly
B. It may be treated with meperidine
C. It may be treated with droperidol
D. It does not occur in the absence of hypothermia

513. ECG changes associated with hyperkalemia include
A. Increased P-wave amplitude
B. Shortened PR interval
C. Narrowed and peaked T waves
D. Increase in U-wave amplitude

514. A 53-year-old woman presents to the preoperative evaluation clinic before a scheduled pancreaticoduodenectomy. She complains of a 6-month history of dyspnea on exertion, fatigue, palpitations, chest discomfort, and occasionally feeling "like she is about to faint." She has a 40-pack-year history of smoking and a long history of COPD. She receives oxygen by nasal cannula at night. Jugular venous distention, bilateral pedal edema, an enlarged pulsatile liver, and a high-pitched, holosystolic murmur at the left lower sternal border radiating to the right lower sternal border are all noted on examination. She has suffered multiple pulmonary emboli in the past year and currently takes warfarin. Which of these findings below is most likely to be revealed upon further evaluation?
A. Absence of P2 heart sounds during auscultation of chest
B. Left axis deviation in 12-lead ECG tracing
C. Enlarged aorta in chest x-ray
D. Partial systolic closure of the pulmonary valve during transesophageal echocardiograph (TEE) evaluation

515. Each of the following is associated with acromegalic patients undergoing transsphenoidal hypophysectomy **EXCEPT**
A. Enlargement of the tongue and epiglottis
B. Narrowing of the glottic opening
C. Nasal turbinate enlargement
D. Continuous positive airway pressure (CPAP) should be used postoperatively because obstructive sleep apnea (OSA) is common

516. Evidence of an anaphylactic reaction to atracurium 1 to 2 hours after the episode could be best established by measuring blood levels of
A. Tryptase
B. Laudanosine
C. Histamine
D. Bradykinin

517. Which of the following findings is **NOT** consistent with a diagnosis of MH?
A. $PaCO_2$ 150 mm Hg
B. MVO_2 50 mm Hg
C. pH 6.9
D. Onset of symptoms an hour after end of operation

518. A 52-year-old business executive undergoes a radical retropubic prostatectomy uneventfully under general isoflurane anesthesia. He takes fluoxetine (Prozac) for depression. Upon discharge, which of the following analgesics would be the best choice for postoperative pain management in this patient?
  A. Oxycodone plus aspirin (Percodan)
  B. Hydrocodone with acetaminophen (Vicodin)
  C. Codeine with acetaminophen (Tylenol No. 3)
  D. Hydromorphone (Dilaudid)

519. Anesthesia is induced in a 50-year-old, 125-kg man for anterior cervical fusion. The patient is placed on a ventilator. Peak airway pressure is noted to be 20 cm H_2O with O_2 saturation 99% on pulse oximeter. An hour later, the peak airway pressure rises to 40 cm H_2O and $PaCO_2$ is 38 mm Hg on infrared spectrometer and on O_2 saturation falls to 88%. Blood pressure and heart rate are unchanged. The **MOST** likely cause of these findings is
  A Mainstem intubation
  B Thrombotic pulmonary embolism
  C Tension pneumothorax
  D Venous air embolism

520. The phase of liver transplantation where the greatest degree of hemodynamic instability is expected is
  A. Induction
  B. Dissection phase
  C. Anhepatic phase
  D. Reperfusion phase

521. After closure of the incision for an open hemicolectomy, an abdominal x-ray is performed in the OR that shows a piece of gauze remaining in the abdomen. The surgeon requests neuromuscular blockade to facilitate retrieval of the retained surgical object. You used rocuronium for the case, which you subsequently reversed with sugammadex at closure. Which of the following statements is most likely true?
  A. Administering cisatracurium would result in a faster-than-normal onset and more potent blockade
  B. No neuromuscular blocking agent other than succinylcholine will be effective at this time
  C. Administering rocuronium or vecuronium would result in the most potent neuromuscular blockade
  D. Sugammadex forms inclusion complexes with benzylisoquinolinium neuromuscular blockers

522. Which of the factors in adults listed below is the strongest independent predictor of PONV in most studies?
  A. Female gender
  B. History of PONV
  C. History of migraines
  D. History of cigarette smoking

523. Near the end of a 3-hour colectomy, the surgeon complains that the patient is not relaxed. Two twitch monitors placed at different locations show only one twitch of a train-of-four. Blood gases are reported to be pH 6.9, CO_2 82, K 4.6. The most appropriate action would be
  A. Administer more vecuronium
  B. Administer bicarbonate
  C. Increase minute ventilation
  D. Administer dantrolene

524. A 22-year-old parturient is anesthetized for an emergency laparoscopic cholecystectomy. She is in the twenty-fourth week of gestation and receives general sevoflurane anesthesia and has received rocuronium for muscle relaxation. Just before emergence, muscle relaxation is reversed with glycopyrrolate and neostigmine. Three minutes later, the fetal heart rate falls to 88 beats/min. The **MOST** likely cause of this is
  A. Fetal head compression
  B. Uteroplacental insufficiency
  C. Fetal hypoxia
  D. Reversal agents

525. A 43-year-old woman with end-stage liver disease is admitted to the ICU. Which therapy is **LEAST** likely to improve symptoms associated with hepatic encephalopathy (HE)?
  A. Amino acid–rich total parenteral nutrition (TPN)
  B. Neomycin
  C. Lactulose
  D. Flumazenil

526. Ketorolac is contraindicated in patients undergoing scoliosis surgery because of
  A. Renal effects
  B. Risk of postoperative hemorrhage
  C. Effects on bone healing
  D. Effects on pulmonary function

527. Genetic records show a patient has glucose-6-phosphate deficiency. Which of the drugs below should be avoided during cholecystectomy?
  A. Propofol
  B. Fentanyl
  C. Benzocaine
  D. Bupivacaine

528. Which of the following factors is the greatest predictor of sleep apneas in an adult?
  A. Neck circumference
  B. Micrognathia
  C. Weight
  D. BMI

529. The greatest number of malpractice claims made against anesthesiologists (according to the ASA closed claims task force) is associated with which adverse outcome?
  A. Eye injury
  B. Brain damage
  C. Nerve damage
  D. Death

530. Resynchronization therapy
  A. Is indicated for short QRS complexes
  B. Is contraindicated in patients with CAD
  C. Requires pacemaker implantation
  D. Is usually accomplished with biphasic defibrillator

531. The underlying feature in patients with syndrome X is
  A. Hypertension
  B. Morbid obesity
  C. Hypoglycemia
  D. Insulin resistance

532. A 65-year-old hospitalized patient is being treated for pain from pancreatic cancer and is well controlled on 30 mg IV morphine per day. What is the equivalent total oral daily dosage of morphine in this patient for discharge planning?
  A. 10 mg
  B. 30 mg
  C. 90 mg
  D. 120 mg

533. A 64-year-old patient is brought to the PACU after a 7-hour cosmetic surgery operation under 1.7% sevoflurane anesthesia for the entire case. Which of the following describes the sevoflurane concentration in the vessel-rich group (VRG), the muscle group (MG), and the fat or vessel-poor group (VPG) immediately after the vaporizer is turned off?
  A. VRG: falling, MG: falling, VPG: rising
  B. VRG: falling, MG: rising, VPG: rising
  C. VRG: rising, MG: falling, VPG: falling
  D. All three compartments (VRG, MG, and VPG) falling

534. You have been asked to see a 13-year-old boy in the preoperative area scheduled for tooth extraction under general anesthesia. The nurse caring for him in the preoperative area has noted that the boy is arguing with his parents and repeatedly stating that he does not want to have surgery. Upon your arrival, the parents say to you, "Don't listen to him; he's just being a baby! He is having his surgery today no matter what he says. We want him to have the surgery." The boy states that he "doesn't need his teeth removed. They're fine!" After some discussion you find out that the boy is nervous about needles. You patiently explain the different methods to establish an IV, and the boy eventually expresses understanding and agrees to proceed. What is the most accurate term for the type of cooperation obtained from your patient?
  A. Informed consent
  B. Distraction
  C. Coercion
  D. Informed assent

535. Which of the following nerves is **NOT** derived from a cranial nerve?
  A. Great auricular
  B. Infraorbital
  C. Supratrochlear
  D. Supraorbital

536. A 45-year-old woman is experiencing progressive mental deterioration over a 6-hour period, 5 days after emergency evacuation of a large subarachnoid hemorrhage and clipping of a middle cerebral artery aneurysm. The **MOST** likely cause for deterioration is
  A. Cerebral edema
  B. Improper placement of the aneurysm clip
  C. Recurrent cerebral hemorrhage
  D. Vasospasm

537. The period of vulnerability after three courses of bleomycin for testicular cancer is
  A. 1 month
  B. 1 year
  C. Lifelong
  D. No vulnerability with just three courses

538. The most common adverse cardiac event in the pediatric population is
  A. Hypotension
  B. Bradycardia
  C. Tachycardia
  D. Bigeminy

539. Each of the following is a predictor of difficulty with mask ventilation **EXCEPT**
  A. Presence of beard
  B. BMI greater than 26
  C. Presence of teeth
  D. Age greater than 55

540. In a patient with compartment syndrome, which of the following signs would be the last to appear?
  A. Pulselessness
  B. Pain
  C. Paresthesia
  D. Paralysis

541. Select the **TRUE** statement regarding the dose per kilogram of body weight and duration, respectively, of local anesthetics for spinals in infants compared with adults.
  A. Greater dose and longer duration
  B. Greater dose and shorter duration
  C. Greater dose and duration is the same
  D. Smaller dose and longer duration

542. A number 6 endotracheal tube indicates which size?
  A. 6-mm internal diameter (ID)
  B. 6-mm external diameter
  C. 6-mm external circumference
  D. 6-mm internal circumference

543. If a patient were to become trapped in the magnetic resonance imaging (MRI) scanner by a metal object and the engineers decided to quench the magnet, the greatest hazard to the patient would be
  A. Heat
  B. Cold
  C. Fire
  D. Noise

544. A 25-year-old black man is brought to the emergency room unconscious. Supplemental oxygen is administered, and a pulse oximeter is placed on his finger and a reading of 98% is recorded. Arterial gas sampling at the same time shows PaO_2 of 190 mm Hg, pH 7.2, and O_2 saturation of 90%. Presence of which of the following could explain the discrepancies between these two readings?
  A. Methemoglobin (HbMet)
  B. Sickle cell hemoglobin
  C. Carboxyhemoglobin (HbCO)
  D. Hemoglobin shifted to right

545. During surgery for correction of scoliosis, somatosensory evoked potential (SSEP) monitoring is employed. An increase in SSEP latency and a decrease in amplitude could be explained by each of the following **EXCEPT**
  A. Anterior spinal artery syndrome
  B. Propofol infusion (200 µg/kg/min)
  C. Hypotension
  D. 2 MAC isoflurane anesthesia

546. In which of the following conditions would the response to atropine be **MOST** pronounced?
  A. Diabetic autonomic neuropathy
  B. Brain death
  C. Status post heart transplant
  D. High (C8) spinal anesthesia

DIRECTIONS (Questions 547 through 566): Each group of questions consists of several numbered statements followed by lettered headings. For each numbered statement, select the ONE lettered heading that is most closely associated with it. Each lettered heading may be selected once, more than once, or not at all.

Questions 547-554:

547. Skin lesions all appear at the same stage and at the same time

548. Ciprofloxacin for 60 days is prophylaxis for exposed patients

549. Not contagious

550. Treatment may include streptomycin, gentamicin, or tetracycline

551. Treatment includes trivalent equine antitoxin

552. Three primary types: cutaneous, gastrointestinal, and inhalation

553. Vaccine may prevent or greatly attenuate symptoms if given within 4 days of exposure

554. Hemorrhagic fever
  A. Smallpox
  B. Anthrax
  C. Plague
  D. Botulism
  E. Ebola virus

Questions 555-560:

555. Decreased FEV1/FVC ratio

556. Decreased total pulmonary compliance

557. Increased TLC

558. Decreased FRC

559. Decreased FEV1, normal FEV1/FVC ratio

560. Increased lung compliance due to loss of elastic recoil of the lung
- **A.** Pulmonary emphysema
- **B.** Chronic bronchitis
- **C.** Restrictive pulmonary disease
- **D.** Pulmonary emphysema and chronic bronchitis
- **E.** Pulmonary emphysema and restrictive pulmonary disease

Questions 561-566:

561. Weakness of all muscles below the knee

562. Footdrop; loss of dorsal extension of the toes

563. Weakness of the muscles that extend the knee

564. Inability to adduct the leg; diminished sensation over the medial side of the thigh

565. Most commonly caused by placement of patient into the lithotomy position

566. Numbness over the lateral aspect of the thigh
- **A.** Sciatic nerve injury
- **B.** Common peroneal nerve injury
- **C.** Femoral nerve injury
- **D.** Obturator nerve injury
- **E.** Lateral femoral cutaneous nerve injury

General Anesthesia
Answers, References, and Explanations

418. (B) Patients with insulin-dependent diabetes and non–insulin-dependent diabetes require special consideration when presenting for surgery. Geriatric-age patients come to the OR in the fasting state and without having taken their morning dose of their oral diabetic agent. Chlorpropamide is the longest-acting sulfonylurea and has a duration of action up to 72 hours. Accordingly, it is prudent to measure serum glucose before inducing anesthesia and periodically during the course of the anesthetic and surgery. Regular insulin has a peak effect 2 to 3 hours after SQ administration and a duration of action approximately 6 to 8 hours and would therefore not cause a serum glucose of 35 mg/dL 24 hours after it was administered *(Flood: Stoelting's Pharmacology & Physiology in Anesthetic Practice, ed 5, pp 751–755).*

419. (D) Dibucaine is an amide-type local anesthetic that inhibits normal pseudocholinesterase by approximately 80%. In patients who are heterozygous for atypical pseudocholinesterase, enzyme activity is inhibited by 40% to 60%. In patients who are homozygous for atypical pseudocholinesterase, enzyme activity is inhibited by only 20%. The dibucaine number is a qualitative assessment of pseudocholinesterase. Quantitative as well as qualitative determination of enzyme activity should be carried out in any patient who is suspected of having a pseudocholinesterase abnormality *(Miller: Basics of Anesthesia, ed 7, p 149).*

420. (D) All hypotension can be broadly broken down into two main categories: decreased cardiac output and decreased systemic vascular resistance. Flow or cardiac output can be further subdivided into problems related to decreased heart rate (i.e., bradycardia versus problems related to decreases in stroke volume). Normal PO2 in mixed venous blood is 40 mm Hg. Increased mixed venous arterial oxygen levels can be due to many conditions, including high cardiac output, sepsis, left-to-right cardiac shunts, impaired peripheral uptake (e.g., cyanide), and decreased oxygen consumption (e.g., hypothermia), as well as sampling error. The other choices in this question all represent conditions whereby cardiac output is diminished and consequently would not be consistent with the data given in the question *(Hines: Co-Existing Disease, ed 7, pp 544–545).*

421. (C) Tracheal capillary arteriolar pressure (25-35 mm Hg) is important to keep in mind in patients who are intubated with cuffed endotracheal tubes. If the endotracheal tube cuff exerts a pressure greater than capillary arteriolar pressure, tissue ischemia may result. Persistent ischemia may lead to destruction of tracheal rings and tracheomalacia. Endotracheal tubes with low-pressure cuffs are recommended in patients who are to be intubated for periods longer than 48 hours because this will minimize the chances for development of tissue ischemia *(Miller: Miller's Anesthesia, ed 8, pp 1665–1667).*

422. (C) Enoxaparin, dalteparin, and ardeparin are LMWHs. Because of the possibility of spinal and epidural hematoma in the anticoagulated patient with neuraxial blockade, caution is advised. The plasma half-life of LMWH is two to four times longer than that of standard heparin. These drugs are commonly used for prophylaxis for deep vein thrombosis. These drugs are also used at high doses for treatment of deep vein thrombosis and (off label) as "bridge therapy" for patients chronically anticoagulated with warfarin (Coumadin). In these patients who are being prepared for surgery, Coumadin is discontinued and LMWH started. With high-dose enoxaparin administration (1 mg/kg twice daily), it is recommended to wait at least 24 hours before administration of a single-shot spinal anesthetic *(Miller: Miller's Anesthesia, ed 8, p 1691; Interventional Spine and Pain Procedures in Patients on Antiplatelet and Anticoagulant Medications: Guidelines From the American Society of Regional Anesthesia and Pain Medicine, the European Society of Regional Anaesthesia and Pain Therapy, the American Academy of Pain Medicine, the International Neuromodulation Society, the North American Neuromodulation Society, and the World Institute of Pain May/June 2015 [www.asra.com]).*

423. (C) In patients receiving buprenorphine, a reduced response to perioperative administration of opioids is expected (choice C) due to high-affinity binding of buprenorphine to the mu and kappa opioid receptor. Indications for buprenorphine have expanded to include addiction and chronic pain, thereby presenting a significant challenge to anesthesiologists. Buprenorphine is a semisynthetic, highly lipophilic derivative of thebaine that acts as a partial agonist (agonist-antagonist) with a long biological half-life (37 hours) and a high binding affinity for the mu and kappa opioid receptors, as well as a prolonged dissociation phase. Its pharmacokinetic and pharmacodynamic properties facilitate an extended duration of action while mitigating the opioid "high" frequently experienced with the administration of a pure agonist. At higher doses a ceiling effect is seen, limiting respiratory depression and reducing the abuse potential. Due to its high binding coefficient, once bound to the opioid receptor, it creates a competitive blockade to further agonism by additional exogenous opioid agonists.

Buprenorphine is clinically available compounded with naloxone as a sublingual film. Bioavailability of buprenorphine when administered sublingually is 30% to 50%, whereas oral bioavailability is limited (10%). In contrast, naloxone has ~0% oral and 3% sublingual bioavailability. When coadministered as intended (sublingual dosing), buprenorphine remains clinically active, whereas naloxone is not bioavailable and hence not active. This difference facilitates a dosing strategy that minimizes risk of inadvertent or intentional IV administration of the two agents because naloxone blocks the onset of buprenorphine via competitive blockade. Interestingly, dosing of naloxone in advance of or coadministered at the time of buprenorphine administration is effective in blocking buprenorphine receptor binding, whereas it is ineffective in antagonizing already bound buprenorphine even in high doses (poor efficacy for rescue antagonism in the setting of buprenorphine overdose).

Incorrect Answers: Although metabolized by the liver (via CYP3A4 isozymes of the cytochrome P450 enzyme system), buprenorphine does **NOT** upregulate the cytochrome P450 system (choice A), and naloxone has minimal sublingual bioavailability (choice B). Buprenorphine provides partial opioid agonism via binding to the mu and kappa receptors, but a ceiling effect is seen, limiting the efficacy of additional doses of this agent. Patients taking buprenorphine will continue to require additional analgesia during surgical procedures unless the surgical site is amenable to regional/neuraxial/local analgesia. The response to exogenous opioid agonists will be reduced regardless of its binding coefficient (affinity) due to avid binding of buprenorphine to the receptor (choice D) *(Miller: Miller's Anesthesia, ed 8, pp 1705–1737; Pergolizzi J, Aloisi AM, Dahan A, et al: Current knowledge of buprenorphine and its unique pharmacological profile. Pain Pract 10:428–450, 2010 [PubMed: 20492579]; Davis JJ, Swenson JD, Hall RH, et al: Preoperative "fentanyl challenge" as a tool to estimate postoperative opioid dosing in chronic opioid-consuming patients. Anesth Analg 101:389–395, 2005 [PubMed: 16037150]; Chern SS, Isserman R, Chen L, et al: Perioperative pain management for patients on chronic buprenorphine: a case report. J Anesth Clin Res 3(250), 2012, doi:10.4172/2155-6148.1000250).*

424. (A) The orally administered prodrug codeine (methylmorphine) must be metabolized to morphine in order to work. About 7% to 10% of white patients have an inactive variant of the enzyme CYP2D6, which is the enzyme needed to metabolize codeine. In these patients, as well as in patients who have the normal enzyme but the enzyme is inhibited (e.g., coadministration of quinidine), codeine does not produce analgesia but morphine will produce the expected analgesia. The CYP2D6 enzyme is also needed to metabolize oxycodone into oxymorphone and hydrocodone into hydromorphone. In addition, some patients have a polymorphism form of CYP2D6 that results in very rapid metabolism of codeine and can result in morphine toxicity *(Miller: Miller's Anesthesia, ed 8, pp 574–575).*

425. (D) Patients who have undergone percutaneous coronary intervention (PCI) with and without stents require dual antiplatelet therapy (usually aspirin and clopidogrel) to prevent restenosis or acute thrombosis at the site of the stent, often for the patient's lifetime. Cessation of these drugs should be reviewed with the patient's cardiologist. In general, if the elective surgical procedure may involve bleeding, the elective procedure is delayed for at least 2 weeks after balloon angioplasty without a stent, 6 weeks after a bare-metal stent, and 12 months after a drug-eluting stent has been placed. Then the clopidogrel is stopped and restarted as soon as possible after the surgery (aspirin is usually continued). In an emergency situation and when the patient is taking clopidogrel, platelet transfusion may be needed (effectiveness of platelets depends on the last dose of clopidogrel—platelets are effective after 4 hours but much better 24 hours after the last dose of clopidogrel) *(Miller: Basics of Anesthesia, ed 7, pp 360–361).*

426. (C) Blood flow to the retina can be decreased by either a decrease in mean arterial pressure or an increase in intraocular pressure. Decreased blood flow and stasis are more likely in patients with glaucoma because of their elevated intraocular pressure. During periods of prolonged hypotension, the incidence of retinal artery thrombosis increases in these patients *(Hines: Stoelting's Anesthesia and Co-Existing Disease, ed 7, pp 301–302; Miller: Basics of Anesthesia, ed 7, p 491).*

427. (D) Naloxone (Narcan) is a competitive inhibitor at all opioid receptors but has the greatest affinity for μ receptors. Its duration of action is relatively short (elimination half-life of about 1 hour). For this reason, one must be vigilant for the possibility of renarcotization when reversing long-acting narcotics. Naltrexone (ReVia) is the N-cyclopropylmethyl derivative of oxymorphone, with a long elimination half-life of 8 to 12 hours. It is currently available only as an oral preparation and is used to block the euphoric effects of injected heroin in addicts who have been previously detoxified. Nalmefene (Revex) is another opioid antagonist that can be administered orally or parenterally and has an extremely long duration of action (elimination terminal half-life of 8.5 hours) *(Miller: Miller's Anesthesia, ed 8, pp 906–907).*

428. (A) In the recovery room, the most common cause of postoperative hypoxemia is an uneven ventilation/perfusion distribution caused by loss of lung volume resulting from small airway collapse and atelectasis. Risk factors for ventilation/perfusion mismatch in the postoperative period include old age, obstructive lung disease, obesity, increased intra-abdominal pressure, and immobility. Supplemental oxygen should be administered to keep the PaO_2 in the 80 to 100 mm Hg range, which is associated with a 95% saturation of hemoglobin. Other measures can be taken to restore lung volume, which include recovering obese patients in the sitting position, coughing, and deep breathing *(Barash: Clinical Anesthesia, ed 8, pp 1544–1549).*

429. (D) Airway obstruction after total thyroidectomy may be caused by a postoperative hematoma, compression of the trachea, tracheomalacia, bilateral recurrent laryngeal nerve damage, or hypocalcemia resulting from inadvertent removal of the parathyroid glands. Although the airway symptoms of hypocalcemia can develop as early as 1 to 3 hours after surgery, they typically do not develop until 24 to 72 hours postoperatively. Because the laryngeal muscles are particularly sensitive to hypocalcemia, early symptoms may include inspiratory stridor, labored breathing, and eventual laryngospasm. Therapy consists of IV administration of calcium gluconate or calcium chloride *(Miller: Basics of Anesthesia, ed 6, p 634; Barash: Clinical Anesthesiology, ed 7, p 1330; Hines: Stoelting's Anesthesia and Co-Existing Disease, ed 7, pp 463–464; Barash: Clinical Anesthesia, ed 8, pp 1334–1335).*

430. (A) Damage to the radial nerve is manifested by weakness in abduction of the thumb, inability to extend the metacarpophalangeal joints, wrist drop, and numbness in the webbed space between the thumb and index fingers. The radial nerve passes around the humerus between the middle and lower portions in the spiral groove posteriorly. As it wraps around the bone, the radial nerve can become compressed between it and the OR table, resulting in nerve injury *(Barash: Clinical Anesthesia, ed 8, pp 814, 957–959).*

431. (C) The ASA introduced a physical status classification system to assess the patient's fitness for surgery. It does not consider the risk of the particular surgical procedure. Initially, there were five classes: ASA I = healthy patient, ASA II = patient with mild systemic disease, ASA III = patient with severe systemic disease, ASA IV = patient with severe systemic disease that is a constant threat to life, ASA V = moribund patient who is not expected to survive without the operation. If the surgery was emergent in nature, the letter "E" followed the ASA class. Later, an ASA VI was added for a patient declared brain dead whose organs are being removed for donor purposes.

   Because many anesthesia providers had trouble classifying patients who had moderate disease or had localized and not systemic disease, examples for each ASA class have been suggested.

   ASA I examples include healthy, nonsmoking, and no or minimal alcohol use.

   ASA II examples include current smoker, social alcohol drinker, pregnancy, obesity (30 < BMI < 40), well-controlled diabetes mellitus or hypertension, mild lung disease.

   ASA III examples include poorly controlled diabetes mellitus or hypertension, COPD, morbid obesity (BMI >40), alcohol dependence or abuse, implanted pacemaker, moderate reduction in EF, end-stage renal disease on dialysis, premature infant <60 weeks' postconceptual age, history of myocardial infarction (MI) >3 months, cerebrovascular accident (CVA), transient ischemic attack (TIA), or coronary artery stents.

ASA IV examples include recent MI (<3 months), ongoing cardiac ischemia, severe reduction of EF, sepsis, disseminated intravascular coagulation (DIC), ARDS, or end-stage renal disease not undergoing dialysis.

ASA V examples include ruptured abdominal/thoracic aneurysm, massive trauma, intracranial bleed with mass effect, ischemic bowel in the face of significant cardiac or multiple-organ failure *(ASA website asahq.org [last approved Oct 15, 2014]; Miller: Basics of Anesthesia, ed 7, p 190; Miller: Miller's Anesthesia, ed 8, pp 1144–1145).*

432. (D) Drugs that block dopamine receptors may cause acute dystonic reactions in some patients. The incidence with droperidol is about 1%. Treatment is the administration of a drug that crosses the blood-brain barrier with anticholinergic properties, such as diphenhydramine or benztropine. Although glycopyrrolate is an anticholinergic drug, it would not be useful in this setting because it does not cross the blood-brain barrier *(Miller: Miller's Anesthesia, ed 8, p 2963; Flood: Stoelting's Pharmacology & Physiology in Anesthetic Practice, ed 5, pp 695–696).*

433. (A) Serotonin or 5-hydroxytryptamine (5-HT) is a monoamine neurotransmitter. Granisetron is a selective 5-hydroxytryptamine 3 (5-HT$_3$) antagonist that is used for its antinauseant and antiemetic effects. Other 5-HT$_3$ antagonists include ondansetron (Zofran), dolasetron (Anzemet), palonosetron (Aloxi), and tropisetron (Navoban). The 5-HT$_3$ receptor is an ion channel consisting of five monomers that form a central pore that can be readily permeated by small cations. The 5-HT$_3$ receptors are located in the brain and the gastrointestinal tract. Serotonin is released from the enterochromaffin cells of the small intestine and stimulates vagal afferent neurons through the 5-HT$_3$ receptors, initiating the vomiting reflex. 5-HT$_3$ antagonists are most effective for chemotherapy and radiation induced nausea and vomiting, as well as PONV. They do not work for motion-induced nausea and vomiting because that is a different pathway. Paroxetine (Paxil) is an SSRI used most commonly as an antidepressant but also used as an anxiolytic agent and in patients with post-traumatic stress disorder (PTSD). Other SSRIs include citalopram (Celexa), fluoxetine (Prozac), and sertraline (Zoloft). Milrinone (Primacor) and inamrinone or amrinone (Inocor) are phosphodiesterase 3 (PDE$_3$) inhibitors that decrease cellular cyclic adenosine monophosphate (CAMP) degradation, which results in increased cyclic AMP in cardiac and smooth muscle myocytes. The increase in cyclic AMP improves cardiac output by increasing inotropy and by decreasing both preload and afterload, which is why these medications are often referred to as inodilators. Cyproheptadine (Periactin) is a histamine 1 (H$_1$) receptor antagonist with antihistamine and antiserotonin properties and is used to decrease the symptoms of allergies. Other H1 receptor antagonists include diphenhydramine (Benadryl), cetirizine (Zyrtec), loratadine (Claritin), meclizine (Antivert), and promethazine (Phenergan) *(Brunton: Goodman and Gilman's The Pharmacologic Basis of Therapeutics, ed 12, pp 351, 405–411, 805, 918–924, 1341–1342; Flood: Stoelting's Pharmacology & Physiology in Anesthetic Practice, ed 5, pp 692–697; Miller: Miller's Anesthesia, ed 8, pp 2965–2967).*

434. (D) Pheochromocytoma is an endocrine tumor (with release of catecholamines) in which 90% of patients are hypertensive, 90% of the tumors originate in one adrenal medulla, and 90% of all pheochromocytomas are benign. This disease is rare (<0.1% of hypertension in adults), but when it occurs, it is often seen with a triad of diaphoresis, tachycardia, and headache in patients with hypertension. Other symptoms include palpitations, tremulousness, weight loss, hyperglycemia, hypovolemia, and in some cases dilated cardiomyopathy and CHF. Death as a result of pheochromocytoma is due to cardiac conditions (e.g., MI, CHF) or an intracranial bleed. In about 5% of cases, pheochromocytomas show an autosomal dominant pattern and may coexist with other endocrine diseases, such as medullary carcinoma of the thyroid and hyperparathyroidism. This combination is called multiple endocrine neoplasia (MEN) type II or IIA (Sipple syndrome). MEN type IIB consists of pheochromocytoma, medullary carcinoma of the thyroid, and neuromas of the oral mucosa. The von Hippel-Lindau disease consists of hemangiomas of the nervous system (i.e., retina or cerebellum), and 10% to 25% of these patients also have a pheochromocytoma. The average-sized pheochromocytoma contains 100 to 800 mg of norepinephrine *(Barash: Clinical Anesthesia, ed 8, pp 1340–1343; Hines: Stoelting's Anesthesia and Co-Existing Disease, ed 7, pp 464–467).*

435. (D) Oral agents that are used to help control hyperglycemia in type 2 diabetic patients (relative β-cell insufficiency and insulin resistance) include four major drug classes:
   1. drugs that stimulate insulin secretion (hypoglycemia is a risk)

    a. sulfonylureas

        i. first-generation (chlorpropamide, tolazamide, tolbutamide)

        ii. second-generation (glimepiride, glipizide, glyburide)

    b. meglitinides (repaglinide, nateglinide)

2. Drugs that decrease hepatic gluconeogenesis (hypoglycemia not a risk)

    a. biguanides (metformin)

3. Drugs that improve insulin sensitivity (hypoglycemia not a risk)

    a. thiazolidinediones (rosiglitazone, pioglitazone)

    b. glitazones

4. Drugs that delay carbohydrate absorption (hypoglycemia not a risk)

    a. α-glucosidase inhibitors (acarbose, miglitol)

    Only drugs that stimulate insulin secretion are a risk for producing hypoglycemia.

    Initial therapy is usually with second-generation sulfonylureas (more potent and fewer side effects than first-generation sulfonylureas) or with a biguanide *(Hines: Stoelting's Anesthesia and Co-Existing Disease, ed 7, pp 451–455; Flood: Stoelting's Pharmacology & Physiology in Anesthetic Practice, ed 5, pp 751–755; Powers AC, D'Alessio D: Endocrine pancreas and pharmacotherapy of diabetes mellitus and hypoglycemia. In: LL Brunton et al., eds. Goodman & Gilman's The Pharmacological Basis of Therapeutics, ed 13, New York, NY: McGraw-Hill).*

436. (C) Although early mild symptoms of alcohol withdrawal can be seen within 6 to 8 hours after a substantial drop in the serum alcohol levels, DTs, which is seen in about 5% of patients, is a life-threatening medical emergency that develops 2 to 4 days after the cessation of alcohol in alcoholics. Symptoms of DTs include hallucinations, combativeness, hyperthermia, tachycardia, hypertension or hypotension, and grand mal seizures. Treatment of severe alcohol withdrawal consists of fluid replacement, electrolyte replacement, and IV vitamin administration with particular attention paid to thiamine. Aggressive administration of benzodiazepines is indicated to prevent seizures (5-10 mg of diazepam every 5 minutes until the patient becomes sedated but not unconscious). β-Blockers are used to suppress overactivity of the sympathetic nervous system, and lidocaine may be effective in the treatment of cardiac dysrhythmias *(Hines: Stoelting's Anesthesia and Co-Existing Disease, ed 7, pp 622–623).*

437. (A) Operations on the trachea may be indicated in patients who have tracheal tumors or in patients who had a previous trauma to the trachea resulting in tracheal stenosis or tracheomalacia. Eighty percent of the operations on the trachea involve segmental resection with primary anastomosis, 10% involve resection with prosthetic reconstruction, and another 10% involve insertion of a T-tube stent. These operations frequently are very complicated and require constant communication between the surgeon and the anesthesiologist. Preoperative pulmonary function tests are indicated in all patients who are to undergo elective tracheal resection. Severe lung disease necessitating postoperative mechanical ventilation is a relative contraindication for tracheal resection because positive airway pressure may cause wound dehiscence *(Miller: Miller's Anesthesia, ed 8, pp 1987–1988).*

438. (B) Hypercalcemia is associated with a number of signs and symptoms, including hypertension, dysrhythmias, shortening of QT interval, kidney stones, seizure, nausea and vomiting, weakness, depression, personality changes, psychosis, and even coma. Generally, patients with total serum calcium levels of 12 mg/dL or less do not require any intervention, with the possible exception of rehydration with saline. Higher calcium levels may be associated with clinical symptoms and should be treated before anesthetizing the patient. Caution should be taken with (rarely used) digitalis administration to any patient who is hypercalcemic because some patients may exhibit extreme digitalis sensitivity (Miller: Miller's Anesthesia, ed 8, p 1794; Barash: Clinical Anesthesia, ed 8, pp 411–412, 1406–1407).

NORMAL CALCIUM LEVELS

	Serum Calcium	**Serum Ionized Calcium**
Conventional units (mEq/L)	4.5-5.5 mEq/L	2.1-2.6 mEq/L
Conventional units (mg/dL)	9.0-11.0 mg/dL	4.25-5.25 mg/dL
SI units (mmol/L)	2.25-2.75 mmol/L	1.05-1.30 mmol/L

439. (D) Red-top eye drops cause mydriasis and should be used with caution in patients with closed-angle glaucoma. Green-top eye drops cause miosis, and the pupillary constriction helps keep the drainage route open in patients with glaucoma and helps prevent an acute attack of glaucoma. Clear or white-top eye drops do not change pupillary size.

440. (D) When reviewing growth curves, the normal 40-week term newborn weighs about 3.5 kg. Infants then double their birth weight by 5 months and triple their weight by 1 year. Therefore the average 1-year-old weighs 10 kg (22 lb). From the age of 1 to 6 years, children gain about 2 kg per year. Thus an average 2-year-old weighs 12 kg, 3-year-old weighs 14 kg, 4-year-old weighs 16 kg, 5-year-old weighs 18 kg, and 6-year-old weighs 20 kg. From age 6 to 10 years, children gain about 3 kg per year *(Davis: Smith's Anesthesia for Infants and Children, ed 9, Appendix B, pp e7–e14)*.

441. (C) PKU is a rare inherited defect in the metabolism of the amino acid phenylalanine. Newborns are routinely screened for PKU by looking for an increased level of phenylalanine in the bloodstream. Patients with PKU should have a diet low in foods that contain phenylalanine.

Patients with mitochondrial myopathies have problems with energy metabolism. Complications of muscle function, such as respiratory failure, cardiac depression, cardiac conduction defects, and dysphagia, may be seen. Neurologic signs and symptoms are often present. Higher doses of vitamins and other supplements such as coenzyme Q are often used.

Most patients with epilepsy are well controlled with antiepileptic medications. However, if the epilepsy is not well controlled, a ketogenic diet is often tried, which can reduce the frequency of seizures in some patients. A ketogenic diet consists of a high-fat, low-carbohydrate, and low-protein diet. Normally the body uses carbohydrates for the energy source, but in a low- carbohydrate diet, fat becomes a main source of energy production. Ketones are formed when the fat is converted into energy. The ketogenic diet predisposes the patient to metabolic acidosis.

Glycogen storage diseases reflect enzyme defects. Hypoglycemia and lactic acidosis can occur with short periods of fasting.

(Cote: A Practice of Anesthesia for Infants and Children, ed 6, pp 568–580; Cottrell, Patel: Neuroanesthesia, ed 6, p 303; Davis: Smith's Anesthesia for Infants and Children, ed 9, pp 1182–1184; Hines: Stoelting's Anesthesia and Co-Existing Disease, ed 7, p 383).

442. (C) Therapies aimed at increasing FRC of the lungs are useful in reducing the incidence of postoperative pulmonary complications. Forced expiratory maneuvers may lead to airway closure, which would be of no benefit for this patient (Miller: Miller's Anesthesia, ed 8, pp 447, 2932–2934).

443. (D) Continuous quality improvement (CQI) programs to improve patient outcomes are often oriented to three components: namely, the process of care (the sequence of care, such as sequence and coordination of activities), the structure of care (the setting where the care was administered), and the outcome of health care (change in the health status of the patient). In the process measure, a protocol, such as the timely administration of antibiotics to decrease surgical site infections or the administration of a beta-adrenergic blocker within 24 hours of admission for an MI, has been implemented. Although following the protocols has generally resulted in performance improvement, clinical outcomes have not consistently improved, and some of the process measures have been rescinded, such as administration of a beta-adrenergic blocker within 24 hours of admission for an MI.

Structural measures to improve outcome, such as having electronic health records (EHRs), appropriate nurse/patient ratios, having physicians in the hospital 24 hours every day for emergencies, and hand washing, are easy to measure. Clearly improved outcomes with these changes are hard to measure.

Postoperative outcomes are affected by many factors; intraoperative care is one of these. There is great variability in patients' underlying health, as well as considerable practice variation, which may greatly impact outcome measures *(Barash: Clinical Anesthesia, ed 8, pp 100–101; Miller: Basics of Anesthesia, ed 7, pp 824–825)*.

444. (B) PEEP is the maintenance of positive airway pressure during the entire ventilator cycle. The addition of PEEP to the ventilator cycle is often recommended when PaO_2 is not maintained above 60 mm Hg, when breathing an FIO_2 of 0.50 or greater. Although not completely understood, PEEP is thought to increase arterial oxygenation, pulmonary compliance, and FRC by expanding previously collapsed but perfused alveoli, thereby decreasing shunt and improving ventilation/perfusion matching. An important adverse effect of PEEP is a decrease in arterial blood pressure caused by a decrease in venous return, left ventricular filling and stroke volume, and cardiac output. These effects are exaggerated in patients with decreased intravascular fluid volume. Other potential adverse effects of PEEP include pneumothorax, pneumomediastinum, and subcutaneous emphysema *(Miller: Miller's Anesthesia, ed 8, pp 3077–3078; Miller: Basics of Anesthesia, ed 7, p 667).*

445. (A) Platelets contain two purinergic receptors (P2Y$_1$ and P2Y$_{12}$). Clopidogrel (Plavix) is a prodrug and an irreversible inhibitor of platelet P2Y$_{12}$ receptors, which blocks the ADP receptors and inhibits platelet activation, aggregation, and degranulation. There is wide interindividual variability for clopidogrel to inhibit ADP-induced platelet aggregation, and some patients are resistant to its effects. Glycoprotein IIb/IIIa inhibitors block fibrinogen binding to platelet glycoprotein IIb/IIIa receptors, which is the final common pathway of platelet aggregation and includes the IV drugs abciximab (ReoPro), eptifibatide (Integrilin), and tirofiban (Aggrastat). Aspirin, naproxen, and ibuprofen inhibit platelet COX-1 and inhibit the release of ADP by platelets and platelet aggregation. Selective COX-2 inhibitors such as celecoxib, parecoxib, and valdecoxib have no effect on platelet function because only COX-1 inhibitors affect platelet function. Direct thrombin inhibitors suppress platelet function and include the parenteral drugs hirudin, argatroban, lepirudin (Refludan), desirudin (Iprivask), bivalirudin (Angiomax), and drotrecogin α (Xigris), as well as the oral drug dabigatran (Pradaxa, Pradax) and ximelagatran *(Hogg K, Weitz JI: Blood coagulation and anticoagulant, fibrinolytic, and antiplatelet drugs. In: Brunton LL, Hilal-Dandan R, Knollmann BC, eds. Goodman & Gilman's The Pharmacological Basis of Therapeutics, ed 13, New York, NY: McGraw-Hill; Miller: Basics of Anesthesia, ed 7, p 359; Flood: Stoelting's Pharmacology & Physiology in Anesthetic Practice, ed 5, pp 656–657).*

446. (B) As a rough approximation, if one divides 150 by the MAC for any given volatile anesthetic, the quotient will be approximately equal to the oil/gas partition coefficient. For example, if one were to divide the MAC of halothane (0.75) into 150, the quotient would be 200, which is very close to the actual oil/gas partition coefficient for halothane (224). Similarly, if one were to divide the MAC of enflurane (1.68) into 150, the quotient would be 89, which is very similar to the oil/gas partition coefficient for enflurane (98). The fact that anesthetics with a high oil/gas partition coefficient (i.e., lipid-soluble agents) have lower MACs supports the Meyer-Overton theory (critical volume hypothesis) *(Flood: Stoelting's Pharmacology & Physiology in Anesthetic Practice, ed 5, pp 107–108).*

447. (A) The HHS developed the Health Insurance Portability and Accountability Act of 1996 (HIPAA) (Public Law 104-191). HIPAA's Privacy Rule set national standards for the protection of an individual's health information by health plans, health care clearinghouses, and health care providers, as well as for the security of the electronic medical record. HIPAA's Security Rule requires certain precautions so that the information is used only for legitimate purposes and only by those with proper authority. HIPAA's Breach Notification Rule requires health care providers and organizations to report any breach to the affected individuals, the HHS, and, in some cases, the media *(hhs.gov website for professionals HIPAA - Public Law 104-191; Miller: Basics of Anesthesia, ed 7, pp 22–23).*

448. (B) The principal feature of Alzheimer disease is progressive dementia. The onset typically occurs after age 60 years and may affect as many as 20% of patients older than age 80 years. In addition to age, other risk factors include history of serious head trauma (e.g., boxing), Down syndrome, and presence of the disease in a parent or sibling. One biochemical feature of this disease is a decrease in the enzyme choline acetyltransferase in the brain. There is a strong correlation between reduced enzyme activity and decreased cognitive function. Interestingly, administration of the anticholinergic drugs scopolamine or atropine (but not glycopyrrolate, which does not cross the blood-brain barrier) causes confusion similar to that seen in the early stages of Alzheimer disease. Conversely, anticholinesterase drugs capable of penetrating the blood-brain barrier, such as donepezil (Aricept), galantamine, rivastigmine (Exelon), and tacrine, are used to treat patients with Alzheimer disease. Physostigmine may have beneficial effects in some patients as well. Scopolamine is therefore a poor choice for premedication in patients with Alzheimer disease *(Butterworth: Morgan & Mikhail's Clinical Anesthesiology, ed 5, pp 619–620; Hines: Stoelting's Anesthesia and Co-Existing Disease, ed 7, p 293).*

449. (A) The likelihood of anesthetic recall under the condition cited above is very unlikely, but not impossible. Risk factors for intraoperative recall include history of previous recall event. Other risk factors include emergency surgery, cesarean section, cardiopulmonary bypass, history of alcohol or opiate abuse, total levothyronine anesthesia (TIVA), and difficult airway. Disputing the patient's claim of a recall event may alienate the individual and make the probability of a lawsuit more likely *(Miller: Basics of Anesthesia, ed 7, pp 816–817).*

450. (A) Complete or almost complete cessation of urine flow suggests a postrenal obstruction. However, at times, pooling of the urine in the dome of the bladder should be considered as a possible cause of oliguria in this patient, in the absence of significant bleeding (Miller: Miller's Anesthesia, ed 8, pp 556–557).

451. (B) D_L is defined as the diffusing capacity of the lung. When a nontoxic, low concentration of carbon monoxide is used for the measurement, it is called D_{LCO}. The normal value of D_{LCO} is 20 to 30 mL/min/mm Hg and is influenced by the volume of blood (hemoglobin) within the pulmonary circulation. Thus diseases associated with a decrease in pulmonary blood volume (i.e., anemia, emphysema, hypovolemia, pulmonary hypertension) will be reflected by a decrease in the D_{LCO}. D_{LCO} is also decreased with oxygen toxicity, as well as pulmonary edema. Conditions associated with an increased D_{LCO} include the supine position, exercise, obesity, and left-to-right cardiac shunts *(Miller: Miller's Anesthesia, ed 8, p 365; Barash: Clinical Anesthesia, ed 8, pp 378, 1033–1034).*

452. (C) Patients undergoing thyroid surgery are at risk for airway obstruction from a number of causes. Postoperative hemorrhage sufficient to cause a large hematoma could compress the trachea and cause airway obstruction because of the close proximity of the thyroid gland to the trachea. Permanent hypoparathyroidism is a rare complication that may cause hypocalcemia, leading to progressive stridor followed by laryngospasm. The most common nerve injury after thyroid surgery is damage to the abductor fibers of the recurrent laryngeal nerve. Unilaterally, this is manifested as hoarseness. Bilateral recurrent laryngeal nerve damage, however, may lead to airway obstruction during inspiration. Selective injury of the adductor fibers of the recurrent laryngeal nerve is a possible complication of thyroid surgery. This injury would leave the vocal cords open because the abductor fibers would be unopposed, placing the patient at great risk for aspiration. The superior laryngeal nerve has an extrinsic branch that innervates the cricothyroid muscle (which tenses the vocal cords) and an internal branch that provides sensory innervation to the pharynx above the vocal cords. Bilateral damage to this nerve would result in hoarseness and would predispose the patient to aspiration, but would not lead to airway obstruction per se *(Miller: Basics of Anesthesia, ed 7, p 469).*

453. (D) MH is a clinical syndrome that may develop rapidly or take hours to manifest, sometimes not occurring until the patient is in the recovery room. Clinical signs include hypertension, tachycardia, respiratory acidosis, metabolic acidosis, muscle rigidity, myoglobinuria, and fever. The diagnosis of MH is unlikely, however, if only one of these signs is manifested. Because MH is a metabolic disorder, one of the first sensitive signs is an increase in the production of CO_2 and concomitant respiratory acidosis. This is the most reliable early sign of the syndrome *(Barash: Clinical Anesthesia, ed 8, pp 479–480, 622–624).*

454. (D) Hyperventilation to $PaCO_2$ of 20 mm Hg or higher for more than 2 hours will result in active transport of HCO_3- out of the central nervous system (CNS). This results in spontaneous breathing at a lower (not higher) $PaCO_2$. The other choices should be included in the differential diagnosis of apnea *(Barash: Clinical Anesthesia, ed 8, pp 370–371; Miller: Basics of Anesthesia, ed 7, pp 62–64, 340).*

455. (B) MVV is a nonspecific pulmonary function test that measures the endurance of the ventilatory muscles and indirectly reflects the compliance of the lung and thorax, as well as airway resistance. A decreased MVV may be caused by impairment to inspiration or expiration. In this patient, FEV1 is normal, which strongly suggests that the ventilatory impairment is during inspiration. A flow-volume loop would be a very useful confirmatory test *(Barash: Clinical Anesthesia, ed 8, pp 1032–1033).*

456. (A) Guidelines for safe discharge of patients from ambulatory surgical centers include stable vital signs, ability to walk without dizziness, controlled pain, absence of nausea and vomiting, and minimal surgical bleeding. The PADSS is a tool for objectively assessing a patient's readiness for discharge from the surgical center and includes these five criteria. Requirements to drink fluids and to void before home discharge are controversial and are not parameters included in the PADSS *(Barash: Clinical Anesthesia, ed 8, pp 1542–1543).*

457. (C) MH is a difficult diagnosis to make on clinical grounds alone. Signs of MH may be fulminant or very subtle. They may occur immediately after induction or may not be manifested until the patient has reached the recovery room or even later. MH is a disorder of metabolism and is associated with hypertension, tachycardia, dysrhythmias, respiratory acidosis, metabolic acidosis, muscular rigidity, rhabdomyolysis, and fever. Contrary to what one might believe based on the name of this disease, fever is typically a late finding. Other diseases that may mimic MH include alcohol withdrawal, acute cocaine toxicity, bacteremia, pheochromocytoma, hyperthyroidism, and neuroleptic malignant syndrome. An elevation in temperature alone with normal blood gases, heart rate, and blood pressure and with no evidence of muscle breakdown would very likely not be due to MH. If a patient had been previously subjected to muscle biopsy and caffeine-halothane contracture testing with negative results, MH would be exceedingly rare, although a false-negative result is possible. A history of a previous anesthetic without MH triggering would be of little reassurance in a patient in whom an MH episode is suspected. It is not uncommon for MH-susceptible individuals not to trigger when a triggering anesthetic is administered initially but to develop fulminant MH with a subsequent anesthetic *(Barash: Clinical Anesthesia, ed 8, pp 622–624).*

458. (D) Asthma is an inflammatory illness that has bronchial hyperreactivity and bronchospasm as a result. Treatment is first directed at the inflammatory component as the underlying problem, reserving bronchodilators for symptomatic use. Because leukotrienes may function as inflammatory mediators, the leukotriene pathway inhibitors such as zileuton and the leukotriene receptor antagonist montelukast (Singulair) are being used for treatment of asthma. Zileuton and montelukast are available only as oral preparations, whereas the other drugs listed are given by inhalation. Fluticasone and triamcinolone are anti-inflammatory corticosteroids. Ipratropium is a quaternary ammonium compound formed by the introduction of an isopropyl group to the N atom of atropine and produces effects similar to those of atropine. One unexpected finding is a relative lack of effect on mucociliary clearance, which makes it useful in patients with airway disease, especially if parasympathetic tone of the airways is increased. Salmeterol is a β2-selective adrenergic drug *(Barnes PJ: Pulmonary pharmacology. In: Brunton LL, Hilal-Dandan R, Knollmann BC, eds. Goodman & Gilman's The Pharmacological Basis of Therapeutics, ed 13, New York, NY: McGraw-Hill; Flood: Stoelting's Pharmacology & Physiology in Anesthetic Practice, ed 5, p 593).*

459. (D) Acute decreases in serum sodium due to absorption of bladder irrigating fluids rarely cause symptoms unless the sodium level drops below 120 mEq/L. At this level, tissue edema may develop and clinical neurologic signs (e.g., restlessness, nausea, confusion, seizures, and coma) or ECG changes (e.g., widening of the QRS complex, elevation of the ST segment, ventricular tachycardia, or ventricular fibrillation) may be manifested. Treatment of mild decreases in serum sodium (i.e., 120-135 mEq/L with no neurologic or ECG changes) is by fluid restriction and/or administration of a diuretic such as furosemide. When the sodium level drops below 120 mEq/L and neurologic symptoms or changes in the ECG develop, sodium chloride administration is needed. To calculate the amount needed, one multiplies the patient's total body water (i.e., 0.6 × body weight = TBW) by the change in sodium desired. In this case the TBW is 60 L (0.6 × 100 kg) and the change of sodium is 10 mEq (120 mEq/L - 110 mEq/L); thus 60 L × 10 mEq/L = 600 mEq. Caution is advised in administering sodium because too rapid administration may lead to demyelinating CNS lesions. The recommended rate of 3% sodium chloride (513 mEq/L) is 1 to 2 mL/kg/hr. Serum sodium levels should be checked at least every hour until the sodium level increases above 120 mEq/L *(Barash: Clinical Anesthesia, ed 8, pp 399–403).*

460. (B) In a patient having convulsive seizures, your first phase is stabilization. You start with the basics (Circulation, Airway, Breathing) and administer oxygen by nasal cannula, face mask, and consider intubation if needed. In addition, you monitor the patient's ECG, start an IV, obtain a blood sugar, and consider a drug screen. If the blood sugar is less than 60 mg/dL, administer glucose. If the seizure does not stop within 5 minutes, anticonvulsant medications are started. First-line medications include a benzodiazepine (e.g., midazolam, lorazepam, or diazepam) and, if a benzodiazepine is not available, phenobarbital. If the seizure continues, a second-line medication such as fosphenytoin, valproic acid, or levetiracetam is administered. If the seizure still continues, either repeat second-line medications or use thiopental, pentobarbital, or propofol. If at any time the seizure stops, symptomatic care is given. Although dexmedetomidine has sedative properties, it has no anticonvulsant activity *(American Epileptic Society - Guideline for the Treatment of Prolonged Seizures in Children and Adults, Feb 9, 2016; Miller: Basics of Anesthesia, ed 7, p 114).*

461. (B) Ketamine is unique among the IV induction agents in that it usually produces cardiac stimulation manifested by increased heart rate, mean arterial pressure, and cardiac output. Ketamine is believed to have a centrally mediated sympathetic nervous system stimulating effect. This effect is, however, not related to dose. In isolated rabbit and canine hearts and in intact dogs, ketamine has been demonstrated to produce myocardial depression. Clinically, however, the myocardial depressant properties of ketamine are overridden by its sympathetic nervous system stimulating properties. When systemic catecholamines have been depleted or when the patient is under deep anesthesia, the myocardial depressant properties of ketamine may predominate *(Flood: Stoelting's Pharmacology & Physiology in Anesthetic Practice, ed 5, p 189)*.

462. (C) In the normal muscle cell, depolarization results in release of calcium from the sarcoplasmic reticulum. The increased intracellular calcium concentration results in muscle contraction. The calcium then is rapidly taken up via calcium pumps back into the sarcoplasmic reticulum, resulting in relaxation. Both the release and reuptake of calcium are energy-requiring processes (i.e., result in the hydrolysis of adenosine triphosphate [ATP]). Dantrolene, the pharmacologic treatment for MH, blocks release of calcium from the sarcoplasmic reticulum without affecting the reuptake process. The defect in MH is thought to be decreased control of intracellular calcium stores, preventing muscle relaxation *(Barash: Clinical Anesthesia, ed 8, pp 622–624)*.

463. (D) Approximately 4% of patients treated with bleomycin develop pulmonary toxicity, which manifests as severe pulmonary fibrosis and hypoxemia. Death from severe pulmonary toxicity occurs in approximately 1% to 2% of patients treated with bleomycin. Patients who are at greater risk for bleomycin-induced pulmonary toxicity include elderly patients, those receiving more than 200 to 400 mg, those with coexisting lung disease, and those recently exposed to bleomycin. In addition, there is evidence that prior radiotherapy and possibly receipt of enriched concentrations of O_2 (i.e., inspired oxygen >30%) during surgery increase risk of pulmonary toxicity. Clinically, patients gradually develop dyspnea, a nonproductive cough, and hypoxemia, and pulmonary function tests typically demonstrate changes in gas flow and lung volumes consistent with restrictive pulmonary disease. If radiographic evidence such as bilateral diffuse interstitial infiltrates appears, pulmonary fibrosis usually is irreversible *(Flood: Stoelting's Pharmacology & Physiology in Anesthetic Practice, ed 5, pp 817–818)*.

464. (C) Head flexion can advance the tube up to 1.9 cm toward the carina and in some cases convert an endotracheal intubation into an endobronchial intubation. Extension of the head has the opposite effect and can withdraw the tube up to 1.9 cm, resulting in extubation of some patients. Turning the head laterally can move the distal tip of the endotracheal tube about 0.7 cm away from the carina. The Trendelenburg position causes a cephalad shift of the mediastinum and can cause the endotracheal tube to migrate distally as well *(Miller: Basics of Anesthesia, ed 7, p 242)*.

465. (C) Sulfur hexafluoride is sometimes injected in the vitreous in patients with a detached retina to mechanically facilitate reattachment. To prevent changes in the size of the gas bubble, the patients should be given 100% O_2 15 minutes before injection of sulfur hexafluoride. If these patients are anesthetized with general anesthesia within 10 days, N_2O should not be given because N_2O can diffuse into the gas bubble, increasing intraocular pressure, and may result in blindness *(Barash: Clinical Anesthesia, ed 8, pp 1390–1391)*.

466. (D) The symptoms of hypocalcemia, which manifest as laryngospasm or laryngeal stridor, usually develop within the first 24 to 96 hours after total thyroidectomy. After the airway is established and secured, the patient should be treated with IV calcium in the form of either calcium gluconate or calcium chloride *(Barash: Clinical Anesthesia, ed 8, pp 409–411)*.

467. (C) Because the circulating levels of T_3 and T_4 regulate TSH release from the anterior pituitary gland by a negative feedback mechanism, a normal plasma concentration of TSH confirms a euthyroid state. The pharmacologic treatment of choice for patients with hypothyroidism is sodium levothyroxine (T_4). triiodothyronine, (T_3) and desiccated thyroid are alternate therapeutic agents *(Barash: Clinical Anesthesia, ed 8, pp 1328–1332)*.

468. (A) Large quantities of irrigating fluid can be absorbed during transurethral resection of the prostate gland because the open venous sinuses in the prostate allow the irrigation fluid to be absorbed. On average, from 10 to 30 mL of fluid per minute are absorbed, and during long cases this can amount to several liters, causing hypertension, reflex bradycardia, and pulmonary congestion. Treatment consists of fluid restriction and a loop diuretic (e.g., furosemide) when the $[Na^+]$ level is greater than 120 mEq/L. Rarely does the amount of fluid absorbed cause significant hyponatremia ($[Na^+] < 120$ mEq/L). In these cases of significant hyponatremia, 3% sodium chloride may be infused slowly IV (in addition to the loop diuretic and fluid restriction) until the sodium level reaches 120 mEq/L *(Barash: Clinical Anesthesia, ed 8, pp 1428–1430)*.

469. (C) Patients who have sustained thermal injuries are at risk for massive potassium release and potential cardiac arrest if succinylcholine is administered 24 hours or more after they sustain the burn, and they remain at risk until the burn has healed. This increased sensitivity to succinylcholine is thought to be related to proliferation of extrajunctional receptors. These same receptors are thought to be related to the increased requirement for nondepolarizing neuromuscular blocking agents in these patients *(Barash: Clinical Anesthesia, ed 8, pp 1522–1523)*.

470. (A) The facial nerve (seventh cranial nerve) runs within the substance of the parotid gland and might become damaged during parotid surgery. The facial nerve innervates the lacrimal, submandibular, and sublingual glands, is sensory to the anterior two thirds of the tongue, and innervates all of the muscle of facial expression (including the orbicularis oculi—close the eyelids; orbicularis oris—purse the lips; frontalis—raise the eyebrows).

The trigeminal nerve (fifth cranial nerve) innervates the muscles of mastication (masseter, temporalis, medial and lateral pterygoids), which are used to clench the teeth *(Orient: Sapira's Art and Science of Bedside Diagnosis, ed 4, pp 533–537; Miller: Basics of Anesthesia, ed 7, pp 489, 497; Miller: Miller's Anesthesia, ed 8, p 2513)*.

471. (D) One gram of hemoglobin can combine with 1.34 mL of O_2. None of the other choices in this question will do as much to increase the O_2-carrying capacity of this patient's blood as a transfusion *(Flood: Stoelting's Pharmacology & Physiology in Anesthetic Practice, ed 5, p 576)*.

472. (A) Many of the drugs commonly administered during surgery and anesthesia have the potential to evoke allergic reactions (e.g., morphine, propofol, local anesthetics, antibiotics, and protamine, as well as other materials used during surgery, such as vascular graft material, chymopapain, and latex). Virtually all drugs administered IV have been reported to cause allergic reactions. Possible exceptions include benzodiazepines and ketamine. An allergic reaction should be considered when there is an abrupt fall in blood pressure accompanied by increases in heart rate that exceed 30% of the control values. Greater than 60% of all drug-induced allergic reactions observed during the perioperative period are attributable to muscle relaxants. Latex allergy is thought to be responsible for 15% of allergic reactions under anesthesia, sometimes including reactions originally attributed to other substances. Patients at risk for latex allergy include health care workers and patients with spina bifida. Although most drug-induced allergic reactions develop within 5 to 10 minutes of exposure, latex signs typically take more than 30 minutes to develop *(Hines: Stoelting's Anesthesia and Co-Existing Disease, ed 7, pp 576–577)*.

473. (C) Decreased levels of pseudocholinesterase have been reported in patients with Huntington chorea. For this reason, the effects of succinylcholine may be prolonged in some of these patients. It has been suggested that the sensitivity to nondepolarizing muscle relaxants is also increased *(Hines: Stoelting's Anesthesia and Co-Existing Disease, ed 7, p 295)*.

474. (A) Normal intraocular pressure is 10 to 22 mm Hg. In general, IV anesthetics, with the possible exception of ketamine, decrease intraocular pressure. In addition, nondepolarizing neuromuscular blockers, inhaled anesthetics, narcotics, carbonic anhydrase inhibitors, osmotic diuretics, and hypothermia decrease intraocular pressure. However, elevation of $PaCO_2$ out of the physiologic range, as seen with hypoventilation as well as arterial hypoxemia, will increase intraocular pressure. Depolarizing neuromuscular blockers, such as succinylcholine, also increase intraocular pressure. This increase in intraocular pressure occurs when succinylcholine is administered IM or IV. Pretreatment with a nondepolarizing muscle relaxant before administering succinylcholine may attenuate the rise in intraocular pressure. The mechanism for the increase in intraocular pressure after succinylcholine use is related to drug-induced cycloplegia rather than contraction of extraocular muscles, as this increase in intraocular pressure will occur even if the intraocular muscles are cut. The greatest increase in intraocular pressure occurs with coughing or vomiting, where the intraocular pressure may increase as much as 35 to 50 mm Hg. The proposed mechanism for the acute increase in intraocular pressure is an increase in venous pressure. There does not appear to be a change in intraocular pressure with changes within normal physiologic ranges in arterial blood pressure or $PaCO_2$ *(Barash: Clinical Anesthesia, ed 8, pp 1377–1378).*

475. (C) The AHI is used to quantify the number of apnea or hypopnea episodes that occur per hour. Apnea is defined as no ventilation for periods of 10 seconds or more. Hypopnea is defined as a 50% decrease in airflow or a decrease sufficient to cause a decrease in oxygen saturation of 4%. An AHI of greater than 30 signifies severe OSA *(Lobato: Complications in Anesthesiology, p 625; Miller: Miller's Anesthesia, ed 8, pp 312–314, 2203).*

476. (B) Andexxa, (coagulation factor Xa [recombinant], inactivated-zhzo) is a specific antidote for direct factor Xa inhibitors. These include rivaroxaban, edoxaban and betrixaban. There is also a specific reversal for Dabigatran, idarucizumab, sold as Praxabind. Enoxaparin can be reversed with protamine, but clopidogrel has no specific reversal agent. (www.fda.gov; *Miller: Basics of Anesthesia, ed 7, pp 387–388).*

477. (A) Measured PaO_2 should be decreased about 6% for each degree Celsius cooler the patient's temperature is than the electrode (37° C). Because the patient is 2° C cooler than the electrode, a 12% decrease (9 mm Hg) would be expected in this patient (77 mm Hg − 9 mm Hg = 68 mm Hg) *(Miller: Basics of Anesthesia, ed 7, pp 338–339).*

478. (A) The two main causes of central cyanosis are decreased arterial oxygen saturation and hemoglobin abnormalities (e.g., methemoglobinemia and sulfhemoglobinemia). Sulfasalazine (Azulfidine) can cause the formation of sulfhemoglobin. Sulfhemoglobin, like methemoglobin, may cause low O_2 saturation in the face of high PaO_2. There is no treatment for sulfhemoglobinemia except to wait for the destruction of the erythrocytes *(Hines: Stoelting's Anesthesia and Co-Existing Disease, ed 7, pp 368–370, 486).*

479. (D) Unfractionated heparin is a mixture of highly sulfated glycosaminoglycans with molecular weights of 5000 to 30,000 daltons. The onset of action of unfractionated heparin is immediate, the plasma half-life is ½ hour to 2 hours, and it can be completely reversed with protamine. Clinically, monitoring of anticoagulation is usually performed with the activated PTT (aPTT) test with a target prolongation of 1.5 to 2 times control. When unfractionated heparin is used for cardiopulmonary bypass, the doses are much higher and it is monitored with the activated clotting time, or ACT test (>400 seconds is usually considered safe for cardiopulmonary bypass). LMWHs are 4000 to 5000 daltons in size, the onset of action is 20 to 60 minutes, the plasma half-life is 4.5 hours, and it can only be partially reversed (65%) with protamine. Monitoring the LMWH's effects is not performed, because the PT and the aPTT tests are most often unaffected. LMWHs have a much lower risk for HIT compared with the unfractionated heparin *(Miller: Basics of Anesthesia, ed 7, p 358; Miller: Miller's Anesthesia, ed 8, pp 1872–1873).*

480. (B) Serum creatinine is inversely proportional to the GFR. With the increase in creatinine by a factor of 4, the GFR is cut in half twice; that is, 120/2 = 60 60/2 = 30 mL/min *(Miller: Miller's Anesthesia, ed 8, pp 558–559; Lobato: Complications in Anesthesiology, p 433).*

481. (A) Trisomy 21 or Down syndrome is the most common human chromosomal syndrome seen. An increased incidence of congenital hypothyroidism occurs. About one fourth of children with Down syndrome and many adults have smaller tracheas than predicted and require an endotracheal tube that is one or two sizes smaller. One should avoid unnecessary flexion or extension of the neck during intubation because occipito-atlantoaxial instability occurs in about 15%-20% of patients. Because subluxation is relatively uncommon, routine neck radiographs for all Down syndrome patients are excessive. More than 40% of Down syndrome children have congenital heart disease (e.g., endocardial cushion defects, ventricular septal defects, tetralogy of Fallot, patent ductus arteriosus). Although some children have hypotonia, an increased incidence of MH has not been reported in these patients *(Hines: Stoelting's Anesthesia and Co-Existing Disease, ed 7, pp 664–666).*

482. (B) Scopolamine is an anticholinergic that may produce mydriasis and cycloplegia. This can result in the inability of a patient's eyes to accommodate *(Flood: Stoelting's Pharmacology & Physiology in Anesthetic Practice, ed 5, p 196).*

483. (D) Neuroleptic malignant syndrome is a potentially fatal disease that affects 0.5% to 1% of all patients being treated with neuroleptic (antipsychotic) drugs. The syndrome develops gradually over 1 to 3 days in young males and is characterized by the following: (1) hyperthermia, (2) skeletal muscle rigidity, (3) autonomic instability manifested by changes in blood pressure and heart rate, and (4) fluctuating levels of consciousness. The mortality from neuroleptic malignant syndrome is 20% to 30%. Liver transaminases and creatine phosphokinase levels are often elevated in these patients. Treatment includes supportive care and administration of dantrolene. This disease may mimic MH because of its many similarities. One difference between neuroleptic malignant syndrome and MH is the fact that nondepolarizing muscle relaxants such as vecuronium or cisatracurium will cause flaccid paralysis in patients with neuroleptic malignant syndrome but not in patients with MH *(Hines: Stoelting's Anesthesia and Co-Existing Disease, ed 7, pp 618, 666–669).*

484. (C) In the setting of vasodilatory shock states (e.g., septic shock, post cardiopulmonary bypass, late stages of hemorrhagic shock), exogenous vasopressin has been reported to be a potent vasopressor. This is thought to be due to dysfunctional baroreceptor reflex–mediated signal in the setting of vasodilatory shock, resulting in reduced secretion of endogenous vasopressin coupled with an overall deficiency of endogenous vasopressin. The administration of vasopressin results in a potent vasoconstrictor response under these circumstances. High doses of vasopressin administered to healthy subjects presumed to have normal plasma levels of vasopressin did not result in a vasopressor effect, further supporting the aforementioned theory. Vasopressin acts on V1 receptors to increase cytosolic calcium levels via the inositol triphosphate (IP3) second messenger system. However, in the pulmonary vasculature vasopressin has been found to cause pulmonary vasodilation via the induction of endothelial nitric oxide release, making vasopressin unique among vasopressors *(Morales DL, et al.: A double-blind randomized trial: prophylactic vasopressin reduces hypotension after cardiopulmonary bypass. Ann Thorac Surg 75:926–930, 2003; Braun EB, Palin CA, Hogue CW: Vasopressin during spinal anesthesia in a patient with primary pulmonary hypertension treated with intravenous epoprostenol. Anesth Analg 99:36–37, 2004).*

485. (C) Remifentanil is an ultrashort-acting narcotic. Chemically it is a derivative of piperidine (like fentanyl), but remifentanil has an ester linkage and is rapidly broken down by nonspecific plasma, as well as tissue esterases. The elimination half-life is less than 20 minutes and is best administered by a continuous infusion. Pseudocholinesterase deficiency or renal or hepatic failure does not affect remifentanil's rapid metabolism *(Barash: Clinical Anesthesia, ed 8, p 516; Flood: Stoelting's Pharmacology & Physiology in Anesthetic Practice, ed 5, p 238).*

486. (D) A term infant with a strong cry and good muscle tone does not require oxygen therapy based on a 5-minute saturation alone. The fetal lungs make a rapid transition from a fluid-filled organ to an air-filled organ. As the zones of atelectasis open, the saturation rises. The table below shows acceptable preductal oxygen saturation as a function of time.

Minutes	Preductal Oxygen Saturation
1	60%-65%
2	65%-70%
3	70%-75%
4	75%-80%
5	80%-85%
10	85%-95%

From Wyckoff M, Aziz K, Escobedo M, et al: 2015 American Heart Association Guidelines Update for Cardiopulmonary Resuscitation and Emergency Cardiovascular Care, Circulation 132:S543–S560, 2015.

487. (C) Anesthesia for extracorporeal shock wave lithotripsy may be accomplished with either general anesthesia or epidural anesthesia. When a patient is submerged in the stainless steel tub, the peripheral vasculature becomes compressed by the hydrostatic pressure, resulting in an increase in preload. Removing the patient from the tank has the opposite effect. In patients who have received epidural anesthesia, there is an increased incidence of hypotension caused by epidural-induced sympathectomy after they emerge from the bath *(Miller: Basics of Anesthesia, ed 7, p 627)*.

488. (A) The most common reason for unexpected hospital admission after outpatient general anesthesia, as well as a prolonged recovery-room stay (for both adults and children), is nausea and vomiting. Two other reasons for a prolonged recovery-room stay are pain and drowsiness *(Barash: Clinical Anesthesia, ed 8, pp 858, 860)*.

489. (A) Cholinergic crisis can be differentiated from myasthenic crisis by administering small IV doses of anticholinesterases. With a cholinergic crisis, there are significant muscarinic effects (e.g., salivation, bradycardia, miosis) and an accentuated muscle weakness. Because this patient's V_T (tidal volume) decreased with the administration of edrophonium, the diagnosis of cholinergic crisis is made. Although atropine may be needed to treat the cholinergic symptoms, muscle weakness will be worse and these patients need to be intubated until the muscle strength returns *(Hines: Stoelting's Anesthesia and Co-Existing Disease, ed 7, pp 521–524)*.

490. (C) Tramadol, a synthetic codeine analog, is a centrally acting analgesic. It can be used for mild to moderate pain but is not as effective as morphine or meperidine for severe or chronic pain. One drawback for tramadol's perioperative use is its high incidence of nausea and vomiting. Its mechanism of action for analgesia is complex. It is a weak μ-receptor agonist, it inhibits serotonin and norepinephrine reuptake, and it enhances serotonin release. Tramadol-induced analgesia is not entirely reversed with naloxone; however, the respiratory depression and sedation can be reversed. Ondansetron, a serotonin antagonist, may interfere with part of tramadol's analgesic action. Because of its low μ-receptor agonist activity, it may be less likely to produce physical dependence than other stronger narcotics. Seizures have been reported in patients receiving tramadol alone. The drug should be used with caution in patients taking drugs that lower the seizure threshold, such as tricyclic antidepressants and SSRIs. It has some monoamine oxidase (MAO) inhibiting activity and should not be used in patients taking MAO inhibitors. Another warning is its use in patients who are depressed or suicidal. Tramadol is not recommended in depressed or suicidal patients because excessive doses, either alone or with other CNS depressants including alcohol, are a major cause of drug-related deaths, with fatalities reported within the first hour of overdosage. Patients who are depressed or suicidal are better managed with nonnarcotic analgesics *(Physicians' Desk Reference 2009, ed 63, pp 2428–2431; Flood: Stoelting's Pharmacology & Physiology in Anesthetic Practice, ed 5, p 241; Yaksh T, Wallace M: Opioids, analgesia, and pain management. In: Brunton LL, Hilal-Dandan R, Knollmann BC, eds. Goodman & Gilman's The Pharmacological Basis of Therapeutics, ed 13, New York, NY: McGraw-Hill; FDA Black Box Warning on Ultram and Suicide Risk)*.

491. (A) The null hypothesis states that there is no difference between two groups of data, while the alternative hypothesis states the opposite or that there is a difference between the groups. The P value is derived from a test statistic and is the probability that we could have observed a difference if in reality the null hypothesis was true and there was not a difference. If the P value is less than a predetermined level of significance (the α value, often set at = 0.05) then the null hypothesis (no difference) is rejected and the differences observed are stated to be statistically significant (P < 0.05). It can then be stated that it is unlikely (calculated to be less than a 1 in 20 probability) that the differences detected in the two groups occurred by random chance or that the null hypothesis was true. When the P value is less than α but there actually is not a difference between the groups, it is called a type 1 error.

On the other hand, if no statistically significant differences are detected (P value $> α$), we accept that the null hypothesis (no difference exists) is true. If we accept the null hypothesis when the alternative hypothesis (there is a difference) is in fact true, a type 2 error has occurred. Type 2 errors are related to the power of the study. Power is the probability of rejecting the null hypothesis (no difference) when a specific alternative hypothesis (difference) is correct. Power is related to the magnitude of the difference to detect, the variability of the data, the α level, and the sample size. Often a power of 0.8 is selected, meaning that we accept an 80% probability that the null hypothesis (no difference) is true or that there is also a 20% chance that a difference does exist but was not observed. Larger sample sizes make it easier to observe that a difference exists and increase the power of an analysis *(Miller: Miller's Anesthesia, ed 8, pp 3250–3251).*

492. (D) In the absence of diuretics, oliguria associated with urine sodium concentration greater than 40 mEq/L and urine osmolality less than 400 mOsm/L is strongly suggestive of intrinsic renal disease (e.g., acute tubule necrosis), whereas prerenal causes have urine sodium concentration less than 20 mEq/L and urine osmolality greater than 400 mOsm/L. Furosemide, mannitol, and dopamine, however, obscure the accurate diagnosis *(Hines: Stoelting's Anesthesia and Co-Existing Disease, ed 7, pp 428–432; Miller: Basics of Anesthesia, ed 7, pp 450–452).*

493. (B) In the United Kingdom, the National Institute of Academic Anaesthesia Health Services Research Centre developed a project called SNAP-1 (Sprint National Anaesthesia Project) with two goals. The first goal was to look at patient satisfaction, and the second goal was to access patient awareness when undergoing anesthesia in nonobstetric adults (>18 years of age). This project was conducted over 2 days and included 15,040 patients in 257 hospitals throughout the UK (May 13-14, 2014). The project used the Brice Questionnaire (developed in the 1970), which consisted of six questions.
   1. What is the last thing you remember before going to sleep?
   2. What is the first thing you remember after waking up?
   3. Do you remember anything between going to sleep and waking up?
   4. Did you dream during the procedure?
   5. Were your dreams disturbing to you?
   6. What was the worst thing about your operation?
   35% of patients reported severe discomfort in at least one domain (thirst 18.5%, surgical pain 11%, drowsiness 10%). Accidental awareness during general anesthesia (AAGA) occurred in 0.12% of patients (1:800). Interestingly, only 5% of patients reported any dissatisfaction with their care *(Miller: Basics of Anesthesia, ed 7, pp 812–813; Walker EMK, et al. Patient reported outcome of adult perioperative anesthesia in the United Kingdom: a cross-sectional observational study. BJA 117:758–766, 2016; www.niaa-hsrc.org.uk).*

494. (C) MAC is the minimum alveolar concentration of anesthetic that will prevent movement of 50% of patients when a skin incision is made at sea level (e.g., San Diego). MAC × 1.3 will prevent movement in 95% of patients. In this question, total gas flow is 4 L/min (1 L/min + 3 L/min). Roughly 75% of the total gas is N_2O. The MAC of N_2O is 104%. The patient is receiving about 0.75 MAC N_2O. The MAC for isoflurane is 1.15. A concentration of 0.85% would represent 0.75 MAC. Because MACs are additive, the total MAC would be 1 *(Miller: Basics of Anesthesia, ed 7, p 89; Barash: Clinical Anesthesia, ed 8, pp 468–470).*

495. (D) Cardiac output increases by about 100 mL/min for each kilogram of weight gained. It is estimated that every kilogram of adipose tissue contains nearly 3000 m of additional blood vessels. The additional cardiac output is due to ventricular dilation and increased stroke volume, as resting heart rates are not increased in obese patients *(Miller: Basics of Anesthesia, ed 7, pp 92–93).*

496. (D) IV anesthetics tend to be lipophilic and after an IV bolus are preferentially partitioned into the highly perfused lipophilic tissues (e.g., brain and spinal cord), which helps to explain the rapid onset of action.

The termination of the anesthetic effect is related to its redistribution into the less perfused and inactive tissues (e.g., muscle and adipose tissue). After a 2 mg/kg bolus dose of propofol into a healthy adult, the peak plasma concentration of 7 to 8 μg/mL is reached in less than 1 minute. The blood level then falls to the therapeutic range of 1.5 to 5 μg/mL by about 2 minutes. Then it takes about 8 minutes to become subtherapeutic. Keep in mind that the therapeutic effect reflects the concentration of the drug at the site of action (e.g., brain for propofol), not the blood concentration. Therefore the awakening time reflects the brain tissue concentration, not the actual blood level *(Barash: Clinical Anesthesia, ed 8, pp 828–831; Miller: Basics of Anesthesia, ed 7, pp 104–106).*

497. (B) Ideally, factor VIII levels should be raised to 100% predicted before elective surgery to ensure that the levels will not fall below 30% intraoperatively. Fifty percent of the normal factor VIII concentration or greater is thought to be necessary for a patient who is to undergo minor surgery; it is 80% to 100% for major surgery. Elimination half-time of factor VIII is 12 hours. This may be accomplished with factor VIII concentrate (preferred) or cryoprecipitate or with fresh frozen plasma in areas with limited resources *(Miller: Basics of Anesthesia, ed 7, p 381).*

498. (A) Hemophilia A is associated with decreased levels of factor VIII. PTT tests the intrinsic coagulation cascade and would be abnormally elevated in all but the mildest disease. A normal PTT is 25 to 35 seconds. Platelet count, PT, and bleeding times are normal (see also explanation to Question 395) *(Miller: Basics of Anesthesia, ed 7, pp 379, 385).*

499. (D) Propofol is a rapidly metabolized, highly fat soluble IV anesthetic. A typical patient will fall asleep with a single dose of 2.0 mg/kg and will awaken in 8 to 10 minutes. As shown in the graph below, the blood level of this drug will begin falling about 1 minute after the dose is injected, yet the cytosol concentration in some tissues will continue to rise for several minutes. This concept is referred to as "redistribution" and is true of all IV anesthetic induction agents because they all share high lipid solubility.

There is an apparent contradiction regarding tissue concentration. If propofol is so fat soluble, wouldn't fat be the first place it would go? The explanation is simple.

The reason the brain intracellular concentration rises so quickly (relative to most other tissues) is because of the high portion of cardiac output the brain receives (25%). At the 1-minute mark, after bolusing, the blood concentration starts falling because the liver and other organs are rapidly metabolizing the drug. Other tissues with relatively poor blood flow continue to take up propofol because uptake is dependent on the concentration gradient. Although the blood level is declining 1 minute after bolus injection, it is still higher than the concentration found in, for example, fat, and the intracellular propofol concentration in fat tissue will continue to rise. It's all about gradient.

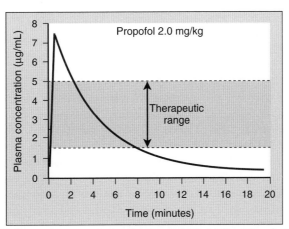

(From Bokoch MP, Eilers H: Intravenous anesthetics. In: Pardo MC, Miller RD, eds. Basics of Anesthesia, *ed 7, Elsevier, 2018, pp 104–122.)*

500. (B) Inferior ischemia is associated with blockage or spasm of the right coronary artery. The right coronary artery supplies blood to the atrioventricular node in 90% of patients. Complete heart block therefore is not unexpected in patients with severe CAD involving the right coronary artery *(Hines: Stoelting's Anesthesia and Co-Existing Disease, ed 7, pp 101–102).*

501. (B) MAC is influenced by a variety of disease states, conditions, drugs, and other factors. Drugs that increase CNS catecholamines, such as MAO inhibitors, tricyclic antidepressants, acute amphetamine ingestion, and cocaine, increase MAC. Other factors that increase MAC include hyperthermia, hypernatremia, patients with natural red hair, and infancy. It is interesting that MAC values are higher for infants than for neonates or older children and adults. Thyroid gland dysfunction, including hyperthyroidism, does not affect the MAC. Factors that lower MAC include narcotics, IV anesthetics, local anesthetics (except cocaine) and other sedatives, age (6% per decade), hypothermia, hypoxia, and severe anemia (e.g., Hgb <5). The following table modified from the references in this question summarizes the impact of various factors on MAC *(Barash: Clinical Anesthesia, ed 7, pp 458–459; Butterworth: Morgan & Mikhail's Clinical Anesthesiology, ed 5, p 164; Miller: Basics of Anesthesia, ed 7, p 86).*

IMPACT OF PHYSIOLOGIC AND PHARMACOLOGIC FACTORS ON MINIMUM ALVEOLAR CONCENTRATION (MAC)

No Change in MAC	Increase in MAC	Decrease in MAC
Duration of anesthesia Type of surgery Hyperthyroidism Hypothyroidism Gender Hyperkalemia	Drugs that increase CNS catecholamines (MAO inhibitors, tricyclic antidepressants, acute amphetamine use, cocaine, ephedrine) Chronic ethanol abuse Hyperthermia Hypothermia Infants Patients with natural red hair	CNS depressants (narcotics, IV anesthetics, chronic amphetamine use) Acute ethanol use Hypernatremia Hyponatremia Increasing age Pregnancy Hypoxia

CNS, central nervous system; MAO, monoamine oxidase.

Data from Barash: Clinical Anesthesia, *ed 7, Lippincott, Williams & Wilkins, 2013, pp 458–459; Butterworth:* Morgan & Mikhail's Clinical Anesthesiology, *ed 5, McGraw Hill, 2013, p 164; Miller:* Basics of Anesthesia, *ed 7, Philadelphia, Elsevier, 2017, p 86.*

502. (B) Long-term lithium therapy in patients with manic-depressive illness may be associated with nephrogenic diabetes insipidus. Hypothyroidism may develop in about 5% of patients because lithium can inhibit the release of thyroid hormones. Lithium is almost 100% renally excreted. Reabsorption occurs at the proximal convoluted tubule and is inversely related to the concentration of sodium in the glomerular filtrate. Consequently, administration of diuretics (mainly thiazide, but to a lesser extent loop diuretics) may lead to the development of toxic lithium levels. Lithium has sedative properties and may reduce the need for IV and inhalational anesthetic agents. It may prolong the duration of action of both pancuronium and succinylcholine, but it is not associated with an exaggerated release of potassium when succinylcholine is administered *(Brunton: Goodman & Gilman's The Pharmacological Basis of Therapeutics, ed 12, pp 448–449; Hines: Stoelting's Anesthesia and Co-Existing Disease, ed 7, pp 617–618; Miller: Basics of Anesthesia, ed 7, p 165).*

503. (D) Carcinoid tumors can arise wherever enterochromaffin cells are present. Most (>70%) originate in the intestine, and about 20% originate in the lung. Of those that originate in the gastrointestinal tract, 50% occur in the appendix, 25% in the ileum, and 20% in the rectum. These interesting tumors were called carcinoid because they were originally believed not to metastasize. We now know this is not true. The hormones released by the nonmetastatic tumors reach the liver by the portal vein and are rapidly inactivated. However, once metastases reach the liver, the released hormones reach the systemic circulation and produce signs and symptoms of the "carcinoid syndrome." Symptoms include cutaneous flushing, abdominal pain, vomiting, diarrhea, hypotension or hypertension, bronchospasm, and hyperglycemia. The natural hormone somatostatin suppresses the release of serotonin and other vasoactive substances from the tumor. Because the half-life is about 3 minutes, somatostatin is given by infusion. Octreotide is a synthetic somatostatin analog with a half-life of 2.5 hours and is given SQ or IV for the prevention and treatment of carcinoid symptoms (e.g., hypotension, hypertension, bronchospasm). However, the treatment of hypotension in patients with carcinoid disease is different because ephedrine, epinephrine, and norepinephrine can release vasoactive hormones from the tumor and make the hypotension worse. Hypotension is best treated with fluids and IV octreotide or somatostatin. Hypertension is treated with deepening the anesthetic and administering octreotide, somatostatin, or labetalol. Bronchospasm is treated with IV octreotide, somatostatin, or nebulized ipratropium. When giving anesthesia to these patients, it is probably wise to avoid drugs that release histamine and other vasoactive hormones that may precipitate symptoms. Propofol or etomidate are good induction agents, followed by maintenance anesthesia with a volatile anesthetic (e.g., isoflurane, sevoflurane, or desflurane) and/or nitrous oxide with oxygen. Vecuronium, cisatracurium, and rocuronium appear to be safe muscle relaxants. Fentanyl, sufentanil, alfentanil, remifentanil, and benzodiazepines are also safe to use. The serotonin antagonist ondansetron is a useful antiemetic *(Miller: Miller's Anesthesia, ed 8, p 1210)*.

504. (A) New diagnostic criteria for sepsis are based on the quick Sequential Organ Failure Assessment (qSOFA) score. A patient exhibiting two of the three criteria below (a SOFA score >2) is associated with an in-hospital mortality of 10%. Lactate is not included in SOFA scoring.
qSOFA Criteria
Respiratory rate teriate
Altered mentation
Systolic blood pressure riaSOFA sc
(Singer M, Deutschman C, Seymour C: The Third International Consensus Definitions for Sepsis and Septic Shock (Sepsis-3). JAMA 315(8):801–810, 2016).

505. (D) The Glasgow Coma Scale has three categories: eye opening, for which a maximum of 4 points can be received; best verbal response, for a maximum of 5 points; and best motor response, for a maximum of 6 points. The higher the score, the better the response; the minimal score for each category is 1. Mild head injury scores are 13 to 15, moderate are 9 to 12, and severe are 3 to 8. This severe head-injured patient is totally unresponsive and would receive a score of 3 *(Miller: Basics of Anesthesia, ed 7, p 729)*.

506. (A) Insulin metabolism involves both the liver and kidneys. Renal dysfunction, however, has a greater impact on insulin metabolism than does hepatic dysfunction. In fact, unexpected prolonged effects of insulin sometimes are seen in patients with renal disease *(Rabkin R, Ryan MP, Duckworth WC: The renal metabolism of insulin. Diabetologia 27:351–357, 1984)*.

507. (B) Most pulse oximeters illuminate tissue with two wavelengths of light: 660-nm red light and 940-nm infrared light. Because carboxyhemoglobin has an absorbance at 660 nm, very similar to O2 hemoglobin, it produces a falsely elevated SaO_2 when present in the blood. Hemoglobin F, bilirubin, and fluorescein dye have no effect on pulse oximetry. Methylene blue, as well as indigo carmine and indocyanine green, lowers the SaO_2 as measured by pulse oximetry. Methemoglobin absorbs red and infrared light equally well and gives saturation readings of 85% (Miller: Basics of Anesthesia, ed 7, p 341).

508. (D) On March 4, 1984, Libby Zion, an 18-year-old college freshman, was admitted with a high fever, dehydration, and chills to a New York hospital and died within a day. The cause of her death was widely believed to be due to a drug interaction between phenelzine, which she had taken for depression, and meperidine, which was used to calm her down. This led to a serotonin syndrome and more agitation. During the night, her temperature rose to 107° F (42° C), and she suffered a cardiac arrest and could not be resuscitated. Cocaine had been detected in her body and may have contributed to her death as well. This case was used to exemplify the fact that the intern and residents taking care of her were overworked, and this eventually led to New York State Department of Health Code, Section 405, known as the Libby Zion Law, which limits the amount of work for residents to 80 hours per week. In 2003 the Accreditation Council for Graduate Medical Education (ACGME) adopted regulations for medical training in the United States. Since then, studies have looked at fatigue and clinical performance. A major peak in vulnerability occurs between 2 AM and 7 AM, with a smaller peak in the midafternoon. Single-occupant MVAs occur more frequently in the morning. Although patient simulation of the effects of sleep deprivation have been studied, psychomotor performance and mood have been affected, but clinical performance was not affected. No difference in mortality rates were seen in the 2 years before compared with the 2 years after the 2003 guidelines were put into effect, and no difference in mortality was noted when large teaching programs (thought to be the most affected) were compared with smaller programs *(Lerner: A Life-Changing Case for Doctors in Training, New York Times, August 14, 2011; Miller: Miller's Anesthesia, ed 8, p 3239; New York State Department of Health Code, Section 405, known as the Libby Zion Law)*.

509. (A) Gabapentin, an anticonvulsant, was developed to be a centrally active γ-aminobutyric acid (GABA) agonist but does not appear to interact with GABA receptors. Its mechanism for producing analgesia is unclear, but it may involve inhibition of voltage-activated calcium channels, as well as potentiating GABA release. Carbamazepine slows the recovery rate of voltage-gated sodium channels, but it also is an anticonvulsant. Carbamazepine is indicated in the treatment of trigeminal neuralgia *(Benzon: Essentials of Pain Medicine, ed 3, pp 123–129; Hemmings: Pharmacology & Physiology, p 200).*

510. (B) In evaluating this patient in heart failure (e.g., rales), one observes that the EF is high (e.g., 80%), after-load is high (e.g., elevated systolic blood pressure), and the heart rate is high (e.g., 120 beats/min). Although he has diffuse rales (often a sign of high preload and fluid overload), this patient is actually dehydrated from his bowel prep, and his left ventricle does not fill properly. To compensate for the low filling volume, the heart rate increases. Patients with heart failure with preserved EF (HFpEF), previously called diastolic heart failure, have signs of left-sided heart failure. To better understand this, think of the heart as a hydraulic pump that you need to not only empty effectively (during systole) but also need to fill effectively (during diastole). So in this case, your main goals are to slow the heart rate to allow the left ventricle adequate time to fill (e.g., with a β-blocker such as esmolol) and to better oxygenate him (e.g., increase the FIO_2 and add PEEP). The diuretic furosemide would exacerbate the situation. Other conditions in which the left ventricle does not fill effectively include less compliant ventricular walls (e.g., thick from long-standing hypertension or aortic valve stenosis, fibrotic walls), less room to fill (e.g., cardiac tamponade), loss of the atrial kick (e.g., atrial fibrillation), and valvular stenosis (e.g., mitral stenosis) *(Miller: Basics of Anesthesia, ed 7, p 196).*

511. (B) Perioperative visual loss associated with nonocular surgery is rare and may result from corneal trauma, retinal artery occlusion, retinal vein occlusion, optic nerve ischemia, or cortical disease. Although overall it is a rare problem, it may develop in up to 1% of prone spinal surgical cases and is most commonly due to ischemic optic neuropathy. The cause is unknown and multifactorial. Associated factors include prolonged intraoperative hypotension, anemia (Hgb <8), large intraoperative blood loss, prolonged surgery, and facial edema. It is more common in males and in patients with peripheral vascular disease, diabetes mellitus, and in tobacco users *(Miller: Miller's Anesthesia, ed 8, pp 3011–3012; Miller: Basics of Anesthesia, ed 7, p 334).*

512. (D) Postoperative shivering or postanesthetic tremor can occur during recovery from all types of general anesthesia. If profound, shivering can increase metabolic rate and O2 consumption (100%-200%) with an associated increase in cardiac output and minute ventilation. Although shivering usually occurs in patients with decreased body temperature, it also may occur in patients with normal body temperature after anesthesia. Postanesthesia shivering is best treated by a combination of supplemental oxygen, rewarming the patient, and/or administering IV meperidine. Other less frequently used pharmacologic treatments include clonidine, magnesium sulfate, calcium chloride, chlorpromazine, droperidol, and other opioids (e.g., butorphanol). Application of radiant heat to the face, head, neck, chest, and abdomen has been shown to eliminate shivering within minutes in postoperative patients, despite low core body temperatures *(Miller: Basics of Anesthesia, ed 7, p 687).*

513. (C) The ECG signs of hyperkalemia include narrowed and peaked T waves (earliest manifestation of hyperkalemia), decrease in P-wave amplitude, prolonged PR interval, and a widened QRS interval. In extreme cases, the ECG can appear as a sine wave as well as cardiac arrhythmias (e.g., sinus arrest, supraventricular tachycardia, atrial fibrillation, premature ventricular contractions, ventricular tachycardia, and ventricular fibrillation). These changes are potentiated by hypocalcemia, and IV calcium can rapidly correct some of these ECG changes. An increase in U-wave amplitude suggests hypokalemia, not hyperkalemia *(Miller: Miller's Anesthesia, ed 8, pp 1205–1206; Miller: Basics of Anesthesia, ed 7, pp 349–351).*

514. (D) This patient's history and physical are strongly suggestive of right-sided heart failure secondary to pulmonary hypertension. The combined effects of hypoxia, inflammation, and loss of capillaries in COPD are thought to result in pulmonary vascular remodeling and, over time, increases in pulmonary arterial pressure. Additionally, this patient may be exhibiting signs of chronic thromboembolic pulmonary hypertension secondary to chronically elevated pulmonary vascular pressures due to excessive embolic burden. The clinical assessment for patients with pulmonary hypertension is notable for the presence of

P2 heart sounds on auscultation, right axis deviation on ECG, partial systolic closure of the pulmonary valve during TEE evaluation, and mean pulmonary arterial pressures exceeding 25 mm Hg at rest or exceeding 30 mm Hg with exercise *(Fischer LG, Van Aken H, Bu H: Management of pulmonary hypertension: physiologic and pharmacologic considerations for anesthesiologists. Anesth Analg 96:1603–1616, 2003; Chaouat A, Naeije R, Weitzenblum E: Pulmonary hypertension in COPD. Eur Respir J 32:1371–1385, 2008).*

515. (D) Enlargement of the tongue and epiglottis predisposes the patient to upper airway obstruction and makes visualization of the vocal cords more difficult. The vocal cords are enlarged, making the glottic opening narrower. In addition, subglottic narrowing may be present as well as tracheal compression from an enlarged thyroid (seen in about 25% of acromegalic patients). This often necessitates the use of a narrower endotracheal tube than one might choose based on the facial enlargement. The placement of nasal airways may be more difficult due to the enlarged nasal turbinates. The use of CPAP is contraindicated after transsphenoidal hypophysectomy *(Hines: Stoelting's Anesthesia and Co-Existing Disease, ed 7, p 472).*

516. (A) There are four types of immune-mediated allergic reactions. Anaphylaxis is a type I IgE-mediated reaction that involves mast cells and basophils. Anaphylactoid reactions appear like anaphylaxis but are not immune mediated. Tryptase is a neutral protease normally stored in mast cells but is released into systemic circulation during anaphylactic but not anaphylactoid reactions. Tryptase levels would need to be measured within 1 to 2 hours of the suspected allergic reaction. Plasma histamine levels return to baseline within 30 to 60 minutes of an anaphylactic reaction. Laudanosine is a normal metabolic product of atracurium metabolism *(Hines: Stoelting's Anesthesia and Co-Existing Disease, ed 7, pp 575–576).*

517. (B) Signs of MH reflect the hypermetabolic state (up to 10 times normal) that develops. Clinical signs include tachycardia, tachypnea, arterial hypoxemia, hypercarbia (e.g., $PaCO_2$ 100-200 mm Hg), metabolic and respiratory acidosis (e.g., pH 6.80-7.15), hyperkalemia, hypotension, muscle rigidity, trismus after succinylcholine administration, and increased body temperature. Mixed venous oxygen tension would be very low. The clinical presentations are quite variable, and some reactions may not develop until the postoperative period *(Hines: Stoelting's Anesthesia and Co-Existing Disease, ed 7, pp 665–667).*

518. (D) The SSRI fluoxetine is one of the most potent inhibitors of the cytochrome P-450 enzymes CYP3A4 and CYP2D6. CYP2D6 facilitates the conversion of codeine to morphine, meaning that the response from a "normal" dose would be less than expected because of decreased conversion. Oxycodone and hydrocodone are metabolized by CYP2D6 to their active form as well, and a "normal" dose of these would give less response than expected. Thus codeine, oxycodone, and hydrocodone would be poor analgesic choices for patients taking SSRIs. CYP3A4 is responsible for the metabolism of fentanyl, sufentanil, and alfentanil. Remifentanil is metabolized by nonspecific plasma esterases *(Miller: Basics of Anesthesia, ed 7, pp 132–133).*

519. (A) Symptoms of a mainstem or bronchial intubation include asymmetric chest expansion, unilateral breath sounds, elevation of peak airway pressures, and ABG abnormalities (e.g., hypoxemia). Frequently, bronchial intubation is intentional (e.g., thoracic surgery with double-lumen endotracheal tubes), but, if undetected with a single-lumen tube, atelectasis, hypoxia, and pulmonary edema may result in time. Peak airway pressures can also increase with many conditions such as airway obstruction (e.g., kinked endotracheal tube, secretions, overinflated cuffs), bronchospasm, increasing VT, increase in chest wall muscle tone (rigid chest with narcotics, coughing), and tension pneumothorax. If a tension pneumothorax develops, associated hypotension usually is present. Pulmonary embolism would not cause the peak airway pressure to rise, as in this case *(Lobato: Complications in Anesthesiology, pp 101–102).*

520. (D) Although hemodynamic instability can occur at any time during liver transplantation, it is during the initial part of the reperfusion phase, when the vascular clamps are removed from the liver graft, when cardiovascular instability is most marked. At this time there can be profound hypotension, reduced cardiac contractility, cardiac arrhythmias, and hyperkalemic cardiac arrest. Epinephrine, atropine, calcium, and sodium bicarbonate, as well as blood products, should be available during this critical part of the surgery *(Miller: Miller's Anesthesia, ed 8, pp 2281–2282; Miller: Basics of Anesthesia, ed 7, p 629–630).*

521. **(A)** Sugammadex is a neuromuscular blocker drug (NMBD) reversal agent that acts by encapsulating and forming inclusion complexes with the aminosteroid types of NMBD, such as rocuronium and vecuronium, in a 1:1 ratio, thereby reversing their effects. Sugammadex does not reverse blockade of succinylcholine or benzylisoquinolinium types of NMBDs such as atracurium and cisatracurium. Therefore administration of succinylcholine is unlikely to be affected by recent administration of sugammadex. Furthermore, for successful neuromuscular transmission to occur, only 25% to 30% of postsynaptic receptors need to be free from blockade. Thus sugammadex reversal may not require 100% reduction in postsynaptic receptor occupation for complete reversal, and any subsequent administration of nonsteroidal NMBD has been reported to have a faster onset and stronger effect *(Naguib M: Sugammadex: another milestone in clinical neuromuscular pharmacology. Anesth Analg 104:575–581, 2007; Bom A, Hope F: Neuromuscular block induced by rocuronium and reversed by the encapsulating agent Org 25969 can be re-established using the non-steroidal neuromuscular blockers succinylcholine and cis-atracurium: A-457. Eur J Anaesth (EJA) 22:120, 2005).*

522. **(A)** PONV is the second most common complaint from patients after surgery (postoperative pain is the number one complaint). Of the many independent predictors of PONV in adult prospective studies, female gender is the strongest predictor for PONV and the need for postoperative antiemetic rescue treatments. It is interesting to note that although patients often experience nausea when smoking their first cigarettes, smokers have a lower incidence of PONV compared with nonsmokers. Other predictors of PONV include nonsmokers, previous history of PONV, history of migraine headaches, use of postoperative narcotics, lengthy surgical procedures, use of nitrous oxide, and the use of volatile anesthetics *(Miller: Miller's Anesthesia, ed 8, pp 2947–2954, Miller: Basics of Anesthesia, ed 7, p 688).*

523. **(D)** Rare muscle diseases can have dramatic anesthetic implications. MH is among the most important manifestations of a muscular disorder. MH is thought to be caused by alterations in calcium control in muscle sarcoplasmic reticulum in response to succinylcholine or potent volatile anesthetics (most likely mediated by mutations of the ryanodine receptor). Because MH is a disorder in muscle metabolism, rigidity during administration of a volatile anesthetic or after succinylcholine use may be the presenting sign. Additionally, administration of any muscle relaxant would not provide muscle relaxation, and succinylcholine would be contraindicated. The patient does have a respiratory and metabolic acidosis and significantly increasing minute ventilation with 100% oxygen, and the use of sodium bicarbonate would be needed; however, stopping the triggering agent and administering dantrolene is most important *(Hines: Stoelting's Anesthesia and Co-Existing Disease, ed 7, pp 665–667; Miller: Basics of Anesthesia, ed 7, p 101).*

524. **(D)** Atropine and scopolamine cross the placenta easily (fetal/maternal ratio of 1.0), whereas glycopyrrolate is poorly transferred across the placenta (fetal/maternal ratio of 0.13). Case reports suggest that although neostigmine crosses the placenta poorly, enough does cross the placenta and can cause fetal bradycardia in utero. That is why it is better to reverse muscle relaxants in pregnant patients for nondelivery surgery with neostigmine and atropine instead of neostigmine and glycopyrrolate *(Suresh: Shnider and Levinson's Anesthesia for Obstetrics, ed 5, pp 50–51).*

525. **(A)** With liver failure, the liver cannot adequately detoxify noxious chemicals. Fifty to seventy percent of patients with end-stage liver disease develop HE. Symptoms vary from mild confusion, drowsiness, and stupor to coma. The etiology of HE is complex. Because an elevation in blood ammonia levels (easily measured) is strongly associated with HE, treatment is aimed at lowering the ammonia level. Other toxins also contribute to HE. To lower the ammonia level, lactulose (which decreases the absorption of ammonia) and neomycin (which reduces the production of ammonia by reducing the ammonia-producing intestinal flora) are commonly administered. Protein restriction is commonly done to decrease ammonia production, so amino acid–rich TPN is not helpful. Flumazenil (a GABA receptor antagonist) has been shown to produce short-duration reversal of the symptoms of HE in some patients and thus suggests that GABA receptors are somehow activated during HE. GABA receptors are responsible for inhibitory neurotransmission in the CNS *(Miller: Basics of Anesthesia, ed 7, p 492; Miller: Miller's Anesthesia, ed 8, p 541).*

526. (C) Ketorolac is one of the few nonsteroidal anti-inflammatory drugs (NSAIDs) approved for parenteral use. Although NSAIDs have analgesic and anti-inflammatory effects without ventilatory depression, they also inhibit platelet aggregation, can produce gastric ulceration, are associated with renal dysfunction, and may impair bone healing. NSAIDs are contraindicated in patients undergoing spinal fusion, where bone healing is essential to a successful surgical procedure, however there is no significant association with NSAID's and poor bone healing in orthopedic procedure not involving the spine. *(Miller: Miller's Anesthesia, ed 8, p 2982; Miller: Basics of Anesthesia, ed 7, p 545; Hemmings: Pharmacology and Physiology for Anesthesia, pp 276–277).*

527. (C) Glucose-6-phosphate dehydrogenase (G6PD) deficiency is an X-linked recessive disorder that predisposes RBCs to breakdown with oxidative stress. It is the most common enzymatic disorder of RBCs with >400 million people worldwide affected. G6PD deficiency appears to protect people from malaria. The half-life of RBCs in patients with G6PD deficiency can be about 60 days, instead of the normal RBC life span of 100 to 120 days. The amount of hemolysis depends on how much G6PD activity is present. The World Health Organization describes five classes of G6PD variants: Class I with <10% G6PD activity (chronic hemolytic anemia), Class II with 10% G6PD activity (intermittent hemolysis), Class III with 10% to 60% G6PD activity (hemolysis develops with stressors), and Class IV and V (nondeficient variant or increased amounts of G6PD with no clinical significance). Hemolysis can be precipitated by certain conditions such as the ingestion of fava beans, hypothermia, acidosis, hyperglycemia, diabetic ketoacidosis, infections, certain antibiotics (e.g., sulfonamides, penicillin), and oxidative stress. The development of methemoglobinemia, where hemoglobin is oxidized from the ferrous to the ferric state (oxygen cannot bind to hemoglobin in the ferric state), leads to oxidative stress. Methemoglobinemia can be produced when the patient is exposed to nitroprusside, benzocaine, large amounts of prilocaine, and silver nitrate. Although methemoglobinemia is often treated with methylene blue, methylene blue is ineffective in patients with G6PD deficiency and can lead to the patient's death. Some anesthetic agents are safe to use, such as midazolam, propofol, codeine, fentanyl, ketamine, bupivacaine and halothane. It may be wise to avoid the inhaled anesthetics (e.g., isoflurane, sevoflurane), which have shown depressed G6PD activity in vitro, but this, as well as the use of lidocaine, is controversial *(Barash: Clinical Anesthesia, ed 8, p 634; Elyassi AR, Rowshan HH: Perioperative management of the glucose-6-phosphate dehydrogenase patient, a review of the literature. Anesth Prog 56 (3):86–91, 2009; Hines: Stoelting's Anesthesia and Co-Existing Disease, ed 7, p 482).*

528. (A) Although many books suggest that obesity is the most common cause of OSA, more recent data suggest that a large neck circumference (>44 cm) reflects pharyngeal fat deposition and is more strongly correlated with OSA than obesity (BMI >30). Other risk factors include male gender, middle age, evening alcohol consumption, or sleep-inducing medications *(Miller: Miller's Anesthesia, ed 8, pp 2203–2204; Miller: Basics of Anesthesia, ed 7, pp 200–201, 854–855).*

529. (D) The ASA closed claims task force lists the leading causes of malpractice claims against anesthesiologists in the 1990s to be death (22%-41%), followed by nerve damage (22%). *(Miller: Miller's Anesthesia, ed 8, p 1256).*

530. (C) Cardiac resynchronization therapy (CRT) is used in patients with heart failure (EF <35%) and ventricular conductive delay (prolonged QRS complex usually is 120-150 msec). The conduction delay creates a mechanical dyssynchrony and worsens the heart failure. CRT requires biventricular pacing, with one lead in the coronary sinus to activate the left ventricle. CRT has nothing to do with breathing. Although CRT has nothing to do with an implantable cardioverter-defibrillator (ICD), many patients may require both because typically a patient with poor left ventricle function is also at risk for sudden death. Most of these patients also have underlying CAD *(Miller: Miller's Anesthesia, ed 8, pp 2078–2079).*

531. (D) Patients with syndrome X (also called metabolic syndrome X) have insulin resistance that leads to elevated levels of insulin and the metabolic changes that occur with elevated insulin levels, except that hypoglycemia does not develop. Associated with it are low levels of high-density lipoproteins, hypertension, and increased plasminogen activator inhibitor-1 levels, which are associated with CAD. Many of these patients are obese *(Miller: Miller's Anesthesia, ed 8, pp 2201–2203).*

532. (C) The parenteral-to-oral conversion for morphine sulfate is 1:3; thus, 30 mg morphine parenterally would be similar to 30 mg $\times$ 3 = 90 mg of morphine orally. The parenteral-to-oral conversion for methadone is 1:2 *(Brunton: Goodman & Gilman's The Pharmacological Basis of Therapeutics, ed 12, p 498).*

533. (A) The VRG comprises only 10% of the body but receives 75% of the cardiac output. Equilibrium with alveolar partial pressure is rapid (8-10 minutes [4 time constants]). After that point, uptake is accounted for by the MG and this equilibrium would be approached in a time frame on the order of 2 to 4 hours. The last compartment to reach equilibrium is the VPG, which includes fat. This equilibrium requires many hours, even days, to be achieved. When the vaporizer is turned off, the alveolar (arterial) partial pressure falls rapidly. The partial pressure in the VRG would also fall, as would the MG. The fat continues to take up volatile anesthetic for hours and actually contributes to recovery. The partial pressure of gas in the VPG at the time the vaporizer is turned off would be lower than the partial pressure in the VRG and MG and thus would initially take up some anesthetic from the higher pressure VRG and MG *(Miller: Miller's Anesthesia, ed 8, pp 639, 654–655).*

534. (D) Minors are not considered capable of giving informed consent to undergo surgical procedures or participate in research; therefore informed consent from the parents is required. This parental permission protects children from assuming risk that may be unreasonable to a capable adult. Informed assent from the minor child is a way to show respect for the child's developing autonomy and requires that the minor understand the procedure, voluntarily agree to proceed, and communicate this to the care providers. Thus informed consent and assent can be intertwined when eliciting cooperation from a pediatric patient and are both likely necessary *(Rossi WC, Reynolds W, Nelson RM: Child assent and parental permission in pediatric research. Theor Med Bioeth 24(2):131–148, 2003; Lewis I, et al: Children who refuse anesthesia or sedation: a survey of anesthesiologists. Pediatr Anesth 17(12):1134–1142, 2007).*

535. (A) All of the nerves listed in this question are derived from the fifth cranial nerve (trigeminal nerve) except the great auricular nerve. The ophthalmic nerve (V1 branch of trigeminal nerve) gives rise to the supratrochlear, infratrochlear, and supraorbital nerves. The infraorbital nerve is a branch of V2 (maxillary branch of the trigeminal nerve). The mental nerve is a branch of V3 (mandibular nerve). The great auricular nerve arises from branches of C2 and C3 spinal nerves and innervates the skin of the outer ear, the mastoid process, and the parotid gland *(Miller: Miller's Anesthesia, ed 8, pp 1722–1724).*

536. (D) Cerebral vasospasm is often associated in patients who have suffered a subarachnoid bleed. Angiographic evidence of vasospasm can be noted in up to 70% of patients; however, clinical vasospasm with detectable ischemia (e.g., mental confusion, lethargy, focal motor, and speech impairments) is detected in about 30% of patients. When clinical vasospasm develops, it usually occurs between 4 and 12 days after the bleed. Although it may resolve spontaneously, it may also progress to coma and death within a few hours or days. Rebleeding tends to occur earlier (i.e., within 24 hours) *(Barash: Clinical Anesthesia, ed 6, pp 1585–1586; Miller: Miller's Anesthesia, ed 8, pp 2178, 3110–3111).*

537. (C) Bleomycin is used primarily in the treatment of Hodgkin lymphoma and testicular tumors. Bleomycin causes oxidative damage to nucleotides, which leads to breaks in DNA. Although the more common side effects of bleomycin use are mucocutaneous, it is the dose-related pulmonary toxicity that is the most serious side effect. Early signs and symptoms of pulmonary toxicity include dry cough, fine rales, and diffuse infiltrates on radiograph. Approximately 5% to 10% of patients will develop pulmonary toxicity, and about 1% will die of this complication. Most believe that the risk of pulmonary toxicity increases with dose (especially total dose >250 mg), patients older than 40 years of age, patients with a creatinine clearance (CrCl) of <80 mL/min, and in patients with prior chest radiation or preexisting pulmonary disease. Although a relationship appears to exist between the use of bleomycin and the use of high concentrations of oxygen, the details are unclear. Currently, it has been suggested to use the lowest concentration of oxygen consistent with patient safety, with a careful evaluation of oxygen saturation with pulse oximetry in any patient who has received bleomycin *(Brunton: Goodman & Gilman's The Pharmacological Basis of Therapeutics, ed 12, pp 1716–1718; Miller: Miller's Anesthesia, ed 8, p 1943).*

538. (B) The most common adverse cardiac event in the pediatric population is bradycardia. An outcome study from the Medical College of Virginia examined the incidence of bradycardia in nearly 8000 children younger than 4 years old. The most common causes of bradycardia were cardiac disease or surgery and inhalation anesthesia, followed by hypoxemia. Of those children who had bradycardia, hypotension occurred in 30%, asystole or ventricular fibrillation in 10%, and death in 8%. Tachycardia, which is common, is not an adverse event *(Davis: Smith's Anesthesia for Infants and Children, ed 8, pp 1232–1236).*

539. (C) Mask ventilation, one of the most basic anesthesia techniques, can be challenging in some patients. Use of mask ventilation in patients who are prone to airway obstruction can be more difficult because of extra airway tissue (i.e., obese patients with a BMI >26), patients without teeth (i.e., tongue is closer to the roof of the mouth, and face conformity may not fit the mask well), and patients who snore (i.e., already have reason for airway obstruction). Mask ventilation can also be more difficult in patients who have a beard (i.e., harder to get a good mask seal), patients whose age is older than 55 years, patients with facial tumors, and patients with facial trauma. Use of an oral airway may be needed in many of these patients *(Miller: Basics of Anesthesia, ed 7, p 246; Miller: Miller's Anesthesia, ed 8, p 1651).*

540. (A) Whenever perfusion to an extremity is inadequate (e.g., trauma or poor perfusion), hypoxic edema develops, producing swelling. When this occurs in a compartment, tissue pressures rise, decreasing capillary perfusion. Symptoms of compartment syndrome include extreme pain unrelieved by analgesics, paresthesias, paralysis, and pallor. Extensive rhabdomyolysis may develop, as well as permanent nerve and muscle injury in the compartment. Because the problem is at the tissue level, pulses and capillary refill may still be present. Treatment includes fasciotomy to relieve the elevated pressure *(Miller: Miller's Anesthesia, ed 8, p 2450).*

541. (B) The amount and distribution of cerebrospinal fluid (CSF) is different in neonates compared with adults. The neonate has about 4 mL/kg of CSF compared with the adult's 2 mL/kg. In addition, almost half of the neonate's CSF is in the spinal subarachnoid space, compared with about a quarter of the adult's CSF in the spinal subarachnoid space. These factors help explain why the dose is greater in neonates and infants and of shorter duration compared with adults *(Miller: Miller's Anesthesia, ed 8, pp 2727–2728).*

542. (A) Endotracheal tube sizes are measured according to the ID. They are available in 0.5-mm ID increments *(Miller: Basics of Anesthesia, ed 7, p 258).*

543. (B) MRI scanners have superconducting electrical currents that produce large magnetic fields (up to 6 m) and are always "on." The presence of any ferromagnetic objects in the room may cause a missile-type injury when the objects are strongly attracted to the scanner. If a patient is pinned into the scanner by a magnetic object that flew into the scanner, the MRI technicians may have to turn off the superconducting magnet. During magnetic shutdown (quench) the scanner will become extremely cold *(Miller: Basics of Anesthesia, ed 7, p 661).*

544. (C) Carbon monoxide is a colorless, odorless gas that binds to hemoglobin with an affinity more than 200 times stronger than oxygen. Inhalation of CO is a major cause of morbidity and mortality in the United States. A dual-wave (660 nm and 940 nm) pulse oximeter is incapable of distinguishing CO hemoglobin from oxyhemoglobin, but the distinction is easily made in the clinical laboratory with a co-oximeter. Significant quantities of methemoglobin would result in a saturation of 85% of the pulse oximeter. The slight right shift from a mild acidemia would be insufficient to account for 90% saturation in the face of a PaO_2 of 190. Furthermore, the pulse oximeter reading would be nearly the same as the co-oximeter value *(Miller: Miller's Anesthesia, ed 8, pp 2679–2680; Miller: Basics of Anesthesia, ed 7, p 341; Hines: Stoelting's Anesthesia and Co-Existing Disease, ed 7, pp 631–632).*

545. (A) The pathway for SSEP monitoring of the lower extremity starts with a stimulus of the posterior tibial nerve, which generates an impulse that passes through the dorsal root ganglion into the dorsal (posterior) columns and then to the dorsal column nuclei. Second-order nerves carry the impulse across the midline to the thalamus, and the impulse travels over third-order nerves to the sensory cortex of the brain. Electrodes in the scalp record the electrical activity in the brain. Severe hypotension or ischemia in any portion of the pathway along which the induced signal is conducted can result in a reduced evoked potential amplitude or increased latency. Volatile anesthetic administration in MAC values greater than 0.5 to 0.75 can produce a similar effect. Barbiturates, benzodiazepines, propofol, and other sedative drugs can likewise interfere with SSEP monitoring. Anterior spinal artery syndrome affects the anterior (motor) portion of the spinal cord and does not interfere with SSEP monitoring *(Miller: Basics of Anesthesia, ed 7, pp 358, 543)*.

546. (D) Diabetic autonomic neuropathy can affect the autonomic nervous system to such an extent that atropine and propranolol would have little effect (because there would be nothing to block). After heart transplantation, the new heart (donor heart) is denervated and will not respond to autonomic nervous system blocking drugs. Brain death by definition is associated with absence of autonomic function. A high spinal would be associated with total sympathectomy, and propranolol would have no effect on heart rate, but the vagus nerve would be unaffected. Atropine would have no effect on a patient with atrial fibrillation and complete heart block *(Hines: Stoelting's Anesthesia and Co-Existing Disease, ed 7, pp 104–105, 456–457; Miller: Basics of Anesthesia, ed 7, pp 630–631)*.

547. (A) Miller: Basics of Anesthesia, ed 7, pp 761–763.

548. (B) Miller: Basics of Anesthesia, ed 7, pp 761–763.

549. (D) Miller: Basics of Anesthesia, ed 7, pp 761–763.

550. (C) Miller: Basics of Anesthesia, ed 7, pp 761–763.

551. (D) Miller: Basics of Anesthesia, ed 7, pp 761–763.

552. (B) Miller: Basics of Anesthesia, ed 7, pp 761–763.

553. (A) Miller: Basics of Anesthesia, ed 7, pp 761–763.

554. (E) There are three categories of biological weapons: A, B, and C. All of the diseases in this question are in the highly contagious Category A agents. Smallpox is caused by a virus (Variola major) and in 1980 was declared extinct by the World Health Organization. The incubation period was 7 to 14 days, and patients with the disease presented with malaise, headache, and fever. Two to 4 days later, a characteristic rash develops where all lesions are at the same stage (papules, vesicles, pustules, and scabs). Exposed patients and health care workers who received a vaccination within 4 days of exposure had greatly attenuated symptoms. Unvaccinated patients who were untreated had a mortality rate of greater than 30%. Patients who previously had been vaccinated had a lower mortality rate. Treatment includes the drug cidofovir.

Anthrax is caused by an aerobic gram-positive spore-forming bacillus (*Bacillus anthracis*) and has three primary forms: cutaneous, gastrointestinal, and inhalational. Weaponized anthrax is mainly an inhalational disease. Inhalational anthrax symptoms occur within 1 to 7 days of exposure and initially look like viral flu (fever, chills, myalgia, and a nonproductive cough). Later on, the patient's mediastinal lymph nodes, where the spores germinate, enlarge, producing a widened mediastinum that can be seen on a chest x-ray film. Treatment is primarily with ciprofloxacin; prophylaxis to exposed personnel includes 60 days of ciprofloxacin. Mortality rate for inhaled anthrax is greater than 80%.

Plague is caused by a gram-negative coccobacillus (*Yersinia pestis*) and has two forms: bubonic and pneumonic. With the more common bubonic plague, there is painful swelling of the lymph nodes (buboes), which can grow to 5 to 10 cm in diameter. The patients develop cyanosis, shock, and gangrene in peripheral tissues (black death). If the lungs become infected then pneumonic plague develops, which, if untreated, has 100% mortality. Treatment is primarily with streptomycin, although gentamicin, tetracycline, and chloramphenicol have been used.

Botulism is caused by the toxin from *Clostridium botulinum*. Because this disease is due to a neuro toxin, it is not contagious. The neurotoxin affects cholinergic neurons and prevents the release of acetylcholine. Symptoms typically develop within 12 to 36 hours of exposure and include acute flaccid paralysis, decreased salivation, ileus, and urinary retention. There are no sensory deficits. With appropriate supportive care and trivalent equine antitoxin, the mortality rate is less than 5%. Without the use of antitoxin, patients may take 2 to 8 weeks to recover. Mortality rate is 5% to 10%.

There are more than 18 hemorrhagic fever viruses, including Ebola virus. The incubation period is 2 to 21 days, and patients present with fever, myalgias, headaches, thrombocytopenia, and hemorrhagic complications (petechiae, ecchymosis). Untreated, the mortality rate for Ebola virus is 90%. Treatment includes the drug ribavirin *(Barash: Clinical Anesthesia, ed 7, pp 1543–1545; Miller: Miller's Anesthesia, ed 8, pp 2501–2502; Miller: Basics of Anesthesia, ed 7, pp 761–763).*

555. (D) Miller: Basics of Anesthesia, ed 7, pp 463–466.

556. (C) Miller: Basics of Anesthesia, ed 7, pp 463–466.

557. (D) Miller: Basics of Anesthesia, ed 7, pp 463–466.

558. (C) Miller: Basics of Anesthesia, ed 7, pp 463–466.

559. (C) Miller: Basics of Anesthesia, ed 7, pp 463–466.

560. (A) Pulmonary function tests can be used to classify patients with chronic pulmonary disease into those with obstructive airway diseases (e.g., asthma, pulmonary emphysema, and chronic bronchitis) and those with restrictive pulmonary diseases (e.g., pulmonary fibrosis, scoliosis). The forced expiratory volume in 1 second or FEV1 is the amount of air expired in 1 second and commonly is expressed as a percentage of the FVC, or FEV1/FVC. The normal FEV1/FVC is 75% to 80%. In the presence of obstructive airway disease, FEV1 of less than 70% has mild obstruction, less than 60% has moderate obstruction, and less than 50% has severe obstruction. Patients with obstructive lung disease also have a normal (asthma) or increase in (bronchitis, emphysema) TLC and FRC. In the presence of restrictive pulmonary disease, FEV1 is reduced, but because FVC is also reduced, the FEV1/FVC is normal. Patients with restrictive disease have a TLC, FRC, and total pulmonary compliance that are reduced. In patients with pulmonary emphysema, lung compliance is increased because the elastic recoil of the lungs is decreased *(Miller: Miller's Anesthesia, ed 8, p 1149; Miller: Basics of Anesthesia, ed 7, pp 463–466).*

561. (A) Miller: Basics of Anesthesia, ed 7, pp 331–333.

562. (B) Miller: Basics of Anesthesia, ed 7, pp 331–333.

563. (C) Miller: Basics of Anesthesia, ed 7, pp 331–333.

564. (D) Miller: Basics of Anesthesia, ed 7, pp 331–333.

565. (B) Miller: Basics of Anesthesia, ed 7, pp 331–333.

566. (E) In many cases of peripheral nerve injuries, the mechanism of injury is largely unknown; however, stretching or compression of the nerves can lead to nerve ischemia and damage. In the lithotomy position, hyperflexion of the hips and/or extension of the knees can aggravate stretch of the sciatic nerve. Also in the lithotomy position, compression of the common peroneal nerve between the head of the fibula and the metal supporting frame can occur. The common peroneal nerve is the most common nerve injured in the lithotomy position. Proper padding between the metal leg braces and positioning of the legs will limit the occurrence of these injuries. The sciatic nerve provides motor function for all the skeletal muscles below the knees and sensory innervation for the lateral half of the leg and most of the foot. Injury to the common peroneal nerve, a branch of the sciatic nerve, causes a footdrop from the impaired ankle dorsiflexion and the loss of foot eversion and toe extension. Injury to the femoral or obturator nerves can occur with excessive retraction during lower abdominal surgery. The obturator nerve can also be injured during a difficult forceps vaginal delivery or by excessive flexion of the thigh to the groin. Injury to the femoral nerve will manifest as decreased extension of the knee (paresis of the quadriceps femoris muscle) and numbness over the anterior aspect of the thigh and medial/anteromedial side of the leg. The inability to adduct the leg and thigh, as well as numbness over the medial side of the thigh, are clinical manifestations consistent with damage to the obturator nerve. Excessive flexion of the hip on the abdomen can cause a neuropathy of the lateral femoral cutaneous nerve (sensory only) resulting in numbness of the lateral aspect of the thigh *(Miller: Miller's Anesthesia, ed 8, pp 1256–1258; Miller: Basics of Anesthesia, ed 7, pp 331–333).*

CHAPTER 7

Pediatric Physiology and Anesthesia

DIRECTIONS (Questions 567 through 642): Each of the questions or incomplete statements in this section is followed by answers or by completions of the statement, respectively. Select the ONE BEST answer or completion for each item.

567. A previously healthy 3.5-kg, 1-month-old infant with a strong family history of sickle cell anemia is brought to the emergency room with an incarcerated inguinal hernia. Which of the following should be carried out before surgery?
- **A.** Hemoglobin electrophoresis
- **B.** Peripheral smear
- **C.** Hematology consultation
- **D.** None of the above

568. In the premature newborn, the glottis is at which level relative to the cervical spine?
- **A.** C3
- **B.** C4
- **C.** C5
- **D.** C6

569. A 5-month-old infant is scheduled for an elective operative reduction of a right inguinal hernia. Spinal anesthesia is performed. The first sign of a high spinal block in this patient would be
- **A.** Decrease in blood pressure
- **B.** Increase in heart rate
- **C.** Decrease in oxygen saturation
- **D.** Asystole

570. What percentage of a term newborn's total body weight consists of water?
- **A.** 45%
- **B.** 60%
- **C.** 75%
- **D.** 90%

571. Which of the following patients is **LEAST** likely to develop retinopathy of prematurity (ROP)?
- **A.** A term infant, 46 weeks' postmenstrual age (PMA), exposed to 100% oxygen for 6 hours
- **B.** A premature infant, 29 weeks' PMA, exposed to a PaO$_2$ of 150 mm Hg for 1 hour
- **C.** A premature infant, 28 weeks' PMA, never exposed to supplemental oxygen
- **D.** A cyanotic infant with tetralogy of Fallot, 34 weeks' PMA, receiving supplemental oxygen

572. A 4-week-old male infant is brought to the emergency room with projectile vomiting. At the time of admission, the patient is lethargic, with a respiratory rate of 16 breaths/min and has had no urine output in the preceding 3 hours. A diagnosis of pyloric stenosis is made, and the infant is brought emergently to the operating room (OR) for pyloromyotomy. The **MOST** appropriate anesthetic management would be
- **A.** Awake intubation after placing an oral gastric tube
- **B.** Inhalation induction with sevoflurane with cricoid pressure after placing an oral gastric tube
- **C.** Awake saphenous IV catheter or an intraosseous needle placement followed by a rapid-sequence induction with ketamine, atropine, and rocuronium after placing an oral gastric tube
- **D.** Postpone surgery

573. Which figure of esophageal atresia (EA) or tracheoesophageal fistula (TEF) is the **MOST** common?

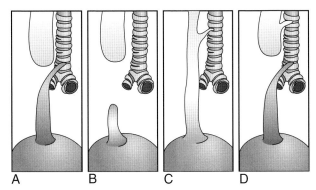

A   B   C   D

Modified from Gross RE: The Surgery of Infancy and Childhood, Philadelphia, Saunders, 1953.

574. The predicted blood volume in a 3-kg term newborn is
- **A.** 100 mL
- **B.** 150 mL
- **C.** 250 mL
- **D.** 300 mL

575. An 11-month-old infant is to undergo a craniosynostosis repair. The surgeon and anesthesiologist agreed to start transfusing blood when the hemoglobin fell to 8 g/dL (hematocrit [Hct] of 24%). Using the transfusion threshold of a hemoglobin of 8, what is the maximum allowable blood loss (MABL) for this 10-kg infant whose initial Hct is 32 and the minimal acceptable Hct is 24?

A. 180 mL
B. 200 mL
C. 320 mL
D. Cannot be calculated without additional information

576. What volume of packed red blood cells (PRBCs) with an Hct of 60 is needed to raise the Hct from 18 to 24 in a 10-kg 11-month-old?

A. 40 mL
B. 80 mL
C. 120 mL
D. Cannot be calculated without additional information

577. Reasons for selecting a cuffed endotracheal tube (ETT) over an uncuffed ETT include all of the following **EXCEPT**

A. Fewer intubations and ETTs are needed
B. Less chance for airway fires
C. Spontaneous breathing is easier
D. Aspiration of gastric contents is less likely

578. An otherwise healthy 4-year-old male patient is undergoing elective tonsillectomy. Before induction of general anesthesia, the patient is breathing at a rate of 20 breaths/min. An inhalation induction is begun with 8% sevoflurane, 50% nitrous oxide, and oxygen. Sixty seconds later, the patient is noted to breathe at a rate of 40 breaths/min, and the heart rate is 160. This rapid respiratory rate with tachycardia most likely represents

A. Severe hypoxia
B. Hypercarbia and early development of malignant hyperthermia (MH)
C. The excitement stage of anesthesia
D. Aspiration of gastric contents

579. A healthy 3-kg, 1-month-old neonate is anesthetized for an inguinal hernia repair. An inhalation induction with sevoflurane is carried out, and the patient is intubated. Before the surgical incision, the systolic blood pressure is noted to be 65 mm Hg and the heart rate is 150 beats/min. The most appropriate intervention for this patient's blood pressure would be

A. Administration of ephedrine
B. Administration of phenylephrine
C. 50-mL fluid bolus
D. None of the above

580. A 5-year-old boy is anesthetized for elective repair of an umbilical hernia. General anesthesia is induced and maintained with sevoflurane, nitrous oxide, and oxygen via an anesthesia mask. At the conclusion of the operation, the patient is taken to the recovery room and subsequently discharged to the outpatient ward. Before discharge, the patient's mother notes that the urine appears dark brown (cola-colored). The most appropriate action at this time would be

A. Discharge the patient with instructions to return if urine color does not normalize
B. Discharge the patient in 3 hours if no other signs or symptoms are manifested
C. Obtain serum creatinine and blood urea nitrogen (BUN) levels and discharge the patient if they are normal
D. Evaluate the patient for MH

581. At what maximum inspiratory pressure should a cuffed ETT leak in a child (leak test)?

A. 5 to 15 cm H_2O
B. 15 to 25 cm H_2O
C. 25 to 35 cm H_2O
D. None of the above

582. A premature newborn delivered at 32 weeks of gestation is brought to the OR 5 days after delivery for repair of a left-sided congenital diaphragmatic hernia (CDH). The newborn has a nasogastric tube in place, is intubated, and is stable with mechanical ventilation at peak airway pressures <25 cm H_2O. 30 minutes after induction of general anesthesia, the anesthesiologist notes significant difficulty with adequate ventilation. The SaO_2 subsequently falls to 65%, and the heart rate decreases to 50 beats/min. What would be the most appropriate step to take at this time?

A. Pull the ETT from the right mainstem bronchus
B. Ventilate with positive end-expiratory pressure (PEEP) and administer furosemide
C. Place a chest tube on the right side after confirming a tension pneumothorax
D. Pull out the ETT, mask ventilate, and reintubate the patient

583. An 8-year-old boy, who weighs 30 kg, was found at the site of a motor vehicle accident (MVA). He has arrived in the OR for exploratory laparotomy. He has not received any sedation or pain medication because he appeared "confused and lethargic." He has a normal blood pressure, is tachycardic with thready distal pulses, and has cold extremities. In spite of a 20 mL/kg fluid bolus, the patient has produced only 5 mL of urine. What is the approximate percentage of blood volume loss in this patient?

A. <20%
B. 25%
C. 40%
D. Cannot determine

584. In a 6-year-old child, the distance an oral ETT should be placed (from the gums to the midtrachea) most often is
   A. 10 cm
   B. 13 cm
   C. 15 cm
   D. 20 cm

585. Which of the following is the most suitable intraoperative replacement fluid for a 3-year-old, 14-kg child who has been NPO for 10 hours and will be undergoing repair of clubfeet?
   A. D_5W
   B. D_5 in 0.2 NaCl
   C. D_5 in 0.45 NaCl
   D. Lactated Ringer solution

586. An otherwise healthy 14-day-old neonate is transported to the OR well hydrated for surgery for a bowel obstruction. A rapid-sequence induction is planned. Compared with the adult dose, the intravenous (IV) dose of succinylcholine administered to this patient should be
   A. Diminished because of the immature nervous system
   B. The same as the adult dose
   C. Decreased because of decreased acetylcholine receptors
   D. Increased because of a greater volume of distribution

587. You receive a call from the preoperative nurse stating that the child you will be caring for with type 1 diabetes mellitus has a preoperative blood glucose value of 300 mg/dL. He has been NPO for the morning and has not had any rapid-onset or short-acting insulin. The child typically uses a total of 30 units of insulin a day. How much rapid-onset or short-acting insulin should you give the child to reduce the blood sugar to 150 mg/dL?
   A. 1 unit
   B. 3 units
   C. 5 units
   D. 10 units

588. A 10-week-old infant born at 31 weeks' gestation is anesthetized for repair of an inguinal hernia. General anesthesia is induced by mask with sevoflurane, an ETT is placed, and anesthesia is maintained with sevoflurane and oxygen. What is the best postoperative pain management for this patient?
   A. Caudal block with 0.25% bupivacaine, 1 mL/kg, and admitted to a pediatric ward for overnight observation
   B. Caudal block with 0.25% bupivacaine, 2 mL/kg, and admitted to a pediatric ward for overnight observation
   C. Oral pain medication (acetaminophen) and discharged home
   D. Fentanyl (1 mL = 50 µg IV), and admitted to a pediatric ward for overnight observation

589. A 6-year-old, 20-kg girl develops pulseless ventricular tachycardia (pVT) after induction of general anesthesia for a tonsillectomy. The anesthesiologist intubates the child, administers 100% oxygen, and starts chest compressions. When the biphasic defibrillator quickly arrives in the OR and is attached to the child, the defibrillator should be charged to what energy level for the initial shock?
   A. 10-20 joules (J)
   B. 20-30 joules (J)
   C. 40-80 joules (J)
   D. 120-200 joules (J)

590. The spinal cord of newborns extends to the
   A. L1 vertebra
   B. L2-L3 vertebrae
   C. L4-L5 vertebrae
   D. S1 vertebra

591. The most common initial symptom of esophageal atresia (EA) or tracheoesophageal fistula (TEF) is
   A. Respiratory distress at delivery (e.g., retractions, tachypnea)
   B. Projectile vomiting
   C. Hypoxia
   D. Coughing and regurgitation during first feeding

592. A 4.5-kg, 3-hour-old newborn with Beckwith-Wiedemann syndrome is scheduled for surgical repair of an omphalocele. Which of the following is **NOT** part of this syndrome?
   A. Large fontanelles
   B. Macroglossia
   C. Polycythemia
   D. Hyperglycemia

593. Which of the following is the **LEAST** appropriate technique for induction of general anesthesia in a newborn for surgical repair of a TEF?
   A. Awake tracheal intubation
   B. Sedated tracheal intubation (e.g., fentanyl)
   C. Inhalation induction with spontaneous ventilation and tracheal intubation
   D. Inhalation induction with cisatracurium as a muscle relaxant and positive-pressure bag and mask ventilation and tracheal intubation

594. A 3-year-old with cough, sore throat, and temperature of 102° F, is scheduled for hydrocele repair. Physical examination reveals wheezing and rhonchi. Chest x-ray reveals small left lower lobe (LLL) infiltrate. The best course of action would be
   A. Administer IV steroids and proceed
   B. Administer acetaminophen and if the temperature goes below 100° F, proceed
   C. Postpone surgery for at least 4 weeks
   D. Proceed, because the temperature will return to normal during anesthesia

595. Which of the following statements regarding teeth is **INCORRECT**?
- **A.** Primary teeth start to erupt around 6 to 9 months of age
- **B.** There are 20 primary teeth, and all are usually present by 3 years of age
- **C.** Permanent teeth start to erupt at 4 years of age
- **D.** There are 32 permanent teeth, and most are present by 12 years of age, except for the third molars, which erupt at 15 to 25 years of age

596. The pulmonary vascular resistance (PVR) in newborns decreases to that of adults by age
- **A.** 1 to 2 days
- **B.** 1 to 2 weeks
- **C.** 1 to 2 months
- **D.** 1 year

597. A 10-month-old infant is undergoing elective repair of a left testicular hydrocele under general anesthesia with isoflurane, nitrous oxide, oxygen, and fentanyl. All of the following are effective and reasonable means of preventing hypothermia in this patient **EXCEPT**
- **A.** Placement of an infrared heater over the operating table and prewarming the OR
- **B.** Covering the OR table with a heating blanket
- **C.** Wrapping the extremities with sheet wadding and covering the head with a cloth cap
- **D.** Ventilating the patient with a Mapleson D circuit at low gas flows (e.g., 50 mL/kg/min)

598. Postoperative mechanical ventilation is common after repair of the following lesions. Which of the following is **MOST** likely to result in central postoperative depression of spontaneous ventilation in a term newborn?
- **A.** Gastroschisis
- **B.** Omphalocele
- **C.** TEF
- **D.** Pyloric stenosis

599. A premature male neonate born at 36 weeks of gestation is scheduled to undergo repair of a left-sided diaphragmatic hernia. Which of the following vessels could be cannulated for preductal arterial blood sampling?
- **A.** Femoral artery
- **B.** Umbilical artery
- **C.** Right radial artery
- **D.** Left radial artery

600. In which of the following patients would the minimum alveolar concentration (MAC) for isoflurane be the greatest?
- **A.** A premature infant 30 weeks' postconceptual age (PCA)
- **B.** Full-term neonate
- **C.** 3-month-old infant
- **D.** 13-year-old adolescent

601. A 40-kg, 10-year-old child sustains a thermal injury to his legs, buttocks, and back. The estimated area involved is 50%. Using only crystalloid fluids, how much fluid should be administered during the first 24 hours after the burn?
- **A.** 2.5 L
- **B.** 5.5 L
- **C.** 8.0 L
- **D.** 10.0 L

602. An otherwise healthy 3-month-old black female infant who had a hemoglobin value of 19 mg/dL at birth presents for elective repair of an inguinal hernia. Her preoperative hemoglobin is 10 mg/dL. Her father has a history of polycystic kidney disease. The most likely explanation for this patient's anemia is
- **A.** Sickle cell anemia
- **B.** Iron deficiency
- **C.** Undiagnosed polycystic kidney disease
- **D.** It is a normal finding

603. The anesthesiologist is called to the emergency room by the pediatrician to help manage a 3-year-old boy with a high fever and upper airway obstruction. His mother stated that earlier that afternoon, he complained of a sore throat and hoarseness. The patient is sitting erect and leaning forward; has inspiratory stridor, tachypnea, and sternal retractions; and is drooling. Which of the following is the **MOST** appropriate management of airway obstruction in this patient?
- **A.** Aerosolized racemic epinephrine
- **B.** Awake tracheal intubation in the emergency room or the OR if time permits
- **C.** Transfer to the OR, inhalation induction, and tracheal intubation
- **D.** Transfer to the OR, IV induction, paralysis with succinylcholine, and tracheal intubation

604. A 2-year-old child with cerebral palsy (CP) and known severe gastroesophageal reflux (with frequent nightly aspiration) and a seizure disorder is scheduled to undergo iliopsoas release under general anesthesia. Which of the following would be the preferred technique for inducing general anesthesia in this patient?
- **A.** Inhalation induction with sevoflurane followed by tracheal intubation
- **B.** IV induction with propofol followed by laryngeal mask airway
- **C.** IV induction with etomidate and vecuronium followed by tracheal intubation
- **D.** Rapid-sequence induction with propofol and succinylcholine followed by tracheal intubation

605. A 7-week-old male infant is admitted to the pediatric intensive care unit (ICU) with a bowel obstruction. His laboratory values are sodium 120 mEq/L, chloride 85 mEq/L, glucose 85 mg/dL, and potassium 2.0 mEq/L. Respiratory rate is 40 breaths/min, heart rate is 220 beats/minute, and blood pressure is 50/32. According to the patient's mother, urine output has been zero for the last 4 hours. The most appropriate initial fluid for resuscitation of this patient would be

A. $D_{2.5}W$ with 0.45 sodium chloride and 20 mEq/L potassium chloride

B. 0.45% sodium chloride

C. 0.9% sodium chloride with 30 mEq/L potassium chloride

D. 0.9% sodium chloride

606. A 24-hour-old, 1200-g neonate, 30 weeks' estimated gestational age (EGA), is noted in the ICU to begin making twitching movements. Blood pressure is 45/30, heart rate is 160, oxygen saturation is 88%, blood glucose is 50 mg/dL, total calcium level is 4 mg/dL, and urine output is 5 mL/hr. The **MOST** appropriate course of action to take at this point would be

A. Administer calcium gluconate (1 mL of 10% solution) over 5 to 10 minutes

B. Administer glucose 200 mg/kg ($D_{10}W$) IV over 5 minutes

C. Hyperventilate with 100% O_2

D. Administer a 10-mL/kg bolus of 5% albumin

607. A Eutectic Mixture of Local Anesthetics (EMLA) cream is a mixture of which local anesthetics?

A. Lidocaine 2.5% and prilocaine 2.5%

B. Lidocaine 2.5% and benzocaine 2.5%

C. Prilocaine 2% and benzocaine 2%

D. Lidocaine 4%

608. Advantages of catheterization of the umbilical artery versus the umbilical vein in a newborn include all of the following **EXCEPT**

A. It allows assessment of oxygenation

B. Hepatic damage from hypertonic infusion is avoided

C. It permits assessment of systemic blood pressure

D. It is easier to cannulate

609. The **TRUE** statement concerning thermoregulation in neonates is which of the following?

A. A significant proportion of their heat loss can be accounted for by their small surface area–to–weight ratio

B. They compensate for hypothermia by shivering

C. The principal method of heat production is metabolism of brown fat

D. Heat loss through conduction can be reduced by humidification of inspired gases

610. A 10-year-old child was climbing a tree and fell, sustaining a lower cervical neck injury. He is unable to move his legs but can move his arms somewhat and is scheduled for an MRI scan. All of the following are signs of neurogenic shock **EXCEPT**

A. Hypotension

B. Narrow pulse pressure

C. Hypothermia

D. Normal heart rate

611. A 5-year-old child undergoing strabismus surgery under general anesthesia suddenly develops sinus bradycardia and intermittent ventricular escape beats but is hemodynamically stable. Which initial therapy is appropriate for treating this arrhythmia?

A. Tell the surgeon to stop pulling on the eye muscle

B. Tell the surgeon to do a retrobulbar block

C. Decrease the depth of the volatile anesthetic

D. Administer atropine

612. Which of the following respiratory indices is increased in healthy neonates compared with healthy adults?

A. Tidal volume (mL/kg)

B. Minute ventilation (mL/kg/min)

C. Functional residual capacity (mL/kg)

D. Pa_{CO_2}

613. A 16-year-old girl with neurofibromatosis is anesthetized for resection of an acoustic neuroma. Each of the following may potentially complicate the anesthetic management of this patient **EXCEPT**

A. Presence of a pheochromocytoma

B. Upper airway obstruction from a laryngeal neurofibroma

C. Intracranial hypertension

D. Increased risk for MH

614. With which of the following congenital anomalies is right-to-left intracardiac shunting of blood from pulmonary hypertension **MOST** likely and difficult to treat?

A. Tracheoesophageal fistula (TEF)

B. Gastroschisis

C. Omphalocele

D. Congenital diaphragmatic hernia (CDH)

615. Which of the following is **NOT CONSISTENT** with an infant who suffers from severe dehydration?

A. 15% weight loss

B. Normal respirations

C. Urine output <0.5 mL/kg/hr

D. Tachycardia

616. Postoperative bleeding following tonsillectomy occurs most commonly

A. By the first 6 hours

B. 6 to 24 hours after surgery

C. On the third postoperative day

D. On the seventh postoperative day

617. A 9-year-old undergoing sinus surgery is treated with an unmeasured amount of 0.5% phenylephrine by the surgeon, and the patient develops a blood pressure of 250/150. The most appropriate treatment for this would be
  A. Administer verapamil
  B. Administer esmolol
  C. Administer labetalol
  D. Administer phentolamine

618. A 5-kg, 3-month-old male infant undergoes a left inguinal herniorrhaphy with a spinal anesthetic. Typically, how long would 1 mL of a 0.5% bupivacaine (5 mg) isobaric solution last?
  A. Less than 30 minutes
  B. 30 to 60 minutes
  C. 60 to 80 minutes
  D. 90 to 100 minutes

619. Which of the following combination of drug and dose used alone is **INCORRECT** for preoperative sedation for an anxious child?
  A. Midazolam 0.1 mg/kg orally
  B. Clonidine 2 to 5 µg/kg orally
  C. Dexmedetomidine 1 to 2 µg/kg nasally
  D. Ketamine 3 to 7 mg/kg intramuscular (IM)

620. Which of the following statements regarding resuscitation of the infant by health care providers is **NOT** correct?
  A. Mouth-to-mouth or mouth-to-nose ventilation at a rate of 12 to 20 breaths/min is performed when breathing is inadequate but an adequate pulse is present
  B. Start chest compressions when the pulse is less than 60 beats/min and there are signs of poor tissue perfusion
  C. Chest compression depth is 1/5 the anteroposterior diameter of the chest (about 1 cm)
  D. Compression-to-ventilation ratio is 30:2 for one-person and 15:2 for two-person cardiopulmonary resuscitation (CPR)

621. All of the following are true statements concerning the physiology of newborns compared with that of adults **EXCEPT**
  A. Newborns have a greater percentage of total body water compared with adults
  B. Newborns have a higher glomerular filtration rate (GFR) than adults
  C. Newborns' hearts are relatively noncompliant compared with adults' hearts
  D. Newborns' diaphragms have a lower proportion of type I muscle fibers (i.e., fatigue-resistant, highly oxidative fibers)

622. Which of the following statements concerning the anatomy of the infant and the adult airway is **INCORRECT**?
  A. The larynx is in a more cephalic position in infants than in adults
  B. The infant's epiglottis is narrower and "omega" shaped, whereas the adult epiglottis is flat and broad
  C. The vocal cords are in a more perpendicular position to the trachea in infants and in a more diagonal position to the larynx and trachea in adults
  D. The narrowest part of the infant and adult larynx is at the level of the cricoid cartilage

623. Which of the following operations would be associated with the **LEAST** incidence of postoperative nausea and vomiting (PONV) in a 5-year-old boy?
  A. Tonsillectomy
  B. Strabismus surgery
  C. Myringotomy tube placement
  D. Orchiopexy

624. Anomalies and features associated with Down syndrome include
  A. Smaller tracheas
  B. Atlanto-occipital instability
  C. Thyroid hypofunction
  D. All of the above

625. Congenital syndromes frequently associated with cardiac abnormalities include all of the following **EXCEPT**
  A. Tracheoesophageal fistula (TEF)
  B. Meningomyelocele
  C. Omphalocele
  D. Gastroschisis

626. Appropriate management of a neonate born with congenital diaphragmatic hernia (CDH) should include
  A. Insertion of an orogastric or nasogastric tube
  B. Expansion of the hypoplastic lung with positive-pressure ventilation
  C. Hyperventilation to keep the $PaCO_2$ below 40 and the pH greater than 7.40
  D. Rapid transport to the OR for surgical correction

627. Select the **TRUE** statement regarding complex regional pain syndrome (CRPS) in children
  A. More common in males than females
  B. Upper extremity is more frequently involved than the lower extremity
  C. Best treated with sympathetic blocks
  D. Often associated with depression and anxiety

628. Which of the following statements regarding perioperative cardiac arrest in children is **NOT** correct?
  A. Cardiac arrest is more common in neonates than in infants or older children
  B. "Equipment related" causes occur in more than 25% of cardiac arrests
  C. Resuscitation is more often successful if the cause is anesthesia related rather than nonanesthesia related
  D. Emergency surgery is associated with greater than four times the chance of a cardiac arrest

629. Which of the following represents the greatest risk for postoperative apnea in an infant?
  A. PCA of 60 weeks
  B. Hemoglobin 10 g/dL
  C. Recovery in the postanesthesia care unit (PACU) after pyloric stenosis repair
  D. 20th weight percentile on growth chart

630. Which of the following statements regarding the Mapleson D breathing circuit is **FALSE**?
  A. It has a proximal fresh gas inflow and a distal overflow valve
  B. With an inspiratory-to-expiratory (I:E) breathing ratio of 1:2, rebreathing is eliminated with spontaneous ventilation when the fresh gas flow is three times the minute ventilation
  C. The Mapleson D circuit requires lower fresh gas flows with spontaneous ventilation compared with controlled ventilation
  D. The Bain circuit is a modification of the Mapleson D circuit

631. Which of the following is **LEAST** likely to reduce the incidence of postoperative apnea in preterm infants undergoing surgery for inguinal hernia repair?
  A. Delaying operation until 60 weeks' PCA
  B. Preoperative correction of anemia
  C. Caffeine administration
  D. Spinal anesthetic with ketamine sedation

632. A 32-week-EGA, 2-kg newborn born a few hours ago is to undergo a repair of his gastroschisis under general anesthesia. Which of the following sizes of uncuffed ETTs should you use, and how far should it be positioned to most likely be properly placed in the trachea (gums to midtrachea distance)?
  A. 2.0-internal diameter (ID) ETT placed at 6 cm
  B. 2.5-internal diameter (ID) ETT placed at 8 cm
  C. 3.0-internal diameter (ID) ETT placed at 10 cm
  D. 3.5-internal diameter (ID) ETT placed at 12 cm

633. Induction of general anesthesia for an elective operation should be delayed how many hours after breastfeeding?
  A. 2 hours
  B. 4 hours
  C. 6 hours
  D. No fasting needed because breast milk is OK

634. In the infant, hypothermia would **LEAST** likely manifest as
  A. Metabolic acidosis
  B. Prolonged duration of action of nondepolarizing muscle relaxants
  C. Hyperglycemia
  D. Impaired coagulation

635. Necrotizing enterocolitis (NEC) has all of the following characteristics **EXCEPT**
  A. Most have thrombocytopenia ($<70,000/mm^3$) and a prolonged prothrombin time (PT) and activated partial thromboplastin time (aPTT)
  B. Commonly associated with decreased cardiac output in the presence of fetal asphyxia or postnatal respiratory complications
  C. Umbilical artery catheters are useful to assess acid-base status
  D. Occurs in 10% to 20% of newborns weighing less than 1500 g

636. Which of the following statements concerning codeine is **INCORRECT**?
  A. Codeine is a weak opioid and is used for the treatment of mild to moderate pain
  B. Peak blood level after oral or IM administration is about 30 minutes
  C. Codeine is metabolized to morphine
  D. Codeine is the postoperative analgesic of choice, after acetaminophen, for the treatment of pain after tonsillectomy in children <12 years of age

637. Which of the following drugs is **LEAST** likely to be used for a 4-year-old receiving proton beam radiation treatment for his medulloblastoma?
  A. EMLA cream
  B. Propofol
  C. Rocuronium
  D. Dexmedetomidine

638. A 5-year-old girl with hemolytic-uremic syndrome (HUS) is brought to the OR for placement of a dialysis catheter. Medical issues typical for this disease include
  A. Thrombocytopenia
  B. Increased intracranial pressure
  C. Pancreatitis
  D. All of the above

639. A 3-year-old child status post resection of Wilms tumor at age 2 years is receiving doxorubicin (Adriamycin) and cyclophosphamide for metastatic disease. The patient is scheduled for placement of a Hickman catheter for continued chemotherapy. Anesthetic concerns related to this patient's chemotherapeutic treatment include each of the following **EXCEPT**
   A. Thrombocytopenia
   B. Inhibition of plasma cholinesterase
   C. Cardiac depression
   D. Pulmonary toxicity

640. Hypotension in children is characterized by a systolic blood pressure
   A. Less than 60 mm Hg for the term neonate (0-28 days old)
   B. Less than 70 mm Hg for infants 1 to 12 months old
   C. Less than 70 mm Hg + (2 × age in years) mm Hg for children 1 to 10 years old
   D. All of the above

641. What percent of the adult's glomerular filtration rate, or GFR, does a 1-year-old possess?
   A. 30%
   B. 50%
   C. 75%
   D. 100%

642. Each of the following results in a reduction of the incidence of postoperative vomiting (POV) in children undergoing strabismus surgery **EXCEPT**
   A. IV hydration of 30 mL/kg/hr
   B. Dexamethasone 0.15-0.5 mg/kg IV
   C. Ondansetron 50 to 200 μg/kg IV
   D. Anticholinergics (atropine 10-20 μg/kg or glycopyrrolate 10 μg/kg)

567. (D) The hemoglobin molecule is encoded by two hemoglobin genes; one gene is inherited from each parent. Each gene encodes two globulin chains, one alpha chain, and one nonalpha chain. The hemoglobin molecule consists of four globulin chains; two of these are alpha chains, and two are nonalpha chains. Normal adult hemoglobin has two alpha and two beta chains.

Sickle cell disease (SCD) describes a group of autosomal recessive red blood cell disorders wherein patients have abnormal hemoglobin, called hemoglobin S (HbS). HbS occurs when there is a single amino acid substitution in the beta chain (valine for glutamic acid). Patients with sickle cell *anemia* have two HbS genes (HbSS) (normal alpha and abnormal beta chain from each parent). Patients with sickle cell *trait* (SCT) have a normal alpha chain and beta chain from one parent and a normal alpha but an abnormal beta chain (HbS) from the other parent. In the United States, about 0.2% of African Americans have sickle cell anemia and 8% to 10% have SCT. Sickling can occur in homozygous patients (HbSS) when HbS changes shape to long helical strands, leading to changes in the RBC shape, which can impede blood flow. Sickling can be precipitated by hypoxia, acidosis, hypothermia, dehydration, and poor perfusion.

Fetal hemoglobin has two alpha and two gamma chains (no beta chains) and does not sickle. At birth, the concentration of hemoglobin F (fetal hemoglobin) is about 80% and decreases to about 40% at 2.5 months, 5% at 6 months, and 2% at 1 year. The predominant hemoglobin in this 1-month-old infant is hemoglobin F, which would initially protect the infant from the manifestations of sickle cell anemia were he or she homozygous for HbS. The patient should, however, be screened for sickle cell anemia at some point in early life if hemoglobin electrophoresis was not done as part of routine newborn screening in at-risk populations. Screening for sickle cell anemia is not a prerequisite for surgery at 1 month of age *(Davis: Smith's Anesthesia for Infants and Children, ed 9, pp 399–401, 1074, 1077, 1160–1163; Hines: Stoelting's Anesthesia and Co-Existing Disease, ed 7, pp 483–484; Miller: Miller's Anesthesia, ed 8, pp 1211–1212).*

568. (A) The glottis of a premature newborn is at the level of C3. In the full-term newborn, the glottis is at the level of C4, and in the adult, the glottis is at the C5-C6 level. The relatively higher (more cephalic) glottis coupled with the relatively larger tongue makes intubation more difficult in the newborn *(Barash: Clinical Anesthesia, ed 8, p 1185).*

569. (C) Spinal anesthesia can be administered safely to children of all ages. Hypotension secondary to a loss of sympathetic tone, common in the adult, is rare in the child younger than 5 years of age, even when the level rises as high as T3. Respiratory depression, including apnea and a decrease in oxygen saturation with associated bradycardia, will likely be the initial signs associated with a total spinal block in the infant *(Barash: Clinical Anesthesia, ed 7, pp 1196–1197; Davis: Smith's Anesthesia for Infants and Children, ed 9, pp 476–477).*

570. (C) The body compartment volumes change with age. Total body water (TBW = extracellular fluid + intracellular fluid) tends to decrease from about 80% of total body weight in preterm newborns to 75% in term newborns and 60% in 6-month-old infants and healthy adults, whereas fat and muscle tend to increase with age. Muscle contains about 75% water, whereas fat contains only 10% water. In addition, the percentage of intracellular fluid and extracellular fluid is different. In adults two thirds of the fluid is intracellular and one third is extracellular, whereas in term newborns only 40% of the fluid is intracellular and 60% is extracellular. These alterations in body composition have implications for the volume of distribution and redistribution of drugs. For example, most antibiotics as well as succinylcholine, which are more water soluble, require a larger initial dose per kg compared with that for adults to achieve the desired blood levels in newborns *(Davis: Smith's Anesthesia for Infants and Children, ed 9, pp 114–115; Miller: Miller's Anesthesia, ed 8, pp 2763–2764).*

571. (A) ROP, formally called retrolental fibroplasia (scar tissue forming behind the lens of the eye), typically occurs in newborns who are born at less than 35 weeks' gestational age (GA). It is a leading cause of childhood blindness worldwide. The risk of ROP is inversely related to age and birth weight, with a significant risk occurring in infants weighing less than 1500 g. ROP occurs in about 70% of infants who weigh less than 1000 g at birth; fortunately, 80% to 90% of these have spontaneous regression of the retinal changes. Post-conceptual age (PCA) is the sum of the GA (the period between conception and birth) and the postnatal age (the time since birth). Because of the difficulty in determining the exact date of conception, the PMA is often used in place of PCA. The risk of ROP is negligible after 44 weeks' PMA. The mechanism for ROP is complex and is related to the process of retinal development and maturation. Under normal circumstances, retinal vasculature develops from the optic disk toward the periphery of the retina. This process typically is completed by 40 to 44 weeks' PMA. Hyperoxia causes constriction of the retinal arterioles, resulting in swelling and degeneration of the endothelium, which disrupts normal retinal development. Vascularization of the retina resumes in an abnormal fashion when normal oxygen conditions return, resulting in neovascularization and scarring of the retina. In the worst-case scenario, this process can lead to retinal detachment and blindness.

Consequently, hyperoxia should be avoided when anesthetizing preterm infants and infants up to 44 weeks' PMA. To reduce the risk of ROP, it is recommended that the oxygen saturation be maintained between 88% and 93% (about PaO_2 50-70 mm Hg) during anesthesia. Monitoring of the oxygen saturation should be preductal (in the right arm), which correlates better with the oxygen saturation going to the brain and the retinal vessels. Although oxygen exposure has been strongly associated with ROP, other factors play a role, including respiratory distress syndrome, mechanical ventilation, hypoxia, hypocarbia, hypercarbia, blood transfusions, sepsis, congenital infections, and vitamin E deficiency. Although rare, newborns with cyanotic congenital heart disease who have never been exposed to supplemental oxygen therapy have also developed ROP *(Davis: Smith's Anesthesia for Infants and Children, ed 9, pp 578, 905–907; Hines: Stoelting's Anesthesia and Co-Existing Disease, ed 7, p 641; Miller: Basics of Anesthesia, ed 7, pp 605–606).*

572. (D) This patient has signs consistent with severe dehydration and needs resuscitation with fluid and electrolytes before surgery. Infantile hypertrophic pyloric stenosis (IHPS) is the most common cause of intestinal obstruction in infancy and is more of a medical emergency than a surgical emergency. Surgery should be delayed until there is thorough evaluation and treatment of the associated fluid and electrolyte imbalances. Typically, the infant presents with nonbilious vomiting soon after feeding, between the third and fifth weeks of age. Soon after a vomiting episode, an "olive"-shaped mass may be felt in the right epigastrium in 50% to 90% of affected infants. Ultrasound is now commonly performed to confirm the diagnosis. Vomiting results in dehydration and electrolyte abnormalities. The loss of gastric hydrochloric acid (HCl) can produce hypochloremia and metabolic alkalosis. The kidneys attempt to maintain pH by exchanging K^+ for H^+ can result in hypokalemia. Fluid resuscitation should be initiated with isotonic saline (20 mL/kg for severe dehydration), followed by 5% dextrose in 0.45% NaCl up to two times maintenance rate. If an IV line catheter cannot be established, an intraosseous needle should be placed. After the infant resumes urine production, potassium (10-40 mEq/L) can be safely added to the IV fluids. Once there has been adequate hydration and correction of the electrolyte and acid-base abnormalities, the patient can more safely undergo anesthesia and surgery. Most infants respond with good urine output and correction of electrolyte abnormalities within 12 to 48 hours. Then surgery can be performed in a less urgent setting. An oral gastric tube is placed before the induction of anesthesia to remove any gastric contents due to the obstruction, regardless of the anesthetic used (general or spinal), in an attempt to minimize the risk of aspiration of gastric contents *(Davis: Smith's Anesthesia for Infants and Children, ed 9, pp 795-797; Hines: Stoelting's Anesthesia and Co-Existing Disease, ed 7, p 647).*

573. (A) EA and TEF result from the failure of the esophagus and trachea to completely separate during development. The incidence is about 1 in 4000 live births. Although each of the listed answers is possible, Figure A, called a Type C TEF (EA with a distal TEF), represents the most common type (about 85%-90% of cases). Because the fetus cannot swallow with EA, there is a higher incidence of maternal polyhydramnios and premature deliveries. Currently, about 40% to 50% of cases are diagnosed prenatally. In the delivery room, one is unable to pass a suction catheter into the stomach, and, if an x-ray is taken, the presence of air in the stomach suggests that a fistula exists between the trachea and the stomach. If it is not detected in the delivery room, the newborn tends to have excessive oral secretions and is unable to feed. About 20% to 50% of patients with EA or TEF have additional congenital defects: congenital heart disease (20%-35%), genitourinary disorders (15%-24%), gastrointestinal disorders (16%-24%), skeletal abnormalities (13%-18%), central nervous system (CNS) disorders (10%), mediastinal disorders (8%), and chromosomal disorders (5.5%). Because of the frequency of associated defects, the term VATER (Vertebral defects, imperforate Anus, TracheoEsophageal fistula, and Renal abnormalities) and VACTERL (VATER with associated Cardiac and Limb anomalies) have been coined and remind us to look for other associated conditions. Figure B (8% of cases) is a Type A TEF (EA without a TEF). Figure C (4% of cases) is a Type E TEF (TEF without an EA) and is also called an H-type TEF. Figure D (1% of cases) is a Type D TEF (EA with a proximal and a distal TEF). Type B (1% of cases; not shown) is a Type B TEF (EA with a proximal TEF) *(Davis: Smith's Anesthesia for Infants and Children, ed 9, pp 597–604; Hines: Stoelting's Anesthesia and Co-Existing Disease, ed 7, pp 643–644; Miller: Basics of Anesthesia, ed 7, pp 602–604).*

574. (C) The estimated blood volume (EBV) in mL/kg for premature infants is 90 to 100 mL/kg, for term infants is 80 to 90 mL/kg, for infants less than a year is 75 to 80 mL/kg, and for older children is 70 to 75 mL/kg. For this 3-kg term newborn, the volume is 80 to 90 mL/kg $\times$ 3 kg = 240 to 270 mL *(Davis: Smith's Anesthesia for Infants and Children, ed 9, pp 413–414).*

575. (B) In patients greater than 4 months of age, transfusion is almost always indicated when the hemoglobin level is <6 g/dL (Hct is <18%), and transfusion is rarely indicated when the hemoglobin level is >10 (Hct is >30), especially if the anemia is acute. In the intermediate hemoglobin range 6 to 10, individualization is needed based on ongoing blood loss as well as evidence of organ ischemia. In this case where blood loss is common, the transfusion threshold of 8 g/dL Hgb was chosen as the indication to start transfusions.

To calculate the MABL, the following formula is commonly used:

$MABL = EBV \times (Hi - Hp)/Hi$
Where EBV = estimated blood volume
Hi = initial Hct
Hp = lowest permissible Hct or target Hct

In this case using 80 mL/kg, the EBV for the 10-kg infant, the EBV = 800 mL.

$MABL = 800\,mL\,(32 - 24)/32 = 200\,mL$

NOTE: Some anesthesiologists put the average Hct (Ha = Hi− Hp) in the denominator of the above MABL formula [i.e., MABL = EBV $\times$ (Hi − Hp)/Ha = 800 mL $\times$ (32 − 24)/28 = 228 mL]. Before infusing blood, the circulating blood volume is usually expanded with crystalloids in a ratio of 3 mL of crystalloid for each mL of blood lost *(Cote: A Practice of Anesthesia for Infants and Children, ed 6, pp 257–259; Davis: Smith's Anesthesia for Infants and Children, ed 9, pp 413–414; Miller: Basics of Anesthesia, ed 7, p 594; Miller: Miller's Anesthesia, ed 8, pp 2784–2785).*

576. (B) If blood loss exceeds the MABL replacement, PRBCs are usually needed. The normal Hct of PRBCs is about 60%. To calculate the volume of PRBCs to be transfused, the following formula is used:

Volume of RBCs = EBV $\times$ (desired Hct − present Hct)/Hct of PRBCs
Where EBV = estimated blood volume

In this case using 80 mL/kg, the EBV for the 10-kg 11-month-old, we have an EBV of 800 mL. In this case the volume to be infused = 800 $\times$ (24 − 18)/60 = 80 mL

In clinical practice, many clinicians use a simpler formula of 10 mL/kg of packed RBCs to raise the hemoglobin about 2 g/dL (Hct 6%) *(Cote: A Practice of Anesthesia for Infants and Children, ed 6, pp 257–259; Davis: Smith's Anesthesia for Infants and Children, ed 9, pp 413–415; Miller: Miller's Anesthesia, ed 8, pp 2784–2785).*

577. (C) Given that cuffed ETTs are often chosen to be a size smaller (i.e., 0.5 mm) than uncuffed ETTs, the lumen is narrower and, therefore, spontaneous breathing is more difficult. Because a smaller ETT can be used with a cuff, fewer intubations are needed to select the correct tube size. Also because of the cuff, less gas leaks from the trachea into the pharynx, allowing administration of lower gas flows with potential cost savings as well as less environmental pollution. The gases are less likely to leak into the pharynx, and this should decrease the chance of an airway fire if high oxygen or nitrous oxide concentrations are used with cautery in the oral cavity. To further decrease the chance of an airway fire, most anesthesiologists would avoid the use of nitrous oxide and would decrease the F_{IO_2} to around 0.30 if oxygen saturations are acceptable. The chance of aspiration of gastric contents with a cuffed ETT is still possible but less likely than with an uncuffed ETT. Other indications for a cuffed over an uncuffed ETT include impaired pulmonary compliance, cardiopulmonary bypass, and the need for controlled mechanical ventilation *(Davis: Smith's Anesthesia for Infants and Children, ed 9, pp 360–362; Miller: Miller's Anesthesia, ed 8, pp 2777–2778)*.

578. (C) Inhalation agents are respiratory depressants. In general, they increase the respiratory rate and decrease the tidal volume (V_T) of respirations and are associated with an increase in $PaCO_2$. When inducing a child with an inhalation agent, especially below the MAC level, the respiratory pattern can vary and include breath holding, excessive hyperventilation, and laryngospasm. The stages of inhalation anesthesia were classically described with ether; similar stages are seen with the newer inhalation agents. However, because the signs are less pronounced with the newer volatile anesthetics, they are rarely described anymore. The classic stages of depth of ether anesthesia include the first stage of anesthesia (analgesia). Patients in the first stage can respond to verbal stimulation, have an intact lid reflex, have normal respiratory patterns and intact airway reflexes, and have some analgesia. The second stage of anesthesia (delirium or excitement stage) is associated with unconsciousness, irregular and unpredictable respiratory patterns (including hyperventilation), nonpurposeful muscle movements, and the risk of clinically important reflex activity (e.g., laryngospasm, vomiting, cardiac arrhythmias). The third stage of anesthesia (surgical anesthesia) is associated with a return to more regular periodic respirations and is the level associated with the achievement of MAC. MAC is noted by the absence of movement (in 50% of patients) in response to a surgical incision. As anesthesia is deepened, stage 4 (respiratory paralysis) is associated with respiratory and cardiovascular arrest. In the case cited in this question, the second stage or excitement stage of anesthesia is demonstrated, which is seen in about 10% of children with a sevoflurane induction. Note: MH triggered by the sole use of volatile anesthetics produces an elevation of carbon dioxide levels with tachypnea and tachycardia, but this is rare during the first 20 minutes of an anesthetic. In this case the tachypnea and tachycardia will usually quickly resolve with continued administration of inhaled agents. If over several minutes the tachycardia and tachypnea worsen, especially with an increase in end-tidal carbon dioxide, then the diagnosis of MH should be considered. Sevoflurane and desflurane seem to be less of a trigger for MH than halothane. Mild hypothermia, propofol, nondepolarizing neuromuscular blockers, and tranquilizers may delay or prevent MH from developing. Succinylcholine (the only depolarizing neuromuscular blocker in use today) often hastens the development of MH in susceptible patients. Although in the unanesthetized patient mild hypoxia can initially be associated with tachypnea and tachycardia, the severely hypoxic patient with high concentrations of sevoflurane is associated with hypopnea or apnea. Aspiration of gastric contents would more likely lead to laryngospasms, wheezing, and hypoxia *(Cote: A Practice of Anesthesia for Infants and Children, ed 6, pp 922–926; Davis: Smith's Anesthesia for Infants and Children, ed 9, pp 106, 207, 212, 1190–1191; Miller: Basics of Anesthesia, ed 7, pp 95–100)*.

579. (D) The hemodynamic indices described in this question are normal for a healthy 1-month-old neonate *(Cote: A Practice of Anesthesia for Infants and Children, ed 6, p 18; Miller: Basics of Anesthesia, ed 7, pp 588–591)*.

AGE-DEPENDENT CARDIOVASCULAR VARIABLES

	Neonate	12-Month- Old	5-Year- Old	Adult (>16 years)
Weight (kg)	3	10	19	70
Oxygen consumption (mL/kg/min)	6-8	5	4	3-4
Systolic blood pressure (mm Hg)	60-75	70-90	80-100	100-125
Heart rate (beats/min)	100-160	80-140	65-120	60-100

580. (D) Dark brown or cola-colored urine (i.e., myoglobinemia) may be caused by rhabdomyolysis, a possible sign of MH, and this patient should be evaluated. More typical signs and symptoms of MH include tachycardia, tachypnea, hypercarbia, hyperkalemia with peaked T waves, acidosis, increased sympathetic activity, irregular heartbeat, mottled cyanotic skin, profuse sweating, and a late sign of increased temperature (>1.5° C over 5 minutes or temperature >38.8° C). Supportive laboratory tests for MH include elevated serum creatinine phosphokinase (CPK; typically >20,000 U/L); myoglobin in the serum and urine; increased serum potassium, calcium, and lactate levels; and a metabolic/respiratory acidosis on an arterial blood gas. If the presumed diagnosis is MH, therapy should be initiated *(Davis: Smith's Anesthesia for Infants and Children, ed 9, pp 1190–1191; Hines: Stoelting's Anesthesia and Co-Existing Disease, ed 7, pp 666–668).*

581. (B) In infants and young children, there should be a small air leak around the ETT at peak inflation pressures of approximately 15 to 25 cm H_2O. The "leak test" is performed by listening with a stethoscope over the larynx for an air leak with airway pressures of 15 to 25 cm H_2O. With a cuffed ETT, the cuff is slowly inflated until the air leak ceases. An air leak within this pressure range allows for adequate ventilation and reduces the incidence of postintubation croup. The most common cause of postintubation croup is a tight-fitting ETT without an air leak at 30 to 40 cm H_2O. Other causes of postintubation croup are multiple or traumatic intubations, frequent head position changes during surgery, position other than supine, coughing on the ETT, neck surgery, and prolonged intubations (>1 hour). To decrease the incidence of postintubation croup, dexamethasone is frequently administered IV at the start of the procedure. If postintubation croup develops, racemic epinephrine (0.5 mL of a 2.25% solution) mixed with 3 to 5 mL of normal saline is administered by nebulizer over 5 to 10 minutes. Because the child may develop "rebound effect" when the racemic epinephrine wears off, patients are typically watched for at least 4 hours. If croup redevelops, the child should be admitted overnight and further therapy given *(Cote: A Practice of Anesthesia for Infants and Children, ed 6, pp 313, 778–780; Davis: Smith's Anesthesia for Infants and Children, ed 9, pp 360–362, 395).*

582. (C) A CDH is the herniation of abdominal viscera into the chest cavity through a defect in the diaphragm and occurs in approximately 1 in every 3000 live births. In about 50% of patients with CDH, other congenital abnormalities are present. Most CDHs occur through a defect in the left side of the diaphragm (>80%) and produce the classic triad of dyspnea, cyanosis, and apparent dextrocardia. Symptoms depend on the degree of herniation and the amount of respiratory compromise. Spontaneous ventilation is usually inadequate, and endotracheal intubation in the delivery room is usually needed (and preferred over mask ventilation, which may push some gas into the stomach, increasing respiratory compromise). Oral or nasogastric tubes are placed early to prevent gastric distention and worsening respiratory compromise. Because CDH is associated with hypoplastic lungs, current ventilatory support aims at maintaining a preductal oxygen saturation of 85% to 95%, using low airway pressures (goal of Peaked Inspiratory Pressures (PIP) <25 cm H_2O) and allowing for moderate permissive hypercarbia ($PaCO_2$ 60-65 mm Hg). Normally the high PVR that babies have in utero quickly decreases to the adult lower PVR after birth, allowing more blood flow to the lungs. If the PVR persists or recurs, the inhalation of nitric oxide, a selective pulmonary artery vasodilator, is often used.

If the patient experiences sudden oxygen desaturation during positive-pressure ventilation, a tension pneumothorax should be suspected (usually on the contralateral side to the CDH); if confirmed, a chest tube should be placed. Because breath sounds are not equal in patients with CDH, auscultation for proper ETT placement is difficult to interpret, and an x-ray would be helpful. Despite intensive treatments, including extracorporeal membrane oxygenation (ECMO), many of these newborns will die in the newborn period. The cause of death is often related to the hypoplastic lungs, poor transition from fetal to adult circulation, and congenital abnormalities. At one time, these patients were rushed to the OR; now they are usually stabilized (sometimes for 5-15 days) and more electively taken to the OR. An ETT in the mainstem would lead to increased airway pressures and a slow decline in oxygen saturation that usually rapidly responds to an elevation in FiO_2. Endotracheal tubes with an obstruction from secretions are usually treated with suctioning of the ETT and not replacement, and PEEP is potentially dangerous and might lead to a tension pneumothorax *(Davis: Smith's Anesthesia for Infants and Children, ed 9, pp 586–597; Hines: Stoelting's Anesthesia and Co-Existing Disease, ed 7, pp 642–643; Miller: Miller's Anesthesia, ed 8, p 2793).*

583. (B) The normal estimated blood volume (EBV) in children over 1 year of age is 70 to 75 mL/kg, and in this previously normal 8-year-old boy who weighs 30 kg, his normal blood volume would be 2100 to 2250 mL. Unlike adults, children maintain stable blood pressure until reaching a 25% to 35% loss of their circulating blood volume. This is related to their high sympathetic tone, which produces profound peripheral vasoconstriction in an effort to maintain blood pressure, making tachycardia an earlier sign of volume depletion than hypotension. Pediatric patients with <20% blood loss are tachycardic with weak thready pulses, have only a slight decrease in urine output, and can be irritable with normal mentation. With 25% blood loss, they are also tachycardic with weak and thready pulses, but urine output is decreased, and they are often confused and lethargic. With 40% blood loss, there is frank hypotension, usually tachycardia, urine output is zero (anuric), and the patient may be comatose. At times, patients with >40% blood loss may be bradycardic due to the marked decrease in the amount of blood returning to the heart for pumping. This patient is most likely approximately 25% depleted and not in the <20% range because his blood pressure is normal with tachycardia, oliguria, and confusion and lethargy *(Davis: Smith's Anesthesia for Infants and Children, ed 9, pp 978–979).*

584. (C) The depth of insertion of an oral ETT from the gums to the midtracheal level is approximately 7 cm for a 1-kg newborn, 8 cm for a 2-kg newborn, 9 cm for a 3-kg newborn, and 10 cm for a typical 3.5-kg term newborn. There are many ways to estimate the appropriate depth of insertion of an oral ETT (in centimeters) for infants and children. One method is using age (e.g., >3 years):

(Age in years)/2 + 12 = tube length inserted
In this 6-year-old child : 6/2 + 12 = 15 cm

Another way is to multiply the internal diameter (ID) size of the ETT by 3. For example, when you use a 5.0 ID size ETT, insert the tube about 15 cm. When using a cuffed ETT, the cuff should be visualized as just passing the vocal cords. If an uncuffed ETT is used, the tube is inserted to the first or second line on the tube at the level of the vocal cords *(Davis: Smith's Anesthesia for Infants and Children, ed 9, pp 360–362; Miller: Basics of Anesthesia, ed 7, p 596).*

585. (D) In elective cases, IV fluids are administered to maintain maintenance fluid requirements, to replace fluid deficits from preoperative fasting, to replenish third space losses, and to replace ongoing fluid losses from the surgical procedure. In emergency cases, fluid may also be needed to restore intravascular volume due to hemorrhage or gastrointestinal or renal losses.

The maintenance IV fluid rate or volume per hour is based on a 4:2:1 rule, where 4 mL/kg is administered for the first 10 kg of weight, 2 mL/kg for the next 10 kg of weight, and 1 mL/kg for any weight over 20 kg. Thus for this 14-kg child, hourly maintenance fluid requirement is [(4 mL × 10 kg) + (2 mL × 4 kg)] per hour = 48 mL/hour.

NPO replacement is often calculated by multiplying the hourly maintenance requirement × number of hours the child has been NPO. Thus for this child, 48 mL/hr × 10 hours = 480 mL. In general, half of the fluid deficit + the hourly maintenance fluid (240 mL + 48 mL) is administered in the first hour of anesthesia, one fourth of the deficit + maintenance fluids for the second hour (120 mL + 48 mL), and one fourth of the deficit + maintenance fluids for the third hour (120 mL + 48 mL); maintenance fluids are administered thereafter (48 mL). However, because the fasted patient conserves fluid, these calculated volumes are higher than required. Replacing the entire fluid deficit with 5% dextrose, 5% dextrose in 0.2% or 5% dextrose in 0.45% NaCl (i.e., hyponatremic fluids) will often produce hyperglycemia as well as hyponatremia in the child, and these fluids are not recommended as replacement fluids. Common practice is to replace fluid deficits and maintenance fluids with either normal saline or lactated Ringer solution and then to evaluate the response.

Third space losses can vary from 1 mL/kg/hr for minor procedures (e.g., strabismus repair) to greater than 15 mL/kg/hr for major abdominal procedures (e.g., gastroschisis repair).

Typically, healthy children older than 1 year of age (or >10-kg weight) do not require supplemental glucose during surgery because their glycogen stores are adequate for the stress of surgery. Glucose solutions are commonly administered to pediatric patients when the development of hypoglycemia is greatest, namely neonates (<6 months of age) and any patient who is critically ill, malnourished, or has hepatic dysfunction. In these infants, 1% to 2.5% dextrose in lactated Ringer solution is administered as a separate piggyback infusion at maintenance rates (5% dextrose in lactated Ringer often leads to hyperglycemia). Keep in mind that it is important to avoid hyperglycemia because hyperglycemia can induce an osmotic diuresis and can worsen neurologic outcome if cerebral ischemia develops.

The most common isotonic solutions used to replace fluid losses are lactated Ringer solution, normal saline, and PlasmaLyte A solution. Most would avoid the use of large amounts of normal saline because there is a risk of developing hyperchloremic metabolic acidosis. Normal saline contains 154 mEq/L of Na^+, which causes the kidney to excrete bicarbonate to preserve electrical neutrality.

As always the clinician should individualize the child's care using the above as a guideline for a starting point in fluid management *(Cote: A Practice of Anesthesia for Infants and Children, ed 6, p 206; Davis: Smith's Anesthesia for Infants and Children, ed 9, p 388; Miller: Basics of Anesthesia, ed 7, pp 593–594; Miller: Miller's Anesthesia, ed 8, pp 2782–2784).*

586. (D) Neonates and infants (<2 years of age) require more succinylcholine per body weight than do older children and adults to produce neuromuscular blockade because the extracellular fluid volume is much greater in neonates and infants. Because succinylcholine is highly water soluble, its volume of distribution is greater. Therefore the recommended dose of succinylcholine in neonates and infants to provide optimal conditions for tracheal intubation is 2 to 3 mg/kg instead of the 1 mg/kg used for adults. See also Question 570 *(Cote: A Practice of Anesthesia for Infants and Children, ed 6, p 146; Davis: Smith's Anesthesia for Infants and Children, ed 9, pp 247–248; Miller: Miller's Anesthesia, ed 8, p 2771).*

587. (B) The usual goal for a child with type 1 diabetes is to maintain a blood glucose value between 100 to 200 mg/dL. On the day of surgery, no rapid-acting or short-duration insulin is administered unless the blood glucose is elevated, especially over 250, before surgery. The "1500 rule" gives you a correction value for each unit of insulin administered. Dividing 1500 by the child's daily insulin dose gives you a correction value. For this child, 1500/30 = 50, which means that each unit of subcutaneously administered insulin will reduce the blood sugar by 50 mg/dL. So 3 units will reduce the sugar from 300 mg/dL to 150 mg/dL. The onset for subcutaneously administered rapid-acting insulin (Lispro or Humalog; Aspart or Novolog; Glulisine or Apidra) is 15 minutes with a peak effect in 30 to 90 minutes and a duration of 3 to 4 hours. For IV or subcutaneously short-acting regular insulin (Humulin R or Novolin R), onset is 30 to 60 minutes and peak effect is in 2 to 3 hours with a duration of 3 to 6 hours. Although drugs can be used to adjust the blood sugar to the level you want, you should also evaluate the reason for such a high preoperative blood sugar and consider the need for surgical intervention that day. Patients with diabetic ketoacidosis tend to have blood sugars >200 mg/dL, ketonemia, ketonuria, and acidemia (pH <7.30 and/or serum bicarbonate <15 mEq/L) *(Cote: A Practice of Anesthesia for Infants and Children, ed 6, pp 629–641; Davis: Smith's Anesthesia for Infants and Children, ed 9, pp 1101–1104).*

588. (A) Apnea spells are defined as cessation of breathing for at least 15 seconds and are often accompanied by bradycardia and/or cyanosis. Postoperative apnea is inversely correlated with both gestational age (GA) at birth and post-conceptual age (PCA). Postoperative apnea is also associated with infants who have had a history of apnea and bradycardia (A&B) spells as well as anemia (Hct <30). Infants (especially former premature newborns) younger than 60 weeks' PCA are at risk for apnea after general anesthesia, although most cases will occur in infants less than 45 weeks' PCA. These patients should be admitted to the hospital and have at least 12 apnea-free hours of monitoring before discharge. This child was born at 31 weeks' EGA and is now 10 weeks old or is 41 weeks' PCA and needs to be admitted. Of the postoperative analgesia plans listed with overnight observation, answer A is the most appropriate. Answers B and D include analgesic doses that are too high. Although caffeine (10 mg/kg) can effectively treat apnea in premature infants, these patients should be admitted for observation and further treatment *(Cote: A Practice of Anesthesia for Infants and Children, ed 6, pp 64–65; Davis: Smith's Anesthesia for Infants and Children, ed 9, pp 394, 463).*

589. (C) The treatment for documented ventricular fibrillation (VF) or pVT is electrical defibrillation as soon as possible. CPR is performed until the defibrillator arrives and defibrillation is attempted. The 2015 American Heart Association guidelines for pediatric defibrillation recommend the first (monophasic or biphasic defibrillator) dose of 2 to 4 J/kg, 4 J/kg for subsequent doses with a consideration of a maximum of 10 J/kg. In this 20-kg child the initial dose is 20 × 2 J/kg = 40 J or 20 × 4 J/kg = 80 J. Automated external defibrillators (AEDs) can be safely used in children 1 to 8 years of age. When using an AED, it is best to use one with a pediatric attenuator system, which decreases the delivered energy to doses appropriate for children, with a common pediatric initial AED dose of 35 to 50 J and 80 to 90 J for subsequent doses *(American Heart Association/American Academy of Pediatrics: Pediatric Advanced Life Support – Provider Manual 2016, pp 26–28, 89–96; Davis: Smith's Anesthesia for Infants and Children, ed 9, pp 1260–1262; Miller: Basics of Anesthesia, ed 7, p 798).*

590. (B)

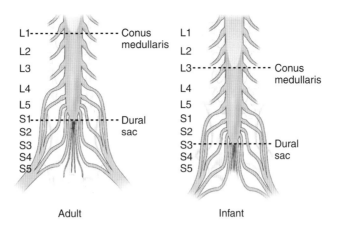

Adult   Infant

Common teaching states that the spinal cord of the newborn ends at L3 and does not reach the adult level of L1 until 1 year of age. Recent data using ultrasound suggest that the spinal cord of newborns ends at L2. The dural sac of newborns extends to S3-S4, and for the adult the dural sac ends at S1-S2. Most pediatric anesthesiologists would perform spinal puncture at the L4-L5 or L5-S1 interspace and would have the child in the sitting position to assist in cerebrospinal fluid (CSF) flow through the needle to ascertain successful placement of the tip of the spinal needle *(Cote: A Practice of Anesthesia for Infants and Children, ed 6, pp 949–953; Davis: Smith's Anesthesia for Infants and Children, ed 9, pp 472–476).*

591. (D) EA and TEF may be suspected prenatally when the mother has polyhydramnios; otherwise it is suspected soon after birth when excessive oral secretions, drooling, or coughing are noted and an oral suction catheter cannot be passed into the stomach. Because the passage of an oral gastric tube is not routine in many centers, the first manifestation of EA occurs when the newborn has trouble breathing (e.g., coughing) and regurgitates with the first feeding. After the diagnosis is made, these patients should be placed in the head-up position and the blind upper pouch of the esophagus should be decompressed with a suction tube immediately to reduce pulmonary aspiration of secretions *(Davis: Smith's Anesthesia for Infants and Children, ed 9, pp 599–602; Hines: Stoelting's Anesthesia and Co-Existing Disease, ed 7, pp 643–644; Miller: Basics of Anesthesia, ed 7, p 602).*

592. (D) An omphalocele develops when the normal gut fails to migrate from the yolk sac into the abdomen and is therefore located at the umbilical cord. The omphalocele may contain the stomach, loops of small and large intestine, and sometimes the liver. Omphaloceles are the most common abdominal wall defect and occur in about 1 in 4000 to 7000 births. 50% to 80% of patients with an omphalocele have associated chromosomal abnormalities (30% have Trisomy 21, 13, or 18), cardiac disease (20%), or other complex syndromes (e.g., pentalogy of Cantrell, exstrophy of the bladder, Beckwith-Wiedemann syndrome). Beckwith-Wiedemann syndrome occurs in about 1 in 10,000 births and is characterized by omphalocele, organomegaly, gigantism, large fontanelles, macroglossia, polycythemia, and profound hypoglycemia. These patients may be very difficult to intubate because of their significant macroglossia. The associated hypoglycemia will require blood glucose evaluations and often dextrose administration *(Cote: A Practice of Anesthesia for Infants and Children, ed 6, pp 863–865; Davis: Smith's Anesthesia for Infants and Children, ed 9, pp 519, 582–586; Miller: Miller's Anesthesia, ed 8, pp 2791–2792).*

593. (D) Preoperatively the newborn for a surgical repair of a TEF should not be fed, the upper pouch should be periodically suctioned, and the newborn should be placed in a 30- degree head-up, prone, or lateral position to decrease the chance of gastroesophageal reflux. Although an "awake" intubation (with no sedation and topical local anesthetic) is considered by some to be the safest technique for establishing an airway, in vigorous newborns this can be challenging, and slight sedation with fentanyl (0.2-0.5 µg/kg) may be needed. Also used is inhalation induction with sevoflurane or ketamine, with the newborn breathing spontaneously. Positive-pressure mask ventilation and paralysis should be avoided because it could force gas into the stomach, potentially making ventilation of the lungs more difficult. If positive-pressure ventilation is needed, the lowest inspiratory pressure should be used. A frequently used technique to facilitate correct placement of the ETT in a patient with a TEF is to advance the tube into a bronchus. While listening over the stomach, slowly withdraw the tube until breath sounds are heard over the stomach, which signifies that the ETT is now above the fistula. The ETT is then advanced until these sounds become diminished (i.e., properly placed just below the TEF). Bronchoscopy is used by some anesthesiologists to make sure only one fistula is present and to help position the ETT. After the ETT is properly positioned, muscle paralysis is used (*Cote: A Practice of Anesthesia for Infants and Children, ed 6, pp 858–859; Davis: Smith's Anesthesia for Infants and Children, ed 9, pp 600–602; Hines: Stoelting's Anesthesia and Co-Existing Disease, ed 7, pp 643–644*).

594. (C) Manifestations of an upper respiratory infection (URI) include (1) mildly sore or scratchy throat; (2) change in feeding or level of activity; (3) cough or sneezing; (4) rhinorrhea (new or change in consistency); (5) nasal congestion; (6) fever higher than 101° F (38.8° C); and (7) inflamed throat or hoarse voice. A child with a URI has an increased incidence of complications during anesthesia, such as laryngospasm, bronchospasm, breath holding, severe coughing, and major oxygen desaturations. If minor surgery is to be performed in the setting of a URI and the case involves ear, nose, and throat (ENT) surgery (e.g., adenotonsillectomy), the surgical procedure may help decrease the incidence of infections, and the case often proceeds. For less urgent or more major surgery (e.g., abdominal, thoracic, or cardiac), postponement for at least 4 weeks usually is advised.

This child has a lower respiratory infection. The planned procedure should be delayed for a period of at least 4 weeks. This child has early manifestations of pneumonia with an LLL infiltrate and should be evaluated by a pediatrician. Keep in mind that a negative chest x-ray may exist in the presence of pneumonia because radiographic changes lag behind the clinical symptoms of a lower respiratory infection.

Children with preexisting reactive airway disease who develop a URI are at higher risk of postoperative complications, and the threshold for postponing surgery should be even lower than for similar patients without comorbidities (*Cote: A Practice of Anesthesia for Infants and Children, ed 6, pp 285–288; Davis: Smith's Anesthesia for Infants and Children, ed 9, pp 1127–1128; Miller: Basics of Anesthesia, ed 7, p 597*).

595. (C) The first set of teeth are called primary teeth (milk or baby teeth) and are usually named by the letters of the alphabet, whereas the secondary or permanent teeth are usually named by numbers. There are 20 primary teeth. The first primary teeth to erupt are the central incisors followed by the lateral incisors at 6 to 9 months of age. At 1.5 to 2 years of age, the remaining primary teeth (cuspid, first molar, and second molar) erupt. The second molars are the last primary teeth to erupt and are often called the 2-year molars. All primary teeth are usually present by 3 years of age. The 32 permanent teeth begin to erupt at about 6 years of age, and most are present by 12 years of age (except the wisdom teeth, or third molars, which erupt at 15 to 25 years of age). Each primary tooth is shed about the time its permanent successor erupts. When caring for children, it is important to check for loose teeth to prevent dislodgement during airway manipulations (*Davis: Smith's Anesthesia for Infants and Children, ed 9, pp 1018–1020*).

596. (C) In the fetus, the fetal circulation includes PVR, which is extremely high. The PVR is 7 to 8 times higher during the third trimester compared with PVR at 24 hours after an uncomplicated birth. In utero, most of the right ventricular output bypasses the lungs and flows into the descending aorta through the ductus arteriosus. The driving force for the high PVR is hypoxia, with PaO_2 values in utero of <20 mm Hg. With the onset of ventilation at birth, the PVR suddenly decreases, enabling blood to flow more easily through the lungs. The combination of increasing PaO_2 values in the pulmonary circulation with breathing as well as a reduction in the mechanical compression of the lungs now filled with air leads to a marked increase in pulmonary blood flow and a decrease in PVR. The increase in PaO_2 not only acts as a pulmonary artery vasodilator (along with the lowering of the $PaCO_2$) but also acts as a vasoconstrictor to the ductus arteriosus (thus further assisting the change from the fetal to the adult circulation). Pulmonary vascular resistance continues to decrease after birth, reaching adult levels by 1 to 2 months of life. In patients with a left-to-right intracardiac shunt, the decrease in PVR leads to an increase in pulmonary blood flow and may result in pulmonary edema and eventual right heart failure (*Davis: Smith's Anesthesia for Infants and Children, ed 9, pp 78–79, 703*).

597. (D) A comprehensive understanding of thermoregulation and a meticulous attention to detail during the anesthetic care of infants are both necessary to minimize intraoperative heat loss. In anesthetized infants, heat loss occurs through the transfer of heat from the patient to the environment in one of four ways: radiation (transfer between objects not in contact), conduction (transfer between objects in contact), convection (transfer to moving molecules such as air and fluid), and evaporation. Of these, radiation and convection account for about 75% of the infant's heat loss. For this reason, placement of an infrared heater over the OR table and prewarming the OR atmosphere are the most effective means of preventing hypothermia in these patients. Covering the OR table with a heating blanket (up to 40° C and covered with a blanket); ventilating the patient with warm, humidified anesthetic gases; wrapping the extremities of the patient with sheet wadding; and covering the patient with a blanket or covering the patient's head with a cloth or plastic cap can also reduce heat loss and help prevent hypothermia. Convective forced-air warmers can help prevent a decrease in body temperature and also have been effective in rewarming hypothermic patients. A Mapleson D breathing circuit is not a circle system and does not preserve heat or moisture. To prevent rebreathing of expired gases, spontaneous breathing flow rates need to be two to three times the minute ventilation, and for controlled ventilation fresh gas flows need to be greater than 90 mL/kg/min. Low flows such as 50 mL/kg/min with Mapleson circuits are inadequate and will result in respiratory acidosis *(Davis: Smith's Anesthesia for Infants and Children, ed 9, pp 150–158, 299–300; Miller: Miller's Anesthesia, ed 8, pp 1627–1628).*

598. (D) Although all of these conditions can produce ventilatory depression in the newborn's postoperative period requiring mechanical ventilation, only pyloric stenosis produces CNS depression of respiration. Patients with pyloric stenosis have protracted vomiting of gastric contents (including HCl) that leads to dehydration, hypochloremic metabolic alkalosis, and hypokalemia (due to the kidneys exchanging potassium ions with hydrogen ions as a compensatory mechanism for the alkalosis). Postoperative ventilatory depression frequently occurs in infants with pyloric stenosis and is related to CSF alkalosis that is worsened by intraoperative hyperventilation of the lungs. Thus these patients should be fully awake with a normal rate and pattern of respiration before extubation is considered. This is one reason infants with pyloric stenosis should be stabilized and hydrated before coming to the OR. The other conditions listed can lead to mechanical, not central, causes of respiratory difficulty in the postoperative period. With gastroschisis and omphalocele, postoperative ventilation for 24 to 48 hours is often needed until respiratory compromise improves (unless the abdominal wall defect is very small). With TEF postoperative ventilation for 24 to 48 hours is commonly needed due to underlying pulmonary conditions (e.g., prematurity, pneumonia, tracheomalacia). In some cases when the esophagus needed to be anastomosed, ventilation is often needed for 5 to 7 days *(Davis: Smith's Anesthesia for Infants and Children, ed 9, pp 582–586, 597–602, 795–797; Hines: Stoelting's Anesthesia and Co-Existing Disease, ed 7, pp 643–647).*

599. (C) Newborns with diaphragmatic hernia have significant respiratory difficulty. In addition to their hypoplastic lungs, persistent pulmonary hypertension is present, producing right-to-left shunting through the patent ductus arteriosus. To more appropriately administer the anesthetic, a preductal (ductus arteriosus) artery should be cannulated to monitor arterial blood gases and blood pressure. The goal is to achieve a preductal oxygen saturation of 85% to 95% with mechanical ventilation and peak inspiratory pressures below 25 to 30 cm H_2O. To assess proper oxygen and carbon dioxide levels for appropriate ventilator settings, the right radial or temporal arteries (which arise from vessels that originate from the aorta proximal to the ductus arteriosus) are utilized. Blood may be shunted through the ductus arteriosus before its closure and may contain lower oxygen and higher carbon dioxide levels with the femoral, umbilical, or left radial arteries. The oxygen saturation monitors should be placed on the right arm as well *(Davis: Smith's Anesthesia for Infants and Children, ed 9, pp 591–592; Hines: Stoelting's Anesthesia and Co-Existing Disease, ed 7, pp 642–643).*

600. (C) MAC is defined as the minimal alveolar concentration at which 50% of patients do not move to a painful stimulus with the use of inhalation anesthetics. Of the currently used volatile anesthetics, isoflurane has been the most studied. The MAC for isoflurane is greatest at age 1 to 6 months (1.87%). The MAC is lower in preterm neonates (<32 weeks' PCA = 1.3%) compared with term neonates (1.4%). The low MAC in the newborns may be related to the immaturity of the CNS and/or related to the elevated levels of progesterone (transferred from mother's blood across the placenta) and β-endorphins. The increase in MAC in the first few weeks after birth seems to be related to the falling progesterone levels in the newborn. After age 3 to 6 months, the MAC of these most volatile anesthetics steadily declines with age, except for a slight increase at puberty.

For reasons that are unclear, the MAC for sevoflurane is similar in neonates and infants younger than 1 year (3.2%). The MAC of sevoflurane decreases with age (neonates to 1 year, 3.2%; 1-12 years, 2.5%; 40-year-old, 2%; after age 40, MAC decreases about 6% per decade) *(Cote: A Practice of Anesthesia for Infants and Children, ed 6, pp 124–126, 852; Davis: Smith's Anesthesia for Infants and Children, ed 9, pp 170, 574; Hines: Stoelting's Anesthesia and Co-Existing Disease, ed 7, p 638).*

601. (C) Several formulas (none ideal) have been used as a guide for initial fluid resuscitation in burn injuries. Intravascular fluid-volume deficits in patients with burn injuries are roughly proportional to the extent and depth of the burn. The Parkland formula is perhaps the most commonly used formula. This formula estimates fluid needs to be 4 mL/kg of crystalloid (lactated Ringer solution or PlasmaLyte) for each percent of body surface area burned over the first 24 hours. Thus in this case: 4 mL/kg × 40 (kg) × 50 (%) = 8000 mL. Approximately two thirds of this fluid should be replaced with isotonic crystalloid solutions during the first 8 hours after the injury; the rest is administered over the next 16 hours.

   The Brooke formula, another fluid replacement estimate, uses a combination of crystalloid (1.5 mL/kg crystalloid × % burn) + colloid (0.45 mL/kg colloid × % burn). This estimate is modified clinically by the patient's clinical response as noted by the vital signs and urine output (normal target urine output of about 1 mL/kg/hr).

   NOTE: In children who weigh less than 10 kg, these formulas are often insufficient, and an additional maintenance fluid load (4 mL/kg of crystalloid) is often added. Because hypoglycemia often occurs in children <20 kg, many add 5% dextrose to the maintenance fluid load *(Cote: A Practice of Anesthesia for Infants and Children, ed 6, pp 827–828; Davis: Smith's Anesthesia for Infants and Children, ed 9, pp 1012–1013; Miller: Basics of Anesthesia, ed 7, p 741).*

602. (D) The most likely explanation for the "falling" hemoglobin level in this patient is that this is a normal physiologic finding. At birth, a full-term infant has a hemoglobin level of approximately 17 to 18 g/dL. After birth, fetal hemoglobin (F) is replaced with adult hemoglobin (A). Because oxygen levels are higher after birth, less total hemoglobin is needed. A *physiologic anemia* occurs by age 8 to 12 weeks, resulting in hemoglobin concentrations of approximately 9 to 11 g/dL. After 3 months, there is a progressive increase in hemoglobin concentration, which reaches levels similar to those in adults by age 6 to 9 months. For premature infants, the anemia is more pronounced (7-9 g/dL), occurs earlier (age 3-6 weeks), and persists longer *(Cote: A Practice of Anesthesia for Infants and Children, ed 6, pp 217–218; Davis: Smith's Anesthesia for Infants and Children, ed 9, pp 401–402).*

603. (C) This history is consistent with an acute life-threatening cause of upper airway obstruction called epiglottitis (or, more appropriately, supraglottitis because other supraglottic structures are involved as well). In the past, *Haemophilus influenzae* type b (Hib) was the cause of most cases of epiglottitis, and the child often presented at 2 to 6 years of age. With widespread immunization against *H. influenzae,* epiglottitis has become much less common, and when it occurs, it often presents in the 6 to 12-year-old child. This condition is a medical emergency that usually starts out as a severe sore throat and rapidly progresses to the "four Ds" (dysphagia, dysphonia, dyspnea, and drooling). It can progress rapidly and cause death within 6 to 12 hours after the onset of symptoms. The child typically is seen sitting up, appears dyspneic with the mouth open, is drooling, and has a high fever and tachycardia. Inspiratory stridor is a late finding and suggests impending complete upper airway obstruction. When suspected, the anesthesiologist and otolaryngologist should be notified and the child immediately transferred to the OR (with the parent, if appropriate) before complete upper airway obstruction ensues. In the OR, general anesthesia should be induced with sevoflurane and oxygen by mask with the child in a sitting position. Sevoflurane is the preferred volatile anesthetic because it is less likely to induce laryngospasm compared with isoflurane or desflurane. IV access should be established as soon as the child is deeply anesthetized. Atropine (0.02 mg/kg) should be considered to block vagally mediated bradycardia induced by direct laryngoscopy. Muscle relaxants are contraindicated because they can cause complete obstruction of the upper airway in these patients. The trachea should be intubated (with an ETT one to two sizes smaller than predicted due to the swelling) under direct laryngoscopy when the depth of anesthesia is sufficient to blunt laryngeal reflexes. The child should then be transferred to an ICU for treatment (antibiotics and supportive care) until clinical signs and symptoms resolve and the airway swelling subsides (increasing air leak around the ETT) and the child is safely extubated. This usually takes 24 to 48 hours. The use of corticosteroids to decrease airway swelling is controversial. Because children who present with epiglottitis are now older with larger airways, selective cases may be carefully monitored without intubation in the ICU *(Cote: A Practice of Anesthesia for Infants and Children, ed 6, pp 780–781; Davis: Smith's Anesthesia for Infants and Children, ed 9, pp 829–830; Hines: Stoelting's Anesthesia and Co-Existing Disease, ed 7, pp 655–657).*

604. (D) CP is the most common movement disorder related to abnormal brain development and occurs in about 1 in every 500 live births. About 80% of cases are acquired prenatally, with 6% occurring with birth complications and about 10% acquired from infections, trauma, or metabolic disturbances. Initially hypotonia is often noted (6-12 months), followed by spasticity. The most common clinical manifestation is skeletal muscle spasticity. It is usually classified according to the extremity affected (e.g., monoplegia – single limb, hemiplegia – one side of the body, diplegia – both lower limbs, tetraplegia or quadriplegia – all 4 limbs) and the characteristics of the neurologic dysfunction (spastic – increased tone, hypotonic – decreased tone, choreoathetoid – involuntary movements, ataxic – generalized truncal and limb ataxia). Many of the children with CP have above average intelligence and can have anxiety similar to that in children without CP. Other manifestations include seizure disorders (30%) and speech deficits. Pulmonary complications (often related to aspiration, recurrent infections, and chronic lung disease) are a common cause of death.

Because of the increased risk of aspiration, the preferred technique for inducing general anesthesia in patients with CP should include a rapid-sequence IV induction. Propofol is the preferred IV induction drug. Etomidate, ketamine, and methohexital are proconvulsants and in patients with underlying seizure disorders should probably be avoided. Even though these patients have skeletal muscle spasticity, there have been no reports of succinylcholine-induced hyperkalemia. The response to nondepolarizing muscle relaxants is normal in most reports; however, some have reported resistance to nondepolarizing muscle relaxants. For a rapid-sequence induction, propofol followed by succinylcholine or rocuronium (fast-onset nondepolarizing drug) is preferred. Vecuronium (as well as atracurium and cisatracurium) tends to be slow in onset and should be avoided for rapid-sequence inductions. Anticonvulsant medications should be continued in the perioperative period. Baclofen is used to reduce spasticity, and although it can cause muscle weakness, the dose of nondepolarizing muscle relaxants should be reduced. Baclofen should **NOT** be discontinued because abrupt discontinuation of baclofen leads to acute withdrawal symptoms. In addition, the MAC level of anesthetic agents tends to be lower. Patients with CP have a normal response to pain *(Cote: A Practice of Anesthesia for Infants and Children, ed 6, pp 562–563; Davis: Smith's Anesthesia for Infants and Children, ed 9, pp 885–886; Hines: Stoelting's Anesthesia and Co-Existing Disease, ed 7, pp 648–650).*

605. (D) The signs (respiratory rate 40 breaths/min, heart rate 220 beats/minute, blood pressure 50/32 and no urine output) described in this patient are consistent with severe dehydration. The serum sodium level can be low, normal, or high with dehydration. Thus the vascular volume should be expanded initially with an isotonic saline solution or a colloid solution (start with 20 mL/kg and repeat as needed) until the patient's vital signs stabilize and the child voids. When the urine output increases, potassium can be added to the IV fluids. Until the body can regulate potassium, administration of potassium before adequate urine output may result in hyperkalemia. Although glucose administration for long procedures may prevent hypoglycemia, D_5W alone or with a crystalloid solution should not be used to replace fluid deficits *(Davis: Smith's Anesthesia for Infants and Children, ed 9, pp 117–119).*

606. (A) Premature newborns (<37 weeks' gestation) have a number of physiologic challenges in the immediate neonatal period, including respiratory, cardiovascular, and metabolic issues (e.g., hypoglycemia, hypocalcemia). In newborns, the mean blood pressure (BP) (50% percentile) is greater than their gestational age (i.e., 24-week newborn mean BP >24; 30-week newborn mean BP >30; 35-week newborn mean BP >35; and 40-week newborn mean BP >40). So for this 30-week newborn, a blood pressure of 45/30 is normal (i.e., above mean BP of 30). An O_2 saturation of 88% is also acceptable because the patient is at risk for ROP (i.e., <44 weeks' PMA). The aim in resuscitating newborns is an oxygen saturation after 10 minutes of 85% to 95%. Preterm infants have very limited calcium reserves and are very susceptible to hypocalcemia. Hypocalcemia is defined as a total calcium level <7 mg/dL in preterm newborns, <8 mg/dL in term newborns, and <8.8 mg/dL in children (or <1.7, 2.0, 2.2 mmol/L, respectively, for preterm, term, and children). Hypocalcemia occurs in about one third of premature newborns born at <36 weeks' GA. Symptoms related to hypocalcemia in the neonatal period include jitteriness, twitching and seizures (generalized or focal, which typically are short-lived but repetitive), prolonged QT interval, and cardiac arrhythmias. Doses vary significantly in the literature from 2 to 4 mg/kg to 10 to 20 mg/kg of elemental calcium administered, with ECG monitoring over 5 to 30 minutes. Each mL of 10% calcium gluconate has 9 mg of elemental calcium, whereas each mL of 10% calcium chloride has about 3 times the elemental calcium/mL or 27 mg of elemental calcium. If IV calcium is needed, most clinicians would replace calcium with calcium gluconate in newborns because calcium chloride is more irritating to veins. In this infant of 1200 g, the starting dose of elemental calcium is (2 mg/kg to 20 mg/kg) × 1.2 kg = 2.4 to 24 mg of elemental calcium. Using 10%

calcium gluconate (9 mg/mL elemental calcium), you would inject between 0.26 mL and 2.6 mL. Bradycardia and occasionally asystole can be seen if it is injected too rapidly. Some of the signs of hypoglycemia are similar to those of hypocalcemia and include jitteriness, seizure, irritability, and hypotension; sometimes apnea is seen when the blood sugar falls below 30 to 40 mg/dL. In the patient described in this question, the glucose has already been measured at 50 mg/dL, which is acceptable for a preterm infant. To treat hypoglycemia symptoms (without seizures), the IV dose of 10% dextrose is 2 mL/kg (200 mg/kg). To treat hypoglycemic seizures, the IV dose is doubled, or 4 mL/kg of 10% dextrose, followed by an infusion of dextrose at 8 mg/kg/min. Glucose monitoring should be performed to guide therapy to maintain a blood sugar above 40 to 50 mg/dL. Hyperventilation can cause alkalosis, which would decrease the unbound fraction of free calcium and make the patient more susceptible to hypocalcemic seizures. Because the urine output and blood pressure are adequate, it is unlikely that the patient needs a fluid bolus to correct hypotension *(Cote: A Practice of Anesthesia for Infants and Children, ed 6, pp 272, 849-850; Davis: Smith's Anesthesia for Infants and Children, ed 9, pp 137-138; Hines: Stoelting's Anesthesia and Co-Existing Disease, ed 7, pp 641-642).*

607. (A) A eutectic mixture occurs when two compounds are mixed and their melting point is lowered. In this case when lidocaine powder and prilocaine powder are mixed, a solution forms. The EMLA cream contains lidocaine (2.5%) and prilocaine (2.5%). When the 5% EMLA cream is applied to dry, intact skin and covered with an occlusive dressing for at least 1 hour, topical anesthesia to a depth of 5 mm is obtained. Four percent liposomal lidocaine (ELA-Max) can also be used and requires only 30 minutes to become effective *(Davis: Smith's Anesthesia for Infants and Children, ed 9, pp 449–450).*

608. (D) Although the umbilical vein is larger and easier to cannulate than the umbilical artery, the umbilical vein will not allow for adequate assessment of arterial blood gases or systemic blood pressure. In emergency situations at birth, the tip of the umbilical venous catheter (3.5 or 5 French catheter) should be placed until you get free flow of blood in the catheter (usually 2-4 cm in the term newborn and less in the preterm newborn). If the health care provider is very experienced in catheter placement, the umbilical vein catheter tip is advanced into the inferior vena cava above the level of the ductus venosus and hepatic veins. If the umbilical venous catheter is improperly advanced, hypertonic solutions might be infused directly into the liver, which might result in hepatic injury.

Careful placement of an umbilical artery catheter is equally important. The tip of the umbilical artery catheter should be placed in a "high position" in the descending aorta above the diaphragm (T7 to T9). All intra-arterial catheters are associated with thrombosis or embolism in these vessels, but fortunately serious injuries are rare. There are usually two arteries and only one vein. If there is difficulty in cannulating one umbilical artery, the other umbilical artery can be used *(Cote: A Practice of Anesthesia for Infants and Children, ed 6, pp 1139–1142; Weiner: American Heart Association/American Academy of Pediatrics Textbook of Neonatal Resuscitation, ed 7, 2016, pp 194–197).*

609. (C) Because of the large surface area–to-weight ratio, the thin layer of insulating subcutaneous fat, and the limited ability to compensate for cold stress, neonates and infants are at greater risk for intraoperative hypothermia than adults. Infants younger than 3 months do not produce heat by shivering; their principal method of thermogenesis is metabolism of brown fat. Heat loss can occur by radiation, conduction, convection, and evaporation. Heat loss through evaporation (not conduction) can be reduced by humidification of inspired gases. Heat loss by conduction (not convection) is reduced with the use of a warming blanket *(Davis: Smith's Anesthesia for Infants and Children, ed 9, pp 150–159; Miller: Miller's Anesthesia, ed 8, p 2763).*

610. (B) Shock is characterized by tissue perfusion inadequate to meet the metabolic demands of vital organs. The four types of shock are hypovolemic (e.g., hemorrhage shock, inadequate fluid intake), cardiogenic shock (e.g., cardiomyopathy), obstructive shock (e.g., cardiac tamponade, tension pneumothorax), and distributive shock. The three main types of distributive shock are septic, anaphylactic, and neurogenic (e.g., spinal injury) shock. In neurogenic shock, the sympathetic nervous system below the injury does not function. The loss of sympathetic compensatory mechanisms results initially in uncontrolled vasodilation (loss of sympathetic vasoconstriction) and prevents tachycardia (loss of sympathetic stimulation to the heart). The primary signs of neurogenic shock are hypotension with a wide pulse pressure, a normal heart rate (sometimes bradycardia), and hypothermia. Other signs of neurogenic shock include increased respiratory rate (diaphragmatic breathing) and hypoxemia as well as motor and sensory losses below the injury. Initial neurogenic shock requiring treatment may last about 1 to 3 weeks before compensatory physiologic mechanisms develop *(American Heart Association/American Academy of Pediatrics: Pediatric Advanced Life Support – Provider Manual 2016, pp 171–195; Hines: Stoelting's Anesthesia and Co-Existing Disease, ed 7, pp 305–307).*

611. (A) The oculocardiac reflex (OCR) is commonly defined as a 10% to 20% decrease in heart rate that is sustained for more than 5 seconds. It can be induced by traction on extraocular muscles, pressure on the eye, orbital hematoma, ocular trauma, or eye pain. It is commonly seen with strabismus operations and may produce a wide variety of cardiac arrhythmias, including sinus bradycardia, nodal bradycardia, ectopic beats, VF, and, rarely, asystole. The initial treatment of this is to stop the stimulus (i.e., tell the surgeon to stop what he or she is doing). This reflex quickly responds, and future similar stimulation typically elicits less of a response. In many cases, no further treatment is necessary. Increasing the depth of general anesthesia may help to block the reflex. In addition you should reassess the adequacy of ventilation, because hypercarbia and hypoxemia decrease the threshold to elicit the OCR. A retrobulbar block will prevent the reflex. Infiltrating lidocaine locally into the recti muscles may be effective in preventing and treating the OCR. Atropine (0.01-0.02 mg/kg) or glycopyrrolate (0.01 mg/kg) can be administered IV if the arrhythmia persists. Some advocate the prophylactic use of atropine or glycopyrrolate during strabismus surgery, especially in children *(Davis: Smith's Anesthesia for Infants and Children, ed 9, pp 902–903; Miller: Basics of Anesthesia, ed 7, p 526).*

612. (B) There is no significant difference in tidal volume (V_T) (mL/kg) between neonates and adults. Neonates have a high O_2 consumption (about twice that of adults). To compensate for the increased oxygen demand, alveolar and minute ventilation are increased. The increase in alveolar ventilation explains the slightly lower $PaCO_2$. Of note, the pH also is slightly lower. The lower functional residual capacity with the increased O_2 consumption places the neonate at an increased risk for hypoxia during general anesthesia if there is any difficulty with ventilation *(Barash: Clinical Anesthesia, ed 7, pp 376, 1181–1182; Cote: A Practice of Anesthesia for Infants and Children, ed 6, pp 15–17; Miller: Basics of Anesthesia, ed 7, pp 588–591).*

AGE-DEPENDENT RESPIRATORY VARIABLES

	Neonate	12-Month- Old	5-Year- Old	Adult
Weight (kg)	3	10	19	70
Respiratory rate (breaths/min)	40–60	18–30	18–28	9–15
Tidal volume (mL/kg)	6–8	6–8	7–8	6–7
Minute ventilation (mL/kg/min)	350	178		91
Functional residual capacity (mL/kg)	27		36	43
Vital capacity (mL/kg)	40		61	57
Total lung capacity (mL/kg)	53		79	86
Oxygen consumption (mL/kg/min)	6–8	5	4	3–3.5
Pao_2 (room air, mm Hg)	60–90	80–100	80–100	80–100
$PaCO_2$ (room air, mm Hg)	30–35	30–40	30–40	30–40
Arterial pH	7.30–7.40	7.35–7.45	7.35–7.45	7.35–7.45

613. (D) Neurofibromatosis (von Recklinghausen disease) is an autosomal dominant genetic disorder characterized by multiple neurofibromas involving the skin, peripheral nervous system, and CNS. The clinical features of this disease are diverse and always progress with time. The anesthetic management of patients with neurofibromatosis can be complicated by the associated clinical manifestations of this disease. For example, a pheochromocytoma may be present in approximately 1% of patients. If this goes unrecognized, severe hypertension can occur during anesthesia. Intracranial tumors occur in 5% to 10% of patients, and signs and symptoms of intracranial hypertension may develop. If intracranial pressure is elevated, efforts to reduce intracranial pressure should be initiated. Finally, airway patency may become compromised by an enlarging laryngeal neurofibroma. Abnormal responses to both depolarizing neuromuscular blocking agents (sensitive or resistant) and nondepolarizing neuromuscular blocking agents (sensitive) have been described. There is no evidence that these patients are at increased risk for MH *(Davis: Smith's Anesthesia for Infants and Children, ed 9, pp 866, 1231; Hines: Stoelting's: Anesthesia and Co-Existing Disease, ed 7, pp 292–293).*

614. (D) The initial decline (from fetal levels) in pulmonary vascular resistance (PVR) and rise in pulmonary blood flow are dependent on adequate function of the endothelial cells in the pulmonary vasculature and their reaction to oxygen levels. Hypoxemia is a primary factor in producing a high PVR. When normal ventilation begins, there is an increase in PaO_2 and a decrease in $PaCO_2$; pulmonary vasoconstriction decreases, and pulmonary blood flow increases. With a CDH, this process does not occur normally because there is associated pulmonary hypoplasia and pulmonary hypertension. Delaying repair of CDH to allow stabilization of pulmonary blood flow, and using nitric oxide (a selective pulmonary vasodilator) and a gentle approach to ventilation (e.g., permissive hypercarbia, high-frequency oscillatory ventilation or the use of extracorporeal membrane oxygenation) have led to improved survival of these newborns.

Patients with each of the other anomalies also are at risk for right-to-left intracardiac shunting, but each one can be readily treated, thus avoiding significant shunting and concomitant hypoxemia. In patients with CDH, shunting is exceedingly difficult to manage because of pulmonary hypertension, pulmonary hypoplasia, and endothelial changes *(Cote: A Practice of Anesthesia for Infants and Children, ed 6, pp 859–860; Davis: Smith's Anesthesia for Infants and Children, ed 9, pp 56, 78, 520–521, 586–590).*

615. (B) Dehydration is often classified as mild, moderate, or severe. The amount of dehydration that children have can be assessed by a variety of observations. For mild dehydration (5% weight loss—fluid deficit of 50 mL/kg) the child would have moist mucous membranes, normal skin turgor, and normal vital signs (e.g., pulse, respirations, and blood pressure), but the urine output would be less than 2 mL/kg/hr. With moderate dehydration (10% weight loss—fluid deficit of 100 mL/kg), the mucous membranes would be dry, skin turgor would be decreased, pulse would be increased and weak, respirations would be deep, blood pressure would be normal to low normal, and urine output would be less than 1 mL/kg/hr. With severe dehydration (15% weight loss—fluid deficit of 150 mL/kg) mucous membranes would be very dry, skin turgor would be greatly decreased, pulse would be greatly increased and feeble, respirations would be deep and rapid, blood pressure would be reduced and orthostatic, and urine output would be less than 0.5 mL/kg/hr. For dehydration treatment, start by expanding the intravascular volume with 20 mL/kg of a balanced salt solution, repeating as needed to reestablish hemodynamic stability. If a total of 60 mL/kg has been infused and hemodynamic stability is not reached, further assessment is needed, including evaluation of the original underestimation of fluid needs and the need for other fluids (e.g., colloid or blood) and assessment for other types of shock (e.g., septic shock requiring antibiotic administration) and possible ongoing fluid loss *(American Heart Association/American Academy of Pediatrics: Pediatric Advanced Life Support – Provider Manual 2016, pp 214–217; Davis: Smith's Anesthesia for Infants and Children, ed 9, pp 117–119).*

616. (A) Postoperative bleeding after a tonsillectomy occurs in 0.1% to 8% of cases. The bleeding is defined as primary if it occurs within 24 hours and secondary if more than 24 hours after surgery. Primary bleeding tends to be more profuse than secondary bleeding. Secondary bleeding (often 5-10 days postoperatively) occurs when the eschar covering of the tonsillar bed sloughs. Because bleeding most often occurs within the first 6 hours after the surgery (75% of bleeding cases), most outpatient units keep patients for at least 6 to 8 hours after the surgery is completed. The amount of bleeding tends to be underestimated because often a large amount of blood is swallowed *(Barash: Clinical Anesthesia, ed 7, pp 1357–1360; Cote: A Practice of Anesthesia for Infants and Children, ed 6, pp 772–774; Davis: Smith's Anesthesia for Infants and Children, ed 9, pp 828–829).*

617. (D) Ear, nose, and throat surgeons often use vasoconstrictors (e.g., phenylephrine, cocaine, or oxymetazoline) to control bleeding in pharyngeal and nasal surgery. For adults, the initial dose of phenylephrine is up to 0.5 mg (4 drops of a 0.25% solution). For children less than 25 kg, the initial dose is up to 20 µg/kg. The maximum recommended dose for cocaine (usually a 4% solution) is 1.5 to 3 mg/kg with a maximum dose of 200 mg. The dose of 0.05% oxymetazoline solution is two to three sprays in each nostril.

When excessive doses are used, severe hypertension and cardiovascular decompensation may develop due to the marked increase in peripheral vascular resistance. This also shifts blood from the peripheral site into the pulmonary vasculature (which is less sensitive to vasoconstrictors) and increases left ventricular filling pressure. In this case the use of labetalol and deepening the anesthesia have been associated with severe pulmonary edema, cardiac arrest, and death. If labetalol or a β-blocker (e.g., esmolol) is used and congestive heart failure develops, consider using high-dose glucagon (5-10 mg) to counteract the loss of cardiac contractility. This may also occur with the use of calcium channel blockers. Baroreceptor-induced bradycardia may not occur in the pediatric patient who has been pretreated with atropine or glycopyrrolate during the anesthetic. The hypertension may be short lived, and deepening the inhalation anesthetic may help; however, treatment of severe hypertension is most effective with direct vasodilators or α-adrenergic receptor antagonists (e.g., phentolamine) *(Davis: Smith's Anesthesia for Infants and Children, ed 9, p 310; Groudine et al: New York State Guidelines on the Topical Use of Phenylephrine in the Operating Room, Anesthesiology 92:859–864, 2000; Miller: Miller's Anesthesia, ed 8, p 2535).*

618. (C) The total volume of CSF varies with age from around 10 mL/kg in term neonates, 4 mL/kg in infants weighing less than 15 kg, 3 mL/kg in children, and 2 mL/kg in adolescents and adults. In children 50% of the CSF is in the spinal subarachnoid space and 50% is in the cerebral space, whereas in adults only 25% of the CSF is in the spinal subarachnoid space and 75% is in the cerebral space. This helps to explain why infants require higher doses of local anesthetic based on weight compared with adults. Tetracaine 0.5% and bupivacaine 0.5% are commonly used drugs for spinal anesthesia in infants. The dose for neonates ($<$5 kg) is 0.5 to 0.8 mg/kg for low to medium levels and 1 mg/kg for higher T2-T4 levels. The duration of action is commonly 60 to 80 minutes. The older the child, the less local anesthetic is needed. For infants and children (5-15 kg) the dose of 0.5% bupivacaine is reduced to 0.4 mg/kg *(Davis: Smith's Anesthesia for Infants and Children, ed 9, pp 476–477; Miller: Miller's Anesthesia, ed 8, pp 2727–2729).*

619. (A) Many children can have general anesthesia induced without premedication, especially if a calm parent is present for induction. However, some children are anxious and may benefit from premedication. Most anesthesiologists choose midazolam orally as the preoperative sedative of choice for routine general anesthetic cases. Most often the oral dose is 0.25 to 1 mg/kg, with onset of sedation occurring at 15 to 30 minutes. Because oral midazolam has a bitter taste for most children, it is often mixed with acetaminophen (which has a more pleasant flavor at an acetaminophen dose of about 10-15 mg/kg) if the commercial strawberry-flavored preparation of midazolam is not available. Midazolam can also be given nasally at 0.2 to 0.3 mg/kg, IM at 0.1 to 0.2 mg/kg, or IV at 0.05 to 0.1 mg/kg. Clonidine can be given as a premedication in a dose of 2 to 5 µg/kg orally or 1 to 2 µg/kg IV. Clonidine tends to taste better than midazolam but takes longer to take effect (30-45 minutes for oral sedation). In addition, clonidine may decrease the need for analgesics in the postoperative period and tends to reduce the incidence of emergence delirium. Dexmedetomidine can be administered orally at 2 to 4 µg/kg, nasally or IM at 1 to 2 µg/kg, or IV at 0.25 to 1 µg/kg. Ketamine has been administered orally at 3 to 10 mg/kg, nasally at 3 to 6 mg/kg, IM at 2 to 10 mg/kg, and IV at 1 to 2 mg/kg. Combinations of sedative medications have also been used, such as midazolam 0.5 mg/kg with ketamine at 3 mg/kg. If the durations of the surgical procedures are short (e.g., bilateral myringotomy and tubes), discharge times are prolonged after preoperative sedation. For intermediate-duration procedures (e.g., adenoidectomy), discharge times are prolonged about 10 minutes. Keep in mind the fact that when the patient is premedicated, propofol infusion rates as well as inhalation concentrations should be reduced *(Cote: A Practice of Anesthesia for Infants and Children, ed 6, pp 42–46; Davis: Smith's Anesthesia for Infants and Children, ed 9, pp 294–296).*

620. (C) The technique for CPR of infants ($<$1 year, excluding newborns) and children (ages 1 year to puberty) is different from that of adults. Puberty is defined here as breast development in females and chest or axillary hair in males. More emphasis has been placed on "push hard and push fast," given that chest compression depth and speed are often inadequate. If only ventilation is needed, the rate for adults is 10 to 12 breaths/min, whereas for children and infants, the rate is 12 to 20 breaths/min. For adults, sternal compressions should be performed with the heel of one hand placed on top of the other hand and compressing the lower half of the sternum at least 5 cm (2 inches). For children, sternal compressions should be performed with the heel of one or two hands compressing the lower half of the sternum at least one third the depth of the chest, or about 5 cm (about 2 inches). For infants, single rescuers compress the sternum with two fingers placed just below the nipple line on the lower half of the sternum and avoiding the lower tip of the sternum. Sternal compressions are performed at least one third the anterior-posterior diameter of the infant's chest, or about 4 cm (1.5 inches). When two rescuers are present, compressions are performed by encircling the infant's chest with both of the rescuers' hands while placing the thumbs together over the lower third of the sternum. The compression rate is the same for adults, children, and infants, that is, approximately 100 to 120 compressions/min. Lay rescuers should not check for pulses in infants or children because they often feel a pulse that is not present. When health care providers palpate for pulses, the brachial artery is preferred in the infant, and the carotid or femoral is preferred in the child. A universal compression-to-ventilation ratio of 30:2 is used for infants, children, and adults by single rescuers; a rate of 15:2 is used for two-person infant or child CPR. For newborns, however, a ratio of 3:1 (90 compressions and 30 ventilations/min) is used *(American Heart Association/American Academy of Pediatrics: Pediatric Advanced Life Support – Provider Manual 2016, pp 15–26; 2015 American Heart Association Guidelines for Update for CPR and ECC, Circulation 132:S519–525, S543–560, 2015).*

621. (B) Body composition changes dramatically during the first year of life. Total body water is about 80% for a term newborn compared with 55% for an adult woman and 60% for an adult man. Drugs that are water soluble (such as succinylcholine and many antibiotics) will need to have a higher mg/kg dose to achieve the desired blood concentrations. With the corresponding lower fat content of the preterm newborn (<5%) and term newborn (10%) compared with the adult (15+%), fat-soluble drugs that depend on redistribution will have a longer clinical effect. The GFR of newborns is low at birth (15%-30% of adult values), increases to about 50% of adult values by 5 to 10 days of life, and then increases at a slower rate until adult values are reached by 1 year of age. This decrease in renal function can delay excretion of drugs that are dependent on renal clearance for elimination. The relatively noncompliant heart of a newborn gives it a limited capacity to deal with a volume load, compared with the adult. An increase in cardiac output is primarily by an increase in heart rate. The preterm newborn has 10%, the term newborn has 25%, and the adult has 55% of type I muscle fibers (i.e., fatigue-resistant, highly oxidative fibers). The lower proportion of type I fibers predisposes the newborn's primary respiratory muscle fibers to fatigue *(Miller: Miller's Anesthesia, ed 8, pp 2759–2764; Miller: Basics of Anesthesia, ed 7, pp 588–592).*

622. (C)

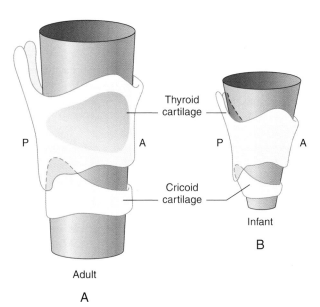

From Fiadjoe JE, Litman RS, Serber JF, Stricker PA, Coté CJ: The pediatric airway. In: Coté J, Lerman J, Anderson BJ, editors: A Practice of Anesthesia for Infants and Children, Elsevier, 2019, pp 297–339.

The anatomy of the infant's airway is different in some respects from that of the adult. The infant head is relatively larger than the adult's head. The larynx is in a more cephalad position in the infant than in the adult (infant's C3-C4, adult's C4-C5). The infant's epiglottis is narrower and "omega" shaped, whereas the adult epiglottis is flat and broad. Because the angle between the base of the tongue and the vocal cords is more acute in infants compared with adults, straight laryngoscope blades are used like curved blades for laryngoscopy in infants. The axis of the vocal cords in the adult is perpendicular to the axis of the larynx and trachea, whereas in the infant the anterior insertion of the vocal cords is lower (caudad) compared with the posterior insertion of the vocal cords. This diagonal position of the vocal cords relative to the axis of the larynx and trachea makes it more likely to have the ETT lodge in the anterior commissure of the vocal cords rather than slide down the trachea when the infant is intubated. The narrowest part of the adult larynx and the infant airway is the same, at the level of the cricoid ring *(Cote: A Practice of Anesthesia for Infants and Children, ed 6, pp 297–301; Davis: Smith's Anesthesia for Infants and Children, ed 9, p 519; Miller: Miller's Anesthesia, ed 8, pp 2760–2761).*

623. (C) Children at highest risk for PONV include those whose surgery lasts more than 30 minutes and those older than 3 years of age (especially adolescents). Before puberty, the incidence of PONV is the same for boys and girls. After puberty the incidence of PONV is higher in girls, in those with a family or patient history of PONV, a history of motion sickness or certain surgical procedures (e.g., strabismus surgery, intraocular procedures, middle ear surgery, testicular surgery, laparoscopic procedures, and endoscopic procedures when gas is insufflated into the bowel), and finally in cases where volatile anesthetics, ± nitrous oxide, and narcotics are routinely needed, such as tonsillectomy, orchiopexy, and herniorrhaphy. Brief procedures with minimal pain, such as myringotomy tube placements, have a low incidence of PONV. In cases where PONV is likely, prophylaxis is recommended *(Cote: A Practice of Anesthesia for Infants and Children, ed 6, pp 1103–1104; Davis: Smith's Anesthesia for Infants and Children, ed 9, pp 903–904, 1084–1085).*

624. (D) Down syndrome (trisomy 21) occurs in 1 in 700 to 800 live births. More than half of trisomy conceptions spontaneously abort. Although variable degrees of mental retardation are common (IQs of 25-85 are typical), many other significant conditions are also present. Congenital cardiac lesions are seen in about half of these patients (complete AV canal, ventricular septal defect (VSD)s, patent ductus arteriosus, Atrial septal defect (ASD)s, tetralogy of Fallot) and commonly necessitate prophylactic antibiotics. Other findings include hearing loss (50%), short neck, small mouth, narrow nasopharynx, large tongue, thyroid hypofunction (15%-20%), atlanto-occipital instability (15%-30%, which is most often asymptomatic), and smaller airways. About 5% to 15% have a seizure disorder requiring anticonvulsants. As many as 65% have associated sleep disorder breathing, including obstructive sleep apnea. Despite these abnormalities, tracheal intubation usually is not difficult in the hands of an experienced anesthesiologist. The size of the ETT used to create an air "leak" with increasing airway pressure should be one to two sizes smaller than normally selected based on age, because of the narrower trachea. For example, in children age 18 months to 8 years, the ETT size is 1 mm smaller *(Davis: Smith's Anesthesia for Infants and Children, ed 9, pp 1211–1213; Hines: Stoelting's Anesthesia and Co-Existing Disease, ed 7, pp 664–666; Miller: Miller's Anesthesia, ed 8, p 1201; Shott: Down syndrome: analysis of airway size and a guide for appropriate intubation, Laryngoscope 110:585–592, 2000).*

625. (D) Congenital cardiac abnormalities frequently occur in association with congenital diaphragmatic hernia (CDH), TEF, meningomyeloceles, and omphaloceles. Gastroschisis is rarely associated with other congenital anomalies, except for intestinal atresia (10% of cases) *(Hines: Stoelting's Anesthesia and Co-Existing Disease, ed 7, pp 642–652).*

626. (A) Newborns with CDH often present with respiratory distress immediately after birth. They often have a flat (scaphoid) abdomen because some of the intestines herniate into the chest (and therefore do not distend the abdomen). Immediate care includes endotracheal intubation for ventilatory support in the delivery room and placement of an orogastric or nasogastric tube to evacuate the stomach. Ventilation of the lungs with a bag and mask may cause more respiratory compromise by producing gastric and intestinal distention and is relatively contraindicated. When ventilating the newborn with CDH, an ETT should be passed. Do not to try to expand the lungs to normal size because the lungs are hypoplastic and prone to rupture, producing a pneumothorax. Although at one time hyperventilation was recommended, more recently improved outcomes have been found when moderate permissive hypercarbia has been used (PaCO$_2$ 60-65 mm Hg range). Rushing the child to the OR does not increase survival. It appears better to stabilize the child and look for associated congenital anomalies (seen in up to 50% of these children) before proceeding with surgery. Associated congenital anomalies include CNS anomalies (e.g., spina bifida, hydrocephalus, anencephaly), cardiovascular (e.g., hypoplastic left heart syndrome, ASDs and VSDs, coarctation, tetralogy of Fallot), gastrointestinal (e.g., malrotation, atresia), and genitourinary (e.g., hypospadias) *(Davis: Smith's Anesthesia for Infants and Children, ed 9, pp 586–597; Hines: Stoelting's Anesthesia and Co-Existing Disease, ed 7, pp 642–643).*

627. (D) Chronic pain is not an uncommon problem in children. Some studies have suggested that 30% to 50% of adolescents have recurrent and chronic pain. As pain becomes a daily occurrence, the children often become depressed and withdraw from daily activities. The most common chronic pain problems involve the extremity, CRPS (33%), diffuse musculoskeletal and back pain (30%-50%), abdominal pain (15%-40%), and headaches (60%). The diagnosis of CRPS is based primarily on the patient's history and physical examination (e.g., edema, changes in skin blood flow, abnormal sudomotor activity in the extremity, abnormal capillary refill, tremor, weakness, abnormal hair growth). There may be a genetic factor because CRPS is rare in African-Americans. CRPS is also rare in preadolescents. Patients with CRPS have regional pain that is not always associated with sympathetic nervous system involvement. When no identifiable provoking trauma is noted, the CRPS is called Type I (previously called reflex sympathetic dystrophy). When an identifiable peripheral nervous lesion is noted, CRPS is called Type II (previously called causalgia). The pain is often described as an intense, burning pain with allodynia and hyperalgesia in the distal extremity (a glove or stocking distribution and does not follow a dermatomal distribution). About 90% of 8- to 16-year-old patients with CRPS are female. Also in children, the lower extremity is more commonly affected than the upper extremity. Treatment is aimed at improving the affected limb function with physical therapy and mobilization of the limb, which not only helps prevent disability but also lessens the pain. Treatment involves not only medication (e.g., nonsteroidal anti-inflammatory drugs, narcotics, anticonvulsants) but also cognitive behavior therapy. In severe cases when the conservative approach is ineffective, nerve blocks are sometimes performed. There does not seem to be an association of nerve blocks and adverse long-term outcome. However, some have suggested that nerve blocks may be a problem because the relief of pain allows the patients to be more passive. If a nerve block is performed, it is for severe uncontrolled pain, which prevents the child from performing physical reconditioning (*Cote: A Practice of Anesthesia for Infants and Children, ed 6, pp 1065–1068; Davis: Smith's Anesthesia for Infants and Children, ed 9, pp 451–453*).

628. (B) Perioperative pediatric cardiac arrest is often defined as the need for CPR during anesthesia care (OR and PACU) and occurs more frequently in patients undergoing cardiac surgery. It is more than four times more frequent in neonates (0-30 days) than in infants or children. Causes of pediatric cardiac arrest vary from study to study, but about 40% are cardiovascular related (e.g., hypovolemia, hemorrhage, hyperkalemia, hypocalcemia, vagal reflexes, embolism, sepsis, central venous catheter complications), and about 30% are respiratory related (e.g., inadequate ventilation, loss of the airway, aspiration, pneumothorax). Medication-related causes of cardiac arrest occur in about 15% to 30% of cases (e.g., inhalation or IV overdosage, succinylcholine-induced dysrhythmia, medication "swaps," high spinal anesthesia, local anesthetic toxicity, allergic reactions, opioid-induced respiratory depression, inadequate reversal of muscle relaxants), and only about 4% are equipment related (e.g., disconnects, stuck valves). About 80% of cardiac arrests due to anesthesia-related episodes are reversed (return of spontaneous circulation, or ROSC, that persists for at least 20 minutes after the arrest). If the cardiac arrest is not anesthesia related, outcome is worse (of these, only about 50%-60% are reversed). Regardless of surgical procedure, children with congenital heart disease have a greater chance of a cardiac arrest. Emergency surgery is associated with greater than four times the incidence of cardiac arrest than elective surgery (*Cote: A Practice of Anesthesia for Infants and Children, ed 6, p 918; Davis: Smith's Anesthesia for Infants and Children, ed 9, pp 1236–1242*).

629. (C) Post-conceptual age (PCA) is the sum of the gestational age (GA) (the period between conception and birth) and the postnatal age (the time since birth). Term infants younger than 44 weeks' PCA are high risk for postoperative apnea and therefore should not be anesthetized as outpatients. By contrast, premature infants older than 60 weeks' PCA are at a much lower risk for postoperative apnea; therefore they can be anesthetized as outpatients if discharge criteria are otherwise met. At 8 to 12 weeks of age, the hemoglobin reaches the physiologic nadir of 10 to 11 g/dL. As the transition from Hgb F to Hgb A occurs, the infants experience the so-called physiologic anemia of infancy. Although anemia has been shown to be an independent risk factor for postoperative apnea, the hemoglobin level that would place an otherwise healthy infant at risk is unclear. Many sources suggest that risk is minimal until the Hct falls below 30% (Hgb <10 g/dL). Lower percentile on the growth curve alone does not appear to increase the risk for postoperative apnea.

   After surgical repair of pyloric stenosis, prolonged emergence from anesthesia is not uncommon, even with minimal narcotic administration. It is thought that these patients require very little opioid analgesia because of perturbations in CSF pH, a consequence of prolonged and persistent emesis. Loss of HCl from the stomach produces a metabolic alkalosis with concomitant CSF alkalosis. Even after correction of the serum alkalosis, the pH in the CSF could still be high because equilibration with the blood may not have been achieved (*Davis: Smith's Anesthesia for Infants and Children, ed 9, pp 36–37, 399–402, 538–539, 795–797, 1327–1328*).

630.

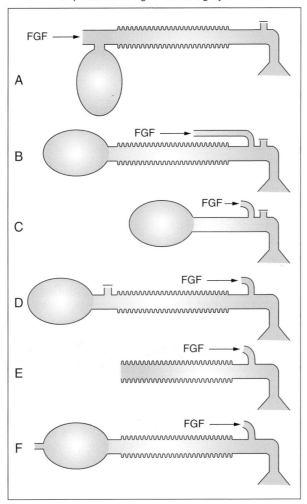

Mapleson A through F Breathing Systems, from Roth P: Anesthesia delivery systems. In: Pardo MC, Miller RD, editors: Basics of Anesthesia, *ed 7, Elsevier, 2018, pp 220–238.*

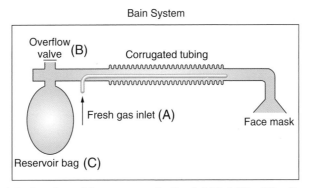

Bain System, from Roth P: Anesthesia delivery systems. In: Pardo MC, Miller RD, editors: Basics of Anesthesia, *ed 7, Elsevier, 2018, pp 220–238.*

(C) The Mapleson systems are all considered semiopen circuits because there is no carbon dioxide absorber in the circuit. Mapleson A, B, and C all have the overflow valve (pop-off valve) close to the mask or ETT. The Mapleson A circuit is more efficient in the spontaneously breathing patient than when controlled ventilation is used. Mapleson D, E, and F are better when controlled ventilation is used, and if they are used for the spontaneously breathing patient, higher fresh gas flows are needed to prevent rebreathing. The Mapleson D system has a proximal fresh gas inflow and a distal overflow valve. To eliminate rebreathing, higher fresh gas flows are needed with spontaneous ventilation than with controlled ventilation. The Mapleson D system is the most commonly used of the Mapleson systems. The Bain circuit is a modification of the Mapleson D circuit, with fresh gas inflow going through the center of the circuit, allowing it to be warmed. The system is lightweight and useful for head and neck surgery involving only a single hose to the ETT *(Davis: Smith's Anesthesia for Infants and Children, ed 9, pp 299–302; Miller: Basics of Anesthesia, ed 7, pp 226–227).*

631. (D) The respiratory center of the newborn's brain is not fully developed at birth. Newborns not uncommonly show two types of pauses in respiration. Periodic breathing exists if the pauses are short (i.e., 5-10 seconds) and not associated with a decrease in heart rate or oxygen saturation. Periodic breathing can be seen in up to 78% of full-term newborns and more commonly in premature newborns. Episodes of central apnea of infancy, also called apnea and bradycardia spells (A&B) spells, are longer, more significant, and less common than periodic breathing. With A&B spells, the respiratory pauses are usually longer than 15 to 20 seconds and are associated with a decrease in heart rate (<100), a decrease in oxygen saturation, cyanosis, and/or pallor. Treatment is usually tactile stimulation for A&B spells, whereas periodic breathing patterns do not need treatment. Untreated A&B spells can be lethal. If tactile stimulation alone is not effective, positive-pressure ventilation is indicated until respirations resume. Postoperative apnea is inversely correlated with both GA at birth and PCA (PCA = GA + chronologic age) up to 60 weeks' PCA. Postoperative apnea is highest in the first 4 to 6 hours but can present up to 12 hours after surgery. Postoperative apnea is also associated with infants who have had a history of A&B spells, as well as anemia (Hct <30). Caffeine has been used as a respiratory stimulant to decrease the incidence and severity of postoperative apnea. Although spinal anesthesia with no sedation has a lower incidence of apnea compared with general anesthesia, the addition of any sedative such as ketamine increases the incidence of apnea more than that observed with general anesthesia.

Controversy exists as to when young infants can be treated as outpatients due to this risk of postoperative apnea. In our practice, healthy full-term infants (>38 weeks' GA) who have not reached 44 weeks' PCA and healthy preterm infants (<38 weeks' PGA) who have not reached 50 weeks are admitted for overnight monitoring. In children with postoperative hypoxemia, hypothermia, anemia, or a history of apnea, individual assessment is needed for admission and monitoring overnight *(Davis: Smith's Anesthesia for Infants and Children, ed 9, pp 37, 538–539, 1327–1328).*

632. (B) There are many charts that show the proper uncuffed ETT size to use and the proper distance from the gums to midtrachea. However, if you remember two rules, you will know what tube to place and the distance for most newborns. Rule 1: Use a 2.5-ID uncuffed ETT for premature newborns <37 weeks' EGA and a 3.0-ID ETT for term newborns. Because it is often difficult to visualize placing the ETT so that the vocal cords are between the single and double lines on the end of the ETT, Rule 2 is helpful. Rule 2: A normal Apgar score is 7 to 10, so place the ETT between 7 and 10 cm from gums to midtrachea in newborns (see table below). Remember always to check for bilateral breath sounds (BBS) to make sure the ETT is in the trachea and not in a left or right mainstem (exceptions: pneumothorax or CDH where BBS are not equal with a properly placed ETT); you should have an air leak <25 cm H_2O. For newborns <27 weeks' EGA and weight <1 kg in size, a 2.0-ID ETT may be needed and placed <7 cm from the gums.

Estimated Gestational Age	Uncuffed ETT Size	Weight	Distance Placed from Gums
27 weeks	2.5 ID	1 kg	7 cm
32 weeks	2.5 ID	2 kg	8 cm
36 weeks	2.5 ID	3 kg	9 cm
40 weeks	3.0 ID	3.3 kg	10 cm

ETT, endotracheal tube; ID, internal diameter in mm.
Data from *Coté CJ: A Practice of Anesthesia for Infants and Children, ed 6, Philadelphia, Elsevier, 2018, pp 311–313; PJ Davis: Smith's Anesthesia for Infants and Children, ed 9, Philadelphia, Elsevier, 2016, pp 360–361; Weiner GM: Textbook of Neonatal Resuscitation (NRP), ed 7, American Academy of Pediatrics, 2011, pp 121–122.*

633. (B) The American Society of Anesthesiologists NPO guidelines are for fasting to reduce the risk of pulmonary aspiration of gastric contents is commonly called "the 2-4-6-8 rule." This applies for otherwise healthy infants (<2 years of age), children (2-16 years of age) and adults.

MINIMUM FASTING PERIODS

Ingested Material	Minimum Fasting Period
Clear fluids (water, Jello, apple or grape juice) (These liquids should not include alcohol)	2 hr
Breast milk	4 hr
Infant formula, nonhuman milk, light meal (no fat)	6 hr
Solid food (toast or cereal) or high-fat meals	8 hr

Data from *American Society of Anesthesiologists Committee. Practice Guidelines for Preoperative Fasting and the Use of Pharmacologic Agents to Reduce the Risk of Pulmonary Aspiration: Application to Healthy Patients Undergoing Elective Procedures.* Anesthesiology *126:376–393, 2017; Miller: Basics of Anesthesia, ed 7, Philadelphia, Elsevier, 2017, p 597.*

634. (C) Although hypothermia has some advantages such as protection against cerebral ischemia and hypoxia, other effects are less desirable. In neonates or infants, the response to hypothermia includes nonshivering thermogenesis (brown fat metabolism) and shivering (mainly in infants >3 months). These increase total body oxygen consumption and produce metabolic acidosis and often hypoglycemia (not hyperglycemia). Hypothermia also can depress ventilation, decrease metabolism of drugs, prolong the duration of action of nondepolarizing muscle relaxants, produce coagulopathies and platelet dysfunction, and increase wound infections. Wound healing can be impaired as a result of impaired immune function, as well as a result of decreased blood supply from vasoconstriction. Therefore monitoring the body temperature and employing maneuvers to minimize or eliminate significant loss of body heat during anesthesia for neonates and small infants are essential during the perioperative period *(Davis: Smith's Anesthesia for Infants and Children, ed 9, pp 162–164; Miller: Miller's Anesthesia, ed 8, pp 1631–1635, 2763).*

635. (C) NEC follows intestinal mucosal injury from ischemia and classically occurs in premature infants and in infants with low birth weight (typically <2500 g). In very-low-birth-weight (VLBW) newborns less than 1500 g, the incidence of NEC is 10% to 20%. NEC carries a high mortality rate (10%-30% if medically treated and a higher mortality rate if surgery is needed). These children may be acidotic, hypoxic, and in shock. Most have thrombocytopenia (50,000-70,000/mm^3), prolonged PT, and prolonged aPTT. NEC is most commonly associated with decreased cardiac output in the presence of fetal asphyxia or postnatal respiratory complications in the early postnatal period. Other factors associated with the pathogenesis of NEC include a history of umbilical artery catheterization, enteral feeding of small preterm infants, bacterial infection, polycythemia, and gram-negative endotoxemia. Although umbilical artery catheters are often used in the newborn period, these should be removed if NEC develops, because they may compromise mesenteric blood flow. Unless there is evidence of intestinal necrosis or perforation, nonoperative therapy should be instituted. This includes cessation of enteral feeding, decompression of the stomach, administration of broad-spectrum antibiotics, fluid and electrolyte therapy, parenteral nutrition, correction of hematologic abnormalities, and in some cases peritoneal drains are placed. Inotropic drugs may be needed in the presence of shock. Postoperatively these infants require ventilator support, and inotropes often are needed for cardiovascular support *(Hines: Stoelting's Anesthesia and Co-Existing Disease, ed 7, pp 647–648; Davis: Smith's Anesthesia for Infants and Children, ed 9, pp 604–611).*

636. (D) Codeine is a weak opioid and is used for the treatment of mild to moderate pain in patients >12 years of age. For codeine (methylmorphine) to exert its mild to moderate analgesic properties, it first must be converted to morphine. The peak blood level for most children age 3 months to 12 years after oral or IM administration of codeine occurs in about 30 minutes. The conversion of codeine to morphine occurs via the CYP2D6 pathway. Individuals have two alleles for CYP2D6, one from each parent. The function of each allele varies from no function to enhanced function. As a result of the alleles' activity, patients can be poor metabolizers (5%-10%), intermediate metabolizers (2%-11%), extensive metabolizers (77%-92%), and ultrarapid metabolizers (1%-2%). Ultrarapid metabolizers may produce 50% to

75% more morphine than "normal or extensive" metabolizers. Although codeine has been useful in treating pain in children and adults for many years, because of several deaths associated with its use in children that are ultrarapid metabolizers, the Food and Drug Administration (FDA) in 2004 published its first warning about codeine use in patients that are rapid metabolizers. In 2013 the FDA reviewed several pediatric deaths and cases of significant morbidity in children who suffered after codeine administration; some pediatric patients were ultrarapid metabolizers, but some were normal extensive metabolizers. On April 21, 2017 the FDA stated that codeine should not be used in children under the age of 12 to treat pain or cough. Similarly, tramadol should not be used in children after tonsillectomy or adenoidectomy. Children age 12 to 18 years of age who are obese or have obstructive sleep apnea should not take codeine or tramadol. In addition, nursing mothers should avoid codeine as well as tramadol because they may pass the drugs to the babies *(Davis: Smith's Anesthesia for Infants and Children, ed 9, pp 235–236; United States Food and Drug Administration, FDA Drug Safety Communication: FDA restricts use of prescription codeine pain and cough medicines and tramadol pain medicines in children; recommends against use in breastfeeding women. April 2017).*

637. (C) It is very important for patients getting proton beam radiation treatments not to move at all during their radiation treatments. Initially a simulation CT scan is made with a fiberglass immobilization cast fitting over the part of the child that will receive the proton beam. Then, after calculations are made, treatment is started. Multiple treatments (commonly around 30) are performed to divide the total radiation dose over several days. Each treatment typically takes about 30 minutes to an hour. When the patient enters the treatment room, several x-rays are initially performed each session to ensure that the patient is in exactly the same position for treatment when the proton beam is used. Several different angles or fields are used to focus the energy on the tumor each treatment day.

Since children often cannot hold perfectly still for the treatments, general anesthesia is often performed. Most commonly the children have central venous access (Port-A-Cath, peripherally inserted central catheter [PICC] line, or Hickman catheter) for treatments, as well as for the associated chemotherapy. If the central access is a Port-A-Cath, it is accessed on Monday about 45 to 60 minutes after EMLA cream is applied over the Port-A-Cath access site for analgesia. The Port-A-Cath then stays accessed for the week and is de-accessed on Friday after the treatment. This is repeated the following Monday until the treatment course is concluded. For general anesthesia, total IV anesthesia (TIVA) is most often used. Typically, propofol along with balanced salt solutions (e.g., saline or lactated Ringer) are administered with the child spontaneously breathing supplemental oxygen by nasal cannula or face mask. If the propofol dose needed to prevent movement is very high (>275 µg/kg/min), dexmedetomidine often is added to the propofol infusion and maintenance IV fluids. Very rarely does muscle paralysis become necessary *(Chantigian: Clinical Experience; Cote: A Practice of Anesthesia for Infants and Children, ed 6, pp 250–254; Davis: Smith's Anesthesia for Infants and Children, ed 9, pp 1047–1048).*

638. (D) HUS is one of the most common acquired causes of acute renal failure in children. Patients present with abdominal cramping, bloody diarrhea, and vomiting; it is often caused by the toxin from *Escherichia coli* O157, but other serotypes may be involved. About 10% of children with bloody diarrhea caused by *E. coli* O157 progress to HUS. HUS is characterized by a triad of microangiopathic hemolytic anemia (Hgb levels around 4-5 g/dL), thrombocytopenia (platelet destruction as well as sequestration of platelets in the liver and spleen), and acute nephropathy. Although the age of children most frequently affected by this disease is between 6 months and 4 years, HUS can occur from the neonatal period through adulthood. Occasionally, CNS abnormalities develop (e.g., decreased levels of consciousness, seizures, and at times cerebral edema and increased intracranial pressure). Pancreatitis is common, and congestive heart failure may develop as a result of fluid overload, hypertension, and myocardial depression from the toxins. Treatment is supportive, and many of these children will require temporary dialysis. The mortality rate is less than 5% *(Hines: Stoelting's Anesthesia and Co-Existing Disease, ed 7, p 496; Miller: Miller's Anesthesia, ed 8, pp 2904–2905).*

639. (D) Wilms tumor, also called nephroblastoma, is the most common abdominal malignancy of children. Children commonly present with increasing abdominal girth and have a palpable mass. About half of the children have hypertension. Peak age of diagnosis is 1 to 3 years. Although it most often occurs in one kidney, it sometimes affects both kidneys. Renal function is usually preserved, but hypertension, often mild, is common (60%). Although metastasis to the lung is common, pulmonary complaints are rare. Fever, hematuria, and anemia are often present. Treatment consists of surgery, radiation, and chemotherapy. Chemotherapeutic drugs used in this tumor include dactinomycin, doxorubicin (Adriamycin), vincristine, and cyclophosphamide (Cytoxan). Bone marrow suppression (e.g., anemia, thrombocytopenia) can occur with all cytotoxic drugs. Because cardiomyopathy can occur with cyclophosphamide (>100 mg/m^2) and with doxorubicin (>220 mg/m^2), preoperative echocardiography should be considered, even in asymptomatic patients. Late cardiac dysfunction may develop 7 to 14 years after treatment. Alkylating agents, such as cyclophosphamide, inhibit plasma cholinesterases, which may affect the metabolism of succinylcholine. Vincristine has several CNS side effects, including peripheral neuropathy, impaired sensorium, and encephalopathy and renal toxicity. Pulmonary fibrosis and/or pneumonitis can occur in patients who have received bleomycin (the patient in this case did not receive bleomycin). Bleomycin pulmonary toxicity may be related to high-inspired oxygen concentrations and excessive fluid administration *(Davis: Smith's Anesthesia for Infants and Children, ed 9, pp 802–803, 1176–1177; Hines: Stoelting's Anesthesia and Co-Existing Disease, ed 7, pp 662–663; Miller: Miller's Anesthesia, ed 8, pp 1216–1217).*

640. (D) All of the answers are correct. Hypotension is based on systolic blood pressures and is correctly described in each of the choices in the question. In addition, for children 10 years of age or older, hypotension is a systolic blood pressure less than 90. In evaluating a low blood pressure, one evaluates the four factors that affect cardiac output: preload, afterload, contractility, and heart rate. Shock occurs when perfusion to vital organs is inadequate to meet the organ's metabolic demands. Shock is often classified as compensated shock (systolic blood pressure in the normal range) or decompensated shock (blood pressure less than the 5th percentile for age) *(American Heart Association/American Academy of Pediatrics: Pediatric Advanced Life Support – Provider Manual 2016, pp 53–54, 171–195).*

641. (D) At birth, the GFR is 15% to 30% of adult values and increases to about 50% by 5 to 10 days of life and to 75% by 6 months. Renal function is complete by 1 year of age. Thus the half-life of medications that are excreted primarily by the kidney is prolonged in children under 1 year of age, and the dosage intervals should be increased *(Cote: A Practice of Anesthesia for Infants and Children, ed 6, p 849; Miller: Basics of Anesthesia, ed 7, p 591; Miller: Miller's Anesthesia, ed 8, p 2762).*

642. (D) Prophylaxis for POV is recommended for patients undergoing strabismus surgery because untreated, the incidence is 40% to 90% of patients. No benefit was demonstrated with the use of anticholinergic medications or with gastric content evacuation before emergence from anesthesia. IV hydration is very important. Recent studies have recommended that "superhydration" with 30 mL/kg/hr of lactated Ringer solution decreases the PONV rate by about half compared with 10 mL/kg/hr fluid use. Prophylaxis and treatment for PONV with dexamethasone 0.15 to 0.5 mg/kg, ondansetron 50 to 200 µg/kg, granisetron 10 to 40 µg/kg, dolasetron 0.35 mg/kg, and droperidol 10 to 75 µg/kg have been successful in reducing PONV. The higher dose of droperidol often leads to prolonged recovery times. After induction (often inhalation based before the IV start), maintenance anesthesia with propofol at 100 to 175 µg/kg/min has decreased PONV as well. Because only mild pain tends to be associated with strabismus surgery, avoiding narcotics or using only a low dose along with acetaminophen and ketorolac is adequate for pain management. The use of nitrous oxide as part of maintenance anesthesia remains controversial *(Cote: A Practice of Anesthesia for Infants and Children, ed 6, pp 799–800; Davis: Smith's Anesthesia for Infants and Children, ed 9, pp 903–907).*

DIRECTIONS (Questions 643 through 725): Each of the questions or incomplete statements in this section is followed by answers or by completions of the statement, respectively. Select the ONE BEST answer or completion for each item.

643. Which of the following drugs does **NOT** pass the placenta easily?
A. Etomidate
B. Ephedrine
C. Atropine
D. Glycopyrrolate

644. A 38-year-old obese patient is receiving subcutaneous low-molecular-weight heparin (LMWH) for thromboprophylaxis. Her epidural for an elective cesarean delivery was placed 14 hours after the heparin was stopped. She developed Horner syndrome on the left side 30 minutes after placement of the epidural. On physical examination, a T4 anesthetic level is noted, but aside from the Horner syndrome no other findings are revealed. The most appropriate course of action at this time would be to
A. Remove the epidural
B. Consult a neurosurgeon
C. Obtain a computed tomographic scan
D. None of the above

645. What percentage of all pregnancies is affected by hypertension?
A. 3%-5%
B. 7%-10%
C. 15%
D. 20%

646. A 16-year-old, anxious, preeclamptic patient in active labor develops back pain after the placement of an epidural for labor analgesia. The pain is severe, and the patient has more weakness of the legs than expected. The most appropriate course of action at this time would be to
A. Inject a higher concentration of a local anesthetic or add intravenous (IV) narcotics
B. Replace the epidural and use epidural narcotics to decrease the motor weakness
C. Reassure her that she will get better with delivery
D. Consult a neurosurgeon

647. Magnesium sulfate ($MgSO_4$) is used as an anticonvulsant in patients with preeclampsia and for fetal neuroprotection and sometimes for short-term tocolysis. $MgSO_4$ may produce any of the following effects **EXCEPT**
A. Sedation
B. Respiratory paralysis
C. Inhibition of acetylcholine (ACh) release at the myoneural junction
D. Hypertension when used with nifedipine

648. Normal fetal heart rate (FHR) is
A. 60 to 100 beats/min
B. 90 to 130 beats/min
C. 110 to 160 beats/min
D. 150 to 200 beats/min

649. Which of the following is the **MOST** likely cause of pregnancy-related deaths in the United States (2011-2013)?
A. Anesthesia complications
B. Hemorrhage
C. Cardiovascular disease
D. Hypertensive disorders of pregnancy

650. Drugs useful in the treatment of uterine atony in an asthmatic patient with severe preeclampsia include
A. Oxytocin (Pitocin) only
B. Ergonovine (Ergotrate) or methylergonovine (Methergine) only
C. 15-Methyl prostaglandin $F_{2\alpha}$ ($PGF_{2\alpha}$) (Carboprost, Hemabate) only
D. All of the above are safe and can be used alone or in combination with the others

651. What is the P_{50} of fetal hemoglobin at term?
A. 12 mm Hg
B. 18 mm Hg
C. 24 mm Hg
D. 30 mm Hg

652. Side effects of terbutaline include all of the following **EXCEPT**
   A. Hypertension
   B. Hyperglycemia
   C. Pulmonary edema
   D. Hypokalemia

653. Cardiac output increases dramatically during pregnancy and delivery. The cardiac output returns to non-pregnant values by how long postpartum?
   A. 12 hours
   B. 1 day
   C. 2 weeks
   D. 6 months

654. A 32-year-old parturient with a history of spinal fusion, severe asthma, and hypertension (blood pressure 180/110) is brought to the operating room wheezing. She needs an emergency cesarean section under general anesthesia for a prolapsed umbilical cord. Which of the following induction agents would be **MOST** appropriate for her induction?
   A. Sevoflurane
   B. Midazolam
   C. Ketamine
   D. Propofol

655. Uterine blood flow at term pregnancy typically increases to about
   A. 100 mL/min
   B. 250 mL/min
   C. 500 mL/min
   D. 750 mL/min

656. Which one of the following statements is **TRUE** regarding human immunodeficiency virus (HIV) infected parturients?
   A. Central neurologic blockade and epidural blood patches increase the chance of neurologic complications
   B. Ninety percent of newborns of untreated HIV-seropositive mothers become infected in utero, during vaginal delivery, or with breastfeeding
   C. The pharmacologic effects of benzodiazepines and narcotics are prolonged in patients taking protease inhibitors
   D. The risk of seroconversion after percutaneous exposure to HIV-infected blood is about 5%

657. Which of the following cardiovascular parameters is decreased at term?
   A. Central venous pressure
   B. Pulmonary capillary wedge pressure
   C. Systemic vascular resistance
   D. Left ventricular end-systolic volume

658. Which of the following signs and symptoms is **NOT** associated with amniotic fluid embolism (AFE)?
   A. Chest pain
   B. Bleeding (disseminated intravascular coagulation [DIC])
   C. Pulmonary vasospasm with severe pulmonary hypertension and right heart failure
   D. Left ventricular failure and pulmonary edema

659. When is the fetus most susceptible to the effects of teratogenic agents?
   A. 1 to 2 weeks of gestation
   B. 3 to 8 weeks of gestation
   C. 9 to 14 weeks of gestation
   D. 15 to 20 weeks of gestation

660. A 28-week estimated gestational age (EGA), 1000-g male infant is born to a 24-year-old mother who is addicted to heroin. The mother admits taking an extra "hit" of heroin before coming to the hospital because she was nervous. The infant's respiratory depression would be best managed by
   A. 0.1 mg/kg naloxone intramuscularly (IM) in the newborn's thigh muscle
   B. 0.1 mg/kg naloxone down the endotracheal tube
   C. 0.4 mg naloxone IM to the mother during the second stage of labor
   D. None of the above

661. Cardiac output is **GREATEST**
   A. During the first trimester of pregnancy
   B. During the third trimester of pregnancy
   C. During labor
   D. Immediately after delivery of the newborn

662. A 1000-g, 27-week EGA boy is born with a heart rate of 80 beats/min. He has slow irregular respiratory efforts, grimaces when a suction catheter is inserted into the mouth and nose for suctioning, and flexes his limbs some but is totally cyanotic. The umbilical cord has only two vessels. The 1-minute Apgar score would be
   A. 3
   B. 4
   C. 6
   D. 7

663. Which of the following respiratory parameters is **NOT** increased in the parturient?
   A. Minute ventilation (MV)
   B. Tidal volume (VT)
   C. Arterial Pa_{O_2}
   D. Serum bicarbonate

664. Which of the following drugs should **NOT** be used during transvaginal oocyte retrieval (TVOR) for assisted reproductive technology (ART)?
   A. Propofol
   B. Ketamine
   C. Midazolam
   D. All are safe and can be used

665. Which of the following conditions is associated with increased bleeding during pregnancy?
   A. Lupus anticoagulant
   B. Factor V Leiden mutation
   C. Protein C deficiency
   D. None of the above

666. What is the **BEST** way to prevent autonomic hyperreflexia in a quadriplegic woman who is to undergo induction of labor? The complete spinal cord lesion occurred 2 years ago.
   A. Only IV drugs should be used; spinal and epidural anesthesia are contraindicated
   B. Spinal or epidural lumbar local anesthetics such as bupivacaine alone are effective
   C. Spinal or epidural narcotics such as fentanyl alone are effective
   D. Autonomic hyperreflexia appears only when the complete spinal cord lesion is below T6, so there is no need to worry

667. A 24-year-old gravida 2, para 1 parturient is anesthetized for emergency cesarean section. On emergence from general anesthesia, the endotracheal tube is removed and the patient becomes cyanotic. Oxygen is administered by positive-pressure bag and mask ventilation. High airway pressures are necessary to ventilate the patient, and wheezing is noted over both lung fields, along with hypoxemia. The patient's blood pressure falls from 120/80 to 90/60 mm Hg, and heart rate increases from 105 to 150 beats/min. The **MOST** likely cause of these manifestations is
   A. Amniotic fluid embolus (AFE)
   B. Mucus plug in trachea
   C. Tension pneumothorax
   D. Aspiration

668. A 29-year-old gravida 1, para 0 woman at 8 weeks of gestation is to undergo an emergency appendectomy under general anesthesia with isoflurane, N_2O, and oxygen. Which of the following is a proven untoward consequence of general anesthesia in the unborn fetus?
   A. Congenital heart disease
   B. Cleft palate
   C. Behavioral defects
   D. None of the above

669. A lumbar epidural is placed in a 24-year-old gravida 1, para 0 parturient with myasthenia gravis (MG) for labor. Select the **TRUE** statement regarding neonatal MG.
   A. The newborn is almost always affected with myasthenia
   B. The newborn is affected by maternal immunoglobulin M (IgM) antibodies
   C. The newborn may require anticholinesterase therapy for up to 4 weeks
   D. The newborn will need lifelong treatment

670. A patient having which of the following conditions is **LEAST** likely to develop DIC?
   A. Severe preeclampsia
   B. Placental abruption
   C. Placenta previa (bleeding)
   D. Dead fetus syndrome

671. A 28-year-old gravida 1, para 0 parturient with Eisenmenger syndrome (pulmonary hypertension with an intracardiac right-to-left or bidirectional shunt) is to undergo placement of a lumbar epidural for analgesia during labor. It may be wise to avoid a local anesthetic with epinephrine in this patient because it
   A. Lowers pulmonary vascular resistance
   B. Lowers systemic vascular resistance
   C. Increases heart rate
   D. Causes excessive increases in systolic blood pressure (SBP)

672. Which of the following patients is **MOST** likely to need an emergency hysterectomy for uncontrolled bleeding at the time of delivery?
   A. Patient undergoing cesarean section after an unsuccessful trial of labor after cesarean (TOLAC)
   B. Patient with quadruplets
   C. Patient with a placenta previa (not bleeding) for an elective repeat cesarean section
   D. Patient with an abdominal pregnancy

673. The **MOST** common injury recorded in the American Society of Anesthesiologists' (ASA's) Closed Claims Project regarding obstetric anesthetic claims is
   A. Pain during anesthesia
   B. Maternal nerve damage
   C. Headache
   D. Aspiration pneumonitis

674. Which of the following statements about chorioamnionitis is **FALSE**?
  A. Chorioamnionitis occurs in about 1% of all pregnancies
  B. Clinical signs include temperature higher than 38° C, maternal and fetal tachycardia, and uterine tenderness
  C. Antibiotics are administered only after delivery, because intrapartum antibiotics may "obscure the results of neonatal blood cultures"
  D. Epidural anesthesia can be safely administered

675. Which of the following statements regarding newborns with thick meconium-stained amniotic fluid is **TRUE**?
  A. Only oral or nasal suctioning with a bulb syringe is needed in newborns that are vigorous
  B. Intubation is required for all such newborns
  C. Antibiotics and steroids are often needed to treat the infection
  D. Respiratory distress syndrome (RDS) is common

676. A 38-year-old primiparous patient with placenta previa and active vaginal bleeding arrives in the operating room with a systolic blood pressure (SBP) of 85 mm Hg. A cesarean section is planned. The patient is lightheaded and scared. Which of the following anesthetic induction plans would be most appropriate for this patient?
  A. Spinal anesthetic with 12 to 15 mg bupivacaine
  B. General anesthetic induction with 2 to 2.8 mg/kg propofol and paralysis with 1 to 1.5 mg/kg succinylcholine
  C. General anesthesia induction with 0.75 to 1 mg/kg ketamine and paralysis with 1 to 1.5 mg/kg succinylcholine
  D. Replace lost blood volume first, then use any anesthetic the patient wishes

677. Which of the following lung volumes or capacities change the **LEAST** during pregnancy?
  A. Tidal volume (V$_T$)
  B. Functional residual capacity (FRC)
  C. Expiratory reserve volume (ERV)
  D. Vital capacity (VC)

678. General anesthesia is induced in a 35-year-old patient for elective cesarean section. No part of the glottic apparatus is visible after two unsuccessful attempts to intubate, but mask ventilation is adequate. The most appropriate step at this point would be to
  A. Wake up the patient
  B. Attempt a blind nasal intubation
  C. Continue mask ventilation and cricoid pressure
  D. Use a laryngeal mask airway

679. Which patients describe their labor pain as being the **MOST** intense?
  A. Primipara patients attending prepared childbirth classes
  B. Primipara patients not attending prepared childbirth classes
  C. Multipara patients attending prepared childbirth classes
  D. Multipara patients not attending prepared childbirth classes

680. Cigarette smoking is associated with an increase of each of the following **EXCEPT**
  A. Spontaneous fetal loss
  B. Placental abruption
  C. Preeclampsia
  D. Sudden infant death syndrome (SIDS)

681. All of the following are **TRUE** regarding the use of nitrous oxide for labor analgesia **EXCEPT**
  A. Significant anxiolysis occurs
  B. Do not need to have an IV line in place
  C. Needs to be administered by anesthesia personnel
  D. Only the patient can hold the mask or mouthpiece

682. When performing a rapid-sequence induction (RSI) for an emergency cesarean delivery, which of the following muscle relaxants is LEAST desirable to use after the IV general anesthetic is administered?
  A. Atracurium
  B. Rocuronium
  C. Succinylcholine
  D. Vecuronium

683. True statements regarding inclusion of intrathecal morphine, fentanyl, or sufentanil in obstetric anesthesia practice include each of the following **EXCEPT**
  A. The chief site of action is the substantia gelatinosa of the dorsal horn of the spinal column
  B. There is no motor and no sympathetic blockade
  C. Pain relief is adequate for the second stage of labor
  D. Lipophilic narcotics are associated with less respiratory depression than nonlipophilic narcotics

684. The **MOST** common side effect of intraspinal narcotics in the obstetric population is
  A. Pruritus
  B. Nausea and vomiting
  C. Respiratory depression
  D. Urinary retention

685. A 110-kg (242-lb), gravida 1, para 0 woman has a blood pressure of 180/95 during an office visit at the 16th week of gestation and 175/90 1 week later. She has some ankle but no facial edema, and no protein detected in her urine. Her serum creatinine is 1.2. These findings would be classified as
A. Preeclampsia
B. Chronic hypertension
C. Chronic hypertension with superimposed preeclampsia
D. Gestational hypertension

686. An epidural is placed into a 32-year-old parturient in active labor receiving magnesium therapy for pre-eclampsia. Five minutes after administration of the test dose, the loading dose of bupivacaine and fentanyl is administered. The patient becomes panic-stricken, wrestles briefly with the reassuring nurses, gasps for air, seizes, and develops cardiovascular collapse. During resuscitation, blood is oozing from the IV sites and a pink froth is noted in the endotracheal tube. The **MOST** likely diagnosis is
A. Amniotic fluid embolism
B. High spinal
C. Intravascular bupivacaine injection
D. Eclampsia

687. Which of the following narcotics has the **LONGEST** duration of action when added during a cesarean section under epidural anesthesia?
A. 50 to 100 μg fentanyl
B. 10 to 20 μg sufentanil
C. 3 to 4 mg morphine
D. 50 to 75 mg meperidine

688. Which of the following is **NOT** increased during pregnancy?
A. Renal plasma flow
B. Creatinine clearance
C. Blood urea nitrogen (BUN)
D. Glucose excretion

689. Which inhalation anesthetic does **NOT** produce uterine relaxation?
A. Isoflurane
B. Sevoflurane
C. Nitrous oxide
D. All produce uterine relaxation

690. Passive diffusion of substances across the placenta is enhanced by all of the following **EXCEPT**
A. Low molecular weight of the substance
B. High water solubility of the substance
C. Low degree of ionization of the substance
D. Large concentration gradient of the drug

691. Cesarean delivery is associated with a blood loss of about
A. 250 mL
B. 500 mL
C. 750 mL
D. 1000 mL

692. Which of the following statements is **CORRECT** in describing differences between fetal and maternal blood during labor?
A. Fetal blood has a lower hemoglobin concentration than does maternal blood
B. Fetal placental blood flow is twice maternal placental blood flow
C. Fetal hemoglobin has a greater affinity for O_2 than does maternal hemoglobin
D. The fetal oxyhemoglobin dissociation curve is shifted to the right of the maternal oxyhemoglobin dissociation curve

693. In general, morbidly obese patients have a higher incidence of all of the following **EXCEPT**
A. Cesarean deliveries
B. Postdural puncture headaches (PDPHs)
C. Preeclampsia
D. Thromboembolic diseases

694. A term infant with good muscle tone and a strong cry has an oxygen saturation of 83%, breathing room air 5 minutes after delivery. The **MOST** appropriate action at this point would be
A. Supplemental increased oxygen concentration with a blender up to 50% by a face mask
B. Spontaneous breathing with 100% oxygen by face mask
C. Positive-pressure ventilation with 100% oxygen
D. Observation

695. Which condition **BEST** describes the third-trimester maternal condition with the following signs and symptoms: new-onset vaginal bleeding that stops, no pain, no fetal distress?
A. Placental abruption
B. Placenta previa
C. Uterine rupture
D. Vasa previa

696. During the second stage of labor, complete pain relief can be obtained with
A. Paracervical block
B. Neuraxial block with fentanyl and morphine
C. Pudendal nerve block
D. Lumbar epidural block with bupivacaine and no narcotic

697. Anesthetic considerations for open fetal surgery include all of the following **EXCEPT**
- **A.** Uterine relaxation is essential
- **B.** Maternal hypotension (mean blood pressure <65 mm Hg) can be treated with phenylephrine or ephedrine
- **C.** Vecuronium at the ED_{95} dose of 0.04 mg/kg should be administered IM or IV by the obstetrician or surgeon if fetal muscle relaxation is needed
- **D.** Normal fetal oxygen saturation is 50% to 70%

698. 15-Methyl $PGF_{2\alpha}$ is administered directly into the myometrium to treat uterine atony in a 28-year-old mother. Possible effects from treatment with this drug include
- **A.** Nausea and vomiting
- **B.** Bronchospasm
- **C.** Hypoxia
- **D.** All of the above

699. Which of the following statements regarding $MgSO_4$ therapy for preeclampsia is **TRUE**?
- **A.** The therapeutic range for serum magnesium is 10 to 15 mEq/L
- **B.** High serum magnesium levels can be estimated by changes in deep tendon patellar reflexes in a patient with an epidural anesthetic loaded for a cesarean section
- **C.** Excessive serum magnesium levels cause widening of the QRS complex
- **D.** As soon as delivery occurs, the chance for eclampsia no longer exists and the magnesium should be reversed so that postpartum bleeding is less likely to occur

700. While moving a parturient from the birthing room to the operating room for an emergency cesarean section for a prolapsed umbilical cord, the patient develops cough, wheezing, and stridor and becomes cyanotic. The trachea is intubated, and food is noted in the pharynx. Appropriate treatment in this patient should consist of
- **A.** Intravenous lidocaine to suppress the cough
- **B.** Glucocorticoids
- **C.** 100% oxygen and positive end-expiratory pressure (PEEP)
- **D.** Saline lavage

701. Aortocaval compression starts to become significant in a normal pregnancy at how many weeks EGA?
- **A.** 10 weeks
- **B.** 15 weeks
- **C.** 20 weeks
- **D.** 25 weeks

702. Which agent is the **MOST** useful for raising the gastric pH just before induction of general anesthesia for emergency cesarean section?
- **A.** Ranitidine
- **B.** Sodium citrate
- **C.** Metoclopramide
- **D.** Magnesium hydroxide and aluminum hydroxide

703. Causes of fetal bradycardia include all of the following **EXCEPT**
- **A.** Maternal smoking of cigarettes
- **B.** Neostigmine and glycopyrrolate reversal of neuromuscular blockers
- **C.** Acidosis
- **D.** Umbilical cord compression

704. Most cases of cerebral palsy (CP) are due to conditions during
- **A.** Antepartum
- **B.** Labor
- **C.** Delivery
- **D.** The first 30 days of life

705. All of the following statements regarding pregnant diabetic patients are true **EXCEPT**
- **A.** Gestational diabetes mellitus (DM) occurs in about 7% of all pregnancies in the United States
- **B.** Insulin readily crosses the placenta and causes larger babies
- **C.** Cesarean section is more common in diabetic pregnancies
- **D.** Diabetic ketoacidosis (DKA) occurs in 1% to 2% of Type 1 DM pregnancies

706. In addition to the postural component of a postdural puncture headache (PDPH), signs and symptoms may include any of the following **EXCEPT**
- **A.** Double vision
- **B.** Hearing changes
- **C.** Neck stiffness
- **D.** Fever

707. Early decelerations may occur in response to
- **A.** Fetal head compression
- **B.** Uteroplacental insufficiency
- **C.** Maternal hypotension
- **D.** Umbilical cord compression

708. Agents that are useful for decreasing the incidence of shivering during cesarean section under regional anesthesia or for treating shivering include all of the following **EXCEPT**
- **A.** Administration of intrathecal local anesthetic with fentanyl and/or morphine
- **B.** Intravenous magnesium sulfate
- **C.** Administration of epidural local anesthetic solutions with epinephrine
- **D.** Intravenous meperidine

709. An umbilical arterial blood gas sample at the time of an emergency cesarean delivery shows a P_{O_2} of 20 mm Hg, a P_{CO_2} of 50 mm Hg, a bicarbonate value of 22 mEq/L, and a pH of 7.25. This shows
  A. Severe hypoxemia
  B. Respiratory acidosis
  C. Metabolic acidosis
  D. Normal values

710. Which is the **MOST** frequent condition requiring blood transfusions during or after a cesarean delivery?
  A. Multiple gestations
  B. Placental abruption
  C. Placenta previa
  D. Postpartum hemorrhage

711. All of the following are appropriate techniques or drug doses to be used in resuscitating a depressed term newborn **EXCEPT**
  A. Begin ventilation with air rather than 100% oxygen
  B. If the heart rate is less than 60 beats/min, start chest compressions (ratio of chest compressions to ventilations is 3:1)
  C. After adequate ventilation and chest compressions, administer 0.1 mg/kg of epinephrine IV
  D. After 10 minutes of no detectable heart rate, it may be reasonable to discontinue resuscitation efforts

712. After a vaginal delivery under epidural anesthesia, a healthy 8-lb baby is born. The 23-year-old now gravida 1, para 1 woman is noted to have a temperature of 38.2° C. A leukocyte count is obtained and is 15,000/mm³. The most appropriate course of action would be to
  A. Get a blood culture
  B. Start antibiotics
  C. Administer a sedative
  D. Observe

713. Compared with a healthy 25-year-old primigravida, which of the following conditions is **NOT** associated with a significantly higher incidence of hypertensive disorders of pregnancy?
  A. Multiple gestations
  B. Cigarette smoking (>1 pack/day)
  C. Obesity
  D. Placental abruption

714. Adverse effects (on the mother) associated with aortocaval compression by the gravid uterus include
  A. Nausea and vomiting
  B. Changes in cerebration
  C. Fetal distress
  D. All of the above

715. Which of the following statements regarding a pregnant patient abusing cocaine is **FALSE**?
  A. Hypertension, arrhythmias, myocardial ischemia, and tachycardia may occur with the rapid-sequence induction of general anesthesia in the acutely intoxicated patient
  B. The minimum alveolar concentration (MAC) for general anesthetics is increased in chronic cocaine addicts
  C. Some states consider in utero drug exposure to be a form of child abuse and require physicians to report these patients
  D. If a vasopressor is needed to treat hypotension, phenylephrine is preferred over ephedrine

716. Each of the following is correct when advising the surgeon to perform infiltration anesthesia for an emergency cesarean delivery when general and neuraxial anesthesia are contraindicated **EXCEPT**
  A. A midline incision is most desirable
  B. The rectus muscle should be injected to provide good skin analgesia
  C. Bupivacaine with bicarbonate is the local anesthetic of choice
  D. Mild sedation with ketamine and midazolam is permissible

717. A 24-year-old primiparous woman is undergoing an elective cesarean section (breech position). After prehydration with 1500 mL of saline, a spinal anesthetic is performed; 5 minutes later, the blood pressure is noted to be 80/40 mm Hg and the heart rate is 110 beats/min. The **BEST** treatment (best fetal pH) after ensuring that adequate left uterine displacement is performed would be
  A. Phenylephrine
  B. Ephedrine
  C. Epinephrine
  D. 1000 mL 5% dextrose in lactated Ringer solution

718. A woman has been admitted for a dilation and evacuation (D&E) at 10 weeks' EGA. She has some persistent bleeding and cramping after the expulsion of some tissue. Her obstetric condition is called
  A. A threatened abortion
  B. An inevitable abortion
  C. A complete abortion
  D. An incomplete abortion

719. Which of the following treatments has proven effective in decreasing the incidence of PDPHs after an accidental dural puncture with an epidural needle?
  A. Bed rest
  B. Prophylactic hydration
  C. Prophylactic epidural blood patch after delivery
  D. None of the above

720. Factors associated with advanced molar pregnancy (i.e., >14 to 16-week size uterus) include all of the following **EXCEPT**
  A. Hypertensive disorders of pregnancy
  B. Hypothyroidism
  C. Acute cardiopulmonary distress
  D. Hyperemesis gravidarum

721. Refractory cardiac arrest is **MOST** likely after the rapid unintentional IV injection of which of the following local anesthetics?
  A. Lidocaine
  B. Bupivacaine
  C. Ropivacaine
  D. Chloroprocaine

722. American Society of Regional Anesthesia (ASRA) guidelines for the treatment of local anesthetic systemic toxicity (LAST) for cardiac arrhythmias include the use of Intralipid and the **AVOIDANCE** of all of the following drugs **EXCEPT**
  A. Vasopressin
  B. β-Blockers
  C. Calcium channel blockers
  D. Low-dose epinephrine (<1 µg/kg)

723. Transient neurologic syndrome (TNS) is **MOST** commonly seen after the spinal anesthetic injection of which local anesthetic?
  A. Lidocaine
  B. Bupivacaine
  C. Prilocaine
  D. Tetracaine

724. You have a well-working T10 labor epidural in a woman with a questionable difficult airway and have just been informed that an urgent cesarean section is needed for a nonreassuring FHR tracing. Which of the following local anesthetics would give you the **SLOWEST** onset of surgical anesthesia?
  A. 3% chloroprocaine with freshly added epinephrine (1:200,000)
  B. 2% lidocaine with freshly added epinephrine (1:200,000)
  C. 2% lidocaine and epinephrine with added bicarbonate
  D. 0.5% levobupivacaine with fentanyl

725. Which local anesthetic has the **SHORTEST** plasma half-life after being injected into the epidural space?
  A. Bupivacaine
  B. Chloroprocaine
  C. Lidocaine
  D. Ropivacaine

643. (D) The fetal/maternal (F/M) drug ratio is a way to quantitatively describe drug transfer across the placenta. Time is also important when considering how much drug crosses into the fetus. Many anesthetic drugs cross the placenta, such as local anesthetics, IV induction agents (e.g., propofol [F/M ratio of 0.7-1.1], etomidate [F/M ratio of 0.5], ketamine [F/M ratio of 0.5]), inhalation agents (e.g., volatile anesthetics and nitrous oxide [F/M ratio of 0.7]), and narcotics (e.g., fentanyl [F/M ratio of 0.4], remifentanil [F/M ratio of 0.9], morphine [F/M ratio of 0.6]) and with time may affect the fetus/newborn. For vasopressors, ephedrine has an F/M ratio of 0.7, whereas phenylephrine has an F/M ratio of 0.2. The ionized neuromuscular blocking agents do not readily cross the placenta (F/M ratios of nondepolarizing drugs are around 0.1-0.2); succinylcholine, a depolarizing muscle relaxant, crosses very poorly as well. The anticholinergic drugs atropine and scopolamine have F/M drug ratios of 1.0 and readily cross the placenta, whereas glycopyrrolate has an F/M drug ratio of 0.1 and poorly crosses the placenta. Because the anticholinesterase agents (neostigmine, pyridostigmine, and edrophonium) cross the placenta to a limited extent but more so than glycopyrrolate, a pregnant patient undergoing nonobstetric surgery in which neuromuscular blocking drugs are being reversed with anticholinesterase agents should have atropine rather than glycopyrrolate used with the anticholinesterase mixture to prevent possible fetal bradycardia (*Chestnut: Chestnut's Obstetric Anesthesia, ed 5, pp 63–69; Suresh: Shnider and Levinson's Anesthesia for Obstetrics, ed 5, pp 47–51*).

644. (D) LMWHs are used for both prophylaxis and treatment of arterial and venous thromboembolism. The elimination half-life of LMWH is 3 to 6 hours after subcutaneous injection in patients with normal renal function. With severe renal insufficiency, the half-life of LMWH can be up to 16 hours. At least 12 hours should elapse before performing any neuraxial techniques (e.g., placement or removal of an epidural catheter) to decrease the likelihood of a spinal hematoma forming after low-dose prophylaxis with LMWH (e.g., enoxaparin 30 mg BID or 40 mg once daily). If high-dose LMWH is used for therapeutic anticoagulation (e.g., enoxaparin 1 mg/kg BID or 1.5 mg/kg once daily), you should wait at least 24 hours to decrease the likelihood of a spinal hematoma forming. A postprocedure dose of enoxaparin should usually be given no sooner than 4 hours after epidural catheter is removed. In all cases, the benefit-risk of thrombosis and bleeding should be made. If the patient has back pain and unexpected neurologic paralysis, a workup for an epidural hematoma should be performed. This case demonstrates a benign condition in which the sympathetic nerve supply to the eye is blocked (Horner syndrome [triad of miosis, ptosis, and anhidrosis]). This occasionally develops after a lumbar epidural anesthetic, even when the highest dermatome level blocked is below T5. It may be related to the superficial anatomic location of the descending spinal sympathetic fibers that lie just below the spinal pia of the dorsolateral funiculus (which is within diffusion range of subanesthetic concentrations of local anesthetics in the cerebrospinal fluid) as well as increased sensitivity to local anesthetics during pregnancy (*Chestnut: Chestnut's Obstetric Anesthesia, ed 5, pp 923–925, 1046–1048; Horlocker: Regional anesthesia in the patient receiving antithrombotic or thrombolytic therapy: American Society of Regional Anesthesia and Pain Medicine Evidence-Based Guidelines (Fourth Edition) Reg Anesth Pain Med 43:263–309, 2018*).

645. (B) Hypertension is defined as a systolic blood pressure (SBP) $\geq$ 140 mm Hg or diastolic blood pressure (DBP) $\geq$ 90 mm Hg on two occasions at least 4 hours apart, while the patient is at bed rest (unless antihypertensive therapy has been started); it occurs in 7% to 10% of all pregnancies worldwide. If the SBP is $\geq$ 160 mm Hg or the DBP is $\geq$ 110 mm Hg, the two readings can be done within a few minutes and antihypertensive medications can be started. Hypertension is a leading cause of maternal death worldwide. Hypertension during pregnancy is divided into four groups: preeclampsia-eclampsia, chronic hypertension (of any cause), chronic hypertension with superimposed preeclampsia, and gestational hypertension. Also see Question 685 (*American College of Obstetricians and Gynecologists Task Force on Hypertension in Pregnancy, November 2013 Website; Chestnut: Chestnut's Obstetric Anesthesia, ed 5, pp 825–829; Suresh: Shnider and Levinson's Anesthesia for Obstetrics, ed 5, pp 437–438*).

646. (D) Epidural hematomas and epidural abscesses are quite rare. Severe back pain and/or leg weakness that is greater than expected (or the recurrence of weakness after partial recovery of a neuraxial block) are presenting symptoms of spinal cord compression. Epidural hematomas can develop within 12 hours of a neuraxial procedure, whereas epidural abscesses usually take days to develop and also present with fever and leukocytosis. These conditions need imaging (e.g., magnetic resonance imaging [MRI]) and neurosurgical consultation. Studies have shown that when spinal cord decompression occurs within 8 hours of the onset of paralysis, neurologic recovery is significantly better than after 8 hours. Although epidural hematoma formation is rare, clotting disorders and perhaps marked difficulty in placing a block could lead to epidural bleeding and hematoma formation. Because the preeclamptic patient may develop a coagulopathy, one should carefully evaluate her coagulation status before initiating a regional block. Most anesthesiologists would evaluate a platelet count in the preeclamptic patient and look for any clinical signs of unexplained bleeding before initiating a regional block. Because an epidural blood patch often is performed with 20 mL of blood, the epidural hematoma that causes spinal cord compression is probably significantly greater *(Chestnut: Chestnut's Obstetric Anesthesia, ed 5, pp 749–750; Suresh: Shnider and Levinson's Anesthesia for Obstetrics, ed 5, p 415).*

647. (D) The normal serum magnesium level is 1.5 to 2 mEq/L, with a therapeutic range of 4 to 8 mEq/L. Note: many laboratories report values in mg/dL (1 mEq/L = 1.2 mg/dL). As magnesium sulfate is administered IV, patients often note a warm feeling in the vein as well as some sedation. With increasing serum levels, loss of deep tendon reflexes occurs at 10 mEq/L (12 mg/dL), respiratory paralysis occurs at 15 mEq/L (18 mg/dL), and cardiac arrest at greater than 25 mEq/L (>30 mg/dL) can occur. Magnesium decreases the release of ACh at the myoneural junction and decreases the sensitivity of the motor endplate to ACh. This can produce marked potentiation of nondepolarizing muscle relaxants. The effect on depolarizing muscle relaxants is less clear, and most clinicians use standard intubating doses of succinylcholine (i.e., 1-1.5 mg/kg) followed by a markedly reduced dose of a nondepolarizing relaxant if needed. Because magnesium antagonizes the effects of α-adrenergic agonists, ephedrine is usually preferred over phenylephrine if a vasopressor is needed to restore blood pressure, along with fluids, after a neuraxial blockade. When a calcium channel blocker, such as nifedipine, is administered along with magnesium, greater hypotension has resulted. The antidote for magnesium toxicity is calcium (which, if needed, should be administered slowly) *(ACOG Committee Opinion: Magnesium sulfate use in obstetrics, Number 652, American College of Obstetricians and Gynecologists, Obstet Gynecol, 127:e52–53, 2016; ACOG Practice Bulletin: Management of Preterm Labor, Number 171, October 2016; Chestnut: Chestnut's Obstetric Anesthesia, ed 5, pp 803–804, 838–839, 848; Suresh: Shnider and Levinson's Anesthesia for Obstetrics, ed 5, pp 282, 448).*

648. (C) Fetal monitors consist of a two-channel recorder for simultaneous recording of FHR and uterine activity. In looking at the FHR, one assesses the baseline rate, the FHR variability, and the periodic changes (accelerations or decelerations) that occur with uterine contractions. The normal FHR varies between 110 and 160 beats/min. See also Answer 703 *(Chestnut: Chestnut's Obstetric Anesthesia, ed 5, pp 150–151; Suresh: Anesthesia for Obstetrics, ed 5, pp 70-75).*

649. (C) Worldwide, hemorrhage (H), infection (I), and hypertensive disorders of pregnancy (preeclampsia [P]), or HIP, account for more than half of all maternal deaths. In the developed world, hypertensive disorders, infection, and hemorrhage account for about one third of maternal deaths. The rate of pregnancy-related mortality in the United States has been increasing from 7.2 deaths per 100,000 live births in 1987, to 14.5 deaths per 100,000 live births in 2000, to 17.3 deaths per 100,000 live births in 2013. The reason for the increase in deaths is unclear but may be related to more pregnant women having chronic health conditions such as hypertension, diabetes, obesity, and heart disease. The causes of pregnancy-related deaths in the United States for the years 2011 to 2013 were cardiovascular disease (15.5%), noncardiovascular disease (14.5%), infection or sepsis (12.7%), hemorrhage (11.4%), cardiomyopathy (11%), thrombotic pulmonary embolism (9.2%), hypertensive disorders of pregnancy (7.4%), cerebrovascular accidents (6.6%), amniotic fluid embolus (AFE) (5.5%), anesthesia complications (0.2%), and unknown causes (6.1%) *(http://cdc.gov – Pregnancy Mortality Surveillance System; Chestnut: Chestnut's Obstetric Anesthesia, ed 5, pp 932–941).*

650. (A) Uterine atony is a common cause of postpartum hemorrhage (2%-5% of all vaginal deliveries). Treatment consists of uterine massage, drugs, and, in some cases, tamponade balloon placement (e.g., Bakri with 300-500 mL normal saline), uterine artery embolization, laparotomy with hemostatic sutures, or, in rare cases, hysterectomy. Drugs commonly used include oxytocin, ergot alkaloids (ergonovine, methylergonovine), prostaglandins (PGE_2, $PGF_{2\alpha}$, 15-methyl $PGF_{2\alpha}$), and misoprostol. Oxytocin (Pitocin) is the first-line drug used for the treatment of uterine atony and may be used in patients with asthma or hypertensive disorders of pregnancy. If oxytocin is given as a large IV bolus, vasodilation and hypotension often result. Oxytocin is often given as 3 units over 30 seconds every 3 minutes for 3 doses or 30 units in 500 mL of fluid over 2 hours or 10 units IM. The ergot alkaloids are associated with a high incidence of nausea and vomiting. They cause vasoconstriction, producing elevations in blood pressure, and are contraindicated in patients with hypertension (and in this case preeclampsia). The dose of Methergine is 0.2 mg IM every 2 to 4 hours up to 5 doses. Ergot alkaloids have also been associated with bronchospasm (rarely) and may not be appropriate in asthmatic patients. Thus the ergot alkaloids are relatively contraindicated in patients with hypertension (such as preeclampsia), coronary artery disease, and asthma. The prostaglandin 15-methyl $PGF_{2\alpha}$ (Carboprost, Hemabate) is the only prostaglandin currently approved for uterine atony in the United States and may cause significant bronchospasm in susceptible patients and is contraindicated in asthmatic patients. The dose of Hemabate is 0.25 mg IM every 15 to 90 minutes up to 2 mg. Other smooth muscle contraction-associated side effects of prostaglandin 15-methyl $PGF_{2\alpha}$ include venoconstriction, as well as gastrointestinal (GI) muscle spasm (nausea, vomiting, and diarrhea). The prostaglandin E_1 misoprostol (Cytotec) has been given (off label) for postpartum hemorrhage. Misoprostol can be given once rectally (800-1000 mcg) or sublingually or orally (600-800 mcg) and is used if oxytocin or ergot alkaloids are ineffective. In some cases, tranexamic acid 1000 mg IV is given if blood loss is expected to be >500 to 1000 mL over anticipated blood loss *(Chestnut: Chestnut's Obstetric Anesthesia, ed 5, pp 589–590, 888–891; Suresh: Shnider and Levinson's Anesthesia for Obstetrics, ed 5, p 321).*

651. (B) Newborns have high hemoglobin levels around 15 to 20 g/100 mL. The term P_{50} denotes the blood oxygen tension (Pao_2) that produces 50% saturation of erythrocyte hemoglobin. The P_{50} value of fetal hemoglobin is 18 mm Hg versus the adult value of 27 mm Hg. Thus fetal hemoglobin has a higher affinity for oxygen than maternal hemoglobin *(Chestnut: Chestnut's Obstetric Anesthesia, ed 5, pp 83–84; Suresh: Shnider and Levinson's Anesthesia for Obstetrics, ed 5, pp 26–27).*

652. (A) Terbutaline is a β-adrenergic agonist with tocolytic properties and can be administered IV and subcutaneously, as well as orally. Side effects are similar to those of other β-adrenergic drugs and include tachycardia, hypotension, myocardial ischemia, pulmonary edema (0.3% incidence), hypoxemia (inhibition of hypoxic pulmonary vasoconstriction), hyperglycemia (30% incidence), metabolic (lactic) acidosis, hypokalemia (39% incidence and due to a shift of potassium from extracellular to intracellular space), anxiety, and nervousness. Electrocardiogram (ECG) changes with ST segment depression and T wave flattening or inversion may occur and typically resolve after stopping the β-adrenergic therapy. Whether these ECG changes reflect myocardial ischemia or hypokalemia is unclear *(Chestnut: Chestnut's Obstetric Anesthesia, ed 5, pp 802–803; Suresh: Shnider and Levinson's Anesthesia for Obstetrics, ed 5, pp 280–286).*

653. (C) The numerous changes that take place in the cardiovascular system during pregnancy provide for the needs of the fetus and prepare the mother for labor and delivery. During the first trimester of pregnancy, cardiac output increases by approximately 30% to 40%. At term, the cardiac output is increased 50% over nonpregnant values. This increase in cardiac output is due to an increase in stroke volume and an increase in heart rate. During labor, the cardiac output increases another 10% to 15% during the latent phase, 25% to 30% during the active phase, and 40% to 45% during the expulsive stage. Each uterine contraction increases the cardiac output by about 10% to 25%. The greatest increase in cardiac output occurs immediately after delivery of the newborn, when the cardiac output can increase to 75% above prelabor values. This final increase in cardiac output is attributed primarily to autotransfusion and increased venous return associated with uterine involution. Cardiac output falls to prelabor values within 2 days after delivery; however, it takes about 2 weeks for the cardiac output to decrease to nonpregnant values *(Chestnut: Chestnut's Obstetric Anesthesia, ed 5, pp 16–18; Suresh: Shnider and Levinson's Anesthesia for Obstetrics, ed 5, pp 1–2).*

654. (D) Asthma occurs in about 4% to 8% of all pregnancies. Although sevoflurane is a good induction agent for asthmatic patients, a rapid-sequence IV induction with endotracheal intubation to secure the airway is preferred. Because midazolam has a slow onset of action, it is not recommended for a rapid-sequence induction. When inducing general anesthesia in an asthmatic patient, it is imperative to establish an adequate depth of anesthesia before placing an endotracheal tube. If the patient is "light," then severe bronchospasm may occur. In patients with asthma, IV induction will work with ketamine or propofol. Ketamine is considered by many as the induction agent of choice due to its mild bronchodilator properties, but because propofol (also a good induction agent in asthmatic patients) does not stimulate the cardiovascular system as ketamine does, propofol would be preferred in this patient with hypertensive disorders of pregnancy. In patients with mild asthma who do not need the accessory muscles of respiration, regional anesthesia should be strongly considered if time permits because it would eliminate the need for endotracheal intubation. In addition, inhaled β2-adrenergic agonist (e.g., albuterol) and IV steroids may be beneficial *(Chestnut: Chestnut's Obstetric Anesthesia, ed 5, pp 1179–1186; Shnider and Levinson's Anesthesia for Obstetrics, ed 5, pp 524–535).*

655. (D) Uterine blood flow increases dramatically from 50 to 100 mL/min before pregnancy to about 700 to 900 mL/min at term (i.e., >1 unit of blood per minute). From 70% to 90% of the uterine blood flow at term goes to the intervillous spaces. Uterine blood flow is related to the perfusion pressure (uterine arterial pressure minus uterine venous pressure) divided by the uterine vascular resistance. Thus factors that decrease uterine blood flow include systemic hypotension, aortocaval compression, uterine contraction, and vasoconstriction *(Chestnut: Chestnut's Obstetric Anesthesia, ed 5, pp 40–42; Suresh: Shnider and Levinson's Anesthesia for Obstetrics, ed 5, pp 23–24).*

656. (C) Central neurologic blockade (i.e., epidural, spinal, or combined spinal-epidural), as well as epidural blood patches, appear to be safe for HIV-infected parturients. Vertical transmission from the mother to the newborn can occur in 15% to 40% when the mother is untreated. With antiretroviral therapy and elective cesarean delivery, the rate of transmission is reduced to about 1% to 2%. The risk of developing HIV after a needlestick injury with HIV-infected blood is 0.3%. (Risk of developing hepatitis B from a needlestick injury with hepatitis B infected blood is 30% and hepatitis C from a needlestick injury with hepatitic C infected blood is 2%-4%.) Patients taking protease inhibitors as part of their drug therapy have inhibition of cytochrome P-450, and both benzodiazepines, as well as narcotics, have prolonged effects *(Chestnut: Chestnut's Obstetric Anesthesia, ed 5, pp 1058–1064; Suresh: Shnider and Levinson's Anesthesia for Obstetrics, ed 5, pp 595–604).*

657. (C) There is no change in central venous pressure, pulmonary capillary wedge pressure, pulmonary artery diastolic pressure, or left ventricular end-systolic volume. Left ventricular end-diastolic volume is increased, as is stroke volume, ejection fraction, heart rate, and cardiac output. Systemic vascular resistance is decreased about 20% *(Chestnut: Chestnut's Obstetric Anesthesia, ed 5, pp 16–19; Suresh: Shnider and Levinson's Anesthesia for Obstetrics, ed 5, pp 1–3).*

658. (A) AFE is a very rare but serious complication of labor and delivery that results from the entrance of amniotic fluid and constituents of amniotic fluid into the maternal systemic circulation. About 10% of maternal deaths are caused by AFE, and two thirds of these deaths occur within 5 hours. Of those patients who survive the AFE, about 50% have significant neurologic dysfunction. For AFE to occur, the placental membranes must be ruptured, and abnormal open sinusoids at the uteroplacental site or lacerations of endocervical veins must exist. The classic triad is acute hypoxemia, hemodynamic collapse (i.e., severe hypotension), and coagulopathy without an obvious cause. More than 80% of these women develop cardiopulmonary arrest. Hemodynamic monitoring often shows a biphasic response; initially pulmonary vasospasm with severe pulmonary hypertension and right heart dysfunction is seen, followed by left ventricular failure and pulmonary edema. DIC occurs in about 66% of cases, and seizures occur about 50% of the time. Recently AFE is believed to be a bit different from a pure embolic event, because findings of anaphylaxis and septic shock also are involved. Bronchospasm, however, is rare (<15%) during an AFE, and chest pain is very rare (2% of patients) *(Chestnut: Chestnut's Obstetric Anesthesia, ed 5, pp 915–920; Hines: Stoelting's Anesthesia and Co-Existing Disease, ed 7, pp 683–684; Suresh: Shnider and Levinson's Anesthesia for Obstetrics, ed 5, pp 333–348).*

659. (B) Organogenesis mainly occurs between the 15th and 56th days (3-8 weeks) of gestation in humans and is the time during which the fetus is most susceptible to teratogenic agents. Although all commonly used anesthetic drugs are teratogenic in some animal species, there is no conclusive evidence to implicate any currently used local anesthetics, IV induction agents, or volatile anesthetic agents in the causation of human congenital anomalies *(Chestnut: Chestnut's Obstetric Anesthesia, ed 5, pp 360–366; Suresh: Shnider and Levinson's Anesthesia for Obstetrics, ed 5, pp 806–809).*

660. (D) Opioid use during pregnancy has escalated dramatically in recent years and parallels the opioid epidemic observed in the general population. Opioid abuse during pregnancy is estimated to occur in about 5% of patients in the United States, most often with the nonprescription use of pain-relieving drugs such as oxycodone. Other opioids include morphine, heroin, methadone, meperidine, and fentanyl. The problems associated with abuse are many and include the drug effect itself and the effects of substances mixed with the narcotics (e.g., talc, cornstarch), as well as infection and malnutrition. Neonatal abstinence syndrome (NAS) or drug withdrawal syndrome has increased from 1.5 cases per 1000 hospital births in 1999 to 6 cases per 1000 hospital births in 2013. NAS is manifested by central nervous system (CNS), GI symptoms of irritability, high-pitched cry, and poor sleep and sucking reflexes that lead to poor feeding. After delivery, respiratory depression as manifested by a low respiratory rate is treated with controlled ventilation but not with naloxone. Naloxone can precipitate an acute withdrawal reaction and should not be administered to patients with chronic narcotic use (mother or newborn). The dose of naloxone to treat narcotic-induced respiratory depression in the nonaddicted newborn *was* 0.1 mg/kg, but more recent data suggest that it may worsen the neurologic damage caused by asphyxia. Animal studies have also raised the question of complications such as pulmonary edema and cardiac arrest, as well as seizures, and current recommendations are to avoid naloxone use in the newborn. Current recommendations are to assist ventilation until the narcotic effects wear off and not to use naloxone (this includes nonaddicted mothers who have just received narcotics during labor) *(ACOG Committee Opinion: Opioid Use and Opioid Use Disorder in Pregnancy, Number 711, August 2017; American Heart Association and the American Academy of Pediatrics: Textbook of Neonatal Resuscitation 2016, ed 7, p 257; Chestnut: Chestnut's Obstetric Anesthesia, ed 5, pp 177, 1209–1213; Suresh: Shnider and Levinson's Anesthesia for Obstetrics, ed 5, pp 253, 693–696).*

661. (D) Immediately after delivery, the cardiac output can increase 75% above prelabor values. This is thought to result from autotransfusion and increased venous return to the heart associated with involution of the uterus, as well as increased blood return as the result of the lithotomy position. See also Answer 653 *(Chestnut: Chestnut's Obstetric Anesthesia, ed 5, pp 16–18; Suresh: Shnider and Levinson's Anesthesia for Obstetrics, ed 5, pp 1–2).*

662. (B) The Apgar score is a subjective scoring system used to evaluate the newborn and is commonly performed 1 minute and 5 minutes after delivery. If the score is less than 7, the scoring is also performed at 10, 15, and 20 minutes after delivery. A value of 0, 1, or 2 is given to each of five signs (heart rate, respiratory effort, reflex irritability, muscle tone, and color) and totaled. In this case the child gets 1 point for heart rate, 1 point for respiratory effort, 1 point for reflex irritability, 1 point for muscle tone, and 0 points for color.

THE APGAR SCORE

Sign	0	1	2	Total This Case
1. Heart rate	Absent	<100	>100	___1___
2. Respiratory effort	Absent	Slow, irregular	Good, crying	___1___
3. Reflex irritability	No	response	Grimace	Cough or sneeze
				___1___
4. Muscle tone	Flaccid	Some flexion	Active motion	___1___
5. Color	Blue or pale	Pink body with blue extremities	Completely pink	___0___
			Sum =	___4___

An Apgar score of 7 to 10 is normal, 4 to 6 is moderate, and 0 to 3 indicates severe depression. Weight, gestational age, and sex are not factors included in the scoring system *(Chestnut: Chestnut's Obstetric Anesthesia, ed 5, Philadelphia, Elsevier, Saunders, pp 168–170; Suresh M: Shnider and Levinson's Anesthesia for Obstetrics, 5 ed, Lippincott Williams & Wilkins, pp 244–246).*

663. (D) The respiratory system undergoes many important changes during pregnancy. Oxygen consumption increases about 20% to 60%. To help supply the needed oxygen for the metabolically active mother and fetus, MV increases about 45% to 50%. The increase in MV is primarily due to an increase in V_T of 40% to 45%, with a slight increase in respiratory rate. The increase in MV produces a fall in the Pa_{CO_2} to approximately 30 to 32 mm Hg, and a respiratory alkalosis develops. To help get the pH back to normal, the serum bicarbonate level falls an average of 4 mEq/L. The arterial Pa_{O_2} increases slightly due to the fall in Pa_{CO_2} (*Chestnut: Chestnut's Obstetric Anesthesia, ed 5, pp 19–22; Suresh: Shnider and Levinson's Anesthesia for Obstetrics, ed 5, pp 6–8*).

664. (D) About 11% of women (age 15-44) have received medical evaluation and treatment for infertility at some time in their lives, with another 6% of married women (age 15-44) unable to get pregnant after 12 months of trying to conceive. In 2015 there were 231,936 ART cycles in the United States (including 4003 cycles using frozen eggs and 45,779 cycles started with the intent of freezing and storing eggs or embryos for potential future use). With fresh nondonor ART cycles, 29% resulted in a pregnancy and 24% resulted in a live birth. The oocytes can be retrieved by laparoscopy or, more commonly now, by the transvaginal oocyte retrieval (TVOR) method. Most anesthetic drugs have been studied and found not to be a problem, including propofol, midazolam, ketamine, alfentanil, fentanyl, remifentanil, and meperidine. When general anesthesia was used (laparoscopic retrieval), isoflurane with and without nitrous oxide was usually used and appeared safe. However, with increased time during general anesthesia, the oocytes retrieved earlier had better fertilization rates than the oocytes obtained near the end of the laparoscopy. It is unclear whether this was due to the anesthetics or to the lowered pH as a result of the carbon dioxide pneumoperitoneum. Etomidate has not been widely used, and patient numbers are too small to recommend its use. When morphine is used in high doses in animal studies, chromosomal abnormalities are very common (25%-33%), and morphine is not recommended for ART procedures. It is recommended to avoid using the dopamine antagonists (e.g., droperidol and metoclopramide) during ART cycles because these drugs induce hyperprolactinemia, which impairs ovarian follicular maturation. A single dose immediately before oocyte retrieval probably is safe. The 5-hydroxytryptamine type 3 (5-HT_3) receptor antagonists (e.g., ondansetron, granisetron) are commonly used as antiemetics, but there is insufficient evidence to recommend their use during ART procedures. The phenothiazines and the antihistamine H_1-receptor antagonists are thought to be preferred because they have been studied without adverse effects (*2015 Assisted Reproductive Technology (ART): Fertility Clinic Success Rates Report, October 2017, cdc.gov; Chestnut: Chestnut's Obstetric Anesthesia, ed 5, pp 326–337; Suresh: Shnider and Levinson's Anesthesia for Obstetrics, ed 5, pp 765–773*).

665. (D) All of the conditions listed in this question, as well as deficiencies of antithrombin III and protein S (a cofactor for protein C), lead to hypercoagulable states. Unless treated with anticoagulation therapy, these conditions will have an increased frequency of thrombosis. These conditions may also cause placental thrombosis and insufficiency, and can increase the incidence of obstetric conditions, such as intrauterine growth restriction, preeclampsia, placental abruption, and intrauterine death. Lupus anticoagulant, also called lupus antibody, is a prothrombotic agent. It gets its name because the presence of these antibodies causes an increase in the activated partial thromboplastin (aPTT) test, as these antibodies interfere with phospholipids used to induce in vitro coagulation. However, in vivo these antibodies interact with platelet membrane phospholipids, increasing adhesions and the aggregation of platelets. Factor V Leiden mutation allows factor V to persist longer in the circulation (not metabolized as rapidly by activated protein C), leading to a hypercoagulable state. Protein C inhibits activated clotting factors V and VIII; thus, during a deficiency state, factors V and VIII persist longer in the circulation, leading again to a hypercoagulable state. During pregnancy, the incidence of thrombosis with protein C deficiency is about 25% unless anticoagulation therapy is administered (*Chestnut: Chestnut's Obstetric Anesthesia, ed 5, pp 951–952, 1048–1049*).

666. (B) Patients with complete spinal cord lesions above T10 do not have pain with labor. However, about 85% of women with complete spinal cord lesions at the T6 and higher level will develop autonomic hyperreflexia (severe headache, hypertension, bradycardia, sweating above the lesion, and facial flushing) during labor and delivery. Autonomic hyperreflexia typically occurs with the contractions and disappears between contractions. An epidural or a spinal with local anesthetics works well to prevent and/or treat autonomic hyperreflexia. Epidural narcotics such as fentanyl alone are not effective (unless the narcotic is meperidine, which has local anesthetic properties in addition to narcotic effects). To check whether the epidural or spinal that is loaded with a local anesthetic is working in a quadriplegic patient, check the reflexes below the expected level of anesthesia (e.g., patellar) before and after the block. If the patellar reflex is present before but not after the block is performed, the block is effective. The local anesthetic concentration needed for labor epidurals (alone without narcotics) typically is 0.25% or higher. If a cesarean section is needed, 2% lidocaine with epinephrine (1:200,000) has been reported to be safe. If a cesarean section is needed with general anesthesia, typical IV anesthetics and inhalation drugs are used except for muscle relaxation, where succinylcholine is contraindicated (hyperkalemic response) and a nondepolarizing muscle relaxant such as rocuronium is preferred (*Chestnut: Chestnut's Obstetric Anesthesia, ed 5, pp 1117–1120; Suresh: Shnider and Levinson's Anesthesia for Obstetrics, ed 5, p 564*).

667. (D) The signs presented in this case—bronchospasm, high airway pressures, hypoxemia, and wheezing, followed by hypotension and tachycardia—make gastric acid aspiration the most likely cause. It is important to note that aspiration can develop not only on induction but *also* on extubation, as in this case. That is why it is so important always to empty the patient's stomach with an orogastric tube after an endotracheal tube is placed in any pregnant patient over 20 weeks' gestation undergoing general anesthesia, and to extubate the patient when she is fully awake and responsive. Morbidity and mortality occurring after gastric acid aspiration are determined by both the amount and the pH of the aspirated gastric material. Based on an animal study in which 0.4 mL/kg with a pH less than 2.5 injected into the right mainstem of one rhesus monkey caused death, many have used that definition (0.4 mL/kg with a pH <2.5) to categorize patients who are "at risk" for significant aspiration morbidity and mortality. Using these values, up to 70% of women who fasted before elective cesarean section are "at risk for aspiration." Recently, it has been noted that the volume needed to cause aspiration in primates should be greater (e.g., 0.8 mL/kg) and the pH less than 2.5. Regardless of the definition of the "patient at risk," when aspiration occurs, it can be lethal. Other signs and symptoms of aspiration include sudden coughing or laryngospasm, dyspnea, tachypnea, the presence of foreign material in the mouth or posterior pharynx, chest wall retraction, cyanosis not relieved by oxygen supplementation, tachycardia, hypotension, and the development of pinky frothy exudates. The onset of these signs and symptoms is usually rapid. Early treatment consists of supplemental oxygen with positive-pressure ventilation, PEEP, or continuous positive airway pressure, and suctioning of the airway can decrease the incidence of mortality from acid aspiration. Mortality seems to be reduced when protective ventilatory strategies are used (i.e., tidal volumes of 6 mL/kg with plateau pressures of <30 cm H_2O are better than if 12 mL/kg and plateau pressures of 50 cm H_2O are used). Conservative compared with liberal fluid management (guided by central venous pressures and/or pulmonary artery wedge pressures) also appears to improve lung function. The use of prophylactic antibiotics and/or steroids has not been helpful. With an AFE, high airway pressures and bronchospasm are not seen, but cardiovascular collapse (including >80% cardiac arrest), DIC (60%), and seizures (>50%) are present. A mucus plug of an endotracheal tube can be associated with high airway pressures and mainly airway issues and would be extremely rare after endotracheal extubation. A tension pneumothorax would be more common during the anesthetic with positive-pressure ventilation and would most likely lead to decreased breath sounds on one side and a deviated trachea; it would not have presenting signs after endotracheal extubation. See Question 658 (*Chestnut: Chestnut's Obstetric Anesthesia, ed 5, pp 669–675; Suresh: Shnider and Levinson's Anesthesia for Obstetrics, ed 5, pp 403–411*).

668. (D) The primary objectives in the anesthetic management of a pregnant woman undergoing general anesthesia for nonobstetric surgery are as follows: to (1) ensure maternal safety; (2) avoid teratogenic drugs; (3) avoid intrauterine fetal asphyxia; and (4) prevent the induction of preterm labor. Premature onset of labor is the most common complication associated with surgery during the second trimester of pregnancy. Performance of intra-abdominal procedures in which the uterus is manipulated is the most significant factor in causing premature labor in these patients. Neurosurgical, orthopedic, thoracic, or other surgical procedures that do not involve manipulation of the uterus do not cause preterm labor. No anesthetic agent or technique has been found to be significantly associated with a higher or lower incidence of preterm labor. Furthermore, there is no evidence that the risk of developing any of the conditions listed in this question is increased for the offspring of patients who receive general anesthesia during pregnancy (*Suresh: Shnider and Levinson's Anesthesia for Obstetrics, ed 5, pp 804–816*).

669. (C) MG is an autoimmune neuromuscular disease in which immunoglobulin G (IgG) antibodies are directed against the ACh receptors in skeletal muscle, causing patients to present with general muscle weakness and easy fatigability. Smooth muscle and cardiac muscle are not affected. About 10% to 20% of newborns born to mothers with MG are transiently affected because the IgG antibody is transferred through the placenta. Neonatal MG is characterized by muscle weakness (e.g., hypotonia, respiratory difficulty) and may appear within the first 4 days of life (80% appear within the first 24 hours). Anticholinesterase therapy may be required for several weeks, until the maternal IgG antibodies are metabolized *(Chestnut: Chestnut's Obstetric Anesthesia, ed 5, pp 1120–1122; Suresh: Shnider and Levinson's Anesthesia for Obstetrics, ed 5, pp 537–539).*

670. (C) Disseminated intravascular coagulation (DIC) is an acquired coagulopathy characterized by excessive fibrin deposition, depression of the normal coagulation inhibition mechanism, and impaired fibrin degradation. The formation of clots causes a depletion of platelets and factors. Laboratory diagnosis of DIC is based on the demonstration of abnormalities in platelet count (i.e., <100,000/mm3), prolonged prothrombin time (i.e., >3 seconds above normal), presence of fibrin degradation products, and fibrinogen level (i.e., ≤1 g/L). DIC is associated with the following obstetric conditions: placental abruption, dead fetus syndrome, AFE, gram-negative sepsis, and severe preeclampsia. Placental abruption is the most common cause of DIC in pregnant patients. If one looks at severe placental abruptions (in which the abruption is large enough to cause fetal death), about 30% of patients will develop DIC within 8 hours of the abruption. Nonobstetric causes of DIC include sepsis and malignancy. Patients with placenta previa who are bleeding do not develop DIC because the blood loss does not induce a coagulopathy *(Barash: Clinical Anesthesia, ed 8, pp 447–449; Chestnut: Chestnut's Obstetric Anesthesia, ed 5, pp 1045–1046; Suresh: Shnider and Levinson's Anesthesia for Obstetrics, ed 5, pp 311–321, 444–445, 574–575).*

671. (B) Eisenmenger syndrome may develop in patients with uncorrected left-to-right intracardiac shunting such as for ventricular septal defect (VSD), atrial septal defect (ASD), or patent ductus arteriosus (PDA). About half of the patients with an unrestricted and unrepaired VSD will ultimately develop Eisenmenger syndrome. In this syndrome, the pulmonary and vascular tone and right ventricular muscle undergo changes in response to the increased blood flow from the left-right shunt, producing severe pulmonary hypertension and eventually a change in the direction of the shunt to a right-to-left or bidirectional type with peripheral cyanosis. The maternal mortality rate is 30% to 50%. When the Eisenmenger syndrome develops, the pulmonary vascular resistance becomes fixed, making this condition not amenable to surgical correction. Survival beyond age 40 years is uncommon. Any event or drug that increases pulmonary vascular resistance (e.g., hypercarbia, acidosis, hypoxia) or decreases systemic vascular resistance will increase the right-to-left shunt, will exacerbate peripheral cyanosis, and may precipitate right ventricular heart failure in these patients. Controversy exists regarding pain management for these patients because pain can elevate pulmonary artery pressures and cause more shunting. Many practitioners prefer a narcotic-based analgesic (spinal or epidural). Because these patients are very dependent on preload and afterload, invasive monitors to monitor intravascular volume (e.g., central venous pressure and arterial catheter) and a pulse oximeter to evaluate the amount of shunting (e.g., a decrease in oxygen saturation may indicate an increase in right-to-left shunting) are helpful to assess the need for aggressive treatment of any fall in preload or peripheral vascular resistance. It should be recalled that centrally administered local anesthetics reduce both preload and afterload. An epidural anesthetic with a slower onset of action may be preferred to a spinal anesthetic with the faster onset of action. Low-dose epinephrine used in an epidural anesthetic can be used to decrease the absorption of local anesthetics but should be used cautiously, if at all, because a further decrease in systemic vascular resistance may result from the β effect of absorbed epinephrine, and an intravascular injection may further elevate pulmonary pressures, exacerbating the right-to-left shunt *(Chestnut: Chestnut's Obstetric Anesthesia, ed 5, pp 975–976; Fleisher: Anesthesia and Uncommon Diseases, ed 6, p 128; Hines: Stoelting's Anesthesia and Co-Existing Disease, ed 7, pp 138–139; Suresh: Shnider and Levinson's Anesthesia for Obstetrics, ed 5, pp 491–492).*

672. (C) The need for a hysterectomy for a planned repeat cesarean delivery is 0.3%, for a successful vaginal birth after cesarean is 0.1%, and for an unsuccessful TOLAC is 0.5%. With multiple gestations, uterine atony is common, and the need for a hysterectomy is sixfold in a normal delivery. However, the patient with placenta previa and a previous scar in the uterus has the highest chance of needing an emergency hysterectomy for uncontrolled bleeding at the time of delivery because of the associated placenta accreta (abnormally adherent placenta). The incidence of placenta accreta in a patient with placenta previa and no previous cesarean section is 3% to 4%, with one previous cesarean section is about 10% to 25%, and with two or more previous cesarean sections is 40% to over 60%. Most patients with placenta accreta will require a cesarean hysterectomy. The average blood loss during an emergency cesarean delivery and needed hysterectomy is 5 to 7 units of blood. Patients with a known placenta accreta should undergo a scheduled preterm cesarean delivery and hysterectomy with the placenta left in situ because any attempt to remove the placenta would likely lead to hemorrhage. Attempts to preserve the uterus with a placenta accreta has been described in select cases when hemodynamic stability is present and there is a very strong desire for a future pregnancy. This may include leaving the placenta in situ for placental involution or for only partial placenta accreta management by curettage and oversewing. With an advanced abdominal pregnancy, a laparotomy with delivery of the fetus is performed. Management of the placenta is controversial: Removal of the placenta can lead to massive hemorrhage, whereas leaving the placenta in situ is associated with an increase in infectious morbidity; however, a hysterectomy is not needed because the fetus is extrauterine *(Chestnut: Chestnut's Obstetric Anesthesia, ed 5, pp 344, 893–895; Suresh: Shnider and Levinson's Anesthesia for Obstetrics, ed 5, pp 147–149, 274–275, 311–321).*

673. (B) According to the ASA's Closed Claims Project for Obstetric Anesthesia Claims (640 claims as of December 2010 report), maternal nerve damage (19%), neonatal brain damage (16%), and maternal death (15%) were the three most frequent claims. Other causes include headache (11%), back pain (10%), neonatal death (9%), emotional distress (8%), maternal brain damage (7%), pain during anesthesia (6%), and aspiration pneumonitis (1%) *(Chestnut: Chestnut's Obstetric Anesthesia, ed 5, pp 776–779).*

674. (C) Chorioamnionitis occurs in about 1% of all pregnancies. It includes the clinical signs and symptoms of infection, temperature higher than 38° C, maternal and fetal tachycardia, uterine tenderness (about 10% of patients), and/or foul-smelling amniotic fluid. Prompt delivery is the cornerstone of therapy. At one time it was thought that antibiotics should be administered only after delivery because antepartum or intrapartum antibiotics may "obscure the results of neonatal blood cultures." However, early antepartum treatment with antibiotics leads to a decrease in maternal and neonatal morbidity, compared with delaying the antibiotics until after delivery, and is currently recommended. Epidural anesthesia has been shown to be commonly used and safe in these patients, preferably after antibiotics have been started. It seems prudent, however, to always individualize care and to weigh the risks versus the benefits of epidural anesthesia in a patient with suspected bacteremia *(Chestnut: Chestnut's Obstetric Anesthesia, ed 5, pp 862–873).*

675. (A) Meconium-stained amniotic fluid occurs in about 5% to 15% of all deliveries. Although intrapartum oropharyngeal and nasopharyngeal suction for all newborns born to mothers with meconium staining has been routine care for many years, current evidence shows no real benefit, and it is no longer recommended. In newborns who are vigorous (i.e., strong respiratory efforts, good muscle tone, and heart rate >100 beats/min), no treatment other than gentle bulb syringe suctioning to clear oral or nasal secretions is needed. Intubation and tracheal suction should be performed only in newborns who are not vigorous, and the decision to intubate and suction does not depend on the consistency of the meconium-stained fluid, as was once recommended. Because meconium is sterile, antibiotics are not needed. Steroids have not been necessary in the treatment of meconium-stained newborns. RDS is a condition that occurs as a result of low levels of pulmonary surfactant in the alveoli. RDS occurs in premature newborns, whereas meconium staining occurs typically in older, often post-term, newborns *(American Heart Association and the American Academy of Pediatrics: Textbook of Neonatal Resuscitation 2016, ed 7, pp 18, 51–53, 139–140; Chestnut: Chestnut's Obstetric Anesthesia, ed 5, pp 156–157, 179–180; Suresh: Shnider and Levinson's Anesthesia for Obstetrics, ed 5, pp 251–252).*

Three Variations of Placenta Previa

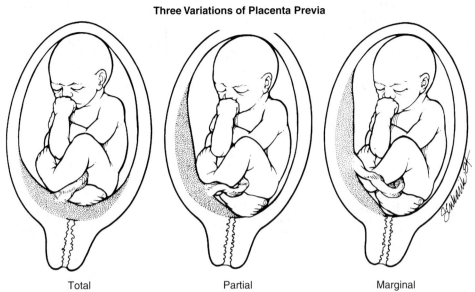

| Total | Partial | Marginal |

From Benedetti TJ: Obstetric hemorrhage. In Gabbe SG, Niebyl JR, Simpson JL, editors: Obstetrics: Normal and Problem Pregnancies, *ed 3, New York, Churchill Livingstone, 1996, p 511.*

676. (C) Placenta previa occurs when the placenta implants on the lower uterine segment so that all (total) or part of the placenta (partial) covers the internal cervical os. A marginal placenta previa occurs when the placenta lies close to but does not cover the internal cervical os. Placenta previa occurs in about 0.5% of all pregnancies and has a maternal mortality of less than 1% but a fetal mortality approaching 20% (primarily because of prematurity and intrauterine asphyxia). Patients typically present with painless vaginal bleeding that stops spontaneously (first bleed). Delivery is cesarean and is often made a few weeks after the "first" bleed, when the baby's lungs are more mature (e.g., after 37 weeks EGA). A later bleed can be uncontrolled and may be accompanied by significant hypovolemia and hypotension. Regional anesthesia is contraindicated in severely hypovolemic patients. Blood should be started when available, but replacing blood loss first to correct intravascular volume before induction of anesthesia may not be practical because bleeding may be faster than replacement is possible (i.e., may be >1 unit/min). A rapid-sequence general anesthetic (assuming acceptable airway) is preferred. Ketamine (0.75-1 mg/kg) as well as etomidate (0.3 mg/kg) supports the cardiovascular system better than propofol. In rare but severe cases of hypovolemic shock, all IV anesthetics may cause the blood pressure to fall further, and succinylcholine alone may be all that is required. In these severe cases, maternal recall should be considered secondary to maternal safety. In cases in which a difficult intubation is likely and the patient is hypovolemic, an infiltration local anesthetic may be best *(Chestnut: Chestnut's Obstetric Anesthesia, ed 5, pp 571, 882–885; Suresh: Shnider and Levinson's Anesthesia for Obstetrics, ed 5, pp 314–316).*

677. (D) At term pregnancy, V_T increases about 40% to 45%, and the inspiratory reserve volume (IRV) increases about 5%. A decrease occurs in both the ERV (20%-25%) and the residual volume (RV; 15%-20%). A capacity is defined as two or more lung volumes. Functional residual capacity (FRC = ERV + RV) is decreased about 15% to 20% and is partly responsible for the rapid fall in maternal oxygenation that occurs with apnea during the induction of general anesthesia. Total lung capacity (TLC = V_T + IRV + ERV + RV) decreases about 5%, whereas vital capacity (VC = V_T + IRV + ERV) remains unchanged *(Chestnut: Chestnut's Obstetric Anesthesia, ed 5, pp 19–21; Suresh: Shnider and Levinson's Anesthesia for Obstetrics, ed 5, pp 6–7).*

678. (A) Evaluation of the airway should be performed before the induction of any general anesthetic. In cases in which an unrecognized difficult airway exists (unable to perform endotracheal intubation in a reasonable period of time), the patient should be awakened if the procedure is purely elective and if the fetus has minimal or no fetal distress (as in this elective case). A regional anesthetic or awake intubation then can be safely performed. In cases of fetal or maternal distress, other options for securing the airway may be necessary *(Chestnut: Chestnut's Obstetric Anesthesia, ed 5, pp 700–701; Suresh: Shnider and Levinson's Anesthesia for Obstetrics, ed 5, pp 382–388).*

679. (B) Labor pain is some of the most intense pain that people can experience. Although there is considerable variability in the amount of intensity of pain during labor, in general primiparous patients have more pain than multiparous patients. Primiparous women who have attended prepared childbirth classes have somewhat less pain than women who have not attended prepared childbirth classes. For women who have experienced labor and delivery, attending prepared childbirth classes does not seem to affect the amount of pain that they experience. Labor pain appears to exceed chronic low back pain, nonterminal cancer pain, phantom limb pain, postherpetic neuralgia, or the pain from a fracture. Patients with causalgia or patients experiencing an amputation of a digit have more pain than the parturient. There appears also to be an association of the increasing amount of pain with increasing cervical dilation. *(Chestnut: Chestnut's Obstetric Anesthesia, ed 5, pp 410–412; Miller: Miller's Anesthesia, ed 8, p 2339).*

680. (C) The prevalence of women smoking during pregnancy was about 16% in the United States in 2010. Cigarettes contain nicotine, carbon monoxide, cyanides, and over 4000 other chemicals. Smoking affects small airway function and mucus secretion, and it impairs ciliary transport in the lungs; smoking also increases atherosclerosis and heart disease. Nicotine increases sympathetic tone (e.g., maternal heart rate, blood pressure, cardiac work). Carbon monoxide can occupy 3% to 15% (or more) of the oxygen-carrying capacity of blood and thus decreases oxygen delivery to tissues. Smoking cessation, even for a short time, may be safer for the fetus. Nonpharmacologic methods are preferred over nicotine patches or nicotine gum to help women stop smoking during pregnancy because studies of nicotine replacement are lacking. Cigarette smoking is associated with an increase in ectopic pregnancies, placental abruption, spontaneous fetal loss, and low-birth-weight babies (with an increased neonatal and infant mortality), as well as SIDS and lower intelligence. Interestingly, the incidence of preeclampsia is 30% to 40% lower among women who are smokers compared with women who are nonsmokers. The reason for this is unclear but may be related to stimulation of nitric oxide release or an inhibition of thromboxane A_2 synthesis. Because smoking irritates the airway, if general anesthesia is needed during pregnancy, desflurane is best avoided, whereas volatile anesthetics, such as sevoflurane, which does not irritate the airway, are preferred *(Chestnut: Chestnut's Obstetric Anesthesia, ed 5, pp 829, 1186–1187, 1201–1202).*

681. (C) In 2012, the U.S. Food and Drug Administration (FDA) approved the use of simple devices for the administration of nitrous oxide as "minimal sedation" for labor analgesia. Inhaled nitrous oxide is used by <1% of patients for labor analgesia in the United States, but its use is more common in other countries such as Canada (43%) and the United Kingdom (62%). These noninvasive devices have demand valves where the patient must initiate the breathing. When inhalation is completed, there is no free flow of anesthetic into the room. The devices also have a scavenging system to decrease exposure to low levels of nitrous oxide. The gas inhaled is typically 50% nitrous oxide and 50% oxygen. The patient must hold the mask or mouthpiece in place without the assistance of a nurse, family member, or labor support person. Typically it takes about 30 to 60 seconds for analgesia to develop, so the patient should initiate inhalation at the start of the uterine contraction and continue breathing the gas until the end of the contraction. This gives the women in labor another analgesic option. The patients have the freedom to move about and do not require the placement of an IV or urinary catheter. It may prove useful for women with disorders of coagulation, chronic pain or anxiety, and a poor response to opioid medications. The quality of analgesia with inhaled nitrous oxide is variable, but less so than with epidural analgesia. Side effects of nitrous oxide for labor analgesia include nausea and vomiting (13%-33%), dizziness (4%), drowsiness (4%), and paresthesias (which are also related to maternal hyperventilation). The incidence of hypoxia appears to be low. Keep in mind that using narcotics or sedatives with nitrous oxide may depress respirations and increase the amount of nausea. Apgar scores of newborn infants whose mothers have used inhaled nitrous oxide appear to be similar to those of infants whose mothers used other forms or no forms of analgesia. Anesthesia personnel are not involved in their use *(Camann W: Inhaled nitrous oxide for labor analgesia: pearls from clinical experience, OBG Manag 30:29–32, 2018; Chestnut: Chestnut's Obstetric Anesthesia, ed 5, pp 452–453).*

682. (A) When performing an RSI for a cesarean section, the patient is preoxygenated, and after you ascertain that intubation should be easy, you inject your IV general anesthetic (e.g., propofol 2.5 mg/kg, ketamine 1-1.5 mg/kg, or etomidate 0.3 mg/kg) followed by a paralytic drug to facilitate oral endotracheal intubation. Thiopental (4-5 mg/kg) is another IV general anesthetic that can be used if it is available (not available in the United States). Paralysis to optimize tracheal intubation conditions can be obtained with either succinylcholine (1-1.5 mg/kg in 30-45 seconds) or rocuronium (1.2 mg/kg in <60 seconds). Vecuronium (0.1 mg/kg) can also be used but is less desirable because it has a slower onset of action of 144 seconds. Atracurium is the least desirable of the listed drugs due to the significant histamine release and resultant hypotension and slow onset of action. Although cisatracurium has little histamine release, it has a very slow onset of action and is not recommended for an RSI induction if succinylcholine, rocuronium, or vecuronium is available *(Chestnut: Chestnut's Obstetric Anesthesia, ed 5, pp 569–577; Miller: Basics of Anesthesia, ed 7, pp 568–571; Miller: Miller's Anesthesia, ed 8, pp 2345–2347).*

683. (C) Intrathecal opiates (e.g., morphine, fentanyl, sufentanil) are very effective in relieving the visceral pain during the first stage of labor. Intrathecal opiates administered alone (except for meperidine, which has local anesthetic properties) do not provide adequate pain relief for second-stage somatic pain *(Chestnut: Chestnut's Obstetric Anesthesia, ed 5, pp 277–282, 465–468; Suresh: Shnider and Levinson's Anesthesia for Obstetrics, ed 5, pp 184–187).*

684. (A) The most common side effect of intraspinal narcotics is pruritus. The next most common side effects are nausea and vomiting, followed by urinary retention and drowsiness. Respiratory depression and headache may occur but are relatively infrequent *(Chestnut: Chestnut's Obstetric Anesthesia, ed 5, pp 283–287; Suresh: Shnider and Levinson's Anesthesia for Obstetrics, ed 5, pp 185–186).*

685. (C) Hypertension during pregnancy is divided into four groups: preeclampsia-eclampsia, chronic hypertension (of any cause), chronic hypertension with superimposed preeclampsia, and gestational hypertension. Preeclampsia-eclampsia is a hypertensive disorder of pregnancy with associated proteinuria ($\geq$300 mg protein per 24-hour urine collection). As of recently (November 2013), the presence of proteinuria is no longer needed for the designation of preeclampsia-eclampsia. The reason for the change is that some patients develop proteinuria late and have their diagnosis and needed treatment delayed. Current definition of preeclampsia-eclampsia is the new onset of hypertension along with proteinuria or, in the absence of proteinuria, new onset of hypertension associated with thrombocytopenia (platelet count <100,000/mL), impaired liver function, new onset of renal insufficiency (serum creatinine >1.1 mg/dL or doubling of serum creatinine in the absence of any other renal disease), pulmonary edema, or new-onset cerebral or visual disturbances. Gestational hypertension, which is isolated new-onset hypertension (after 20 weeks) that resolves by 12 weeks postpartum, is a retrospective diagnosis. Preeclampsia-eclampsia rarely occurs before the 20th week of pregnancy, except in patients with gestational trophoblastic neoplasms (e.g., molar pregnancy). The incidence of preeclampsia is significantly higher in parturients with a hydatidiform mole, multiple gestations, obesity, polyhydramnios, or diabetes and occurs more commonly with the first pregnancy. Mothers with preeclampsia during their first pregnancy have a 33% chance of having preeclampsia in subsequent pregnancies. Preeclampsia can progress to eclampsia (preeclampsia accompanied by a seizure not related to other conditions). Eighty percent of the seizures occur before or during delivery; 85% of the remaining 20% will have the seizure within the first 24 hours after delivery. Approximately 5% of untreated parturients with preeclampsia will develop eclampsia. HELLP syndrome (*H*emolysis, *E*levated *L*iver enzymes, and *L*ow *P*latelet count) is a variant of preeclampsia. Chronic hypertension is persistent hypertension before, during, and after pregnancy (e.g., >6 weeks postpartum). Chronic hypertension with superimposed preeclampsia occurs when a patient with chronic hypertension develops preeclampsia. Also see Question 645 *(American College of Obstetricians and Gynecologists Task Force on Hypertension in Pregnancy, November 2013 Website; Chestnut: Chestnut's Obstetric Anesthesia, ed 5, pp 825–826; Suresh: Shnider and Levinson's Anesthesia for Obstetrics, ed 5, pp 437–438).*

686. (A) AFE is a rare condition (5 per 100,000 live births). It presents in a variety of ways but often in a dramatic way, with acute hypoxemia, cardiovascular collapse, DIC, and, in about 50% of cases, a seizure. Patients with a high spinal or epidural may complain of dyspnea, but they also have marked weakness and would certainly not be able to wrestle or struggle with their health care providers. Patients experiencing an intravascular injection of local anesthetic present with CNS signs of toxicity (light-headedness, visual or auditory disturbances, muscular twitching, convulsion, coma) or, at higher levels, cardiovascular collapse. Magnesium overdosage is also associated with muscle weakness. The typical eclamptic seizure is tonic–clonic. Patients with eclampsia do not complain of dyspnea, although an associated aspiration may produce similar symptoms. See Question 658 *(Chestnut: Chestnut's Obstetric Anesthesia, ed 5, pp 915–920; Suresh: Shnider and Levinson's Anesthesia for Obstetrics, ed 5, pp 333–348).*

687. (C) Epidural fentanyl (50-100 μg) and epidural sufentanil (10-20 μg) each have a duration of action for about 2 to 4 hours. Epidural meperidine (50-75 mg) has an intermediate duration of action of 4 to 12 hours, whereas epidural morphine (3-4 mg) has the longest duration of action, of 12 to 24 hours *(Chestnut: Chestnut's Obstetric Anesthesia, ed 5, pp 566–567).*

688. (C) The renal system undergoes dramatic anatomic (increase in kidney size as well as dilation of the ureters) and functional changes in pregnancy. Renal plasma flow increases about 75% to 85%, and glomerular filtration rate (GFR) increases about 50% and is reflected by an increase in clearance of urea, creatinine, and uric acid. Because of the increased clearance, we see a decrease in BUN to 8 to 9 mg/dL, serum creatinine to 0.5 to 0.6 mg/dL, and serum urate to 2.0 to 3.0 mg/dL. Glucosuria is common and is attributed to both the increase in GFR and a reduced renal tubular resorption of glucose *(Chestnut: Chestnut's Obstetric Anesthesia, ed 5, p 27; Miller: Miller's Anesthesia, ed 8, p 2348).*

689. (C) All volatile halogenated anesthetic agents (e.g., halothane, enflurane, isoflurane, desflurane, sevoflurane) cause a dose-related relaxation of uterine smooth muscle. With anesthetic concentrations of 0.2 MAC, the decrease in uterine activity is slight, and these agents have been used for inhalation analgesia during labor. At 0.5 MAC, uterine relaxation is more significant, but the uterine response to oxytocin remains intact. Nitrous oxide does not affect uterine activity *(Chestnut: Chestnut's Obstetric Anesthesia, ed 5, pp 452–454; 575–576; Suresh: Shnider and Levinson's Anesthesia for Obstetrics, ed 5, pp 156–157, 176–177).*

690. (B) Passive diffusion is the primary means for the placental transfer of drugs. Factors that promote diffusion of drugs across placental membranes include decreased maternal protein binding (although some believe that this is not very important because of rapid diffusion of drugs from protein), low molecular weight (<500 Da), high lipid solubility (low water solubility), a low degree of ionization, and a large concentration gradient across the membranes. Highly ionized drugs, such as neuromuscular drugs, do not pass the placenta in significant amounts *(Chestnut: Chestnut's Obstetric Anesthesia, ed 5, pp 63–65; Suresh: Shnider and Levinson's Anesthesia for Obstetrics, ed 5, pp 19–23).*

691. (D) The average blood loss associated with a vaginal delivery is about 600 mL and after a cesarean delivery is about 1000 mL *(Chestnut: Chestnut's Obstetric Anesthesia, ed 5, pp 24–25).*

692. (C) The fetus has several compensatory mechanisms for dealing with low O_2 pressures (umbilical vein P_{O_2} approximately equal to 30 mm Hg when the mother is breathing room air) to which it is exposed. These include a higher hemoglobin concentration (15-20 g/dL) and the presence of fetal hemoglobin, which has a greater affinity for oxygen (the fetal oxyhemoglobin dissociation curve is shifted to the left of the maternal oxyhemoglobin dissociation curve). At term, maternal blood flow through the placenta (700 mL/min) is about double the fetal blood flow through the placenta (300-360 mL/min). Fetal blood has a lower pH than maternal blood, which may be related to the higher Pa_{CO_2} levels seen in fetal blood *(Suresh: Shnider and Levinson's Anesthesia for Obstetrics, ed 5, pp 22–27).*

693. (B) A pregnant woman is considered overweight when her body mass index (BMI) is 25.0 to 29.9 kg/m^2 and obese when the BMI is greater than 30 kg/m^2. The World Health Organization (WHO) defines three grades of obesity: Class I = BMI 30 to 34.5 kg/m^2, Class II as BMI 35 to 39.9 kg/m^2, and Class III as BMI $\geq$ 40 kg/m^2. The obese patient is at increased risk for several comorbid diseases, including obstructive sleep apnea (OSA), diabetes, hypertension, gallbladder disease, chronic back pain, and coronary artery disease. During pregnancy, the obese patient has an increased chance of gestational diabetes, hypertensive disorders of pregnancy, preterm delivery, deep vein thrombosis, pulmonary thromboembolism, respiratory depression, wound infections, postpartum hemorrhage, cesarean deliveries, and death (reviews note that about 50% or more of pregnant women who die are overweight or obese). The increased incidence of cesarean deliveries may relate to an increase in abnormal presentations, fetal macrosomia, meconium staining, late decelerations in the FHR, and dysfunctional labor.

Anesthetic challenges include increased risk of aspiration, difficulty finding adequate venous access, difficulty with mask ventilation, difficulty with endotracheal intubation, difficulty in performing regional anesthesia, operative positioning, and prolonged surgery. Interestingly, obese and morbidly obese patients appear to have a lower incidence of PDPHs. Etiology for the lower incidence of PDPHs is unclear *(Chestnut: Chestnut's Obstetric Anesthesia, ed 5, pp 1141–1153; Miller: Miller's Anesthesia, ed 8, p 2349; Suresh: Shnider and Levinson's Anesthesia for Obstetrics, ed 5, pp 428, 580–592).*

694. (D) Normal healthy term newborns breathing room air take a while for the oxygen saturations to rise to normal 90% to 95% levels. In caring for the newborn who is not breathing, bag and mask ventilation with room air is now recommended, with targeted preductal oxygen saturation (right hand or wrist) increases of about 5% for each minute of the first 5 minutes of life, starting at 1 minute oxygen saturation of 60% to 65% (at 2 minutes 65%-70%, at 3 minutes 70%-75%, at 4 minutes 75%-80%, at 5 minutes 80%-85%). After 5 minutes, oxygen saturation more slowly increases to 85% to 95% by 10 minutes of life. If higher concentrations of oxygen are needed to reach the targeted oxygen saturations (especially in preterm newborns <32 weeks), a blender for oxygen and air can be used. For this newborn, an oxygen saturation of 83% at 5 minutes is appropriate, and observation only is needed *(American Heart Association and the American Academy of Pediatrics: Textbook of Neonatal Resuscitation 2016, ed 7, pp 33–57; American Heart Association: Part 13: Neonatal Resuscitation, Circulation 132: S543–S560, 2015)*

695. (B) Second- and third-trimester obstetric hemorrhage is not uncommon in obstetrics. Placenta previa (where the placenta is partially or completely covering the cervical os) is suspected when painless vaginal bleeding occurs during the second or third trimester. This first episode of bleeding is usually not associated with maternal shock or fetal distress and is expectantly managed if the bleeding stops and the fetus is immature. However, with a second or third episode of vaginal bleeding, the bleeding may continue and delivery may be indicated. Placental abruption (separation of the placenta from the uterine wall after 20 weeks' EGA and before delivery) is more typically associated with abdominal pain and can be associated with fetal distress. Bleeding with placenta abruption may be revealed or concealed behind the placenta. Uterine rupture usually presents with severe abdominal pain and fetal distress. Vasa previa refers to a condition where the fetal blood vessels are unsupported by the umbilical cord or placental tissue and cross over the cervical os. When the fetal membranes rupture, a tear in a fetal blood vessel may develop, leading to fetal exsanguination *(Chestnut: Chestnut's Obstetric Anesthesia, ed 5, pp 882–888; Hines: Stoelting's Anesthesia and Co-Existing Disease, ed 7, pp 679–683; Suresh: Shnider and Levinson's Anesthesia for Obstetrics, ed 5, pp 312–317).*

696. (D) The first stage of labor starts with the onset of labor and ends with complete cervical dilation (10 cm). It is visceral pain, associated with uterine contractions and dilation of the cervix, and is transmitted via the autonomic nervous system through the sympathetic fibers that pass through the paracervical region and enter the CNS at T10-L1 segments. The second stage of labor includes these pathways and adds the somatic fibers of the birth canal that are transmitted via the pudendal nerve entering the CNS at S2-S4. Neuraxial block (spinal and/or epidural) with only narcotics can be useful for first-stage pain; however, the somatic pain is not well treated with narcotics alone. A local anesthetic–induced lumbar epidural block with or without narcotics can produce complete anesthesia during both first and second stage of labor pain. If a low spinal or saddle block is performed with local anesthetics (covering only sacral areas), the uterine contraction pain still will be felt. Paracervical blocks block only the first-stage pain. Pudendal blocks block the somatic component during the second stage but not the visceral pain of uterine contractions *(Chestnut: Chestnut's Obstetric Anesthesia, ed 5, pp 412–415, 459–480, 518–527; Suresh: Shnider and Levinson's Anesthesia for Obstetrics, ed 5, pp 119–133).*

697. (C) Anesthetic considerations for open fetal surgery include administering anesthesia for the mother and the child, giving excellent uterine relaxation, maintaining an adequate maternal blood pressure, providing muscle relaxation to the fetus if needed, and preventing postoperative premature labor. Uterine relaxation is needed to prevent uterine contractions, with possible separation of the placenta from the uterine wall. High-dose volatile anesthetics (e.g., 2 or 3 MAC) can provide excellent maternal anesthesia, as well as uterine relaxation and anesthesia for the fetus. If additional anesthesia is needed or when a lower concentration of volatile anesthetic is administered, maternally administered IV narcotics can be used (e.g., remifentanil infusions at a dose of 0.1 μg/kg/min) or a fetal IM injection of fentanyl (up to 10-20 μg/kg) can be performed. If one chooses to use a lower dose of volatile anesthetics, nitroglycerin infusion may be needed to keep the uterus from contracting. Maternal hypotension (mean blood pressure <65) is not uncommon and is treated with more left uterine tilt, fluids, and, if needed, phenylephrine or ephedrine. Monitoring the fetal oxygen saturation reveals normal values of 50% to 70%; values less than 50% signal impaired placental perfusion (e.g., maternal hypotension, cord compression). If the obstetrician needs the fetus to be paralyzed, then a neuromuscular blocking drug can be given directly into the fetus because placental transfer of muscle relaxants is poor. The dose of muscle relaxant, however, must be larger when the fetus is in utero compared with the fetus after delivery (newborn of the same weight) because the blood volume of the fetus in utero includes the fetal blood volume as well as the placental blood volume. Typically the IM dose is about four to six times the effective dose in 95% of subjects (ED_{95}) or for vecuronium is 0.2 to 0.3 mg/kg. Magnesium sulfate may be started to decrease the chance of premature labor at the end of the surgery as the volatile anesthetic concentration is decreased or the nitroglycerin infusion is discontinued. One should recall that the magnesium sulfate potentiates neuromuscular blocking drugs significantly. In many cases of fetal surgery, the mother may also receive an epidural for postoperative analgesia *(Chestnut: Chestnut's Obstetric Anesthesia, ed 5, pp 135–141; Suresh: Shnider and Levinson's Anesthesia for Obstetrics, ed 5, pp 792–799).*

698. (D) 15-Methyl PGF2α (carboprost, Hemabate) can be used for the treatment of refractory uterine atony (after oxytocin is administered and uterine massage has been performed). It works by increasing contractions of smooth muscle. The dose is 0.25 mg injected IM or directly into the uterine wall, repeated as needed every 15 to 90 minutes with a maximum total dose of 2 mg (8 doses). It has several important side effects, such as bronchospasm, ventilation-to-perfusion mismatch with an increase in intrapulmonary shunting, hypoxemia, and increased blood pressure. It is contraindicated in patients with asthma and relatively contraindicated in patients with pregnancy-induced hypertension. Other side effects include GI spasms (e.g., nausea, vomiting, and diarrhea) *(Chestnut: Chestnut's Obstetric Anesthesia, ed 5, p 891; Suresh: Shnider and Levinson's Anesthesia for Obstetrics, ed 5, p 321).*

699. (C) International consensus states that magnesium sulfate ($MgSO_4$) is the anticonvulsant of choice in the preeclamptic patient. In addition to its anticonvulsant effect, $MgSO_4$ has many other actions on skeletal and cardiac muscles. $MgSO_4$ is usually started as an IV bolus of 6 g over 20 minutes followed by an infusion of 2 g/hr (provided that kidney function is normal). Clinical monitoring for toxicity is performed looking at deep tendon reflexes, and blood levels are often performed and reported in either mEq/L or mg/dL (1 mEq/L = 1.22 mg/dL). The therapeutic range for serum $MgSO_4$ is 4 to 8 mEq/L (4.8-9.6 mg/dL). In an unanesthetized patient, a loss of deep tendon reflexes occurs at 10 mEq/L (12 mg/dL), respiratory arrest occurs at 15 mEq/L (18 mg/dL), and cardiac arrest occurs at 25 mEq/L (30 mg/dL). As long as deep tendon reflexes are present, significant toxicity is unlikely. In a patient with an epidural or spinal anesthetic loaded for a cesarean section, the patellar reflex is often depressed by the local anesthetic; estimation of deep tendon reflexes should be done with the biceps tendon (unless a total spinal develops). ECG changes, including PR interval prolongation and QRS complex widening, occur at serum levels of 5 to 10 mEq/L (6-12 mg/dL), sinoatrial and atrioventricular block at 15 mEq/L (18 mg/dL), and cardiac arrest at levels greater than 25 mEq/L (30 mg/dL). The treatment for magnesium toxicity is calcium. The dose of 1 g of calcium gluconate (10 mL of a 10% solution) can be administered slowly over at least 2 minutes to treat high magnesium levels. Rapid administration may take away the anticonvulsant effects, so careful slow titration is recommended. About 60% of eclamptic seizures occur before delivery. Most postpartum seizures develop in the first 24 hours after delivery, but eclamptic seizures may occur as late as 22 days after delivery *(Miller: Miller's Anesthesia, ed 8, p 2348; Suresh: Shnider and Levinson's Anesthesia for Obstetrics, ed 5, 448–449).*

700. (C) Three different aspiration syndromes have been described in the general population: aspiration of particulate matter causing mainly mechanical airway obstruction, aspiration of acid fluid causing aspiration pneumonitis (Mendelson syndrome), and aspiration of gram-positive, gram-negative, and anaerobic bacteria (e.g., bowel obstruction) causing aspiration pneumonia. Symptoms of aspiration pneumonitis include coughing, tachypnea, tachycardia, bronchospasm, and hypoxemia. Treatment is supportive and includes the Heimlich maneuver if a large foreign body is lodged in the trachea (which is unlikely in the fasting laboring patient), endotracheal intubation, suctioning the airway to remove particulate material, administration of increased concentrations of oxygen, and application of PEEP to achieve oxygenation goals as needed. Coughing is due to the airway irritation and is most effectively decreased with muscle paralysis. Intravenous lidocaine is not effective. Use of saline or bicarbonate lavage does not decrease lung damage and can worsen hypoxemia. Glucocorticoids or other anti-inflammatory drugs have not been effective in limiting the inflammation and may increase the risk of secondary bacterial infection *(Chestnut: Chestnut's Obstetric Anesthesia, ed 5, pp 671–675; Suresh: Shnider and Levinson's Anesthesia for Obstetrics, ed 5, pp 403–405).*

701. (C) Aortocaval compression typically is not a problem until about 18 to 20 weeks' gestation, when the uterus is large enough to compress the aorta and vena cava when the patient assumes the supine position. If the uterus is larger than normal (e.g., multiple gestations or polyhydramnios), then aortocaval compression may appear earlier. See also Question 714 *(Chestnut: Chestnut's Obstetric Anesthesia, ed 5, p 340; Suresh: Shnider and Levinson's Anesthesia for Obstetrics, ed 5, p 5).*

702. (B) Cimetidine and ranitidine are H_2-receptor antagonists that will increase gastric pH but take at least 30 minutes to work. Metoclopramide is not an antacid but may be useful by increasing the lower esophageal sphincter tone. Only liquid antacids raise gastric pH quickly. Sodium citrate, a clear nonparticulate antacid (0.3 M sodium citrate), is preferred over particulate antacids (aluminum hydroxide, magnesium trisilicate, magnesium hydroxide) because clear nonparticulate antacids cause less pulmonary damage if aspirated. Sodium citrate 30 mL neutralizes 255 mL of HCl with a pH of 1.0. Neutralization of gastric acid occurs rapidly (i.e., <5 minutes) and will last up to an hour *(Chestnut: Chestnut's Obstetric Anesthesia, ed 5, pp 675–677; Suresh: Shnider and Levinson's Anesthesia for Obstetrics, ed 5, pp 407–408).*

703. (A) Causes of fetal bradycardia (FHR <110 beats/min) include hypotension, excessive uterine activity, hypoxemia, acidosis, complete heart block, and some drugs. Atropine readily crosses the placenta but at low doses does not seem to cause fetal tachycardia; at high doses, it may produce tachycardia. The combination of neostigmine, which crosses the placenta slightly, and glycopyrrolate, which does not cross the placenta well, has been associated with fetal bradycardia, which is why neostigmine with atropine is preferred when reversing neuromuscular blockers if a fetus is present. Fetal bradycardias are often associated with early decelerations (head compression with vagal stimulation), late decelerations (fetal hypoxemia with vagal stimulation or myocardial failure), and variable decelerations (umbilical cord compressions with vagal stimulation). Causes of fetal tachycardia (FHR >160 beats/min) include infection, fever, maternal cigarette smoking, fetal paroxysmal supraventricular tachycardia, and some drugs (ritodrine, terbutaline, atropine) *(Chestnut: Chestnut's Obstetric Anesthesia, ed 5, pp 68, 150–159; Suresh: Shnider and Levinson's Anesthesia for Obstetrics, ed 5, pp 69–73, 843).*

704. (A) CP is a nonprogressive disorder of the CNS arising from lesions in the brain that occurred during development (in utero 75%, at birth 10%, soon after birth 15%). CP is associated with impairment of motor function. Mental retardation may or may not be present and is not an essential diagnostic criterion. The cause is unknown and most likely multifactorial. Associated conditions include maternal mental retardation (now called intellectual disability), birth weight of less than 2000 g and fetal malformations, breech presentation (but not breech vaginal delivery), severe proteinuria during the second half of pregnancy, third-trimester bleeding, and gestational age less than 32 weeks, but many other factors may play a role. It occurs in about 2 per 1000 live births. At one time, FHR monitoring was thought to be able to prevent CP, but this has not happened. In fact, among patients with new-onset late deceleration patterns, the false-positive rate is 99% if used to predict the development of CP. This is not to say that intrapartum asphyxial insults do not cause damage; they might, and they probably account for some cases of CP. There is also a very weak association of low Apgar scores and CP; in fact, most children who develop CP had a 5-minute Apgar score that was normal *(Chestnut: Chestnut's Obstetric Anesthesia, ed 5, pp 193–197; Miller: Miller's Anesthesia, ed 8, p 2337; Suresh: Shnider and Levinson's Anesthesia for Obstetrics, ed 5, pp 68–69).*

705. (B) Seven to eight percent of the adult population in the United States has DM. Type 1 DM (about 10% of diabetics) is a T-cell–mediated autoimmune disease where the patients have an absolute deficiency in insulin secretion. Type 2 DM (about 90% of diabetics) occurs primarily in obese individuals and is associated with an inadequate release of insulin or insulin resistance in target tissues. Type 1 DM occurs in 1 of every 700 to 1000 gestations. Gestational diabetes, which occurs only during pregnancy, is currently seen in about 7% of all pregnancies in the United States. Although substantial advances in the obstetric and anesthetic management of diabetic parturients have been made, maternal and fetal mortality is still higher in these patients than in parturients without diabetes. DKA occurs primarily in Type 1 DM patients and has decreased from 9% to currently around 1% to 2% of Type 1 DM pregnancies. One important goal of insulin therapy in diabetic patients is to avoid both hyperglycemia and hypoglycemia. In general, insulin requirements in Type 1 DM patients initially decrease during early pregnancy to their lowest requirement by around 16 to 18 weeks (10%-20% reduction in dose), then increase above pre-pregnant values around 26 weeks to reach values that are highest at term (50% above prepregnant dose). The dose requirements then rapidly decrease at the time of delivery. Insulin does not readily cross the placenta and therefore does not have any direct effects on glucose metabolism in the fetus. Glucose, how-ever, readily crosses the placenta. Preeclampsia and large-for-gestational-age fetuses occur more frequently in parturient women with diabetes. Because of fetal macrosomia, cesarean section is more com-mon in diabetic than nondiabetic patients *(Chestnut: Chestnut's Obstetric Anesthesia, ed 5, pp 1003–1012; Suresh: Shnider and Levinson's Anesthesia for Obstetrics, ed 5, pp 462–472).*

706. (D) PDPHs are positional headaches (exacerbated by sitting or standing and relieved with recumbency) that usually present within 48 hours of a dural puncture (but could take up to a week to present) and typ-ically resolve in 2 to 14 days. They are bilateral and typically located in the frontal or occipital regions. In one prospective series of nonobstetric patients with PDPH, symptoms included nausea (60%), vomit-ing (24%), neck stiffness (43%), ocular changes (photophobia, diplopia, difficulty in accommodation) (13%), and auditory changes (hearing loss, hyperacusis, tinnitus) (12%). Although postpartum seizures have been associated with PDPH, other etiologies are more likely. Seizures, lethargy, fever, nuchal rigid-ity, focal neurologic deficits (other than listed above), and a unilateral location suggest other headache etiologies *(Chestnut: Chestnut's Obstetric Anesthesia, ed 5, pp 713–721; Suresh: Shnider and Levinson's Anesthesia for Obstetrics, ed 5, pp 425–430).*

707. (A) There are several periodic FHR patterns. Accelerations in FHR in response to fetal movement signify fetal well-being. Decelerations are a decrease in FHR of at least 15 beats/min that last at least 15 sec-onds. *Early decelerations* are decreases in FHR that are usually less than 20 beats/min and occur con-comitantly with uterine contractions. Typically they are smooth and are mirror images of the uterine contractions. They are not associated with fetal compromise and are caused by head compression, which produces a vagal slowing of the FHR. *Late decelerations* are decreases in FHR that occur 10 to 30 seconds after the onset of a contraction and end 10 to 30 seconds after the end of a contraction. They are due to uteroplacental insufficiency and can result whenever uterine blood flow decreases. The delayed onset is due to the time required to sense a low oxygen tension. The decrease in FHR may be a vagal reflex (mild cases) or may be due to direct myocardial depression from hypoxia (severe cases). Typically, in severe cases, beat-to-beat variability is decreased or absent as well. *Variable decel-erations* are abrupt decreases in FHR that vary in shape, depth, and duration from contraction to contraction. They are thought to be due to transient umbilical cord compression. A *sinusoidal pattern* is a regular smooth wavelike pattern with no short-term variability. It may be caused by severe fetal anemia or may result from the maternal administration of narcotics *(Chestnut: Chestnut's Obstetric Anesthesia, ed 5, p 101; Suresh: Shnider and Levinson's Anesthesia for Obstetrics, ed 5, pp 71–73, 245).*

708. (C) Shivering occurs in 15% to 20% of all normal vaginal deliveries. The frequency increases from 20% to 85% of patients receiving epidural or spinal anesthesia for cesarean deliveries. The postulated rea-son is that neuraxial anesthesia impairs centrally mediated peripheral vasoconstriction and shivering thresholds and allows greater environmental heat loss (core to peripheral heat redistribution). Intra-thecal narcotics (e.g., especially fentanyl with morphine) and epidural narcotics (e.g., fentanyl, sufen-tanil, meperidine, butorphanol), when added to local anesthetics, decrease the incidence of maternal shivering. Intravenous meperidine (25 mg), clonidine (75 μg), ketanserin (10 mg), magnesium sul-fate (30 mg/kg), or dexmedetomidine decrease the incidence of shivering. Warming the epidural anesthesia solution to body temperature has no effect on the incidence of shivering; however, adding epinephrine to the local anesthetic appears to increase the frequency of shivering *(Chestnut: Chestnut's Obstetric Anesthesia, ed 5, pp 483, 588–589, 646).*

709. (D) The values listed in the question are normal umbilical cord values. The chart is modified from values listed in the references *(Ostheimer: Manual of Obstetric Anesthesia, ed 2, pp 350–352: Chestnut's Obstetric Anesthesia, ed 5, pp 170–171; Suresh: Shnider and Levinson's Anesthesia for Obstetrics, ed 5, p 246).*

NORMAL VALUES FOR UMBILICAL CORD BLOOD

Cord Blood	pH	Pco$_2$ (mm Hg)	Po$_2$ (mm Hg)	Bicarbonate (mEq/L)
Arterial	7.25	50	20	22
Venous	7.35	40	30	20

From Chestnut DH, et al: Chestnut's Obstetric Anesthesia: Principles and Practice, *ed 4, Philadelphia, Mosby, 2009, pp 161–162.*

710. (D) For all obstetric-related admissions, the incidence of transfusion of blood is less than 1%. The most common reason for transfusion was postpartum hemorrhage. Estimates suggest that about one third of transfusions were not appropriate with current guidelines *(Chestnut: Chestnut's Obstetric Anesthesia, ed 5, pp 888–902).*

711. (C) Resuscitation guidelines continue to evolve. About 10% of newborns require some resuscitation to assist breathing at birth, whereas about 1% will need extensive resuscitation. If the newborn appears to be term, has good muscle tone, and is breathing or crying, the baby can remain with the mother and can have initial care performed on mother's chest or abdomen. Initial care consists of drying the newborn, providing warmth, and clearing secretions if needed. If the newborn appears depressed, next open the airway, clear out any remaining oral secretions, then stimulate the newborn by rubbing a towel to completely dry the newborn. If after a minute there is an obvious need for more extensive treatment (e.g., the heart rate is less than 100 beats/min or the newborn is gasping or apneic), then positive-pressure ventilation is started and oximetry and ECG monitoring are suggested. In term newborns, resuscitation is started with air rather than with 100% oxygen. However, preterm newborns (<32 weeks' gestation) may need air blended with oxygen to reach adequate oxygen saturations (e.g., at 10 minutes after delivery, the oxygen saturation should be 85%-95%). The oximetry probe should be placed preductally (i.e., on the right wrist) to assess oxygenation. If, after the first minute of life, the heart rate is less than 100 beats/min, one should ensure adequate positive-pressure mask ventilation and consider endotracheal intubation (or the use of a laryngeal mask). The ventilation rate should be 40 to 60 breaths per minute. If the heart rate is now less than 60 beats/min after at least 30 seconds of good positive-pressure ventilation, endotracheal intubation should be performed and 100% oxygen should be used. Chest compressions should then begin (with a chest compression-to-ventilation ratio of 3:1). At this point the newborn receives 30 breaths and 90 compressions/min (e.g., one and two and three and breath). If the newborn is known to have a cardiac etiology, then a higher compression-to-ventilation ratio should be considered (e.g., 15:2). If the heart rate is less than 60 beats/min after chest compressions and positive-pressure ventilation have been started for at least 30 seconds, consider administering epinephrine. The correct dose is 0.01 to 0.03 mg/kg IV or intraosseous (IO) and can be given every 3 to 5 minutes if needed. If the newborn is intubated and IV or IO access has not yet been achieved, consider administering a higher dose of epinephrine such as 0.05 to 0.1 mg/kg down the endotracheal tube (the higher dose is used because blood levels are unpredictable after endotracheal instillation). In a newborn with blood loss, volume expansion is needed and can be achieved with normal saline, Ringer lactate, or type O Rh-negative blood. The initial dose is 10 mL/kg. There is little evidence of any benefit with volume expansion in the absence of blood loss. If after 10 minutes there is no detectable heart rate, it may be appropriate to discontinue resuscitation (although many factors can contribute to continuing resuscitation beyond 10 minutes) *(American Heart Association and the American Academy of Pediatrics: Textbook of Neonatal Resuscitation 2016, ed 7, pp 33–193; American Heart Association; Part 13: Neonatal Resuscitation, Circulation 132:S543–S560, 2015).*

712. (D) Although epidural anesthesia often causes a fall in body temperature (due to the vasodilation and redistribution of body heat and loss to the environment), some women develop a rise in body temperature even though there is no evidence of infection. This rise in body temperature of greater than 38° C (100.4° F) usually occurs only when the epidural was used for at least 4 to 5 hours (frequency of 1%-36% of patients). The etiology of this rise in temperature in some women is unclear but includes three main factors (thermoregulatory, effect of systemic opioids, and inflammation). Epidural anesthesia may decrease sweating and the hyperventilation associated with labor, as well as shivering, which may increase body temperature. The use of IV systemic opioids may decrease the incidence of fever. Inflammation may play an important role because maternal temperatures are similar in women with or without epidural anesthesia when histologic examination of the placentas reveals the absence of placental inflammation. It may be that the temperature rise was merely an association with obstetric factors such as nulliparity with prolonged labor, more frequent cervical examinations, prolonged rupture of membranes, or early chorioamnionitis. The prepregnant blood leukocyte count of $6000/mm^3$ rises during pregnancy to 9000 to $11,000/mm^3$. During labor the leukocyte count increases to $13,000/mm^3$, and during the first postpartum day is on average $15,000/mm^3$ *(Chestnut: Chestnut's Obstetric Anesthesia, ed 5, pp 25, 867–871).*

713. (B) Although the cause of hypertensive disorders of pregnancy is not known, many factors are associated with a higher frequency of hypertensive disorders of pregnancy. Factors include nulliparous woman, age (especially <20 years and >40 years), family history of hypertensive disorders of pregnancy or a previous history of hypertensive disorders of pregnancy, some chronic medical conditions (e.g., hypertension, diabetes, obesity, thrombotic vascular disease, systemic lupus erythematosus), some obstetric conditions (e.g., placental abruption, intrauterine growth restriction, fetal death), and conditions in which the uterus is rapidly enlarging (e.g., multiple gestations, polyhydramnios, hydatidiform mole). Although smoking is associated with more adverse pregnancy outcomes (e.g., ectopic pregnancies, placenta previa, placental abruption, FHR abnormalities, low birth weight, respiratory impairment in the newborn, and sudden infant death syndrome (SIDS)), there appears to be a 30% to 40% lower incidence of hypertensive disorders of pregnancy in women who smoke. The protective effect appears to be dose related, with heavy smokers having a lower frequency than those who smoke fewer cigarettes. In addition, women who are more physically active have a lower frequency of hypertensive disorders of pregnancy than sedentary women *(Chestnut: Chestnut's Obstetric Anesthesia, ed 5, pp 827–829; Suresh: Shnider and Levinson's Anesthesia for Obstetrics, ed 5, pp 683, 688–689).*

714. (D) Aortocaval compression, as its name suggests, produces both compression of the aorta (increase in afterload) as well as compression of the vena cava (decrease in venous return). The patient's response is variable. Although some women have no symptoms, up to 15% of pregnant patients at term will, over several minutes in the supine position, develop hypotension and bradycardia (also called the supine hypotension syndrome). Some women will actually show an increase in brachial artery blood pressure due to the increase in afterload. These women may have a condition referred to as concealed hypotension (blood pressure above the compression that is adequate but blood pressure below the compression that is reduced). Because the blood supply to the uterus is distal to the aortic compression and uterine blood flow is decreased, the fetus may develop fetal distress. Other signs and symptoms of aortocaval compression include nausea, vomiting, pallor, sweating, and changes in cerebration. See also Question 701 *(Chestnut: Chestnut's Obstetric Anesthesia, ed 5, pp 18–19; Suresh: Shnider and Levinson's Anesthesia for Obstetrics, ed 5, pp 5–6).*

715. (B) Cocaine can produce life-threatening complications that are usually related to the accumulation of catecholamines, and patients may present with the classic signs of toxemia (i.e., hypertension and proteinuria) as well as chest pain. The typical half-life of cocaine is 30 to 90 minutes, but the acute effects can last as long as 6 hours. Because some states consider in utero cocaine exposure a form of child abuse that requires physicians to report positive drug tests in pregnant women, many patients who use cocaine have no prenatal care. Urine tests may be positive for 24 to 72 hours after cocaine use (depending on the amount used). Life-threatening events are more common with general than regional anesthesia. The most frequent problem with induction of general anesthesia is severe hypertension. Arrhythmias, myocardial ischemia, and tachycardia may also occur with the induction of general anesthesia. Labetalol and nitroglycerin have been used to treat these conditions. The MAC level is increased in patients who are acutely intoxicated, whereas patients chronically abusing cocaine have a lower MAC (due to the depletion of catecholamines). These patients are at risk for hypotension, which is commonly seen after the induction of regional anesthesia for cesarean section. Ephedrine may not be an effective vasopressor in these catecholamine-depleted patients. Phenylephrine, a direct-acting drug, is a better vasopressor *(Chestnut: Chestnut's Obstetric Anesthesia, ed 5, pp 1204–1207; Suresh: Shnider and Levinson's Anesthesia for Obstetrics, ed 5, pp 690–692).*

716. (C) In cases of emergency cesarean section when general anesthesia is contraindicated (e.g., poor airway when one questions one's ability to intubate and/or ventilate the patient) and neuraxial anesthesia is contraindicated (e.g., severe hypovolemia or coagulopathy), emergency infiltration anesthesia is acceptable. All of the choices are correct except the choice of a local anesthetic. As the surgeon will be injecting a fair volume of local anesthetic (often 100 mL), and as bupivacaine has a slow onset and potentially dangerous cardiac toxicity with large doses, bupivacaine is a poor choice. A dose of 0.5% lidocaine (plasma half-life of 90 minutes) is often used because it is readily available and relatively safe. Chloroprocaine may be safer because it also has a fast onset and its plasma half-life is extremely short (23 seconds). Both midazolam and ketamine may lead to some amnesia for the patient, which may be advantageous in this emergency situation; however, too much of the IV drugs could obtund the patient and may lead to aspiration of gastric contents. A good coach at the head of the bed may be invaluable for reassuring the patient as to the care *(Chestnut: Chestnut's Obstetric Anesthesia, ed 5, pp 577–578).*

717. (A) The most common complication after a spinal or epidural anesthetic is placed is systemic hypotension. Because the cardiac output is influenced by four main factors (preload, afterload, contractility, and heart rate and rhythm), treatment is directed at these factors. First, consider more left uterine displacement (which can increase venous return and preload). Next, administer more IV fluids (without dextrose such as lactated Ringer or saline solution) to increase preload if the amount of fluid used to prehydrate the patient before the block is thought to be inadequate. In this case the amount of prehydration with saline is an appropriate amount, but a little more non-dextrose containing fluid may be helpful. Intravenous fluids with dextrose are used only for maintenance fluids and should not be used to prevent or treat hypotension from regional anesthesia because the fluid load with dextrose causes significant maternal and fetal hyperglycemia and hyperinsulinemia. After delivery, the sugar supply for the newborn stops but the insulin response continues, often causing fetal hypoglycemia after delivery. It should be noted that 5% albumin solutions are expensive and are not recommended for routine use to treat hypotension. Vasopressors and/or drugs that increase cardiac contractility are commonly needed to increase afterload. Initial laboratory studies with pregnant ewes suggested that ephedrine was a better choice than phenylephrine or other α-adrenergic agonists when looking at changes in uterine blood flow. In these initial studies, the blood pressure was raised from normal to higher levels, and ephedrine was the drug of choice because phenylephrine decreased uterine blood flow, whereas ephedrine did not. However, raising a normal pressure to higher levels is not the same thing as raising a low blood pressure to normal. In more recent human studies looking at ephedrine and phenylephrine use, no difference was noted in the prophylactic or therapeutic use of these drugs for maternal hypotension. It was also noted that maternal bradycardia was more common with maternal phenylephrine administration, whereas maternal tachycardia was more common with maternal ephedrine administration; also, neonatal arterial pH was slightly higher when phenylephrine was used compared with ephedrine. Why this occurs is unclear but may be related to ephedrine's ability to cross the placenta, causing β-adrenergic stimulation in the newborn (F/M blood ratio is 0.7 for ephedrine and 0.2 for phenylephrine). In this patient who has left uterine displacement, adequate IV hydration, and a heart rate of 110 beats/min, phenylephrine would be the preferred vasopressor. If the mother has hypotension with bradycardia, ephedrine might be a better choice. Epinephrine is rarely needed but should be available and used when there is severe hypotension that is not responsive to phenylephrine or ephedrine, especially when there is associated fetal bradycardia *(Chestnut: Chestnut's Obstetric Anesthesia, ed 5, pp 480–481, 580–583; Suresh: Shnider and Levinson's Anesthesia for Obstetrics, ed 5, pp 50, 135–136, 174).*

718. (D) A *threatened abortion* is defined as uterine bleeding without cervical dilation before 20 weeks' gestation. Bleeding may be accompanied by uterine cramps or backache. Half of these cases will go on to spontaneously abort. An *inevitable abortion* has cervical dilation and/or rupture of membranes and will spontaneously abort. A *complete abortion* occurs when there is complete expulsion of the fetus and the placenta, and in these cases there is no need for a dilation and curettage (D&C). If there is only partial expulsion of tissue, as in this case, an *incomplete abortion* has occurred, and this requires a D&E to remove the remaining fetal or placental tissue. In these cases the cervix has usually dilated some and the patient usually can be managed with some mild sedation, because the most painful part of a D&E is cervical dilation. A paracervical block can be most useful for pain control during the procedure if the cervix needs to be dilated. A fetal death that is unrecognized for several weeks is called a *missed abortion,* and if this occurs at an advanced gestational age, DIC may occasionally result. A *habitual* or *recurrent abortion* refers to the occurrence of three or more consecutive spontaneous abortions *(Chestnut: Chestnut's Obstetric Anesthesia, ed 5, pp 345–348).*

719. (D) Accidental dural punctures with an epidural needle occur in about 1% of epidural attempts, and about a half of these patients develop a postdural puncture headache. Several techniques have been tried in an attempt to decrease the incidence of PDPHs but without success. Lying horizontally is helpful in relieving PDPHs, but prophylactic bed rest has not decreased the incidence of PDPH. Although avoidance of dehydration is recommended, excessive fluid intake has not been shown to decrease the incidence of PDPH. Epidural blood patches have proven successful in treating PDPH. However, the prophylactic injection of blood into the epidural space after the epidural block has worn off does not appear to significantly decrease the incidence of headaches but may decrease the duration of the headache. Keep in mind that the injection of blood through a contaminated epidural catheter may increase the risk of infection because blood is an excellent culture medium. For treatment, however, epidural blood patches are very successful, with better success rates if performed several hours after delivery compared with immediately after the delivery. Perhaps the leakage of cerebrospinal fluid into the epidural space dilutes the blood, making the patch weaker. Caffeine has been suggested by some studies to decrease the incidence of PDPHs, but other studies show no prophylactic benefit *(Chestnut: Chestnut's Obstetric Anesthesia, ed 5, pp 724–726; Suresh: Shnider and Levinson's Anesthesia for Obstetrics, ed 5, pp 431–434).*

720. (B) Earlier diagnosis of complete molar pregnancies has decreased the incidence of medical complications. However, excessive uterine size occurs in up to one half of patients with a complete molar pregnancy and is associated with a high incidence of medical complications. Medical complications when the uterine size is greater than 14 to 16 weeks' gestational size include ovarian theca-lutein cysts (4%-50%), hyperemesis gravidarum (15%-30%), hypertensive disorders of pregnancy (11%-27%), anemia (hemoglobin <10 g/dL) (10%-54%), acute cardiopulmonary distress (6%-27%), malignant sequelae (metastasis) (4%-36%), and hyperthyroidism (1%-7%) *(Chestnut: Chestnut's Obstetric Anesthesia, ed 5, pp 351–354).*

721. (B) Several cases of maternal cardiac arrest have occurred in pregnant women who were administered bupivacaine (Marcaine, Sensorcaine). Typically, the patients received an unintentional IV bolus of 0.75% bupivacaine intended for the epidural space. They had a brief grand mal seizure followed by cardiovascular collapse. Successful treatment was often prolonged and involved basic resuscitation (intubation, ventilation with 100% oxygen, cardiac compression with left uterine tilt, defibrillation, epinephrine, vasopressin, atropine), as well as rapid delivery of the fetus (if possible within 4-5 minutes). Delivery of the fetus makes successful resuscitation of the mother more likely. Incremental small injections of local anesthetic looking for toxicity should decrease the chance for cardiovascular collapse. Bupivacaine 0.75% now is considered contraindicated for use in the epidural space of parturients. Both levobupivacaine (Chirocaine) and ropivacaine (Naropin) were developed to have a long duration of action, like bupivacaine, but with less cardiac toxicity. Although these compounds have less cardiac toxicity than bupivacaine, they are more cardiac toxic than lidocaine (intermediate duration of action) and chloroprocaine (short duration of action) *(Chestnut: Chestnut's Obstetric Anesthesia, ed 5, pp 266–267; Miller: Miller's Anesthesia, ed 7, pp 932–934; Suresh: Shnider and Levinson's Anesthesia for Obstetrics, ed 5, pp 108–109).*

722. (D) Treatment of the pregnant patient who develops cardiovascular collapse from LAST consists of positioning the patient with left lateral displacement and preparing for an emergency cesarean delivery. Consider delivery of the infant if the mother cannot be resuscitated within several minutes because delivery of the infant makes it easier to resuscitate the mother. Current (2017) ASRA guidelines for LAST for a patient with cardiovascular collapse include the following:
- Stop injecting the local anesthetic.
- Get help (Call for lipid emulsion, alert nearest cardiopulmonary bypass team because resuscitation may be prolonged).
- Manage airway (Ventilate with 100% oxygen, avoid hyperventilation, and place an advanced airway device if necessary).
- Control seizures (Benzodiazepines are preferred and avoid large doses of propofol, especially in hemodynamically unstable patients).
- Treat hypotension and bradycardia; if pulseless, start CPR.
- Start IV lipid emulsion (Intralipid 20%) therapy (initial bolus of Intralipid is 1.5 mL/kg over 2-3 minutes, or about 100 mL in an adult). The bolus dose is followed by a continuous infusion of 0.25 mL/kg (ideal body weight)/hr. You can repeat the bolus dose one or two times for persistent

cardiovascular collapse and then double the rate in a continuous infusion rate if the blood pressure remains low. Continue the infusion for at least 10 minutes after cardiovascular stability is attained. The upper limit of Intralipid (20%) is 10 mL/kg over 30 minutes.

- Continue to monitor the patient for at least 4 to 6 hours after a cardiovascular event and at least 2 hours after a limited CNS event.
- AVOID the use of vasopressin, calcium channel blockers, β-blockers, and other local anesthetics.
- If you need epinephrine, the dose should be reduced to ≦ 1 µg/kg epinephrine.
- Report LAST to www.lipidrescue.org

(Chestnut: Chestnut's Obstetric Anesthesia, ed 5, pp 486–487; The Third American Society of Regional Anesthesia and Pain Medicine Practice Advisory on Local Anesthetic Systemic Toxicity Executive Summary 2017, Reg Anesth Pain Med 43:113–123, 2018; www.lipidrescue.org).

723. (A) TNS, formerly called transient radicular irritation (TRI), occurs most commonly after spinal anesthesia with lidocaine (Xylocaine). Symptoms include back pain that develops after the block resolves and radiates to the buttocks and legs. The pain is not associated with motor or sensory loss or electromyographic changes. It can be severe, requiring hospital admission of outpatients, and typically resolves within 1 to 4 days. It appears to occur more commonly when outpatients are operated on in the lithotomy position and appears to be less likely when patients are pregnant *(Chestnut: Chestnut's Obstetric Anesthesia, ed 5, p 756; Suresh: Shnider and Levinson's Anesthesia for Obstetrics, ed 5, pp 112–113).*

724. (D) When dealing with an urgent cesarean section in a patient with a well-functioning labor epidural, raising the level of anesthesia is often chosen. Of the commonly used local anesthetics, 3% 2-chloroprocaine with epinephrine 1:200,000 and 2% lidocaine with epinephrine 1:200,000 have much faster onsets of action than bupivacaine or levobupivacaine, which have relatively slow onsets of action. Because of the slow onset of action of bupivacaine or levobupivacaine, they are not recommended to raise an existing labor analgesic level for an urgent cesarean delivery. Alkalinization of the local anesthetic with bicarbonate shifts more of the local anesthetic molecules to the nonionized and more lipid-soluble form for a faster onset (and a more solid block); however, it does take a little time to mix the solution. Typically, 1 mL of 8.4% sodium bicarbonate (1 mEq/mL) is added to each 10 mL of 3% 2-chloroprocaine with epinephrine 1:200,000 or 2% lidocaine with epinephrine 1:200,000, and those solutions in a dose of 15 to 20 mL can usually raise a labor epidural to cesarean levels in <5 minutes. If you do not add the bicarbonate to 2% lidocaine with epinephrine 1:200,000, the onset time is twice as long, or about 10 minutes. Fentanyl can be added (75-100 µg) to the local anesthetic solution for a more solid block and for some postoperative analgesia *(Chestnut: Chestnut's Obstetric Anesthesia, ed 5, pp 568–569; Suresh: Shnider and Levinson's Anesthesia for Obstetrics, ed 5, pp 171–173).*

725. (B) The blood level of a local anesthetic is based on the absorption of the local anesthetic into the bloodstream and on the local anesthetic's metabolism. Ester local anesthetics (e.g., procaine, chloroprocaine, and tetracaine) undergo metabolism by pseudocholinesterase and other plasma esterases, whereas amide local anesthetics (e.g., lidocaine, mepivacaine, prilocaine, bupivacaine, levobupivacaine, ropivacaine, and etidocaine) are not metabolized in the bloodstream but require liver metabolism and have much longer half-lives. If chloroprocaine (Nesacaine) is injected directly into plasma, the in vitro half-life is 11 to 21 seconds in maternal plasma and 43 seconds in fetal plasma. After an epidural injection, where there is absorption of local anesthetic from the injection site as well as metabolism, the maternal half-life for chloroprocaine is <7 minutes, for lidocaine is 110 to 120 minutes, for ropivacaine is 5 to 6 hours, and for bupivacaine is 10 to 12 hours *(Chestnut: Chestnut's Obstetric Anesthesia, ed 5, pp 263–265; Suresh: Shnider and Levinson's Anesthesia for Obstetrics, ed 5, pp 105–108).*

CHAPTER 9

Neurologic Physiology and Anesthesia

726. A 59-year-old man with a subarachnoid hemorrhage (SAH) is admitted to the intensive care unit (ICU). His serum sodium is 115 mEq/L, 24-hour urine sodium collection is 350 mmol, and central venous pressure (CVP) is 1 mm Hg. The **MOST** likely cause of these findings is
    A. Acute tubular necrosis (ATN)
    B. Diabetes insipidus (DI)
    C. Cerebral salt-wasting syndrome (CSWS)
    D. Syndrome of inappropriate antidiuretic hormone (SIADH)

727. Intracranial hypertension is defined as a sustained increase in intracranial pressure (ICP) above
    A. 5 to 10 mm Hg
    B. 15 to 20 mm Hg
    C. 25 to 30 mm Hg
    D. 30+ mm Hg

728. Calculate cerebral perfusion pressure (CPP) from the following data: blood pressure (BP) 100/70, heart rate (HR) 65 beats/min, cardiac output 5 L/min, CVP of 5 cm/H_2O, and ICP 15 mm Hg
    A. 60 mm Hg
    B. 65 mm Hg
    C. 70 mm Hg
    D. 75 mm Hg

729. Which of the following statements about cerebrospinal fluid (CSF) in a healthy adult is **FALSE**?
    A. CSF volume is about 150 mL
    B. CSF pressure is about 10 mm Hg
    C. CSF volume turns over 4 times a day
    D. Specific gravity of CSF is higher than the specific gravity of plasma

730. By what percentage does cerebral blood flow (CBF) change for each mm Hg *decrease* in $PaCO_2$ in a previously normotensive patient with a severe brain injury?
    A. 2% to 4% increase
    B. 2% to 4% decrease
    C. 7% to 10% decrease
    D. 7% to 10% increase

731. Which of the following intravenous (IV) anesthetic induction agents is relatively contraindicated in patients with intracranial hypertension?
    A. Propofol
    B. Etomidate
    C. Ketamine
    D. Thiopental

732. The term *cerebral steal* refers to a situation that occurs in the brain when
    A. Blood flow has resumed after a period of ischemia
    B. Blood flow is directed from a normal region of the brain to an ischemic region
    C. Vasoparalysis exists with hypercarbia
    D. The Robin Hood phenomenon exists

733. A 62-year-old patient is scheduled to undergo resection of a large frontal lobe intracranial tumor under general anesthesia. Preoperatively, the patient is alert and oriented, and has no focal neurologic deficits. Within what range should $PaCO_2$ be maintained during surgery?
    A. 15 and 20 mm Hg
    B. 30 and 35 mm Hg
    C. 40 and 45 mm Hg
    D. 45 and 50 mm Hg

734. A 32-year-old patient is anesthetized for resection of a supratentorial tumor. Preoperatively, the patient is lethargic and disoriented. Which of the following is **MOST** likely to adversely alter ICP?
    A. 5% Dextrose in water
    B. Normal saline
    C. Lactated Ringer solution
    D. 5% Albumin

735. A 22-year-old patient is anesthetized for resection of a temporal lobe tumor. Preoperatively, he is lethargic and confused. After induction of general anesthesia, which of the following would be the **MOST** appropriate drug to control systemic arterial BP (160/100) during direct laryngoscopy and tracheal intubation?
  A. Esmolol
  B. Nitroprusside
  C. Hydralazine
  D. Isoflurane

736. Normal global cerebral blood flow (CBF) is
  A. 25 mL/100 g brain tissue/min
  B. 50 mL/100 g brain tissue/min
  C. 75 mL/100 g brain tissue/min
  D. 100 mL/100 g brain tissue/min

737. CBF remains constant between cerebral perfusion pressure (CPP)s of
  A. 25 and 125 mm Hg
  B. 25 and 200 mm Hg
  C. 40 and 250 mm Hg
  D. 50 and 150 mm Hg

738. All of the following are true concerning vagal nerve stimulator (VNS) placement for the treatment of medically refractory seizures **EXCEPT**
  A. Patients should not take their anticonvulsant medications before the surgery
  B. Placement is usually performed under general anesthesia
  C. The electrode array is placed around the left vagus nerve
  D. Hoarseness occurs about 50% of the time

739. Select the **FALSE** statement concerning autonomic hyperreflexia.
  A. Distention of a hollow viscus below the level of the spinal cord transection can elicit autonomic hyperreflexia
  B. Up to 85% of patients with a spinal cord transection above the T5 dermatome will exhibit autonomic hyperreflexia
  C. Propranolol alone is especially effective in treating hypertension associated with autonomic hyperreflexia
  D. Spinal anesthesia can be effective in preventing autonomic hyperreflexia

740. What is the normal cerebral metabolic rate for oxygen (CMRO$_2$) per minute?
  A. 0.5 mL of oxygen/100 g brain tissue/min
  B. 2.0 mL of oxygen/100 g brain tissue/min
  C. 3.5 mL of oxygen/100 g brain tissue/min
  D. 7.5 mL of oxygen/100 g brain tissue/min

741. A 14-year-old girl with severe scoliosis is to undergo spine surgery. Anesthesia is maintained with propofol, remifentanil, and N$_2$O 50% in O$_2$. Neurologic function of the spinal cord is monitored by somatosensory evoked potentials (SSEPs). In reference to the SSEP waveform, spinal cord ischemia would be manifested as
  A. Increased amplitude and increased latency
  B. Decreased amplitude and increased latency
  C. Decreased amplitude and decreased latency
  D. Increased amplitude and decreased latency

742. For each 1° C decrease in body temperature, how much will cerebral metabolic rate (CMRO$_2$) be diminished?
  A. 2%
  B. 4%
  C. 6%
  D. 10%

743. A 24-year-old carpenter is treated for a closed head injury sustained 3 days earlier after falling from a roof. He has been hemodynamically stable. Despite aggressive efforts to pharmacologically reduce ICP, he is now unconscious and unresponsive to painful stimuli. All of the following are clinical criteria consistent with a diagnosis of brain death in this patient **EXCEPT**
  A. Persistent apnea for 10 minutes
  B. Absence of pupillary light reflex
  C. Persistent spinal reflexes
  D. Decorticate posturing

744. A 60-year-old man is to undergo posterior fossa surgery in the sitting position. Which of the following is the **MOST** sensitive means of detecting venous air embolism (VAE)?
  A. Esophageal stethoscope
  B. End-tidal CO$_2$
  C. Transesophageal echocardiography (TEE)
  D. Precordial Doppler

745. When intracranial hypertension exists, the main initial compensatory mechanism from the body is
  A. Decreased production of CSF
  B. Increased absorption of CSF in the spinal arachnoid villi
  C. Shifting of CSF from intracranial to spinal subarachnoid space
  D. Reduction of cerebral blood volume (CBV) due to compression of intracranial arteries

746. Administration of vecuronium during spinal surgery may interfere with monitoring of
  A. Dorsal columns
  B. Corticospinal tract
  C. ECoG (Electrocorticography)
  D. Bispectral index

747. Patients can be safely imaged in the magnetic resonance imaging (MRI) scanner with conventional versions of which of the following monitors?
  A. Pulmonary artery catheter with cardiac output probe
  B. Foley catheter with temperature probe
  C. Electrocardiography (ECG) electrodes
  D. Arterial line

748. What is the minimum quantity of intracardiac air that can be detected by a precordial Doppler?
  A. 0.25 mL
  B. 5.0 mL
  C. 10 mL
  D. 25 mL

749. Which of the following drugs at high doses **CANNOT** produce an isoelectric electroencephalogram (EEG)?
  A. Etomidate
  B. Isoflurane
  C. Midazolam
  D. Propofol

750. Which of the following statements is **FALSE** concerning cerebral blood flow (CBF)?
  A. CBF is coupled with metabolic demand
  B. CBF is 10% to 20% of the cardiac output during the first 6 months of life
  C. CBF peaks at 55% of the cardiac output between 2 and 4 years of age
  D. CBF decreases to 35% of the cardiac output at 10 years of age

751. A 67-year-old patient is scheduled to undergo posterior fossa surgery in the sitting position under general anesthesia. A multiorifice central venous catheter is inserted from the right basilic vein and advanced toward the heart. Intravascular ECG (with the exploring electrode attached to the V lead) is used to aid in placement of the catheter. After the catheter is advanced 40 cm, the tracing shown in the figure is noted on the ECG.

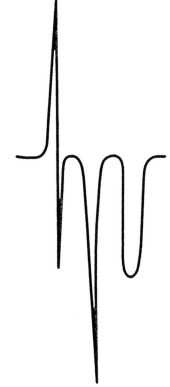

From Miller RD: Anesthesia, *ed 3, New York, Churchill Livingstone, 1990, p 1745.*

At this time the anesthesiologist should
  A. Advance the catheter 3 cm
  B. Advance the catheter slightly
  C. Leave the catheter in the present position
  D. Withdraw the catheter 3 cm

752. At what level of cerebral blood flow (CBF) does the EEG start to show signs of cerebral ischemia?
  A. 5 mL/100 g brain tissue/min
  B. 10 mL/100 g brain tissue/min
  C. 20 mL/100 g brain tissue/min
  D. 25 mL/100 g brain tissue/min

753. What effect does cerebral ischemia have on CBF autoregulation?
  A. CBF autoregulation is abolished and becomes passively dependent on CPP
  B. CBF autoregulation is ablated at low CPPs but remains intact at high CPPs
  C. CBF autoregulation is ablated at high CPPs but remains intact at low CPPs
  D. The CBF autoregulatory curve is shifted to the right

754. Which of the following is the **MOST** rapid maneuver available for lowering ICP in a patient with a large intracranial mass?
   A. Mannitol, 1 g/kg IV
   B. Methylprednisolone, 30 mg/kg IV
   C. Hyperventilation to 25 mm Hg Pa_{CO_2}
   D. Furosemide, 1 mg/kg IV

755. What effect does propofol have on the CO_2 responsiveness of the cerebral vasculature?
   A. Propofol attenuates the effect of hypocarbia on CBF
   B. Propofol attenuates the effect of hypercarbia on CBF
   C. Propofol augments the effect of hypocarbia on CBF
   D. Propofol does not affect CO_2 reactivity at a dose used clinically

756. Cerebral autoregulation is **MOST** likely to remain intact
   A. Immediately after cerebral aneurysm rupture
   B. In a patient with traumatic brain injury (TBI) and a Glasgow Coma Scale (GCS) score of 3
   C. With total IV anesthesia (TIVA) anesthetic using propofol
   D. With 2.5% end-tidal sevoflurane anesthesia

757. A 72-year-old patient undergoing resection of an astrocytoma in the sitting position suddenly develops hypotension. Air is heard on the precordial Doppler ultrasound. Each of the following therapeutic maneuvers to treat VAE is appropriate **EXCEPT**
   A. Discontinue N_2O
   B. Apply jugular venous pressure
   C. Implement positive end-expiratory pressure (PEEP)
   D. Administer epinephrine to treat hypotension

758. Which of the following is the **LEAST** likely sequela of venous air embolism (VAE) during posterior fossa surgery in the upright position?
   A. Increase in pulmonary dead space
   B. Bronchoconstriction
   C. Stroke
   D. Pulmonary hypotension

759. A 30-year-old anxious patient is to undergo Electrocorticography (ECoGH) monitoring to identify epileptogenic foci during seizure surgery. All of the following drugs may make it easier to identify the epileptogenic foci **EXCEPT**?
   A. Alfentanil (20 mcg/kg)
   B. Dexmedetomidine (1 mcg/kg over 10 minutes)
   C. Etomidate (0.2 mg/kg)
   D. Methohexital (20-50 mg)

760. How long after a stroke should surgery be deferred for an elective surgical procedure?
   A. 1 week
   B. 6 weeks
   C. 6 months
   D. 1 year

761. A 13-year-old boy is anesthetized with a propofol infusion and remifentanil infusion for scoliosis repair. SSEP monitoring is conducted during the procedure. Which of the following structures is **NOT** involved in conveyance of the stimulus from the posterior tibial nerve to the cerebral cortex?
   A. Corticospinal tract
   B. Medial lemniscus
   C. Ipsilateral dorsal column of the spinal cord
   D. Thalamus

762. A 19-year-old woman with scoliosis is undergoing surgery with Harrington rod placement under general anesthesia with SSEP monitoring. General anesthesia is administered with desflurane, nitrous oxide, and fentanyl. After completion of spinal instrumentation, the SSEP monitoring is equivocal and a wake-up test is undertaken. Four thumb twitches are present with a train-of-four ratio (TOF) of 0.9 when the nerve stimulator attached to the ulnar nerve is activated. The volatile anesthetic and nitrous oxide have been discontinued for 15 minutes, and the patient is asked to move her hands and feet. After repeated commands, the patient still does not move her hands or feet. The most appropriate intervention at this time would be
   A. 3 mg neostigmine plus 0.6 mg glycopyrrolate IV
   B. 0.04 mg naloxone IV
   C. 0.1 mg flumazenil IV
   D. Reduce the distraction on the rods

763. A 75-year-old patient is undergoing craniotomy for resection of a large astrocytoma. During administration of isoflurane anesthesia, the BP is 110/80 and the arterial blood gas sampling reveals a Pa_{CO_2} of 30 mm Hg. At this time, this patient's global CBF would be approximately
   A. 15 mL/100 g brain tissue/min
   B. 25 mL/100 g brain tissue/min
   C. 35 mL/100 g brain tissue/min
   D. 45 mL/100 g brain tissue/min

764. A 24-year-old patient is brought to the ICU after sustaining a closed head injury in a motor vehicle accident. Each of the following would be useful in managing intracranial hypertension in this patient **EXCEPT**
   A. Corticosteroids
   B. Propofol
   C. Hyperventilation to a Pa_{CO_2} of 35 mm Hg
   D. Osmotic diuretics

765. A 30-year-old patient with a spontaneous SAH from a ruptured intracranial aneurysm is to undergo surgery. This patient does not have signs of concomitant cerebral vasospasm. Preoperative treatment may include any of the following **EXCEPT**
  A. Induced hypertension (to 20% above baseline)
  B. Sedation
  C. Administration of antiepileptic drugs
  D. Administration of nimodipine

766. Which of the following frequency ranges is seen on the EEG in the normal awake patient?
  A. Delta (<4 Hz)
  B. Theta (4-7 Hz)
  C. Alpha (8-13 Hz)
  D. Beta (>13 Hz)

767. A 75-year-old patient with signs and symptoms of an SAH is brought to the emergency room for evaluation. T-wave inversion, a prolongation of the QT interval, and U waves are noted on the preoperative ECG. Appropriate action at this point would be to
  A. Begin infusion of nitroglycerin
  B. Check serum calcium and potassium
  C. Administer esmolol
  D. Place a pulmonary artery catheter

768. Which of the following pharmacologic agents would have the **LEAST** effect on transcranial motor evoked potentials (MEPs)?
  A. Isoflurane
  B. Nitrous oxide
  C. Etomidate
  D. Fentanyl

769. A 75-year-old man with medically refractory Parkinson disease is to undergo deep brain stimulation (DBS). Each of the following statements about DBS is true **EXCEPT**
  A. DBS device can be placed with patients awake, slightly sedated, or with general anesthesia
  B. Dexmedetomidine is most often used for sedation and analgesia
  C. Midazolam is contraindicated for sedation
  D. Patients will need anticonvulsants for the associated seizures in over 50% of patients

770. CMR and CBF are decreased by
  A. Dexmedetomidine
  B. Seizure
  C. Hyperthermia
  D. Ketamine

771. Which of the following statements is **FALSE** concerning the blood supply to the central nervous system?
  A. 70% of the brain's blood supply comes from the right and left internal carotid arteries; the remaining 30% comes from the two vertebral arteries
  B. Each internal carotid artery divides into three branches: the anterior cerebral artery, the posterior communicating artery, and the middle cerebral artery
  C. The vertebral arteries connect directly to the posterior communicating arteries, forming the circle of Willis
  D. The spinal cord gets its blood supply from one anterior spinal artery and two posterior spinal arteries

772. A 65-year-old patient is brought to the ICU after sustaining a cervical spine injury with quadriplegia during a motor vehicle accident. In the first 24 hours after the injury, the patient is at risk for
  A. Hypothermia, hypotension
  B. Tachycardia
  C. Stress response with hypertension and hyperventilation
  D. Autonomic hyperreflexia

773. Signs and symptoms of intracranial hypertension include
  A. Papilledema
  B. Headache
  C. Nausea and vomiting
  D. All of the above

774. A 79-year-old man with a history of transient ischemic attacks is scheduled to undergo a carotid endarterectomy under general anesthesia with EEG monitoring. Which of the following would be appropriate in the anesthetic management of this patient?
  A. Initiation of deliberate hypotension (after induction of anesthesia) to reduce bleeding
  B. Hyperventilation of the lungs to a $Paco_2$ of 30 mm Hg to reduce ICP
  C. Injection of local anesthetic around the carotid body to prevent bradycardia
  D. Induction of anesthesia with propofol

775. Anesthetics that decrease ICP include
  A. Fentanyl
  B. Nitrous oxide
  C. Propofol
  D. All of the above

776. Therapy that is useful in the treatment of cerebral vasospasm after an SAH includes all of the following **EXCEPT**
  A. BP elevation
  B. Hemodilution
  C. Diuretics (e.g., furosemide)
  D. Calcium channel blockers (e.g., nimodipine)

777. All of the following are associated with acromegalic patients undergoing transsphenoidal hypophysectomy **EXCEPT**
   A. Enlargement of the tongue and epiglottis
   B. Narrowing of the glottic opening
   C. Difficulty in placing nasal airways
   D. Increased postoperative use of continuous positive airway pressure (CPAP) because obstructive sleep apnea (OSA) is more common

778. The CBF autoregulatory curve is shifted to the right by
   A. Hypoxia (PaO_2 <50 mm Hg)
   B. Volatile anesthetics
   C. Hypercarbia
   D. Chronic hypertension

779. Cerebral autoregulation is abolished by
   A. Hyperbaric pressure of 4 atmospheres (breathing room air)
   B. Cardiopulmonary bypass with a core temperature of 27° C
   C. Chronic hypertension
   D. 3% Isoflurane

780. Etomidate does all of the following **EXCEPT**
   A. Abolishes CO_2 reactivity of cerebral blood vessel tone
   B. Reduces CMR
   C. Increases both SSEP amplitude and latency
   D. Reduces CBF

781. Following a motor vehicle accident, a 25-year-old man with head trauma is brought to the operating room for repair of facial lacerations and fractures. The patient is cooperative but extremely micrognathic and weighs 150 kg (330 lb). Acceptable techniques for securing the airway include
   A. Blind nasal intubation
   B. Direct laryngoscopy after rapid-sequence induction
   C. Awake fiberoptic intubation
   D. Laryngeal mask airway

782. After resection of a grade II astrocytoma in a 60-year-old patient, the serum sodium is 127 mEq/L, urine sodium is 25 mEq/L, and the BP is 120/80. Therapy could include which of the following?
   A. Intranasal or IV vasopressin (DDAVP)
   B. 500 mL 3% saline over 30 minutes
   C. Chlorpropamide
   D. Demeclocycline

783. A 48-year-old, 110-kg man with a supratentorial astrocytoma is scheduled for a craniotomy for tumor debulking. His wife states he has been somnolent and confused. On examination he is noted to be hyperventilating and sleepy, but arousable, and hypertensive. Useful measures for his anesthetic include
   A. Morphine to decrease his tachypnea
   B. Esmolol to reduce a hypertensive response to intubation
   C. Hyperventilation to 20 mm Hg
   D. 10 cm H_2O PEEP to reduce atelectasis

784. If, during an MRI scan, a patient were to become trapped in the scanner by a large (50 kg) metallic object, the appropriate course of action would be to
   A. Stop the scan immediately to release the magnet
   B. Summon enough people to pull the object away
   C. Interrupt electrical power for 60 seconds to release the magnetic force
   D. Quench the magnet

785. A 45-year-old man is undergoing a posterior cervical decompression in the sitting position. Induction of anesthesia and tracheal intubation are uneventful. Anesthesia is maintained with N_2O 50% in O_2, and sevoflurane. Suddenly, air is heard on the precordial Doppler ultrasound. Other observations consistent with VAE include
   A. Decreased $PaCO_2$
   B. Decreased CVP
   C. Decreased pulmonary arterial pressure (PAP)
   D. Decreased end-tidal CO_2

786. In patients with head injuries and increased ICP, hyperventilation is typically limited to a $PaCO_2$ of 25 to 30 mm Hg because additional hyperventilation
   A. Is virtually impossible
   B. Causes brain ischemia due to a rightward shifting of the oxyhemoglobin dissociation curve
   C. May be associated with a worsening of neurologic outcome
   D. Could result in paradoxical cerebral vasodilation

787. A 28-year-old man arrives in the emergency department by ambulance after being hit by a car while riding his motorcycle. He was not wearing a helmet and sustained a head injury. His oxygen saturation is 99% breathing spontaneously, with a nasal airway in his right nostril and a face mask applied and 5 liters/min of oxygen flowing. Blood pressure is 130/85, and heart rate is 100. He is unresponsive to speech and makes only incomprehensible sounds. When a painful stimulus is applied to his sternum, he opens his eye to the pain and flexes his elbows, wrists, and fingers and extends his legs. What is his GCS score?

   A. 11
   B. 9
   C. 7
   D. 5

726. (C) Patients with SAH often develop many associated changes, including an elevated ICP, rightward shift in the lower limits of the autoregulatory curve, vasospasm, hypovolemia, and hyponatremia. Hyponatremia has two common neurologic etiologies, CSWS and SIADH. Patients with CSWS, as in this case, have a triad of hyponatremia (serum sodium 115 mEq/L; normal serum sodium level is 135-145 mEq/L), intravascular volume contraction (CVP of 1 mm Hg; normal CVP range is 3-8 mm Hg), and high urine sodium (350 mmol/24 hr; normal range for a urine sodium collection is 40-117 mmol/24 hr). CSWS is thought to be related to the release of brain natriuretic peptide, leading to excess urinary sodium excretion as noted with an elevated 24-hour urine sodium sample. CSWS is treated with volume replacement using isotonic sodium chloride solution; the aim is to have the patient normovolemic or slightly hypervolemic because hypovolemia can aggravate cerebral vasospasm (the major cause of death from SAH).

In contrast, hyponatremia associated with SIADH is due to renal retention of free water (rather than renal loss of sodium) and is often treated with fluid restriction. Accordingly, the quantity of sodium collected over the 24-hour period and CVP should be relatively normal in SIADH patients.

DI occurs when there is a decrease in release of antidiuretic hormone (ADH) from the posterior pituitary (neurogenic DI) or when there is a decrease in sensitivity of the renal tubules to AHD (nephrogenic DI). DI is associated with hypo-osmolar urine and high serum sodium (>145 mEq/L) and high serum osmolality. Osmolality is a measure of the number of dissolved solute particles in a solution. Serum osmolality = $(2 \times (Na + K)) + (BUN/2.8) + (glucose/18)$; with a normal range of 285 to 295 mOsm/L. Neurogenic DI may develop in patients with basilar skull fractures or severe head injury involving the hypothalamus or posterior pituitary. ATN results in acute kidney injury and is associated with oliguria with retention of urea and other nitrogenous waste products (*Cottrell: Cottrell and Patel's: Neuroanesthesia, ed 6, pp 222–227, 416; Hines: Stoelting's Anesthesia and Co-Existing Disease, ed 7, pp 65, 283–286, 473–474; Miller: Miller's Anesthesia, ed 8, pp 2177–2178, 2189*).

727. (B) The normal ICP is 5 to 15 mm Hg (or 7-20 cm H_2O). As measured in the supine position, intracranial hypertension is defined as a sustained increase in ICP above 15 to 20 mm Hg. Elevated ICP frequently is the final stage of a pathologic cerebral insult (e.g., head injury, intracranial tumor, subarachnoid hemorrhage (SAH), metabolic encephalopathy, or hydrocephalus).

The intracranial contents consist of three compartments: brain parenchyma (80%-85%), blood (5%-10%), and CSF (5%-10%) with a normal combined volume of approximately 1200 to 1500 mL. Because none of these components is compressible, an increase in the volume of any of these components requires a compensatory decrease in the volume of one or both of the other components to avoid the development of intracranial hypertension (*Hines: Stoelting's Anesthesia and Coexisting Disease, ed 7, p 268; Miller: Basics of Anesthesia, ed 7, pp 514–515*).

728. (B) CPP is equal to mean arterial pressure (MAP) minus the ICP or CVP, whichever is greater. In some institutions, CVP and/or ICP is measured in cm H_2O; to convert from cm H_2O to mm Hg, multiply the amount of cm of H_2O by 0.74 (i.e., 10 cm H_2O pressure = 7.4 mm Hg).

CPP = MAP − (ICP or CVP, whichever is greater)

MAP equals the diastolic blood pressure + 1/3 of the pulse pressure. Pulse pressure equals the systolic blood pressure minus the diastolic blood pressure. In this case the Pulse pressure is (100 mm Hg -70 mm Hg) / 3 = 10 mm Hg. Thus the MAP = 70 mm Hg = 10 mm Hg = 80 mm Hg. Since the ICP is greater than the CVP the CPP = 80 mm Hg (MAP) − 15 mm Hg (ICP) = 65 mm Hg. (*Cottrell: Cottrell and Patel's Neuroanesthesia, ed 6, p 277; Miller: Basics of Anesthesia, ed 7, p 513*).

729. (D) The CSF volume in infants is about 40 to 60 mL, in young children is 60 to 100 mL, in older children is 80 to 120 mL, and in adults is 100 to 160 mL. CSF pressure in children is about 3.0 to 7.5 mm Hg, whereas in adults the pressure is normally 4.5 to 13.5 mm Hg. The rate that CSF is formed is 0.35 to 0.40 mL/min or 500 to 600 mL/day, which in the average adult yields a turnover of four times a day. The specific gravity of CSF is about 1.007, whereas the specific gravity of plasma is higher at 1.025 (*Cottrell: Cottrell and Patel's Neuroanesthesia, ed 6, pp 59–60; Hemmings Jr: Pharmacology and Physiology for Anesthesia, p 130*).

730. (B) Carbon dioxide is a powerful modulator of cerebral vascular resistance. CO_2 readily crosses the blood-brain barrier (BBB) and changes in the blood Pa_{CO_2} levels rapidly changes the extracellular brain fluid pH, which affects vascular tone. Hyperventilation of the lungs causes the blood Pa_{CO_2} level to be reduced. A lower Pa_{CO_2} level in the blood will equilibrate with the lower CO_2 level in the extracellular fluid of the brain, resulting in an increase in the pH of the extracellular brain fluid, which causes vasoconstriction of the cerebral blood vessels and reduces cerebral blood flow (CBF) and cerebral blood volume (CBV). Similarly, a decrease in extracellular brain pH from an elevation in CO_2 will result in vasodilation of the cerebral blood vessels and an increase in CBF. When the patient is normotensive, there is a linear response of CBF, with changes in Pa_{CO_2}. For each mm Hg decrease (or increase) in Pa_{CO_2}, there is a decrease (or increase) by approximately 2% to 4% of CBF. In general for a normotensive patient, reducing the Pa_{CO_2} from 40 to 20 mm Hg reduces CBF in half, whereas increasing the Pa_{CO_2} from 40 to 80 mm Hg doubles the CBF. This response breaks down at extremes.

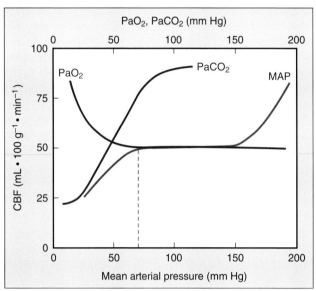

From Lemkuil BP, Drummond JC, Patel PM: *Central nervous system physiology: cerebrovascular. In: Hemmings HC Jr, Egan TD, editors:* Pharmacology and Physiology for Anesthesia, *Saunders, 2013, pp 123–136.*

CO₂ reactivity is preserved in most patients with severe brain injury; thus hyperventilation can rapidly lower the intracranial pressure (ICP) through a reduction in CBF and CBV. Although the effects of hyperventilation on CBF, CBV, and ICP are almost immediate, the effect wanes after 6 to 18 hours of hyperventilation, when the brain's extracellular pH gradually returns to normal by the slow exchange of HCO_3^- across the BBB (*Cottrell: Cottrell and Patel's Neuroanesthesia, ed 6, pp 26–27, Hemmings Jr: Pharmacology and Physiology for Anesthesia, p 126; Miller: Miller's Anesthesia, ed 8, pp 392–393; Rivera-Lara L et al: Cerebral autoregulation-oriented therapy at the bedside: a comprehensive review, Anesthesiology 126:1187–1199, 2017*).

731. (C) Of the choices listed in this question, ketamine is the only IV anesthetic that is not recommended for patients with intracranial hypertension because it increases cerebral metabolic rate (CMR), CBF, CBV, and ICP. However, the increase in ICP can be attenuated by induced hypocarbia or by the prior administration of thiopental or a benzodiazepine. Barbiturates (such as thiopental or methohexital), propofol, and etomidate all decrease CMR, CBF, CBV, and ICP and can be used for IV anesthesia in patients with elevated ICP. One potential advantage of etomidate over barbiturates and propofol is that etomidate does not produce significant cardiovascular depression. Although not as pronounced as the barbiturates, propofol, etomidate, benzodiazepines such as midazolam also reduce to a lesser amount the CMR and CBF. Flumazenil, a benzodiazepine antagonist, has been reported to reverse the effect of midazolam on CMR, CBF, CBV, and ICP. Consequently, flumazenil should be avoided in midazolam-anesthetized patients known to have intracranial hypertension. Generally speaking, the opioid anesthetics, such as morphine and fentanyl, cause either a minor reduction or have no effect on CBF and CMR (*Cottrell: Cottrell and Patel's Neuroanesthesia, ed 6, pp 79–83; Miller: Basics of Anesthesia, ed 7, p 514*).

732. (C) During acute focal cerebral ischemia, regional vasoparalysis develops. Under these circumstances, autoregulation and the reactivity of the cerebrovasculature to CO_2 is impaired in the ischemic areas. In the nonischemic areas of the brain where blood vessels are responsive to changes in CO_2, hypercarbia induces local vasodilation, allowing blood to be diverted to those nonischemic areas, "stealing" the blood from the ischemic areas (cerebral steal). Similarly, if hyperventilation is produced, the nonischemic blood vessels from the normal regions of the brain will contract and blood flow will be diverted from the normal region of the brain to the ischemic areas (inverse steal, or the "Robin Hood effect" of robbing from the rich and giving to the poor). Thus choices B and D are synonymous incorrect responses. Tight control of systemic arterial BP is important in managing patients with focal ischemia because cerebral perfusion is highly dependent on mean arterial BP. The term *luxury perfusion* (or hyperperfusion) is used to describe the return of CBF to a region of the infarcted brain where there is blood flow but decreased oxygen uptake by the metabolically inactive infarcted brain tissue *(Cottrell: Cottrell and Patel's Neuroanesthesia, ed 6, pp 30–34).*

733. (B) The normal intracranial components consist of brain tissue, blood, and CSF. When the tumor grows, there is more tissue in the skull and the two compensatory mechanisms to prevent an increase in ICP are a reduction CSF volume and a reduction in the CBV. Factors that may affect the delivery of adequate perfusion and oxygenation to the brain include hypotension, anemia, hypoxemia, hypercapnia (which can increase CBF, CBV, and ICP), and severe hypocarbia.

To help prevent an increase in ICP, mild hypocarbia is often induced. With severe hypocarbia (i.e., $PaCO_2$ reduced below 20 mm Hg), cerebral ischemia has been reported in both normal humans and laboratory animals. When the $PaCO_2$ is <20 mm Hg, it is likely that cerebral ischemia is caused by a leftward shift of the oxyhemoglobin dissociation curve (produced by the severe respiratory alkalosis) and possibly by intense cerebral vasoconstriction. The leftward shift of the oxyhemoglobin dissociation curve increases the affinity of hemoglobin to bind O_2, which reduces the ability of O_2 to be released from the hemoglobin to diffuse across the capillary bed. This effect combined with decreased CBF (caused by hypocarbia) can result in cerebral ischemia. Because there is little additional benefit in terms of reducing CBV and ICP in most patients who are asymptomatic with brain tumors, it is recommended to limit acute hyperventilation of the lungs to a $PaCO_2$ level of 30 to 35 mm Hg. Within this range there is a mild reduction in ICP and a minimal risk of cerebral ischemia. Reducing the $PaCO_2$ below 30 mm Hg has not been shown to give addition benefits and may cause cerebral ischemia (as noted above).

As an aside, hyperventilation-induced respiratory alkalosis can precipitate hypokalemia. Specifically, serum potassium decreases 0.6 mEq/L for each 0.1-unit increase in pH. Thus overly aggressive hyperventilation should be avoided to decrease the possibility of hypokalemia-induced cardiac arrhythmias *(Cottrell: Cottrell and Patel's Neuroanesthesia, ed 6, pp 189–193; Miller: Basics of Anesthesia, ed 7, p 518; Miller: Miller's Anesthesia, ed 8, pp 2163–2164).*

734. (A) In general, administering 5% dextrose in water (D_5W) is contraindicated in neurosurgical patients with intracranial hypertension for two reasons. First, D_5W easily passes through the BBB. Once in the brain tissue, glucose is rapidly metabolized, leaving only free water, which causes cerebral edema. Second, hyperglycemia is associated with increased severity of neurologic damage in patients with cerebral ischemia. The etiology of hyperglycemia-induced worsening of neurologic injury is associated with simple biochemical processes.

$$\text{Aerobic: glucose} + \text{oxygen} \rightarrow 6\,CO_2 + 6\,H_2O + 36\,ATP\ (\text{energy efficient})$$

$$\text{Anaerobic: glucose} \rightarrow 2\,\text{lactate} + 2\,H^+ + 2\,ATP\,(\text{energy inefficient})$$

Both lactate and H^+ are harmful to compromised neurons and glia. Furthermore, in the setting of hyperglycemia, the anaerobic reaction is forced to the right, resulting in additional accumulation of these toxic metabolites, thereby worsening neurologic outcome. The only indications for the use of D_5W are to prevent and to treat hypoglycemia or hypernatremia.

The two most common crystalloid solutions used in neuroanesthesia are normal saline (0.9% NaCl) and lactated Ringer solution. Many neuroanesthesiologists alternate between normal saline (308 mOsm/L, which can produce hyperchloremic metabolic acidosis when large amounts are administered) and lactated Ringer solution (273 mOsm/L, which can produce a relatively hypo-osmolar state). The osmolarity of plasma is 285 to 295 mOsm/L. 5% albumin can also be used with controversial improvement in neurologic outcome compared with crystalloid fluid *(Cottrell: Cottrell and Patel's Neuroanesthesia, ed 6, pp 152–162, 174; Miller: Basics of Anesthesia, ed 7, pp 396–399, 518; Miller: Miller's Anesthesia, ed 8, pp 2172–2173).*

735. (A) Systemic vasodilators such as sodium nitroprusside, nitroglycerine, hydralazine, adenosine, and calcium channel blockers, as well as volatile anesthetics, are all capable of further elevating the ICP when the BP is elevated. Esmolol is a cardioselective β_1-adrenergic receptor antagonist with rapid onset and short duration of action due to hydrolysis by red blood cell esterases. Plasma cholinesterases and red cell membrane acetylcholinesterase do not play a role in its degradation. Esmolol effectively blunts the sympathetic response to direct laryngoscopy and tracheal intubation, yet is devoid of deleterious effects on CBV or ICP. In addition, propofol, barbiturates (e.g., thiopental, methohexital), and etomidate (but not ketamine) can decrease ICP by decreasing the CMR and CBF *(Miller: Miller's Anesthesia, ed 8, pp 394–396, 2126; Cottrell: Cottrell and Young's Neuroanesthesia, ed 6, pp 75–83).*

736. (B) The adult brain normally weighs about 1350 g and receives about 15% of the cardiac output. Normal global cerebral blood flow (CBF) is approximately 45 to 55 mL/100 g brain tissue/min. Cortical CBF (gray matter) is approximately 75 to 80 mL/100 g brain tissue/min, and subcortical CBF (mostly white matter) is approximately 20 mL/100 g brain tissue/min. Factors that regulate CBF include $PaCO_2$, PaO_2, CMR, cerebral profusion pressure (CPP), autoregulation, and the autonomic nervous system (see the figure in answer 730 above) *(Hemmings Jr: Pharmacology and Physiology for Anesthesia, pp 124–128; Cottrell: Neuroanesthesia, ed 6, pp 23–24; Miller: Miller's Anesthesia, ed 8, p 388, Box 17-1).*

737. (D) Cerebral blood flow (CBF) autoregulation is the intrinsic capability of the cerebral vasculature to adjust its vascular resistance to maintain CBF constant over a wide range of BPs. This cerebral autoregulation helps to protect the brain against hypoperfusion when the BP is low and against hyperemia when the BP is elevated. As the BP decreases, the blood vessels can dilate to maintain CBF up to a point where the blood vessels are maximally dilated. Similarly, as the BP increases, the blood vessels can constrict to maintain CBF to the point where the vessels are maximally constricted. Above or below the limits of CBF autoregulation, CBF is dependent on BP. In normotensive healthy adults, lower and upper limits of autoregulation are CPPs of 50 to 150 mm Hg. Because cerebral perfusion pressure (CPP) equals mean arterial BP minus the ICP (when CVP is normal) or ICP (CPP = MAP − ICP) and because ICP is normally around 10 mm Hg, we say cerebral autoregulation is maintained with mean arterial pressures between 60 and 160 mm Hg in the healthy adult. These values can change under certain conditions; for example, vasoconstricting medications (e.g., epinephrine) may limit cerebral vasodilation, and vasodilation drugs (e.g., volatile anesthetics) may limit cerebral vasoconstriction *(Hemmings Jr: Pharmacology and Physiology for Anesthesia, pp 126–128; Cottrell: Neuroanesthesia, ed 6, pp 23–24).*

738. (A) VNS has been used to treat medically refractory epilepsy and medically refractory severe depression. The mechanism of action is unclear but may involve stimulation of the limbic system, locus ceruleus, and amygdala. Patients should continue to take their anticonvulsant medications before surgery because the goal is primarily to reduce the frequency of seizures. VNS tends to produce about a 50% or more reduction in the frequency of seizures in about 50% of patients after 18 months of stimulation. The electrode array is placed around the left vagal nerve because placement around the right vagal nerve leads to sinus node stimulation, with the resultant bradycardia. The electrical generator is usually placed in the left infraclavicular area. After the electrode and generator are connected, the system is tested. Because left vagal nerve stimulation may rarely (<1%) lead to bradycardia and occasionally asystole, the anesthesiologist should be notified when the system is to be tested. If bradycardia develops, stimulation is stopped and, occasionally, atropine is needed. Then the stimulator's output is adjusted. Placement is usually performed under general endotracheal tube anesthesia. Postoperative complications include hoarseness (50% of the time due to nerve injury, fatigue, or device cardiovascular malfunction), superior laryngeal nerve injury, cough, dyspnea, hematoma, and seizures *(Cottrell: Cottrell and Patel's Neuroanesthesia, ed 6, p 305; Jaffe; Anesthesiologist's Manual of Surgical Procedures, ed 5, pp 80–83).*

739. (C) Autonomic hyperreflexia (also called mass reflex) is a neurologic disorder that occurs in association with resolution of spinal shock and a return of spinal cord reflexes. It begins to appear 2 to 3 weeks after the spinal cord injury in approximately 85% of patients with a spinal cord transection above the T5 dermatome. Cutaneous or visceral stimulation (such as distention of the urinary bladder or rectum, or uterine contractions during labor) below the level of the spinal cord transection initiates afferent impulses that are transmitted to the spinal cord at this level, which subsequently elicits reflex sympathetic activity over the splanchnic nerves. Because modulation of this reflex sympathetic activity from higher centers in the central nervous system is lost (as a result of the spinal cord transection), the reflex sympathetic activity below the level of the injury results in intense generalized vasoconstriction and hypertension. Bradycardia occurs secondary to activation of baroreceptor reflexes arising from the carotid or aortic sinus. In contrast, it is difficult to elicit this reflex in patients with a spinal cord transection below the T10 dermatome. Deep general anesthesia can block this reflex. Treatment of autonomic hyperreflexia is with α-adrenergic receptor antagonists (e.g., phentolamine), direct-acting vasodilators (e.g., nitroprusside, fenoldopam, or nitroglycerin), and deep general or epidural and/or spinal anesthesia.

Patients with autonomic hyperreflexia should NOT be treated initially with propranolol or other β-adrenergic receptor antagonists for three reasons. First, bradycardia can be potentiated by $β_1$-adrenergic receptor blockade; second, $β_2$-adrenergic receptor blockade in skeletal muscle will leave the α-adrenergic properties of circulating catecholamines unopposed, thereby causing a paradoxical hypertensive response; and third, a combination of unopposed α-mediated vasoconstriction coupled with $β_1$-adrenergic negative inotropy could result in congestive heart failure.

In obstetric patients who have a complete spinal cord transection above the T5 dermatome and are in labor, epidural anesthesia can be very effective in blocking the reflex due to labor contractions or an overdistended bladder. Because it is hard to know whether the epidural catheter is properly placed in a patient with no sensory feelings below the lesion, checking for a deep tendon patellar reflex before injecting the local anesthetic and seeing the patellar reflex disappear are confirmation of an effective epidural level and dose. One must, however, use a concentration of local anesthetic high enough to block the reflex, such as 0.25% to 0.5% bupivacaine or 1% to 2% lidocaine *(Datta, Ostheimer: Common Problems in Obstetric Anesthesia, pp 390–399; Cottrell: Cottrell and Patel's Neuroanesthesia, ed 6, p 380; Miller: Miller's Anesthesia, ed 8, pp 382–383).*

740. (C) The brain is basically an obligate aerobe, as it cannot store oxygen. Under normal circumstances, there is a substantial safety margin in that the delivery of oxygen is considerably greater than demand. Oxygen consumption is approximately 3 to 3.8 mL of oxygen/100 g brain tissue/min. With a normal brain weight of 1350 g, oxygen consumption equals about 40 to 50 mL of oxygen per minute. Whole-brain oxygen consumption represents about 20% of total-body oxygen utilization. The CBF is about 50 mL/100 g brain tissue/min, or about 675 mL of blood/min, which is approximately 12% to 15% of the cardiac output *(Barash: Clinical Anesthesia, ed 8, pp 1007–1008; Miller: Miller's Anesthesia, ed 8, pp 387–390).*

741. (B) SSEPs are voltage signals that appear in the cerebral cortex in response to electrical stimulation of peripheral nerves. Electrical stimulation is commonly a current of 20 to 50 mA, stimulus duration of 50 to 250 microseconds, and a frequency of 1 to 6 Hz, using surface electrodes above the nerves or with fine-needle electrodes. Peripheral nerves that are commonly used include the median nerve (C6-T1) and ulnar nerves (C8-T1) at the wrist, the common peroneal nerve at the knee (L4-S2), and the posterior tibial nerve (L4-S2) at the ankle. The impulse elicited by electrical stimulation of a peripheral nerve ascends the peripheral nerve, the ipsilateral dorsal column of the spinal cord, decussates in the medulla oblongata, and is ultimately recorded on the contralateral somatosensory cortex of the brain. Recording electrodes are placed and include a limb electrode proximal to the stimulating electrode to assure that the electrical stimulus is applied to the nerve, an electrode over the cervical spine (for arm or leg stimulus) or lumbar spine (leg stimulus) to assure the electrical stimulus has been transmitted from the peripheral nerve to the spinal cord, and electrodes placed over the contralateral sensory (parietal) cortex on the scalp.

SSEPs are composed of negative and positive voltage deflections with specific latencies and amplitudes. Typically, general anesthesia is induced first, the patients are paralyzed unless concomitant MEPs are also used, and baseline recordings of latency and amplitude are established before surgical manipulation because the characteristics of SSEP waveforms change with recording circumstances (e.g., the latency becomes greater and the amplitude becomes smaller as the distance between the neural generator and the recording electrode is increased). Ischemia, hypothermia, neurologic injury, or transection of a neural pathway (i.e., surgical causes) will result in a decrease in signal amplitude and/or increase in signal latency. Alternatively, such changes may result from medications administered by the anesthesia care team (e.g., isoflurane, sevoflurane, desflurane, propofol, barbiturates, benzodiazepines). Should signal decay occur during surgery, it is imperative for the anesthesiologist to have a systematic approach to elucidate the etiology of signal change. More specifically, nonsurgical causes should be promptly ruled out (e.g., was a medication recently administered or dose changed, hypothermia, hypotension, anemia, hypoxemia) *(Cottrell, Neuroanesthesia, ed 6, pp 114–116; Miller: Miller's Anesthesia, ed 8, pp 1497–1521).*

742. (C) The $CMRO_2$ is proportional to neuronal activity and decreases approximately 6% to 7% per 1° C of temperature reduction. Complete suppression of the EEG can occur at about a body core temperature of 18° to 20° C. Although profound hypothermia (27° C or lower) can allow the brain to survive long periods without perfusion, many complications can occur, including myocardial depression, arrhythmias, and coagulopathies, as well as slower metabolism of medications. When the body rewarms, increased oxygen consumption and cardiac output can occur as a result of shivering.

Although initial studies of mild hypothermia (32°-34° C) have suggested improved neurologic outcome in patients who sustained cardiac arrest, more recent studies show no benefit of mild hypothermia to patients with temperatures <36° C *(Cottrell: Cottrell and Patel's Neuroanesthesia, ed 6, p 9; Hemmings Jr: Pharmacology and Physiology for Anesthesia, pp 125–126; Miller: Miller's Anesthesia, ed 8, pp 391–392).*

743. (D) Brain death is defined as irreversible cessation of brain function (both cerebral and brainstem). It is extremely important to identify and reverse any factors that can mimic the clinical or laboratory criteria for brain death, such as hypothermia, hypotension, drug intoxication (hypnotic sedatives and major tranquilizers, neuromuscular blockade), or metabolic encephalopathy. Clinical criteria for brain death can be divided into those that are related to cortical function and those that are related to brainstem function. Absence of cortical function is manifested by lack of spontaneous motor activity, consciousness, and purposeful movement in response to painful stimuli. Absence of brainstem function is manifested by the inability to elicit reflexes, such as the pupillary response to light and the corneal, oculocephalic, oculovestibular, oropharyngeal (e.g., gag), and respiratory reflexes (e.g., cough). For example, in patients without brainstem function, there is no increase in heart rate when atropine is administered intravenously (due to absence of native vagal tone from the brainstem), and there is no respiratory effort during apnea, even when the $PaCO_2$ is greater than 60 mm Hg. Confirmatory tests include flat EEG and absence of blood flow to the brain with angiography. An apnea test is usually the last test performed. Spinal cord reflexes and spontaneous movements may be present in brain-dead patients; in patients who will undergo organ donations, muscle paralysis may be needed.

The GCS score of 3 is included with brain death (score of 1 for Eye – does not open eyes; score of 1 for Verbal – makes no sounds; score of 1 for Motor – no movement). Decorticate posturing (upper extremities are flexed, lower extremities are extended) and the more severe decerebrate posturing (both arms and legs are extended with internal rotation) are signs of severe brain damage but are not consistent with the diagnosis of brain death (see also Question 787 regarding GCS) *(Barash: Clinical Anesthesia, ed 8, p 1459; Miller: Miller's Anesthesia, ed 8, pp 2317–2326; Misulis: Netter's Concise Neurology, pp 75–77).*

744. (C) VAE occurs when air is entrained into open veins in the presence of negative intraluminal pressures (i.e., negative with respect to atmospheric pressure). During posterior fossa surgery performed with the patient in the sitting position, VAE is common. Current devices used to detect VAE include TEE, precordial Doppler ultrasound, pulmonary artery catheter, infrared spectrometer to monitor changes in end-tidal CO_2 ($PECO_2$) and end-tidal nitrogen (PEN_2), right atrial catheter, and esophageal stethoscope (to listen for a "mill wheel" cardiac murmur). The most sensitive means of diagnosing VAE is the TEE; the least sensitive is the esophageal stethoscope. About 10% to 30% of patients having posterior fossa surgery in the sitting position will have evidence of VAE using end-tidal CO_2 monitoring, 40% using precordial Doppler monitoring, and 50% to 100% using TEE monitoring. VAE is less frequently detected using TEE for patients undergoing cervical laminectomy (about 25%). Although the incidence of VAE is relatively high, clinically significant VAE is in the range of 0.5% to 3%. Significant VAE can result in reduced cardiac output and profound hypoxia. Because the safety of using TEE for prolonged surgery in patients with neck flexion in the sitting position is not well established, many clinicians use the precordial Doppler to monitor for significant VAE. The precordial Doppler is currently the standard of care for VAE monitoring *(Cottrell: Cottrell and Patel's Neuroanesthesia, ed 6, pp 213–218; Miller: Miller's Anesthesia, ed 8, pp 2169–2170; Miller: Basics of Anesthesia, ed 7, pp 328–329, 519).*

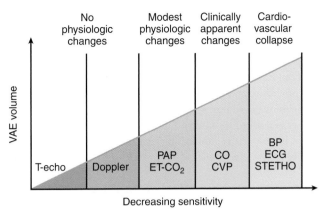

From Miller RD: Miller's Anesthesia, *ed 7, Philadelphia, Saunders, 2011, p 2014, Figure 63-11.*

745. (C) Intracranial pressure (ICP) is determined by the pressure contribution of three volume compartments: brain parenchyma 80% to 90%, CSF 5% to 10%, and blood 5% to 10%. Under normal circumstances, ICP is maintained within the normal range (5-15 mm Hg) over a wide range of intracranial volumes (ICVs) due to the following three compensatory mechanisms: (1) translocation of CSF from the intracranial to spinal subarachnoid space; (2) translocation of intracranial blood (primarily venous) to systemic circulation; and (3) reabsorption of CSF across arachnoid villi into the dural venous sinus and, ultimately, into systemic circulation.

Once these compensatory mechanisms are exhausted, small increases in intracranial volume (ICV) result in large increases in ICP (i.e., a situation of increased intracranial elastance), which leaves the brain vulnerable to ischemia and herniation. CSF production is fairly constant (0.35-0.40 mL/min) regardless of ICP *(Cottrell: Cottrell and Patel's Neuroanesthesia, ed 6, pp 189–190; Miller: Basics of Anesthesia, ed 7, pp 514–515; Miller: Miller's Anesthesia, ed 8, p 2159–2161, Figure 70-3).*

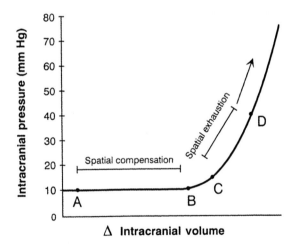

746. (B) Postoperative neurologic dysfunction is a rare but serious complication of spinal reconstructive surgery. In cases where spinal cord dysfunction is more likely to occur (e.g., scoliosis reconstruction), intraoperative spinal cord monitoring is used to identify ischemia and ideally allow the surgeon time to modify the procedure to reverse any spinal cord dysfunction.

Somatosensory evoked potentials (SSEPs) involve repetitive stimulation of the extremity and monitoring the signals at the level of the scalp. SSEPs are used to monitor the dorsal columns of the spinal cord. As this area is sensory, neuromuscular blockers such as vecuronium do not affect SSEP monitoring.

Motor evoked potentials (MEPs) monitoring is used to monitor corticospinal tracts (motor pathways) that are not assessed with SSEPs. Neuromuscular blockers, such as vecuronium, interfere with MEP monitoring and should not be used.

ECoG monitoring is used to identify epileptogenic foci during seizure surgery, or to assess cerebral cortical integrity during carotid endarterectomy. The ECoG is altered by drugs that affect the seizure threshold (e.g., benzodiazepines, as well as volatile anesthetics).

The bispectral index monitor (BIS) uses processed EEG signals to measure level of consciousness. The information obtained can be used to help titrate anesthetic medications to an adequate depth of anesthesia for the surgical procedure and to decrease intraoperative awareness.

Another monitoring technique used during spinal reconstruction is the wake-up test (the patient is awakened during the surgery and asked to move his legs). It is done only when other monitors are not available or when significant intraoperative monitoring suggests injury (*Miller: Basics of Anesthesia, ed 7, pp 358–360, 543, 815–816; Miller: Anesthesia, ed 8, pp 1330–1331, 1497–1505, 1527–1528*).

747. (D) The MRI scanner has no ionizing radiation and does not use radioactive substances but is potentially dangerous because of the strong magnetic field. The most obvious is the risk of projectiles traveling toward the patient. Objects made of iron, nickel, and cobalt are strongly pulled by the constant magnetic force. A more insidious but equally dangerous hazard is represented by indwelling devices, such as pacemakers, infusion pumps, deep brain neurostimulators, cochlear implants, ferromagnetic orthopedic prostheses, and ferromagnetic aneurysm clips. Nonferromagnetic aneurysm clips are MRI compatible. The interactions between these and the magnetic field can be harmful or even lethal for the patient under some circumstances, due to heating of the metal or to movement as a result of the magnetic field. Finally, the antenna effect of the MRI scanner can induce heat in wires that are in close proximity to the patient. For this reason, pulmonary artery catheters and urinary catheters with temperature wires embedded in them cannot be used in patients undergoing MRI scanning. Standard conventional pulse oximeters and ECG wires are also unacceptable because they have ferromagnetic wires, but special MRI-compatible pulse oximeter probes with fiberoptic "cables" can be safely used, as can "wireless" ECG patches. Arterial lines do not pose a problem in the scanner because no wires come into contact with the patient. A long section of nonmagnetic fluid-filled tubing from the arterial catheter (or a CVP catheter) passes through a small channel in the wall of the MRI room to the MRI control room, where the transducer (which contains metallic parts) can be connected to a monitor (*Cottrell: Cottrell and Patel's Neuroanesthesia, ed 6, pp 91–99; Miller: Basics of Anesthesia, ed 7, pp 661–662*).

748. (A) Except for the transesphageal echocardiography (TEE), the Doppler ultrasound is the most sensitive device for detection of intracardiac air. Under ideal circumstances, as little as 0.25 mL of intracardiac air can be detected by a precordial Doppler ultrasound transducer placed over the right side of the heart (second or third intercostal space to the right of the sternum adjusted to maximal audible sounds from the right atrium). In contrast, TEE can detect even smaller volumes of intracardiac air. Symptoms from venous air embolism (VAE) depend on the amount and the rate of air uptake. The amount of air needed to cause clinically significant VAE is much greater than that detected by Doppler or TEE (e.g., 50 mL has been aspirated from a right-sided catheter in patients who have had hypotension, cardiac arrhythmias, and other ECG changes). To cause an air lock within the right side of the heart, a cumulative gas volume estimated at 5 mL/kg rapidly entrained is needed (*Cottrell: Cottrell and Patel's Neuroanesthesia, ed 6, pp 213–215; Miller: Basics of Anesthesia, ed 7, p 519*).

749. (C) Even at high doses, dexmedetomidine, ketamine, benzodiazepines (e.g., diazepam, midazolam), and opioids (e.g., alfentanil, fentanyl, remifentanil) cannot produce an isoelectric EEG. However, at high doses, barbiturates (thiopental, methohexital, pentobarbital), etomidate, propofol, and volatile anesthetics (e.g., desflurane, isoflurane, sevoflurane) can produce an isoelectric EEG. At subhypnotic doses, etomidate and methohexital can cause epileptiform EEGs (*Miller: Miller's Anesthesia, ed 8, pp 1511–1513*).

750. (D) Cerebral blood flow (CBF) is coupled with cerebral metabolic rate (CMR). CBF is 10% to 20% of the cardiac output at birth to 6 months of life, peaks at 55% of the cardiac output between 2 and 4 years of age (CBF values >100 mL/100 g brain tissue/min), and then settles to adult values of 15% of the cardiac output by 7 to 8 years of age (CBF values of 50 mL/100 g brain tissue/min) (*Cottrell: Cottrell and Patel's Neuroanesthesia, ed 6, pp 337–338*).

751. (D) A multiorifice right atrial catheter is used to aspirate air that has been embolized from the venous system into the right side of the heart during episodes of VAE (e.g., most commonly placed for sitting neurosurgical procedures). Multiorifice catheters are more effective than single-orifice catheters in aspirating air. To be effective, the catheter must be accurately placed at the junction of the superior vena cava and right atrium because air has a tendency to localize at this junction. The tip of the catheter should be at or 2 cm below the sinoatrial (SA) node and the proximal port 1 to 3 cm above the SA node.

Several methods can be used to ensure that the catheter tip is accurately positioned at this junction. For example, a chest x-ray film can be obtained. However, there may be difficulty in interpreting the position of the tip of the catheter, and the catheter could migrate after the x-ray film is obtained. A technique frequently used to accurately place a multiorifice catheter at the junction of the superior vena cava and right atrium is an intravascular ECG. An adapted conductive connector is attached to the CVP catheter, and the central line is flushed with $NaHCO_3$ for better electrical conduction; the catheter will be used as the right arm lead. Some centers use lead II, whereas other centers use lead V of the ECG for monitoring during placement. The catheter is often initially placed in the mid-right atrium level, where a biphasic P wave is noted, as shown in the figure of this question, which indicates that the tip of the catheter is in the midatrial position and should be withdrawn slightly until there is a large negative downward configuration of the P wave using lead V and the P wave and QRS complex are similar in size. Then the catheter should be withdrawn 1 cm until the P wave is slightly smaller than the QRS complex; then the catheter is secured. For proper placement, some clinicians note the change from the CVP pressure tracing to the right atrial (RA) pressure tracing when not using an intravascular lead.

An alternative technique to confirm proper positioning of a long-arm CVP is to use a TEE *(Cottrell: Cottrell and Patel's Neuroanesthesia, ed 6, pp 216–217).*

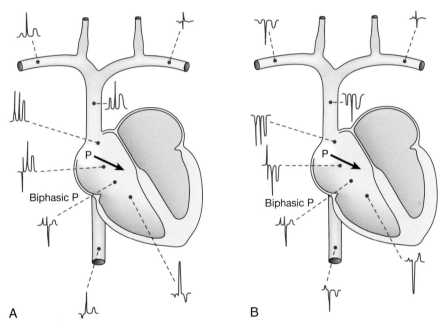

Biphasic P

Biphasic P

A

B

From Schlichter RA, Smith DS: Anesthetic management for posterior fossa surgery. In: Cottrell JE, Patel P, editors: Cottrell and Patel's Neuroanesthesia, ed 6, Elsevier, 2017, pp 209–211.

752. (C) Critical CBF is the CBF below which EEG evidence of cerebral ischemia begins to appear (EEG slowing). Normal CBF is 50 mL/100 g brain tissue/min. Cerebral ischemia starts to appear when the CBF falls to 20 mL/100 g brain tissue/min. At 15 mL/100 g brain tissue/min, the EEG becomes isoelectric. Below 15 mL/100 g brain tissue/min, membrane failure and neuronal death may develop with time. Because volatile anesthetics reduce CMR and can increase CBF due to their cerebral vasodilating properties at normotensive levels, volatile anesthetics may have some neuroprotective properties *(Miller: Miller's Anesthesia, ed 8, pp 401–415).*

753. (A) CBF autoregulation is easily impaired and modified by numerous factors, such as cerebral vasodilators (including nitroglycerin, nitroprusside, calcium channel blockers, hydralazine, volatile anesthetics), severe hypercapnia, inflammation, traumatic brain injury (TBI), intracranial surgery, chronic hypertension, and cerebral ischemia. Cerebral ischemia abolishes CBF autoregulation, with CBF becoming passively dependent on the CPP *(Cottrell: Cottrell and Young's Neuroanesthesia, ed 6, pp 30–31; Miller: Basics of Anesthesia, ed 7, pp 512–514).*

754. (C) Ways to decrease ICP include elevating the head, hyperventilation, avoiding constriction around the neck, avoiding PEEP and excessive airway pressures, CSF drainage, hyperosmolar solutions, diuretics, IV anesthetics (e.g., propofol), and surgery. Hypocarbia (associated with hyperventilation) will rapidly cause vasoconstriction, thereby reducing CBF, CBV, and ICP. Hyperventilation is the technique that will most rapidly decrease ICP in patients with an intracranial mass. Remember that lowering the CO_2 content will also reduce CBF and that if the blood flow is low enough, it can cause cerebral ischemia.

Although mannitol (0.25-2 g/kg) can decrease brain swelling, it can cause a transient increase in ICP due to vasodilation of the cerebral blood vessels. Because of this transient increase in ICP, mannitol is not used unless other methods to decrease brain volume and ICP have been considered. The effects of a brain tumor are due to the mass of the tumor, as well as the swelling of the tissues around the tumor. Steroids have a dramatic effect on reducing the swelling and can decrease ICP, but the process takes hours. Furosemide reduces CSF formation and decreases ICP. Furosemide can be used alone in doses of 1 mg/kg or with lower doses (5-20 mg) combined with mannitol (0.25-1 g/kg) to produce a brisk urine flow (2-3 liters over 2 hours is common) *(Cottrell: Cottrell and Young's Neuroanesthesia, ed 6, pp 84, 175–176, 190; Miller: Miller's Anesthesia, ed 8, pp 2163–2165).*

755. (D) The cerebrovascular response to changes in Pa_{CO_2} is preserved after the administration of propofol, as well as with other IV anesthetics (barbiturates, etomidate, and ketamine), even at doses that produce burst suppression on the EEG. Thus the elevated ICP can be reduced by hyperventilation in patients anesthetized with IV anesthetics. CO_2 responsiveness is also preserved with volatile anesthetics at clinical levels of anesthesia. At high concentrations of volatile anesthetics and lower BPs, CO_2 reactivity is attenuated *(Cottrell: Cottrell and Patel's Neuroanesthesia, ed 6, pp 80–81; Miller: Miller's Anesthesia, ed 8, pp 396–398, 404).*

756. (C) Cerebral autoregulation can be impaired under certain conditions, including acute ischemia, inflammation, brain tumors, arteriovenous malformations, subarachnoid hemorrhage (SAH), intracranial surgery, and traumatic brain injury (TBI). Volatile anesthetics above 1 minimum alveolar concentration (MAC) impair cerebral autoregulation; however, in low doses (i.e., below 1 MAC), autoregulation is maintained. TIVA with propofol does not impair cerebral autoregulation *(Cottrell: Cottrell and Patel's Neuroanesthesia, ed 6, pp 28–32; Miller: Basics of Anesthesia, ed 7, p 513; Miller: Miller's Anesthesia, ed 8, pp 396–403, 2176–2187, 3099).*

757. (C) The general approach to treating patients following VAE is (1) stop further air entrainment, (2) aspirate entrained air, (3) prevent expansion of existing air, and (4) support cardiovascular function. Cessation of subsequent air entrainment is achieved by flooding the surgical field with irrigation fluid. Additionally, noncollapsible veins can be sealed using electrocautery, vessel ligation, or placement of wax on cut bone edges. Neck veins can be compressed as a means of increasing jugular venous pressure, which mitigates or prevents further air entry and helps localize the source of air. A multiorificed right atrial catheter, placed before the event, is the most effective means of aspirating air. To prevent expansion of the VAE, nitrous oxide is immediately discontinued. Some neuroanesthesiologists avoid use of N_2O in any instance where there is a chance of VAE. Cardiovascular function is supported using inotropes, vasopressors, and IV fluids as indicated. If possible, lowering the patient's head would decrease the pressure gradient and decrease the chance of more VAE. Of the response options provided, PEEP is the least correct answer. Approximately 20% to 30% of humans have a probe patent foramen ovale. Initiation of PEEP may increase the risk of paradoxical embolism or decrease venous effluent from the calvarium, resulting in increased CBV and ICP *(Cottrell: Cottrell and Patel's Neuroanesthesia, ed 6, p 218; Miller: Miller's Anesthesia, ed 8, p 2170–2172).*

758. (D) The risk of VAE exists whenever the operative field is above the level of the right atrium. Clinically significant VAE occurs in about 0.5% to 3% of patients operated on in the sitting position. Using TEE, 50% to 100% of patients undergoing neurosurgical procedures in the sitting position have detectable VAE. VAE occurs when air enters the venous circulation and travels to the right atrium, where it continues into the right ventricle and passes into the lungs, causing an increase in pulmonary dead space, impairment of gas exchange (e.g., decreased oxygen absorption and CO_2 retention), and a decrease in end-tidal CO_2. Air in the pulmonary arteries can increase pulmonary vascular resistance and pulmonary artery pressures and can cause right heart strain and dysrhythmias. Air can also pass right to left through a patent foramen ovale (20%-30% of patients have a patent foramen ovale) and may lead to stroke or, if air finds its way into coronary arteries, myocardial infarction and cardiac arrest. Reflex bronchoconstriction may be caused by microvascular bubbles and by the release of inflammatory mediators from endothelial cells, resulting in hypoxemia. Initially, VAE can cause systemic hypertension, but as larger amounts of air are entrained, systemic hypotension and death from cardiovascular collapse can result *(Miller: Basics of Anesthesia, ed 7, pp 328–329; Cottrell: Cottrell and Patel's Neuroanesthesia, ed 6, pp 213–218).*

759. (B) Most patients who undergo ECoG monitoring to localize the epileptogenic foci during seizure surgery receive general endotracheal anesthesia. Some select patients can undergo this procedure with local anesthesia (with mild sedation). The ECoG monitoring is altered by many anesthetic drugs. If during the intraoperative EEG recordings seizure spikes are not obtained, then remifentanil, alfentanil, etomidate, methohexital, or ketamine (>4 mg/kg) can be administered to promote the iatrogenic activation of epileptiform discharges. Alfentanil can provoke abnormal EEG spike activity in over 80% of these patients, compared with 50% when methohexital is administered. Controversy exists as to whether the foci elicited with these pharmacologically induced seizures correspond to the patient's native epileptiform foci.

If the patient is undergoing an awake craniotomy, dexmedetomidine is widely used. Dexmedetomidine gives analgesia, some sedation, and anxiolysis and does not affect ECoG monitoring or the iatrogenic activation with other drugs. Dexmedetomidine does not activate epileptiform foci.

Although propofol is a useful IV anesthetic, it does depress ECoG recordings. Propofol can be used for induction of general anesthesia and, if initially infused during the case, should be discontinued for 20 to 30 minutes before ECoG monitoring. Benzodiazepines are excellent anticonvulsants and should not be used if ECoG monitoring is to be performed.

The epileptic potential of isoflurane, desflurane, or halothane used alone is very low. Enflurane (rarely used today) can cause epileptiform seizures in both epileptics and nonepileptics and should not be used in patients with epilepsy unless the procedure is to identify the seizure foci with ECoG monitoring. Sevoflurane, however, has been reported to cause electrical spikes in both epileptic and nonepileptic patients as the concentration of sevoflurane is increased, especially when accompanied by hyperventilation. Nitrous oxide use in epileptics is relatively benign, but, rarely, convulsions and spike-and-wave activity on the EEG have been reported when nitrous oxide is used with volatile anesthetics.

For general anesthesia and ECoG monitoring, a common anesthetic includes propofol and a muscle relaxant for induction and endotracheal intubation, followed by maintenance anesthesia with low concentrations of sevoflurane, isoflurane, or desflurane with nitrous oxide. After the craniotomy is performed and the surface or deep electrodes are placed, the volatile anesthetic is discontinued or markedly decreased, increased amounts of opioids (e.g., remifentanil) are administered, and muscle paralysis is maintained; nitrous oxide, if used, can be continued. Because the anesthetic is "lightened," the patient is advised that he may have a short period of awareness. After about 20 to 30 minutes to lower the concentrations of the volatile anesthetic, ECoG monitoring is begun. Normocapnia or mild to moderate hyperventilation (PaCO$_2$ 30-35 mm Hg) is often used. If there is difficulty in finding the seizure location, remifentanil, alfentanil, methohexital, or etomidate can be used to promote epileptiform discharges *(Cottrell: Cottrell and Patel's Neuroanesthesia, ed 6, pp 300–305; Jaffe; Anesthesiologist's Manual of Surgical Procedures, ed 5, pp 83–87; Miller: Miller's Anesthesia, ed 8, pp 408–409).*

760. (B) In patients who have had a stroke as a result of occlusive vascular disease, there is a loss of the normal vasomotor responses to changes in PaCO$_2$ and arterial BP in the areas of ischemia (i.e., vasomotor paralysis), as well as disruption of the BBB. Although the risk of extending the area of infarction has not been extensively studied, most would recommend waiting approximately 4 to 6 weeks for stabilization of the vasomotor responses to BP and PaCO$_2$, and for stabilization of the BBB. During this time, complete evaluation of the extent and cause of the stroke should be performed (e.g., occlusive disease versus embolic disease) as well as an evaluation for concomitant cardiovascular system diseases (e.g., cardiac arrhythmias such as atrial fibrillation or ischemic heart disease) that may be present. It is recommended that anesthesia for elective surgical procedures be postponed for at least 4 weeks, and preferably 6 weeks, after a stroke to minimize the risk of a subsequent stroke *(Miller: Miller's Anesthesia, ed 8, pp 418, 1127).*

761. (A) SSEPs are used to monitor peripheral sensory nerve pathway function. They are commonly used during spinal procedures to identify mechanical or ischemic injury. The peripheral nerve (e.g., median nerve at the wrist, common peroneal nerve at the knee, posterior tibial nerve at the ankle) is electrically stimulated. The impulse elicited by electrical stimulation of a peripheral nerve ascends the ipsilateral dorsal column of the spinal cord, then synapses in the dorsal column nuclei at the cervicomedullary junction; these fibers *cross* and travel through the contralateral medial lemniscus to the thalamus, which then projects the sensory impulses to the sensory cortex contralateral to the side of stimulation.

The signals are recorded as a plot of voltage versus time and are composed of negative and positive voltage deflections, with specific amplitudes (peak to adjacent trough) and latencies (time from stimulation to peak). In general, the earlier deflections represent impulses and synapses within the spinal cord or brainstem, whereas the later impulses represent thalamic and/or cortical synapses. Extraction of SSEPs from the background EEG is accomplished by computerized signal averaging for summation. A 50% reduction in amplitude or a 10% increase in latency is considered significant, although at times smaller changes may be significant. SSEPs do not evaluate the integrity of the ventral or lateral spinothalamic tracts or the corticospinal tract. The corticospinal tract is readily eliminated from the answer set because it is a motor (rather than sensory) pathway *(Cottrell: Cottrell and Patel's Neuroanesthesia, ed 6, pp 114–116; Miller: Miller's Anesthesia, ed 8, p 1497–1499; Miller: Basics of Anesthesia, ed 7, p 358).*

762. (B) During scoliosis surgery, spinal cord monitoring for cord ischemia is performed most commonly with an SSEP monitor. SSEP monitoring accesses pathways that carry proprioception and vibratory sensations (dorsal column of the spinal cord) supplied by the posterior spinal artery. SSEP does not monitor motor pathways. MEP monitoring is a better monitor of motor pathways but often is not used because muscle relaxants are usually needed during the surgery, making MEP monitoring difficult to interpret. In cases where the monitoring is equivocal or not available, a wake-up test is performed. The differential diagnosis for a nonmoving patient during a wake-up test includes the presence of neuromuscular blockade, inadequate volatile or nitrous oxide washout, or the presence of opiates or sedative hypnotic medications. There are also a few other extremely rare central causes, such as stroke. In this patient the SSEP monitoring is equivocal, and a wake-up test is to be performed. Because the patient's neuromuscular blockade has worn off (as noted by the TOF ratio of 0.9), there is no need to use neostigmine plus glycopyrrolate to reverse neuromuscular blockade further. In addition, the volatile anesthetic and nitrous oxide have largely been washed out, making a trial of low-dose naloxone a reasonable option. An initial small dose (e.g., 0.04 mg) may be all that is needed to reverse the effects of the narcotic. If this dose is not effective, it should be repeated. If the patient is awake enough to squeeze her hands but failed to move her feet to verbal commands, spinal cord ischemia is suggested, so distraction on the rod is released one notch at a time and the wake-up test repeated until movement of the legs is noted *(Barash: Clinical Anesthesia, ed 8, p 1444; Miller: Basics of Anesthesia, ed 7, p 545).*

763. (C) Arterial CO_2 tension ($PaCO_2$) has a profound physiologic effect on CBF and CBV. At the normal $PaCO_2$ of 40 mm Hg, CBF is 50 mL per 100 g brain tissue per minute. Between $PaCO_2$ values of 20 and 40 mm Hg, CBF decreases 1 to 2 mL per 100 g of brain tissue per min for each 1 mm Hg decrease in $PaCO_2$ from a $PaCO_2$ of 40 mm Hg. Between $PaCO_2$ values of 40 and 80 mm Hg, CBF increases 1 to 2 mL per 100 g of brain tissue per min for each 1 mm Hg increase in $PaCO_2$ from a $PaCO_2$ of 40 mm Hg. This change in blood flow lasts about 6 to 8 hours due to a compensatory change in bicarbonate concentration. Because this patient's $PaCO_2$ is 10 mm Hg below normal, CBF would be decreased 10 to 20 mL to approximately 30 to 40 mL per 100 g of brain tissue per min *(Cottrell: Cottrell and Young's Neuroanesthesia, ed 6, pp 26–27; Miller: Miller's Anesthesia, ed 8, p 392–393; Miller: Basics of Anesthesia, ed 7, pp 513–514).*

764. (A) The main goals in treating patients with severe brain trauma revolve around normalizing ICP (below 20 mm Hg) and achieving a mean BP greater than 80 mm Hg, a CPP between 50 and 70 mm Hg, and an adequate oxygen delivery (PaO_2 >90% saturation or PaO_2 >60 mm Hg with a minimum hematocrit of 30%). Maintaining a CPP >70 mm Hg was a former standard but is no longer recommended due to an increased risk of adult respiratory distress syndrome (ARDS).

ICP is determined by the relationship between the cranial vault (formed by the skull), volume of brain tissue, volume of CSF, and CBV.

Studies evaluating the effectiveness of corticosteroids in the setting of head injury, or global or focal brain ischemia, have demonstrated either no improvement or a worsening of neurologic outcome. The prophylactic use of anticonvulsant medications does not prevent post-traumatic seizures.

Provided ventilation is not depressed, all IV anesthetics, with the exception of ketamine, cause some degree of reduction in CMR, CBF, CBV, and ICP. As an aside, regarding IV anesthetics, barbiturates are thought to be the "gold standard" for anesthetic-mediated brain-protective therapy in animal models of focal or incomplete global brain ischemia. However, this has yet to be proven in humans.

In the setting of TBI, mild hyperventilation is an acceptable intervention, usually to a $PaCO_2$ of 35 mm Hg. If there is any evidence of transtentorial herniation, hyperventilation to a $PaCO_2$ level of 30 mm Hg is started, along with barbiturate therapy. However, the Brain Trauma Foundation now advises against aggressive hyperventilation because the data suggest worsening of outcomes associated with $PaCO_2$ values below 25 to 30 mm Hg.

Both IV osmotic (e.g., 0.25-1 g/kg of mannitol, or 3% or 7.5% hypertonic saline solutions) and loop diuretics (e.g., 0.5-1 mg/kg of furosemide) are effective in reducing ICP.

Provided the patient is hemodynamically stable, elevation of the head above the level of the heart facilitates effluent of blood from the calvarium, which results in decreases in CBV and ICP *(Barash: Clinical Anesthesia, ed 8, pp 1499–1502; Brain Trauma Foundation and the American Association of Neurological Surgeons Guidelines: J Neurotrauma 2007:24:S1–106; Cottrell: Cottrell and Patel's Neuroanesthesia, ed 6, pp 326–331).*

765. (A) After an SAH, patients may experience cerebral vasospasm (25% of patients) as well as rebleeding, intracranial hypertension, and seizures. If the patient is NOT experiencing cerebral vasospasm, hypertension should be avoided to minimize aneurysmal wall tension, thereby mitigating the risk of re-rupture and further hemorrhage. In contrast, had this patient been experiencing cerebral vasospasm, induced hypertension would have been an appropriate therapeutic intervention to decrease cerebral ischemia. Because patients often relate that the clinical symptom of headache is the "worst headache of my life," narcotics and benzodiazepines maybe cautiously administered to reduce pain and anxiety without causing respiratory depression (respiratory depression produces an elevation of $PaCO_2$ and increases ICP). Systemic hypertension is avoided, in part, by the administration of analgesic and sedative medications. Antiepileptic drugs often are administered in an attempt to prevent or mitigate seizures. Calcium channel blockers (e.g., nimodipine) are used to avert adverse sequelae of cerebral vasospasm (also see explanation to Question 776) *(Cottrell: Cottrell and Patel's Neuroanesthesia, ed 6, pp 222–229, 252–253; Hines: Stoelting's Anesthesia and Co-Existing Disease, ed 7, pp 284–286).*

766. (D) The EEG records the electrical activity of the brain and has many uses, including the ability to identify consciousness, stages of sleep, unconsciousness, coma, seizure activity, dementia, encephalitis, brain ischemia (in the absence of significant changes in anesthetic depth), and brain death. When evaluating the EEG, one looks at the frequency, the amplitude, and the location of the leads on the head. The usual awake patient has a frequency on the beta range (high frequency and low amplitude) common with that of the alert patient. With eye closure, the frequency of the EEG is in the alpha frequency (slower but with higher amplitude). When slower frequencies are produced (theta and delta), the brain is depressed. The sleeping patient may show many frequency ranges: slower frequencies with deep natural sleep and higher frequencies with light sleep or during rapid eye movement (REM) sleep, where the EEG appears activated and the eye muscle electromyogram appears on the EEG. A flat or isoelectric EEG pattern can be seen with drug intoxication (e.g., barbiturate coma, high volatile anesthetics in the 1.5-2 MAC range) or severe hypothermia, as well as with brain death. When looking at the entire head pattern, one looks for symmetry. Regional asymmetry is seen with brain tumors, epilepsy, cerebral ischemia, or ischemia. During carotid surgery, cerebral hypoperfusion indicates the need for a shunt placement *(Cottrell: Cottrell and Patel's Neuroanesthesia, ed 6, p 149; Miller: Miller's Anesthesia, ed 8, pp 1491–1494; Miller: Basics of Anesthesia, ed 7, p 101).*

767. (B) SAH is associated with ECG changes (>40% of patients) that are largely reversible and felt to be related to localized catecholamine stimulation in response to the bleeding. The ECG changes include sinus bradycardia, sinus tachycardia, atrial fibrillation, atrial flutter, atrioventricular (AV) dissociation, ventricular tachycardia, and ventricular fibrillation. Morphologic changes include T-wave inversion, diffuse ST elevation, ST segment depression, appearance of U waves, prolonged QT interval (often >550 msec), and, rarely, Q waves. ECG changes tend to recede within 72 hours from the hemorrhage. There does not appear to be a correlation of the ECG changes with echocardiographic examination. Left ventricular function and regional wall abnormalities occur in <18% of cases. Mildly elevated troponin levels (less than seen in myocardial infarction) have also been reported in patients with SAH. Although they have historically been considered functionally insignificant neurogenic phenomena, there is increasing evidence that these changes may be a sign of underlying myocardial ischemia. However, even if myocardial ischemia is present, it seems to have a minimal effect on patient outcome (i.e., morbidity and mortality).

Because electrolyte abnormalities (e.g., hypokalemia or hypocalcemia) may contribute to the etiology of the ECG changes, it would probably be most appropriate to quantify these electrolytes before initiating other therapies or canceling emergency surgery. There is no evidence that the administration of β-blockers (e.g., esmolol. metoprolol) alters the outcome of these patients. Nitroglycerin is a potent cerebral vasodilator that could have a deleterious effect on ICP in patients with increased ICP. Although a pulmonary artery catheter is sometimes placed in patients with cardiac disease, a patient with an SAH does not need one, because the problem is neurogenic and not cardiac in origin *(Cottrell: Cottrell and Patel's Neuroanesthesia, ed 6, pp 225–226; Miller: Miller's Anesthesia, ed 8, pp 2178–2179, 3112).*

768. (D) MEPs are used to monitor the integrity of motor pathways in the nervous system during neurosurgical, orthopedic, or major vascular (e.g., procedures that involve cross-clamping of the thoracic aorta) surgery. MEPs are more sensitive than SSEPs for detecting ischemia. Electrical or magnetic stimulation of the motor cortex produces an evoked potential that is propagated via descending motor pathways and can be recorded from the spinal column, peripheral nerve, or the muscle itself.

Inhalational anesthetics (e.g., volatile anesthetics, nitrous oxide) have the most profound effect on monitoring. If monitoring with MEPs is to be done, inhalation anesthetic concentrations should be ≤0.5 MAC. Propofol's effects on MEPs are less compared with inhalation anesthetics, making TIVA preferred over inhalation anesthesia for maintenance of anesthesia. Ketamine and etomidate may improve MEP monitoring and may be used with lower doses of propofol. Opioids (e.g., fentanyl, sufentanil) have little, if any, effect on MEP monitoring. Neuromuscular blocking drugs will abolish the MEPs if all neuromuscular twitches are absent *(Barash: Clinical Anesthesia, ed 8, pp 1009–1011, 1444; Cottrell: Cottrell and Patel's Neuroanesthesia, ed 5, pp 120–123; Miller: Miller's Anesthesia, ed 8, pp 1518–1519).*

769. (D) DBS can be used for patients with medically refractory Parkinson disease to improve their quality of life. By stimulating certain parts of the brain, symptoms of bradykinesia, rigidity, tremor, and severe dyskinesia can be improved. The DBS device has three components: an intracranial electrode, a pulse generator, and a cable to connect them. Preoperatively, the medications used to treat Parkinson disease are often held for 8 to 24 hours so brain recordings may more accurately localize the area of the brain to be stimulated. Typically, patients are placed in a stereotactic head frame, and computerized tomography (CT) or MRI is performed to locate the part of the brain for electrode placement. In some cases, frameless stereotactic surgery is performed, with external scalp markers for reference. This is followed by the placement of burr holes and insertion of the electrode about 1 cm from the target area to be stimulated. With brain monitoring, the electrode is carefully advanced toward the target area. Most commonly, placement is done on awake or lightly sedated patients where stimulation of the device can be tested. Dexmedetomidine is used for sedation and analgesia during final electrode placement. Propofol and opioids (e.g., fentanyl or remifentanil) are often used in addition to dexmedetomidine when the burr holes are performed and when electrodes are first inserted into the brain. Benzodiazepines (e.g., midazolam) are avoided because they interfere with the brain monitoring and location process. In some centers or when patients cannot be still for the placement of the electrodes, general anesthesia is used, with testing performed after the patient is awakened. Because placement is done in patients in the sitting position, precordial Doppler is often used to detect the occurrence of VAEs. Intraoperative surgical-related complications include bleeding (about 0.5%-6%), seizures (0.8%-4.5%), and VAEs (4.5%). Most of the intraoperative seizures are self-limiting and require only small doses of propofol (e.g., 20 mg). Once the seizure has ended and the patient has recovered and is stable, the procedure is continued. If the patient has a DBS device implanted and requires a surgical procedure, the DBS device should be turned off for the surgery, then restarted in the postanesthesia care unit *(Cottrell: Cottrell and Patel's Neuroanesthesia, ed 6, pp 317–324; Jaffe; Anesthesiologist's Manual of Surgical Procedures, ed 5, pp 72–76).*

770. (A) Most IV anesthetics (dexmedetomidine, benzodiazepines, etomidate, propofol and thiopental) decrease both CMR and CBF, with the exception of ketamine, which increases both CMR and CBF. When there is increased neural activity (e.g., seizures or hyperthermia), CBF and CMR also increase. When BP is normal, volatile anesthetics (e.g., desflurane, halothane, isoflurane, and sevoflurane) cause a simultaneous, dose-dependent increase in CBF but a decrease in CMR (i.e., volatile anesthetics "uncouple" global CBF and CMR). Administered alone, nitrous oxide can increase both CMR and CBF. When nitrous oxide is administered with IV anesthetics, the effect on CBF is markedly diminished *(Cottrell: Cottrell and Patel's Neuroanesthesia, ed 6, pp 75–82; Miller: Miller's Anesthesia, ed 8, pp 396–407).*

771. (C) The common carotid arteries come off of the aortic arch and divide into the internal and external carotid arteries. The internal carotid artery supplies about 70% of the blood supply to the brain (anterior circulation). The internal carotid artery divides into three branches: the anterior cerebral artery, the posterior communicating artery, and the middle cerebral artery. The vertebral arteries originate from the subclavian arteries and supply 30% of the blood supply to the brain (posterior circulation). The vertebral arteries form the basilar artery. The vertebral arteries do not connect directly to the posterior communicating artery. The basilar artery has several branches, including the right and left posterior cerebral artery, which connects to the right and left posterior communicating artery from the carotid arteries. The right and the left anterior cerebral artery are connected by the anterior communicating artery. The circle of blood vessels is called the circle of Willis. This circle is incomplete in about 20% of patients.

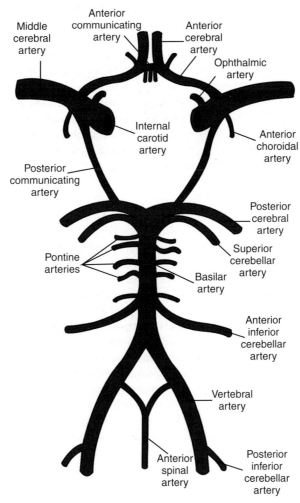

From Meng L, Flexman A: Central nervous system disease. In: Pardo MC Jr, Miller RD, editors: Basics of Anesthesia, ed 6, Elsevier, 2018, pp 511–523.

    The spinal cord gets its blood supply from one anterior spinal artery and two posterior spinal arteries. The anterior spinal artery receives its blood supply from six to eight radicular arteries that are derived from the aorta. The largest radicular artery is called the artery of Adamkiewicz and supplies the spinal cord from T8 to the conus medullaris terminus *(Barash: Clinical Anesthesia, ed 8, pp 1003–1007; Miller: Basics of Anesthesia, ed 7, p 512).*

772. (A) Acute complete spinal cord injury produces a state of spinal shock (flaccid muscle paralysis, loss of deep tendon reflexes, loss of sensation, and a sympathectomy below the level of the injury). With cervical and upper thoracic injuries, respiratory impairment develops as a result of the loss of intercostal muscle activity. With an upper cervical lesion that damages the phrenic nerve (origin C3-C5), there would be diaphragmatic impairment as well. With complete lesions above C3, the patient cannot ventilate. If the lesion is above T4-T6, the sympathectomy results in hypotension (due to a decrease in systemic arterial tone as well as venous vascular tone) and often bradycardia (resulting from a loss of the T1-T4 sympathetic innervation). This pathophysiologic process typically lasts 1 to 3 weeks as some compensatory mechanisms develop after the injury. Thermoregulation is lost, resulting in poikilothermia, because the hypothalamic thermoregulatory center is unable to communicate with the peripheral sympathetic pathways. In the cool environment of the hospital, spinal cord injury patients are unable to have vasoconstriction below the level of injury and thus may experience hypothermia.

About 85% of patients with spinal cord injuries cephalad to T5-T6 develop a condition called autonomic hyperreflexia, or acute generalized sympathetic hyperactivity. Autonomic hyperreflexia is elicited by cutaneous or visceral stimulation of the spinal cord below the level of injury and by the inability of the higher centers of the nervous system to control sympathetic function. This is often manifested by vasoconstriction below the lesion, with severe hypertension and reflex bradycardia (vagus nerve is still intact); at times, pulmonary edema can result from the severe increase in afterload. Above the lesion, vasodilation with nasal stuffiness often occurs. Autonomic hyperreflexia does not occur immediately after the injury, but starts to develop 2 to 3 weeks after the injury *(Cottrell: Cottrell and Patel's Neuroanesthesia, ed 6, pp 177–181, 370–382; Hines: Stoelting's Anesthesia and Co-Existing Disease, ed 7, pp 305–309).*

773. (D) Signs and symptoms of intracranial hypertension include headaches that awaken the patient at night, morning headaches, nausea and vomiting, altered level of consciousness, blurred vision, papilledema, seizure activity, personality changes, and coma. Additionally, patients may manifest a constellation of clinical signs referred to as Cushing triad (i.e., systemic hypertension, bradycardia, and irregular breathing pattern) *(Hines: Stoelting's Anesthesia and Co-Existing Disease, ed 7, pp 268–270; Miller: Miller's Anesthesia, ed 8, pp 1201–1202, 2159).*

774. (D) Carotid endarterectomies are most commonly performed under general anesthesia; however, some perform this procedure under regional anesthesia (e.g., superficial cervical plexus block).

Arterial BP and $PaCO_2$ should be maintained in the normal ranges for each patient because the vasculature within ischemic regions of the brain has lost the ability to autoregulate CBF and respond to changes in $PaCO_2$. Marked reductions in arterial BP may reduce CBF (especially via collateral channels) to ischemic brain tissue, and deliberate hypotension is not recommended. Although many clinicians advocate raising the mean BP to enable better blood flow to the brain via the other carotid artery and the vertebral blood vessels, most evidence suggests that the routine elevation of BP may cause cerebral hemorrhage or cerebral edema in the area of the brain where autoregulation is lost and can cause more stress to the heart muscle that may lead to cardiac ischemia.

Theoretically, if $PaCO_2$ is increased from normal, cerebral blood vessels surrounding the region of ischemia that retain normal CO_2 responsiveness will dilate, diverting regional CBF (rCBF) away from the ischemic brain tissue (i.e., steal phenomenon). Conversely, if the $PaCO_2$ is reduced from normal, the cerebral blood vessels surrounding the ischemic brain tissue will constrict, diverting rCBF to ischemic areas of the brain (inverse steal phenomenon, or Robin Hood effect). Hyperventilating the lungs in an attempt to produce the inverse steal phenomenon is not recommended because the actual effect may be unpredictable; supportive evidence in humans that this is beneficial is lacking.

The carotid sinus (not carotid body) baroreceptor reflex can be blunted by IV injection of atropine or by local infiltration of the area of the carotid sinus with a local anesthetic.

Currently, general anesthesia is most commonly induced with propofol and supplemented with narcotics. After neuromuscular blockade is achieved, the patient's trachea is intubated, and general anesthesia is maintained with either volatile anesthetics or TIVA with propofol as the main anesthetic, supplemented with an opioid (e.g., fentanyl or remifentanil). Nitrous oxide is commonly used to reduce the concentration of volatile anesthetics or IV anesthetics *(Cottrell: Cottrell and Patel's Neuroanesthesia, ed 6, pp 277–278, 285–289).*

775. (C) In general, all volatile anesthetics (e.g., isoflurane, sevoflurane, and desflurane) are potent direct cerebral vasodilators that produce dose-dependent increases in CBF, CBV, and, ultimately, ICP when concentrations exceed 0.6 MAC. The order of vasodilator potency is approximately halothane » enflurane > isoflurane = sevoflurane = desflurane. Opioids have little, if any, effect on CMR, CBF, or ICP (provided minute ventilation is maintained). The effect of N_2O on CBF, CBV, and ICP is controversial. In a number of animal and human studies, N_2O increased CBF by 35% to 103%. Conversely, in other animal studies, N_2O was consistently found to have only minimal effects on CBF. Differences between species may be one factor contributing to these conflicting results. Because N_2O appears to increase CBF and CBV in humans, it seems prudent to discontinue N_2O in patients in whom intracranial hypertension is not responsive to other therapeutic maneuvers. Propofol and barbiturates are potent cerebral vasoconstrictors and can decrease ICP (*Cottrell: Cottrell and Patel's Neuroanesthesia, ed 6, pp 75–83; Hines: Stoelting's Anesthesia and Co-Existing Disease, ed 7, pp 270–275; Miller: Miller's Anesthesia, ed 8, pp 397–407*).

776. (C) Cerebral vasospasm is a leading cause of major morbidity and mortality in patients who have survived an initial SAH. A decrease in level of consciousness followed by focal neurologic signs is an early sign of cerebral vasospasm. After an SAH, the incidence and severity of cerebral vasospasm have been reported to correlate with the amount and location of blood in the calvarium. Angiographic evidence of vasospasm has been noted in up to 70% of SAH patients. However, clinically significant vasospasm occurs in about 20% to 30% of SAH patients. If cerebral vasospasm develops, about 50% of patients die or are left with major neurologic deficits. The incidence of vasospasm peaks approximately 7 days after SAH and is seldom seen after 2 weeks. If vasospasm does develop, it usually lasts 3 to 7 days.

Calcium channel blockers (e.g., nimodipine) decrease the morbidity and mortality associated with vasospasm, but investigators have been unable to demonstrate any significant change in the incidence or severity of vasospasm. This suggests that the beneficial effects of nimodipine may be related to inhibition of primary and secondary ischemic cascades, rather than to direct cerebral vasodilation. Treatment of vasospasm also includes "triple H therapy" (*H*ypervolemia, induced *H*ypertension, and *H*emodilution) and cerebral angioplasty in patients refractory to more conservative treatment. The rationale for induced hypervolemia (or maintaining normovolemia) and hypertension is that ischemic regions of brain have impaired autoregulation, and thus CBF is perfusion pressure dependent. Hemodilution (to a hematocrit 25%-30%) is thought to increase blood flow through the cerebral microcirculation (because of improved rheology and reactive hyperemia). Taken together, BP reductions and diuretic use are incorrect responses to this condition (*Cottrell: Cottrell and Patel's Neuroanesthesia, ed 6, pp 227–229*).

777. (D) Acromegaly develops as a result of excessive production of growth hormone (GH) after the growth plates have fused. If the excessive GH develops before fusion of the growth plates, the patient develops gigantism. Most often, excessive GH secretion is due to a benign anterior pituitary adenoma. In addition to excessive bony growth (e.g., enlargement of the hands and feet, mandible), there is enlargement of the tongue and epiglottis, predisposing the patient to upper airway obstruction and making visualization of the vocal cords more difficult. The vocal cords are enlarged, producing a narrower glottic opening. In addition, subglottic narrowing may be present, as well as tracheal compression from an enlarged thyroid (seen in about 25% of acromegalic patients). This often necessitates the use of a narrower endotracheal tube than one might choose based on the facial enlargement. The placement of nasal airways may be more difficult due to the enlarged nasal turbinates. Associated conditions include skin thickening, diabetes mellitus (insulin resistance), hypertension, heart failure, and OSA. The use of CPAP is contraindicated after transsphenoidal hypophysectomy due to the transsphenoidal approach to removing the adenoma (*Cottrell: Cottrell and Patel's Neuroanesthesia, ed 6, p 461; Fleisher: Anesthesia and Uncommon Diseases, ed 6, p 417; Hines: Stoelting's Anesthesia and Co-Existing Disease, ed 7, pp 472–473*).

778. (D) The CBF autoregulatory curve describes the way blood flow to the normal brain is maintained. Blood flow is maintained at 50 mL/100 g brain tissue/min when the mean BP is between 60 and 160 mm Hg. To maintain blood flow, blood vessels can dilate to a point where the blood vessels are maximally dilated (at 60 mm Hg mean BP); then CBF would decrease at lower pressures. Similarly, at higher mean BPs, the blood vessels can constrict to a point where they are maximally constricted (mean BP of 160 mm Hg mean BP); then CBF would increase at higher pressures. Because blood with a low PaO_2 contains less oxygen, a fall in the PaO_2 below 50 mm Hg causes the cerebral blood vessels to dilate, allowing more blood and oxygen to flow to the brain when the BP is above a mean BP of 60 mm Hg (i.e., when the blood vessels can still dilate). Volatile anesthetics as well as hypercarbia produce cerebral vasodilation, which decreases the ability of blood vessels to constrict (thus CBF would increase at a mean BP of less than 160 mm Hg). Chronic hypertension, as well as vasoconstrictor medications, shifts the CBF autoregulatory curve to the right (i.e., making it more difficult to dilate the cerebral blood vessels). The clinical significance of this observation is that CBF could decrease and cerebral ischemia could occur at a higher mean systemic arterial BP in patients with chronic uncontrolled hypertension compared with normotensive patients. Chronic antihypertensive therapy to control systemic BPs within the normal range may restore normal CBF autoregulation (see the figure for answer 730 above) (*Cottrell: Cottrell and Patel's Neuroanesthesia, ed 6, pp 19–30; Miller: Basics of Anesthesia, ed 7, pp 512–514*).

779. (D) Cerebral autoregulation is disturbed in a number of diseases (e.g., acute cerebral ischemia, mass lesions, trauma, inflammation, prematurity, neonatal asphyxia, and diabetes mellitus). The final common pathway of dysfunction, in its most extreme form, is termed "cerebral vasomotor paralysis." CBF is maintained at PaO_2 between 50 and 200 mm Hg. Hyperoxia (e.g., PaO_2 >500 mm Hg) decreases CBF by about 10% to 15%; however, increasing the atmospheric pressure when breathing room air up to 4 atmospheres of pressure has little effect on CBF (hypoxia below PaO_2 of 50 mm Hg does affect autoregulation). During normothermic and moderate hypothermic (i.e., approximately 27° C) cardiopulmonary bypass, autoregulation as well as CO_2 reactivity is well preserved (even though CMR and CBF is reduced due to the reduced metabolic needs). Chronic uncontrolled hypertension causes a rightward shift of the autoregulation curve toward higher upper and lower CPP limits. Autoregulation is impaired by volatile anesthetics due to cerebral vasodilation (e.g., desflurane, isoflurane, sevoflurane). At greater than 2 MAC, autoregulation is abolished *(Cottrell: Cottrell and Patel's Neuroanesthesia, ed 6, pp 27–30; Miller: Basics of Anesthesia, ed 7, pp 512–514; Miller's Anesthesia, ed 8, pp 401–402)*.

780. (A) Etomidate at standard induction doses of 0.2 to 0.3 mg/kg has minimal cardiovascular side effects and can help maintain CPP. Because etomidate is painful when injected, has a high incidence of postoperative nausea and vomiting, and causes adrenocortical suppression, it is used mainly in patients with limited cardiovascular reserve. Etomidate at induction doses of general anesthesia produces a 30% to 50% reduction in CBF and CMR. ICP also decreases with etomidate. Intravenous etomidate does not disturb cerebral autoregulation or CO_2 reactivity. Etomidate increases both amplitude and latency during SSEP monitoring *(Cottrell: Cottrell and Patel's Neuroanesthesia, ed 6, p 80; Miller: Basics of Anesthesia, ed 7, pp 117–118)*.

781. (C) Nasal intubation should be avoided in patients with suspected basal skull fractures (e.g., tympanic cavity hemorrhage, otorrhea, petechiae on the mastoid process known as Battle's sign, or petechiae around the eyes known as panda sign) or severe facial fractures. Because approximately 10% of high-speed motor vehicle accident head injury patients have associated cervical spine injuries, it is prudent to assume that all head injury patients have coexisting cervical spine injury until proved otherwise. Additionally, the patient described in this question may have abnormal airway anatomy because of extreme micrognathia, facial injuries, and obesity. Taken together, direct laryngoscopy with rapid-sequence induction is probably not an acceptable technique for securing this patient's airway because intubation and mask ventilation cannot be guaranteed due to his anatomy and need for inline stabilization of the neck. In contrast, awake intubation by direct, video, or fiberoptic laryngoscopy or performance of tracheostomy is considered an appropriate technique for tracheal intubation of this patient. Mask and laryngeal mask airway (LMA) techniques may provide a patent airway but do not ensure protection of the airway against aspiration of gastric contents *(Cottrell: Cottrell and Patel's Neuroanesthesia, ed 6, pp 328–333)*.

782. (D) The normal serum sodium level is 135 to 145 mEq/L (mild hyponatremia is 130-134 mEq/L, moderate hyponatremia is 120-130 mEq/L, and severe hyponatremia is <120 mEq/L). The normal urine sodium level is 20 mEq/L. This patient has moderate hyponatremia and is unable to excrete dilute urine, as noted by the urine sodium greater than 20 mEq/L. These laboratory findings are consistent with SIADH. SIADH may result from a variety of causes, including central nervous system lesions, pulmonary infections, hypothyroidism, and drugs (e.g., chlorpropamide, narcotics). Patients with SIADH have an expanded blood volume due to fluid retention but excrete excessive amounts of sodium. ADH is also known as vasopressin, and because the patient has an excessive amount of vasopressin released, giving more vasopressin would make the clinical situation worse. After identifying the cause, treatment is started and usually consists mainly of water restriction. With severe hyponatremia (i.e., Na <120 mEq/L and signs of mental confusion), aggressive treatment with hypertonic sodium chloride may be needed; however, too much and too rapid infusion, as in choice B, may induce central pontine myelinolysis and may cause permanent brain damage. With severe hyponatremia, the dose of 200 to 300 mL of a 3% solution of sodium chloride is usually administered over several hours. The antibiotic demeclocycline interferes with ADH at the level of the renal tubules to produce dilute urine and is sometimes used for the treatment of SIADH. Tolvaptan is a selective, competitive vasopressin antagonist and is also sometimes used. Desmopressin acetate (DDAVP) is used to treat patients with complete DI, whereas chlorpropamide is used to treat incomplete DI. In contrast to SIADH, patients with DI have a lack of ADH and have high output of poorly concentrated urine and hypernatremia *(Barash: Clinical Anesthesia, ed 8, pp 400–403, 1018; Cottrell: Cottrell and Patel's Neuroanesthesia, ed 6, p 417; Miller: Miller's Anesthesia, ed 8, pp 1787–1790)*.

783. (B) This patient has several signs consistent with elevated ICP: hypertension, hyperventilation, and somnolence. Use of morphine premedication is ill advised because it would sedate him further, blunt his hyperventilation, and thus raise ICP. Anesthesia is often induced with propofol to produce a rapid onset of general anesthesia without further increasing the ICP. Most clinicians would use a nondepolarizing muscle relaxant for muscle paralysis to assist with intubation because succinylcholine may be associated with an increase in ICP. The use of esmolol before intubation may blunt the hyperdynamic response to laryngoscopy and prevent a further increase in ICP.

Hyperventilation is an effective maneuver for lowering ICP in the short term. As discussed in the explanations to Questions 733 and 764, $PaCO_2$ levels in the range of 30 to 35 mm Hg suffice for this, and there is no evidence that additional hyperventilation has any added therapeutic benefit.

Use of PEEP can promote impairment of venous drainage as well as raise ICP in patients with intracranial hypertension *(Cottrell: Cottrell and Patel's Neuroanesthesia, ed 6, pp 80–83; Hines: Stoelting's Anesthesia and Co-Existing Disease, ed 7, pp 268–275; Miller: Basics of Anesthesia, ed 7, pp 514–515).*

784. (D) MRI scanners contain powerful magnets that range from 0.5 to 5 Tesla (5000-50,000 G). By contrast, the Earth's magnetic field is 0.5 G. Certain metal objects are magnetic (e.g., iron, nickel, and cobalt) and, if brought into the scanner room, can become dangerous projectiles that fly toward the middle of the magnet, where the patient is located. Small items can be pulled away, but larger items may not be removable, even with a winch, and thus require a magnet shut-down, a process known as a quench. Nonmagnetic metals such as aluminum, titanium, copper, and silver are used for MRI-compatible equipment such as IV poles and special MRI-compatible anesthesia machines.

Attempting to pull the object described in this question away from the magnet would be nearly impossible; even if it could be successfully carried out, there would be great risk. For example, if the grip were lost and the object released, it could fly toward the patient inside the scanner. Stopping the scan or cutting the power to the magnet for 60 seconds does not release the magnetic force.

MRI magnets are always on. Quenching (turning off the magnet) is an expensive process that causes the cooling medium (liquid helium) to boil off and vent to the outside. This gas is cold and can lead to cold injuries to anyone exposed. Because the helium gas displaces air, it lowers the oxygen concentration in the room and may lead to asphyxiation. During this process, the coils become resistive and cease superconducting, thereby diminishing magnetic field strength *(Miller: Basics of Anesthesia, ed 7, pp 661–662).*

785. (D) Progressive entrainment of air into the pulmonary microcirculation reduces lung perfusion and increases pulmonary vascular resistance and alveolar dead-space ventilation. Early clinical signs include an increase in pulmonary artery pressures (pulmonary vascular resistance increases) and a decrease in end-tidal CO_2 (CO_2 cannot be eliminated, and $PaCO_2$ increases). As larger amounts of air are absorbed, there is a rise in CVPs, and cardiac output starts to fall, along with a fall in systemic BP. With severe VAE, cardiovascular collapse can develop *(Cottrell: Cottrell and Patel's Neuroanesthesia, ed 6, pp 213–214; Miller's Anesthesia, ed 8, pp 2169–2170).*

786. (C) In patients with normal brain function, cerebral ischemia does not develop unless the $PaCO_2$ is <20 mm Hg. Hyperventilation, and the resulting respiratory alkalosis, causes a leftward (not rightward) shifting of the oxyhemoglobin dissociation curve. In doing so, hemoglobin undergoes a conformation change, making it more reluctant to release oxygen at the tissue level. Hyperventilation-induced respiratory alkalosis can precipitate hypokalemia as well as hypocalcemia. Specifically, serum potassium decreases 0.6 mEq/L for each 0.1-unit increase in pH. With the respiratory alkalosis, the negative charge on albumin allows more calcium to bind and, if the calcium levels are low enough, can lead to paresthesia and tetany. Thus overly aggressive hyperventilation should be guarded against to avoid electrolyte perturbations that may result in cardiac arrhythmias. Hyperventilation also causes cerebral blood vessels to constrict, which can decrease CBF in the brain-injured patient (especially in the first 48-72 hours of injury), and excessive reduction in $PaCO_2$ <25 to 30 mm Hg may worsen outcome. In most cases, other methods to reduce ICP should be undertaken; in rare cases, hyperventilation may be necessary *(Miller: Miller's Anesthesia, ed 8, pp 2163–2164, 2185).*

787. (C) The GSC is a neurologic examination used to assess patients with head injuries. The total score is based on points for the best of three responses: eye opening (maximum 4 points), verbal response (maximum 5 points), and motor response (maximum 6 points). The score ranges from 3 to 15. GCS <8 = deep coma, severe head trauma, poor outcome. GCS 9 to 12 = moderate injury. GCS >13 = mild injury *(Barash: Clinical Anesthesia, ed 8, pp 1500–1501; Cottrell: Cottrell and Patel's Neuroanesthesia, ed 6, pp 326–327; Miller: Miller's Anesthesia, ed 8, p 729).*

	Score	This patient's score:
Eye-Opening		
Spontaneously	4	
Opens to speech	3	
Opens to pain	2	2
No response	1	
Verbal Response		
Oriented, conversing	5	
Answers are confused	4	
Inappropriate but recognizable words	3	
Incomprehensible sounds	2	2
No verbal response	1	
Motor Response		
Obeys verbal commands	6	
Localizes painful stimulus	5	
Withdrawal from painful stimulus	4	
Decorticate (upper extremity flexed, legs extended)	3	3
Decerebrate (upper extremity extended, legs extended)	2	
Flaccid (no response)	1	
	TOTAL =	7

CHAPTER 10

Anatomy, Regional Anesthesia, and Pain Management

DIRECTIONS (Questions 788 through 897): Each of the questions or incomplete statements in this section is followed by answers or by completions of the statement, respectively. Select the ONE BEST answer or completion for each item.

788. Which of the following is the best example of neuropathic pain?
- **A.** Postherpetic neuralgia (PHN)
- **B.** Fibromyalgia
- **C.** Chronic hip pain
- **D.** Lumbar facet joint pain

789. Which of the following techniques is **LEAST** effective in the treatment of pruritus from administration of neuraxial opiates?
- **A.** Nalbuphine 5 mg intravenous (IV)
- **B.** Dexmedetomidine 30 µg IV
- **C.** Diphenhydramine 50 mg IV
- **D.** Propofol 10 mg IV

790. The **MAXIMUM** dose of lidocaine containing 1:200,000 epinephrine that can be administered to a 70-kg patient for most major regional anesthetic techniques (and excluding spinal and IV regional) is
- **A.** 100 mg
- **B.** 200 mg
- **C.** 500 mg
- **D.** 1000 mg

791. Which of the following concentrations of epinephrine corresponds to a 1:200,000 mixture?
- **A.** 0.5 µg/mL
- **B.** 5 µg/mL
- **C.** 50 µg/mL
- **D.** 0.5 mg/mL

792. A 62-year-old fit patient with no comorbidities other than osteoarthrosis receives a spinal anesthetic for hip replacement. He takes nonsteroidal anti-inflammatory drugs (NSAIDs) and consumes coffee daily. The operation takes less than 1 hour and is uneventful. In the postanesthesia care unit (PACU) the patient complains of thirst and receives a caffeinated sugar-rich beverage and is discharged to floor. In his room he eats lunch and visits with family. After the spinal wears off, 3 hours after arrival to floor, the most likely observation will be
- **A.** Blood sugar greater than 200 mg/dL
- **B.** Nausea and vomiting
- **C.** Severe headache
- **D.** Urinary retention

793. Which of the following is the **EARLIEST** sign of lidocaine toxicity from a high blood level?
- **A.** Shivering
- **B.** Nystagmus
- **C.** Light-headedness and dizziness
- **D.** Tonic-clonic seizures

794. An analgesic effect similar to the epidural administration of **2.5 mg** of morphine could be achieved by which dose of intrathecal morphine?
- **A.** 0.05 mg
- **B.** 0.1 mg
- **C.** 1 mg
- **D.** Morphine should not be injected into the intrathecal space

795. Which of the following peripheral nerves is **MOST** likely to become injured in patients who are under general anesthesia?
- **A.** Ulnar nerve
- **B.** Median nerve
- **C.** Radial nerve
- **D.** Common peroneal nerve

796. Which of the following is the **MOST** important disadvantage of interscalene brachial plexus block compared with other approaches?
- **A.** Large volumes of local anesthetics required
- **B.** Frequent sparing of the ulnar nerve
- **C.** Frequent sparing of the musculocutaneous nerve
- **D.** High incidence of pneumothorax

797. A 68-year-old woman is to undergo lower-extremity surgery under spinal anesthesia. Which of the following statements concerning the immediate physiologic response to the surgical incision is **TRUE**?
- **A.** The cardiovascular (CV) response to stress will be blocked, but the adrenergic response will not
- **B.** The adrenergic response to stress will be blocked, but the CV response will not
- **C.** Both the adrenergic and CV responses will be blocked
- **D.** Neither the adrenergic nor the CV response will be blocked

798. The "snap" felt just before entering the epidural space represents passage through which ligament?
   A. Posterior longitudinal ligament
   B. Ligamentum flavum
   C. Supraspinous ligament
   D. Interspinous ligament

799. The common element thought to be present in cases of cauda equina syndrome after continuous spinal anesthesia is
   A. Use of microcatheter
   B. Maldistribution of local anesthetic
   C. Administration of lidocaine
   D. Addition of epinephrine

800. When performing a single-shot spinal anesthetic, the level of block for motor, sensory, and sympathetic blocks differs often by at least two dermatomes. Which of the following sequences is correct from the highest to the lowest level of block?
   A. Sensory, sympathetic, motor
   B. Sympathetic, sensory, motor
   C. Sympathetic, motor, sensory
   D. Sensory, motor, sympathetic

801. A 95-year-old woman has persistent and prolonged thoracic pain after a herpes zoster infection. Which of the treatments below would be the **LEAST** efficacious in the treatment of her pain?
   A. Oral amitriptyline
   B. Oral clonidine
   C. Topical capsaicin ointment
   D. Topical lidocaine patch

802. The deep peroneal nerve innervates the
   A. Lateral aspect of the dorsum of the foot
   B. Entire dorsum of the foot
   C. Web space between the great toe and the second toe
   D. Medial aspect of the dorsum of the foot

803. The correct arrangement of local anesthetics in order of their ability to produce cardiotoxicity from most to least is
   A. Bupivacaine, lidocaine, ropivacaine
   B. Bupivacaine, ropivacaine, lidocaine
   C. Ropivacaine, bupivacaine, lidocaine
   D. Lidocaine, ropivacaine, bupivacaine

804. Allodynia is defined as
   A. Spontaneous pain in an area or region that is anesthetic
   B. Pain initiated or caused by a primary lesion or dysfunction in the nervous system
   C. An increased response to a stimulus that is normally painful
   D. Pain caused by a stimulus that does not normally provoke pain

805. The primary mechanism by which the action of tetracaine is terminated when used for spinal anesthesia is
   A. Systemic absorption
   B. Uptake into neurons
   C. Hydrolysis by pseudocholinesterase
   D. Hydrolysis by nonspecific esterases

806. Complex regional pain syndrome (CRPS) type I (reflex sympathetic dystrophy [RSD]) is differentiated from CRPS type II (causalgia) by knowledge of its
   A. Etiology
   B. Chronicity
   C. Type of symptoms
   D. Rapidity of onset

807. The primary determinant of local anesthetic potency is
   A. pKa
   B. Molecular weight
   C. Lipid solubility
   D. Protein binding

808. Which of the following would have the **GREATEST** effect on the level of sensory blockade after a subarachnoid injection of hyperbaric 0.75% bupivacaine?
   A. Patient age
   B. Addition of epinephrine to the local anesthetic solution
   C. Patient weight
   D. Patient position

809. Which of the following local anesthetics would produce the **LOWEST** concentration in the fetus relative to the maternal serum concentration during a continuous lumbar epidural?
   A. Ropivacaine
   B. Bupivacaine
   C. Lidocaine
   D. Chloroprocaine

810. Severe hypotension associated with high spinal anesthesia is caused primarily by
   A. Decreased cardiac output secondary to decreased preload
   B. Decreased systemic vascular resistance
   C. Decreased cardiac output secondary to bradycardia
   D. Decreased cardiac output secondary to decreased myocardial contractility

811. Select the one **TRUE** statement concerning phantom limb pain.
   A. The incidence of phantom limb pain increases with more distal amputations
   B. Most amputees do not experience phantom limb pain
   C. Nerve blocks may be used to decrease the incidence of phantom limb pain
   D. Traumatic amputees have a much higher incidence of phantom limb pain than nontraumatic amputees

812. Which of the following is **TRUE** regarding IV regional anesthesia (Bier block)?
- **A.** Useful for postoperative pain in extremity surgery
- **B.** Can be used for extremity surgeries lasting 2 to 3 hours
- **C.** Bupivacaine is the drug of choice for prolonged blocks
- **D.** Lidocaine is most commonly used

813. Select the **FALSE** statement regarding spinal anatomy and spinal anesthesia.
- **A.** The addition of phenylephrine to lidocaine will prolong spinal anesthesia
- **B.** A high thoracic sensory block will result in total sympathetic blockade
- **C.** The largest vertebral interspace is L5-S1
- **D.** The dural sac extends to the S4-S5 interspace

814. Four days after a left total hip arthroplasty, an obese 62-year-old woman complains of severe back pain in the region where the epidural was placed. Over the ensuing 72 hours, the back pain gradually worsens and a severe aching pain that radiates down the left leg to the knee develops. The **MOST** likely diagnosis is
- **A.** Epidural abscess
- **B.** Epidural hematoma
- **C.** Anterior spinal artery syndrome
- **D.** Meralgia paresthetica

815. Which of the following choices is **NOT** consistent with a limb affected by complex regional pain syndrome (CRPS)
- **A.** Allodynia
- **B.** Dermatomal distribution of pain
- **C.** Atrophy of the involved extremity
- **D.** Hyperesthesia

816. The **MAIN** advantage of neurolytic nerve blockade with phenol versus alcohol is
- **A.** Denser blockade
- **B.** Blockade is permanent
- **C.** The effects of the block can be evaluated immediately
- **D.** The block is less painful

817. A 75-year-old man is scheduled to undergo elective orchiectomy for prostate cancer. The patient has selected spinal anesthesia. What is the minimum dermatomal level that must be achieved to carry out this operation?
- **A.** T4
- **B.** T10
- **C.** L3
- **D.** S1

818. The artery of Adamkiewicz **MOST** frequently arises from the aorta at which spinal level?
- **A.** T1-T4
- **B.** T5-T8
- **C.** T9-T12
- **D.** L1-L4

819. Which local anesthetic has the longest elimination half-time ($T_{1/2}$)?
- **A.** Bupivacaine
- **B.** Lidocaine
- **C.** Mepivacaine
- **D.** Ropivacaine

820. Important landmarks for performing a sciatic nerve block (classic approach of Labat) include
- **A.** Iliac crest, sacral hiatus, and greater trochanter
- **B.** Iliac crest, coccyx, and greater trochanter
- **C.** Posterior superior iliac spine, coccyx, and greater trochanter
- **D.** Posterior superior iliac spine, greater trochanter, and sacral hiatus

821. A 76-year-old female patient is undergoing a carotid endarterectomy under a deep cervical plexus nerve block. Which of the following complications would be **LEAST** likely with this unilateral block?
- **A.** Unilateral phrenic nerve paralysis
- **B.** Subarachnoid injection
- **C.** Blockade of the spinal accessory nerve
- **D.** Vertebral artery injection

822. A retrobulbar block anesthetizes each of the following nerves **EXCEPT**
- **A.** Ciliary nerves
- **B.** Cranial nerve III (oculomotor nerve)
- **C.** Cranial nerve VII (facial nerve)
- **D.** Cranial nerve VI (abducens nerve)

823. Which of the following muscles of the larynx is innervated by the external branch of the superior laryngeal nerve?
- **A.** Vocalis muscle
- **B.** Thyroarytenoid muscles
- **C.** Posterior cricoarytenoid muscle
- **D.** Cricothyroid muscle

824. All of the following agents are acceptable for use in a Bier block **EXCEPT**
- **A.** 0.5% Lidocaine
- **B.** 0.5% Mepivacaine
- **C.** 0.25% Bupivacaine
- **D.** 0.5% Prilocaine

825. The stellate ganglion lies in closest proximity to which of the following vascular structures?
- **A.** Common carotid artery
- **B.** Internal carotid artery
- **C.** Vertebral artery
- **D.** Aorta

826. Which of the following structures in the antecubital fossa is the **MOST** medial?
- **A.** Brachial artery
- **B.** Radial nerve
- **C.** Tendon of the biceps
- **D.** Median nerve

827. During placement of an epidural in a 78-year-old patient scheduled for a total knee arthroplasty, the patient complains of a sharp, sustained pain radiating down his left leg as the catheter is inserted to 2 cm. The **MOST** appropriate action at this time would be to
   A. Leave the catheter at 2 cm, and give a test dose
   B. Give a small dose to relieve pain, then advance 1 cm
   C. Withdraw the catheter 1 cm, then give a test dose
   D. Withdraw the needle and catheter, then reinsert in a new position

828. Cutaneous innervation of the plantar surface of the foot is provided by the
   A. Sural nerve
   B. Posterior tibial nerve
   C. Saphenous nerve
   D. Deep peroneal nerve

829. A 32-year-old army officer is unable to oppose the left thumb and left little finger after an 8-hour exploratory laparotomy under general anesthesia. He had an IV induction through a peripheral IV and had a second IV placed in the antecubital fossa after he was asleep. Damage to which of the following nerves would **MOST** likely account for this deficit?
   A. Radial
   B. Ulnar
   C. Median
   D. Musculocutaneous

830. A 57-year-old patient is scheduled for hemorrhoidectomy. The patient has a history of mild chronic obstructive pulmonary disease, hypertension, and traumatic foot amputation from a tractor accident. His only hospitalizations were for two suicide attempts related to phantom limb sensations 10 years ago. He takes phenelzine (Nardil), thiazide, and potassium. Which of the following anesthetic techniques would be **MOST** appropriate for this patient?
   A. Spinal anesthetic with 0.5% hyperbaric bupivacaine
   B. Epidural anesthetic with 0.5% bupivacaine
   C. Local infiltration with lidocaine and epinephrine, sedation with propofol and meperidine
   D. General anesthesia with propofol, succinylcholine, nitrous oxide, and fentanyl

831. If the recurrent laryngeal nerve were transected bilaterally, the vocal cords would
   A. Be in the open position
   B. Be in the closed position
   C. Be in the intermediate position (i.e., 2-3 mm apart)
   D. Not be affected unless the superior laryngeal nerve were also injured

832. A 63-year-old woman undergoes total knee arthroplasty under spinal anesthesia. Two days later she complains of a severe headache. Pain intensity is not related to posture. The **LEAST** likely cause of this headache is
   A. Caffeine withdrawal
   B. Viral illness
   C. Migraine
   D. Postdural puncture headache (PDPH)

833. What is the **CORRECT** order of structures (from cephalad to caudad) in the intercostal space?
   A. Nerve, artery, vein
   B. Vein, nerve, artery
   C. Vein, artery, nerve
   D. Artery, nerve, vein

834. Which of the following types of regional anesthesia is associated with the **GREATEST** serum concentration of lidocaine?
   A. Intercostal
   B. Epidural
   C. Brachial plexus
   D. Femoral nerve block

835. Differences in which of the following local anesthetic properties account for the fact that the onset of an epidural block with 3% 2-chloroprocaine is more rapid than 2% lidocaine?
   A. Protein binding
   B. pKa
   C. Lipid solubility
   D. Concentration

836. A 69-year-old man with a history of diabetes mellitus and chronic renal failure is to undergo placement of a dialysis fistula under regional anesthesia. During needle manipulation for a supraclavicular brachial plexus block, the patient begins to cough and complain of chest pain and shortness of breath. The **MOST** likely diagnosis is
   A. Angina
   B. Pneumothorax
   C. Phrenic nerve irritation
   D. Intravascular injection of local anesthetic

837. Each of the following statements is true concerning a femoral nerve block **EXCEPT**
   A. The femoral nerve primarily arises from the second to the fourth lumbar nerve roots
   B. The femoral nerve provides sensation to the anterior and medial aspect of the thigh
   C. The femoral nerve lies lateral to the femoral artery and femoral vein
   D. Proper needle placement produces sartorius muscle contraction without patellar movement when electrically stimulated

838. If a needle is introduced 1.5 cm inferior and 1.5 cm lateral to the pubic tubercle, to which nerve will it lie in close proximity?
  A. Obturator nerve
  B. Femoral nerve
  C. Lateral femoral cutaneous nerve
  D. Ilioinguinal nerve

839. The **MOST** common complication associated with a supraclavicular brachial plexus block is
  A. Blockade of the phrenic nerve
  B. Intravascular injection into the vertebral artery
  C. Blockade of the recurrent laryngeal nerve
  D. Pneumothorax

840. Which portion of the upper extremity is **NOT** innervated by the brachial plexus?
  A. Posterior medial portion of the arm
  B. Elbow
  C. Lateral portion of the forearm
  D. Medial portion of the forearm

841. Which section of the brachial plexus is blocked with a supraclavicular block?
  A. Roots/trunks
  B. Trunks/divisions
  C. Cords
  D. Branches

842. A celiac plexus block would **NOT** effectively treat pain resulting from a malignancy involving which of the following organs?
  A. Uterus
  B. Stomach
  C. Pancreas
  D. Gallbladder

843. A healthy 27-year-old woman stepped on a nail and is to undergo débridement of a wound on her right great toe. She is anxious about general anesthesia but agrees to an ankle block with mild sedation. Which nerves must be adequately blocked in order to perform the surgery?
  A. Deep peroneal, posterior tibial, saphenous, sural
  B. Deep peroneal, saphenous, superficial peroneal, sural
  C. Deep peroneal, posterior tibial, superficial peroneal, sural
  D. Deep peroneal, superficial peroneal, posterior tibial, saphenous

844. A 54-year-old man is administered morphine via patient-controlled analgesia (PCA) pump after a left total hip arthroplasty. The pump is programmed to deliver a maximum dose of 2 mg every 15 minutes (lockout time) as needed for patient comfort. The total maximum dose that can be delivered in 4 hours is 30 mg. On the first day the patient receives 15 doses every 4 hours by pressing the delivery button every 15 to 18 minutes. How should his pain control be further managed?
  A. Discontinue the PCA pump and administer intramuscular morphine
  B. Increase the lockout time from 15 to 25 minutes
  C. Change the analgesic from morphine to meperidine
  D. Increase the dose to 3 mg every 15 minutes as needed up to a total maximum dose of 40 mg every 4 hours

845. The mechanism of low-frequency transcutaneous electrical nerve stimulation (TENS) units in relieving pain is
  A. Direct electrical inhibition of type A-δ and C fibers
  B. Depletion of neurotransmitter in nociceptors
  C. Hyperpolarization of spinothalamic tract neurons
  D. Activation of inhibitory neurons

846. Epidural use of which of the following opioids would result in the **GREATEST** incidence of delayed respiratory depression?
  A. Sufentanil
  B. Fentanyl
  C. Morphine sulfate
  D. Hydromorphone

847. A 21-year-old patient reports tingling in her thumb during her cesarean section under epidural anesthesia. To which dermatomal level would this correspond?
  A. C5
  B. C6
  C. C7
  D. C8

848. Which of the following would hasten the onset and increase the clinical duration of action of a local anesthetic, and provide the **GREATEST** depth of motor and sensory blockade when used for epidural anesthesia?
  A. Increasing the volume of local anesthetic
  B. Increasing the concentration of local anesthetic
  C. Increasing the dose
  D. Placing the patient in the head-down position

849. Select the **FALSE** statement concerning neurolytic nerve blocks.
   A. Destruction of peripheral nerves can be followed by a denervation hypersensitivity that is worse than the original pain
   B. Neurolytic blocks should be reserved for patients with short life expectancies
   C. Neurolytic blockade with phenol is permanent
   D. Intrathecal neurolysis may be an effective management for certain pain conditions

850. Transient neurologic symptoms (TNS) after spinal anesthesia are associated with each of the following **EXCEPT**
   A. Lidocaine
   B. Lithotomy position
   C. Ambulatory anesthesia
   D. Concentration of local anesthetic injected

851. After you select the appropriate ultrasound transducer, you can adjust several factors to optimize the image for regional anesthesia. Which of the following descriptions is **FALSE?**
   A. Frequency—higher-frequency ultrasound use is better for viewing deep structures
   B. Depth—adjusted to limit the centimeters of viewing area on the monitor
   C. Gain—increased gain produces increased brightness
   D. Frequency—higher-frequency ultrasound use produces better image resolution

852. Each of the following is associated with an increased incidence of PDPHs **EXCEPT**
   A. Younger adults
   B. Early ambulation
   C. Pregnancy
   D. Large needle size

853. Each of the following items describes pain in the abdominal viscera **EXCEPT**
   A. Pain is transmitted via the vagus nerve
   B. The nerve fibers are type C
   C. Pain is characterized by a dull aching or burning sensation
   D. Distention of the transverse colon causes more pain than surgical transection

854. Which of the following blocks has the **LONGEST** duration of action when bupivacaine with epinephrine is administered?
   A. Axillary
   B. Epidural
   C. Infiltration
   D. Spinal

855. All of the following statements concerning a psoas compartment block are true **EXCEPT**
   A. Compartment block is used to provide unilateral anesthesia to the proximal aspect of the thigh and hip
   B. Stimulation of the quadriceps muscle demonstrates good needle placement
   C. Complete leg anesthesia can be obtained when combined with a sciatic nerve block
   D. Continuous catheters are not used because the amount of drug infused would lead to toxicity

856. A 35-year-old woman receives a popliteal block for ankle and foot surgery. Which other nerve must be blocked in order to have complete anesthesia of the foot?
   A. Superficial peroneal nerve
   B. Sural nerve
   C. Saphenous nerve
   D. Posterior tibial nerve

857. The most common complication of a celiac plexus block is
   A. Hypotension
   B. Seizure
   C. Retroperitoneal hematoma
   D. Constipation

858. The occipital portion of the skull receives sensory innervation from
   A. Spinal accessory nerve (nerve XI)
   B. Facial nerve (nerve VII)
   C. Ophthalmic branch of trigeminal nerve (nerve V)
   D. Cervical plexus

859. Each of the following is a potential complication of thoracic paravertebral blocks **EXCEPT**
   A. Pneumothorax
   B. Epidural spread of local anesthetic
   C. Hypertension
   D. Total spinal

860. After placement of an epidural catheter in a 55-year-old patient for total hip arthroplasty, an entire epidural dose is administered into the subarachnoid space. Physiologic effects consistent with subarachnoid injection of large volumes of local anesthetic include all of the following **EXCEPT**
   A. Hypotension and bradycardia
   B. Respiratory depression
   C. Constricted pupils
   D. Possible cauda equina syndrome

861. A 49-year-old type 1 diabetic patient with a long history of burning pain in the right lower extremity receives a spinal anesthetic with 100 mg of procaine with 5% dextrose. The patient reports no relief in symptoms but has complete bilateral motor blockade. What diagnosis is consistent with this differential blockade examination?
  A. Diabetic neuropathy
  B. Central pain
  C. Myofascial pain
  D. Complex regional pain syndrome (CRPS) I (RSD)

862. An 18-year-old man has a seizure during placement of an interscalene brachial plexus block with 0.5% bupivacaine. The anesthesiologist begins to hyperventilate the patient's lungs with 100% O_2 using an anesthesia bag and mask. The rationale for this therapy includes all of the following **EXCEPT**
  A. The therapy helps to prevent and treat hypoxia
  B. Hyperventilation decreases blood flow and delivery of local anesthetic to the brain
  C. Hyperventilation elevates the seizure threshold
  D. Hyperventilation induces alkalosis and converts local anesthetics to the protonated (ionized) form, which is less likely to cross the cell membranes

863. Para-aminobenzoic acid is a metabolite of
  A. Mepivacaine
  B. Ropivacaine
  C. Bupivacaine
  D. Procaine

864. Which statement concerning peripheral nerve structure and function is **FALSE?**
  A. Both nonmyelinated and myelinated nerves are surrounded by Schwann cells
  B. The speed of propagation of an action potential along a nerve axon is greatly enhanced by myelin
  C. Generation of an action potential is an "all-or-nothing" phenomenon
  D. Myelination renders nerves less sensitive to local anesthetic blockade

865. A 42-year-old woman with a morbid fear of general anesthesia receives an interscalene block for shoulder arthroscopy consisting of 20 mL 0.5% ropivacaine. Much of her arm, shoulder, and hand are numb, but the patient complains of pain as the incision is made at the upper portion of the shoulder. The most appropriate next step is to
  A. Repeat block
  B. Perform intercostobrachial block
  C. Perform superficial cervical plexus block
  D. Perform a deep cervical plexus block

866. According to the 2016 American Society of Regional Anesthesia and Pain Medicine (ASRA) practice advisory on infectious complications of regional anesthesia and pain medicine, the **MOST** important action to maintain aseptic technique and prevent cross-contamination during regional anesthesia techniques is
  A. Wearing a surgical gown
  B. Hand washing
  C. Using soap and water instead of alcohol-based antiseptics
  D. Using povidone-iodine (e.g., Betadine) instead of alcohol-based chlorhexidine to scrub

867. A 75-year-old woman with a history of pulmonary embolism is scheduled for a right lower lobectomy for lung cancer. She is receiving dalteparin (Fragmin) for deep vein thrombosis (DVT) prophylaxis. How long after her last dose should one wait before placement of a thoracic epidural?
  A. 12 hours
  B. 24 hours
  C. 72 hours
  D. No waiting is necessary since the dose for prophylaxis is low

868. How long should a patient be off clopidogrel (Plavix) before a central neuraxial block is performed?
  A. 24 hours
  B. 7 days
  C. 14 days
  D. No waiting necessary

869. Addition of bicarbonate to local anesthetics results in
  A. Delayed onset of action
  B. Reduced toxicity
  C. Increased duration of action
  D. Reduced pain with skin infiltration

870. Through which of the following would a spinal needle **NOT** pass during a midline placement of a subarachnoid block in the L3-L4 lumbar space?
  A. Supraspinous ligament
  B. Interspinous ligament
  C. Posterior longitudinal ligament
  D. Dura mater

871. What epidural dose of bupivacaine will give sensory analgesia similar to 10 mL of 2% lidocaine?
  A. 5 mL of 0.25%
  B. 10 mL of 0.25%
  C. 5 mL of 0.5%
  D. 10 mL of 0.5%

872. Each of the following additives to a spinal anesthetic possesses analgesic properties **EXCEPT**
A. Clonidine
B. Hydromorphone
C. Epinephrine
D. All of the above have analgesic properties

873. Which of the following local anesthetics is inappropriately paired with a clinical application because of its properties or toxicity?
A. Tetracaine, topical anesthesia
B. Bupivacaine, IV anesthesia
C. Prilocaine, infiltrative anesthesia
D. Chloroprocaine, epidural anesthesia

874. Discharge criteria from the PACU would be reached **FASTEST** after a 20- to 30-mL volume of which of the following epidurally administered local anesthetics?
A. 3% 2-Chloroprocaine
B. 2% Lidocaine
C. 0.75% Ropivacaine
D. 0.5% Levobupivacaine

875. A caudal block (performed under sevoflurane general anesthesia) with 0.25% bupivacaine and 1:200,000 epinephrine is planned for postoperative analgesia after bilateral inguinal hernia repair in a 5-month-old patient. Each of the following would be consistent with an intravascular injection **EXCEPT**
A. Systolic blood pressure increase by greater than 15 mm Hg
B. Heart rate decrease by greater than 10 beats/min
C. Ventricular extrasystoles
D. Increase in T-wave amplitude >25% over baseline

876. Which is **NOT** a potential complication of a stellate ganglion block?
A. Recurrent laryngeal nerve paralysis
B. Subarachnoid block
C. Brachial plexus block
D. Increased heart rate

877. Discontinuation of which of the following antiplatelet medications, for 14 days, would be necessary before a spinal could be safely administered?
A. Aspirin
B. Clopidogrel
C. Ticlopidine
D. Abciximab (GPIIb/IIIa)

878. Three days after knee arthroscopy under spinal anesthesia, a 55-year-old patient complains of double vision and difficulty hearing. The other likely finding would be
A. Headache
B. Fever
C. Weakness in legs
D. Mental status changes

879. Which of the following statements is **TRUE** concerning transversus abdominis plane (TAP) block?
A. Ultrasound is useful in finding the intercostal nerves
B. The local anesthetic is injected directly into the transversus abdominis muscle
C. The subcostal, ilioinguinal, and iliohypogastric nerves are blocked
D. 10 mL of local anesthetic is all that is needed for good spread

880. Which of the following nerves can be electrically stimulated at the ankle to produce flexion of the toes?
A. Posterior tibial nerve
B. Saphenous nerve
C. Deep peroneal nerve
D. Superficial peroneal nerve

881. Which motor response from peripheral nerve stimulation is **INCORRECTLY** paired with the appropriate nerve?
A. Musculocutaneous nerve—flexion of the forearm at the elbow
B. Radial nerve—extension of all digits as well as the wrist and forearm
C. Ulnar nerve—abduction of the thumb
D. Median nerve—flexion of the wrist, pronation of the forearm

882. During an airway examination, a 53-year-old patient mentions that his right thumb tingles and then becomes numb if he extends his head for more than a few seconds. This symptom **MOST** likely represents a(n)
A. Unstable C-spine
B. Lhermitte's phenomenon
C. C6 nerve root irritation
D. C8 radiculopathy

883. When performing an interscalene block with a peripheral nerve stimulator, you note diaphragmatic movement. You should now
A. Inject the local anesthetic, as the needle is in an appropriate location
B. Redirect the needle in an anterior direction
C. Redirect the needle in a posterior direction
D. Advance the needle about 0.5 cm more and inject

884. During placement of an interscalene block, the patient becomes hypotensive, bradycardic, apneic, and cyanotic. The **MOST** likely cause is
A. Vertebral artery injection
B. Phrenic nerve blockade
C. Total spinal
D. Stellate ganglion block

885. The reason that ropivacaine is marketed as pure S enantiomers is because the S form is associated with
   A. Increased potency
   B. Longer duration
   C. Reduced cardiac toxicity
   D. Reduced incidence of anaphylaxis

886. Nerves that originate from the sacral plexus include each of the following **EXCEPT**
   A. Femoral nerve
   B. Tibial nerve
   C. Sciatic nerve
   D. Common peroneal nerve

887. The only technique shown to prevent anesthetic-related nerve injury during placement of peripheral nerve blocks is
   A. Ultrasound-guided regional technique
   B. Transarterial technique
   C. Nerve stimulator
   D. None of the above

888. An axillary block is performed on a healthy 19-year-old athlete. A 30-mL quantity of 0.75% bupivacaine is injected incrementally. Five minutes after the bupivacaine injection, the patient has a seizure and experiences CV collapse. Which of the measures below is **NOT** indicated?
   A. Begin chest compressions at 100 per minute
   B. Ventilate with 100% oxygen
   C. Bolus propofol to bind local anesthetic
   D. Infuse 20% lipid emulsion

889. The structure **MOST** likely to be blocked during placement of an interscalene block in addition to the brachial plexus is the
   A. Phrenic nerve
   B. Vertebral artery
   C. Recurrent laryngeal nerve
   D. Vagus nerve

890. All of the following are symptoms of a developing epidural hematoma **EXCEPT**
   A. Radicular back pain
   B. Bowel and bladder dysfunction
   C. Motor deficits
   D. Fever

891. In addition to C nerve fibers, which nerve fibers carry pain impulses?
   A. A-alpha (Aα)
   B. A-beta (Aβ)
   C. A-delta (Aδ)
   D. B

892. An intradural mass lesion at the tip of a drug infusion catheter is **LEAST** likely to present as
   A. Increasing pain
   B. Development of numbness in T8 dermatomal pattern
   C. Hypopnea
   D. Perianal numbness

893. A healthy 25-year-old man is anesthetized for a sagittal split osteotomy. Anesthesia is induced with propofol, hydromorphone, and vecuronium and maintained with 2.1% sevoflurane and 50% N_2O. After induction, the nose is prepped with 4% lidocaine and 1% phenylephrine, and the patient is intubated through the right naris. Before emergence, the surgeon performs a bilateral inferior alveolar nerve block. The patient is reversed with neostigmine and glycopyrrolate. When the patient awakens, he is noted to have an 8-mm pupil on the right and a 3-mm pupil on the left. Results of physical examination are otherwise unremarkable. The most likely explanation for the dilated pupil is
   A. Right stellate ganglion block
   B. Accidental introduction of lidocaine into right eye
   C. Accidental introduction of phenylephrine into right eye
   D. Glycopyrrolate

894. Which statement concerning local anesthetics is **CORRECT?**
   A. The un-ionized form of a local anesthetic binds to the nerve membrane to actually block conduction
   B. If one node of Ranvier is blocked, conduction will be reliably interrupted
   C. The presence of myelin enhances the ability of a local anesthetic to block nerve conduction
   D. Local anesthetics block transmission by inhibiting the voltage-gated potassium ion channels

895. Postdural puncture headaches (PDPHs)
   A. Usually occur immediately following dural puncture
   B. Are relieved 8 to 12 hours after an epidural blood patch is performed
   C. Occur more frequently in nonpregnant patients compared with pregnant patients
   D. Can be associated with neurologic deficits

896. Which of the following procedures for treatment of chronic pain requires localization of the epidural space with an epidural needle as part of technique?
   A. Radio-frequency ablation of a lumbar facet joint
   B. Spinal cord stimulation
   C. Percutaneous disk decompression
   D. Vertebroplasty

897. Each of the following drugs has been used to treat neuropathic pain. Selective inhibition of serotonin and norepinephrine reuptake is the mechanism of which drug?

A. Duloxetine
B. Mexiletine
C. Gabapentin
D. Carbamazepine

DIRECTIONS (Questions 898 through 901): Please match the structure below with the letter that corresponds to it in the ultrasound image.

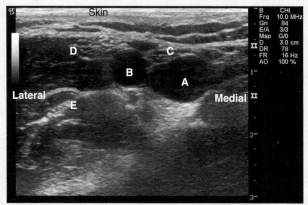

Modified from Hebl J: Mayo Clinic Atlas of Regional Anesthesia and Ultrasound-Guided Nerve Blockade, *New York, Oxford University Press, 2010, Figure 12A.*

898. Musculocutaneous nerve

899. Axillary artery

900. Axillary vein

901. Ulnar nerve

DIRECTIONS (Questions 902 through 914): Each group of questions consists of several numbered statements followed by lettered headings. For each numbered statement, select the ONE lettered heading that is most closely associated with it. Each lettered heading may be selected once, more than once, or not at all.

---

902. Phrenic nerve

903. Cardiac accelerator fibers

904. Pudendal nerve

905. Pain fibers to the uterus

906. Inhibitory presynaptic fibers to the gastrointestinal tract
    A. C3-C5
    B. T1-T4
    C. T5-T12
    D. T10-L1
    E. S2-S4

907. Sensory innervation of the mucous membranes of the nose

908. Main sensory innervation to superior and inferior parts of the hard and soft palate

909. Sensory innervation of the larynx above the vocal cords

910. Sensory innervation below the vocal cords to the carina

911. Sensory innervation to posterior third of the tongue

912. Sensory innervation to the pharyngeal walls and the tonsils

913. Motor innervation to the intrinsic muscles of the larynx, except cricothyroid muscle

914. Motor innervation to the cricothyroid muscle
    A. Trigeminal nerve
    B. Glossopharyngeal nerve
    C. Internal branch of the superior laryngeal nerve
    D. External branch of the superior laryngeal nerve
    E. Recurrent laryngeal nerve

788. (A) Neuropathic pain is persistent pain that occurs following damage or disease of the somatosensory nervous system. Three unique characteristics of neuropathic pain are spontaneous pain (absence of a stimulus), hyperalgesia (exaggerated pain to a mild painful stimulus) and allodynia (pain that occurs with a nonpainful stimulus such as light touch). The forms of neuropathic pain include PHN, diabetic peripheral neuropathy (DPN), Complex regional pain syndrome (CRPS), human immunodeficiency virus neuropathy, and phantom limb pain. Fibromyalgia is chronic widespread musculoskeletal pain accompanied by other symptoms such as excessive fatigue, sleep disturbances, and trouble with memory but may have a partial peripheral neuropathic component. Nociceptive pain, also called physiologic pain, has two main types: radicular pain (e.g., disk herniation) and somatic pain (e.g., facet or hip joint arthritic pain) *(Barash: Clinical Anesthesia, ed 8, pp 1611–1618; Miller: Basics of Anesthesia, ed 7, pp 770–776).*

789. (B) The treatment of pruritus, the most common side effect of neuraxial opiates, is primarily with opioid antagonists, mixed opioid agonist–antagonists, and antihistamine drugs (by their sedating effects). Nalbuphine is a mixed opioid agonist–antagonist; diphenhydramine has antihistamine properties. Propofol at very low doses (e.g., 10 mg) has been useful to treat pruritus, not only induced by neuraxial opiates but also the pruritus associated with cholestatic liver disease. Propofol does not affect analgesia, whereas opioid antagonists and mixed agonist–antagonists may reverse some or all of the analgesia, depending on dose. Dexmedetomidine is a highly selective α_2-receptor agonist that has a faster onset and shorter duration of action compared with clonidine. Dexmedetomidine has analgesic properties, can potentiate neuraxial analgesia when injected spinally, and can perhaps decrease the incidence of pruritus by reducing the amount of opioid dose used. It does not treat pruritus *(Miller: Miller's Anesthesia, ed 8, pp 2986–2987).*

790. (C) The maximum dose of local anesthetics containing 1:200,000 epinephrine that can be used for major nerve blocks in a healthy 70-kg adult is lidocaine, 500 mg; mepivacaine, 500 mg; prilocaine, 600 mg; bupivacaine, 225 mg; levobupivacaine, 225 mg; and ropivacaine, 250 mg *(Miller: Miller's Anesthesia, ed 8, p 1043).*

791. (B) 1:200,000 means: 1 g/200,000 mL = 1000 mg/200,000 mL = 1,000,000 mcg/ 200,000 mL = 5 mcg/mL *(Miller: Basics of Anesthesia, ed 7, p 147).*

792. (D) Postoperative urinary retention is common and may affect up to 70% of patients. The patient described in this question has several risk factors for urinary retention: male gender, age greater than 50, joint replacement surgery, and spinal anesthetic. The spinal anesthetic weakens detrusor muscle function through inhibition of S2-S4. The urge to urinate is also blocked until sensory function returns. A patient with free access to water and other fluids will continue to consume these, while the bladder becomes overly distended, sometimes as much as 1000 mL. Bladder volumes can be measured noninvasively, and catheterization should be considered if volume is greater than 500 mL and patient has no urge, or is unable, to void *(Miller: Basics of Anesthesia, ed 7, pp 298–299, 686).*

793. (C) Toxic reactions to local anesthetics are usually due to intravascular or intrathecal injection or to an excessive dosage. The initial symptoms of local anesthetic toxicity from high blood levels (inadvertent IV injection or excessive dosages) are light-headedness and dizziness, and numbness of the tongue. Patients also may note perioral numbness and tinnitus. Progressive central nervous system (CNS) excitatory effects include visual disturbances (difficulty focusing), auditory disturbances (tinnitus), shivering, muscular twitching, and, ultimately, generalized tonic-clonic seizures. CNS depression can ensue, leading to respiratory depression or arrest. Higher levels can lead to cardiovascular (CV) collapse. To help prevent excessively high levels of local anesthetic, common practice is to aspirate for blood and inject the local anesthetic slowly and incrementally, looking for signs of toxicity (and, if appropriate, adding epinephrine to use as an intravascular marker as noted by an increase in heart rate and blood pressure) *(Miller: Miller's Anesthesia, ed 8, pp 1048–1052).*

794. (B) The site of action of spinally administered opiates is the substantia gelatinosa of the spinal cord. Epidural administration is complicated by factors related to dural penetration, absorption in fat, and systemic uptake; therefore, the quantity of intrathecally administered opioid required to achieve effective analgesia is typically much smaller. Lipid-soluble opioids (e.g., fentanyl) have a faster onset of action but a shorter duration of action compared with the more water-soluble opioids (e.g., morphine). A dose of 1 to 5 mg of epidural morphine is approximately equal to an intrathecal dose of 0.1 to 0.3 mg of morphine. Onset time for epidural administration is 30 to 60 minutes with a peak effect in 90 to 120 minutes. Onset time for intrathecal administration is shorter than for epidural administration. Duration of 12 to 24 hours of analgesic effect can be expected by either route with morphine *(Miller: Miller's Anesthesia, ed 8, pp 2983–2984, Table 98-4; Suresh: Shnider and Levinson's Anesthesia for Obstetrics 5ᵗʰ ed, pp 185–187).*

795. (A) The principal mechanism of peripheral nerve injury is ischemia caused by stretching or compression of the nerves. Anesthetized patients are at increased risk for peripheral nerve injuries because they are unconscious and unable to complain about uncomfortable positions that an awake patient would not tolerate and because of reduced muscle tone that facilitates placement of patients into awkward positions. The ulnar nerve in particular is vulnerable because it passes around the posterior aspect of the medial epicondyle of the humerus. The ulnar nerve may become compressed between the medial epicondyle and the sharp edge of the operating table, leading to ischemia and possible nerve injury, which may be transient or permanent *(Miller: Basics of Anesthesia, ed 7, pp 330–333).*

796. (B) The major disadvantage of the interscalene block for hand and forearm surgery is that blockade of the inferior trunk (C8-T1) is often incomplete. Supplementation of the ulnar nerve often is required. The risk of pneumothorax is quite low, but blockade of the ipsilateral phrenic nerve occurs in up to 100% of blocks. This can cause respiratory compromise in patients with significant lung disease. Horner syndrome from blockade of the stellate ganglion can occur in 70% to 90% of patients if large volumes of local anesthetic are injected *(Miller: Miller's Anesthesia, ed 8, pp 1724–1727).*

797. (C) Surgical trauma includes a wide variety of physiologic responses. General anesthesia has no or only a slight inhibitory effect on endocrine and metabolic responses to surgery. Regional anesthesia inhibits the nociceptive signal from reaching the CNS and, therefore, has a significant inhibitory effect on the stress response, including adrenergic, CV, metabolic, immunologic, and pituitary. This effect is most pronounced with procedures on the lower part of the body and less with major abdominal and thoracic procedures. The variable effect is probably due to unblocked afferents (i.e., vagal, phrenic, or sympathetic *(Miller: Miller's Anesthesia, ed 8, pp 3139–3141).*

798. (B) The structures that are traversed by a needle placed in the midline before the epidural space are as follows: skin, subcutaneous tissue, supraspinous ligament, interspinous ligament, and ligamentum flavum. The ligamentum flavum is tough and dense, and a change in the resistance to advancing the needle is often perceived and, to many, feels like a "snap." The anterior and posterior longitudinal ligaments bind the vertebral bodies together. See also explanation and diagram in Question 870 *(Miller: Miller's Anesthesia, ed 8, pp 1685–1688).*

799. (B) The symptoms of cauda equina syndrome include low back pain, bilateral lower-extremity weakness, saddle anesthesia, and loss of bowel and bladder control. Pooling of local anesthetics in dependent areas of the spine within the subarachnoid space has been identified as the causative factor in cases of cauda equina syndrome. Microlumen catheters (27-gauge and smaller) may enhance the nonuniform distribution of solutions within the intrathecal space, but cauda equina syndrome has been associated with the use of larger catheters, 5% lidocaine with dextrose, and 2% lidocaine, as well as 0.5% tetracaine *(Barash: Clinical Anesthesia, ed 8, p 1199).*

800. (B) Differential nerve blockade is a complex process with both peripheral nerve blocks and central nerve blocks. With spinal anesthesia, the sympathetic nerve block may be anywhere between two and six dermatomes higher than the sensory block, as noted by pinprick. Sensory block is two to three dermatomes higher than the motor block. However, with epidural anesthesia, the sympathetic and sensory blocks tend to be at the same dermatome level and are higher than the motor block *(Barash: Clinical Anesthesia, ed 8, p 923).*

801. (B) Acute herpes zoster is due to the reactivation of the varicella-zoster virus. Acute treatment includes symptomatic pain treatment and antiviral drugs (e.g., acyclovir, famciclovir, or valacyclovir). It is typically a benign and self-limiting disease in patients younger than 50 years of age. As one gets older, the incidence of postherpetic neuralgia (PHN), defined as pain persisting for more than 3 months after resolution of the rash, increases. The incidence of PHN is about 30% to 50% in patients older than 50 years, although current vaccination to varicella-zoster will hopefully decrease incidence over time. Treatment of established PHN has been shown to be resistant to interventions and, thus, can be difficult. However, proven therapies include tricyclic antidepressants, anticonvulsants, opioids, topical local anesthetics (e.g., 5% lidocaine patch), topical capsaicin, and TENS. Sympathetic blocks can provide excellent analgesia but are most useful during the more acute stages of the disease rather than during the late chronic stages. Sympathetic blocks in the acute stages may decrease the incidence of PHN. Oral clonidine, which is used to treat hypertension and opioid withdrawal, has not been shown to be an effective treatment for PHN *(Barash: Clinical Anesthesia, ed 8, p 1616)*.

802. (C) The deep peroneal nerve innervates the short extensors of the toes and the skin of the web space between the great and second toe. The deep peroneal nerve is blocked at the ankle by infiltration between the tendons of the anterior tibial and extensor hallucis longus muscles *(Barash: Clinical Anesthesia, ed 8, p 962)*.

803. (B) CNS toxicity from local anesthetics generally parallels anesthetic potency (e.g., bupivacaine is four times as potent as lidocaine, and ropivacaine is three times as potent as lidocaine). CV toxicity occurs at a higher blood level than CNS toxicity. For bupivacaine and ropivacaine, CV toxicity occurs at two times the CNS dose, whereas for lidocaine, the CV toxicity occurs at seven times the CNS toxicity levels, making lidocaine the least cardiotoxic and bupivacaine the most cardiotoxic of the listed local anesthetics *(Miller: Miller's Anesthesia, ed 8, pp 1049–1050)*.

804. (D) The International Association for the Study of Pain (IASP) has defined several pain terms. Anesthesia dolorosa refers to spontaneous pain in an area or region that is anesthetic. Neuropathic pain is pain initiated or caused by a primary lesion or dysfunction in the nervous system. Dysesthesia is an unpleasant abnormal sensation, whether spontaneous or evoked. Hyperalgesia is an increased response to a stimulus that is normally painful. Allodynia is pain caused by a stimulus that does not normally provoke pain *(Barash: Clinical Anesthesia, ed 8, p 1563)*.

805. (A) Ester local anesthetics are hydrolyzed by cholinesterase enzymes that are present mainly in plasma and, in a smaller amount, in the liver. Because there are no cholinesterase enzymes present in cerebrospinal fluid (CSF), the anesthetic effect of tetracaine will persist until it is absorbed into systemic circulation. The rate of hydrolysis varies, with chloroprocaine being fastest, procaine intermediate, and tetracaine the slowest. Toxicity is inversely related to the rate of hydrolysis; tetracaine is, therefore, the most toxic of the three esters listed in this question *(Flood: Stoelting's Pharmacology and Physiology in Anesthetic Practice, 5th ed, p 290)*.

806. (A) CRPS type I, formally referred to as reflex sympathetic dystrophy, or RSD, is a clinical syndrome of continuous burning pain, usually occurring after minor trauma. Patients present with various sensory, motor, autonomic, and trophic changes. CRPS type II (causalgia) exhibits the same features of RSD, but there is a preceding nerve injury *(Barash: Clinical Anesthesia, ed 8, pp 1048–1049, 1617)*.

807. (C) The potency of local anesthetics is directly related to their lipid solubility. In general, the speed or onset of action of local anesthetics is related to the pKa of the drug. Drugs with lower pKa values have a higher amount of nonionized molecules at physiologic pH and penetrate the lipid portion of nerves faster (an exception is chloroprocaine, which has a fast onset of action that may be related to the higher concentration of drug used) *(Miller: Basics of Anesthesia, ed 7, p 142)*.

808. (D) Many factors have an effect on the sensory level after a subarachnoid injection. The baricity of the solution and the patient position (e.g., lateral, sitting, prone) are the most important determinants of sensory level. The other listed options have little to no effect on sensory level. Patient height also has little effect on sensory level *(Miller: Miller's Anesthesia, ed 8, pp 1693–1694)*.

809. (D) Chloroprocaine is an ester local anesthetic that is rapidly metabolized by pseudocholinesterase. With the epidural injection of chloroprocaine, very little drug is available to cross the placenta, because the half-life is about 45 seconds in the mother (and that which crosses is also rapidly metabolized, making fetal effects essentially nonsignificant). The amide local anesthetics (e.g., ropivacaine, bupivacaine, lidocaine) undergo liver metabolism and have relatively long half-lives, but with prolonged epidural administration may accumulate in the fetus *(Miller: Miller's Anesthesia, ed 8, p 2344)*.

810. (A) Hypotension with a high spinal anesthesia is related to sympathetic blockade, venodilation (decreases preload), arterial dilation (decreases afterload), and a decrease in heart rate (cardioaccelerator fibers T1-T4 blockade and a fall in right atrial filling that affects the intrinsic chronotropic stretch receptors). With a high spinal, the decrease in venous dilation is the predominant cause of hypotension *(Miller: Miller's Anesthesia, ed 8, pp 1688–1690)*.

811. (C) The incidence of phantom limb pain is estimated to be up to 80% after an amputation. This pain may be immediate but, in many cases, will develop within a few days of the amputation. The pain also may not be present all the time but only a few days a month. The incidence of phantom limb pain does not differ between traumatic and nontraumatic amputees. The incidence of phantom pain increases with more proximal amputation. About 50% of patients will have a decrease in pain over time; the rest have no change or an increase in pain with time. Although very difficult to treat, nerve blocks are commonly used in the perioperative setting to decrease the incidence of phantom limb pain. Oral agents such as opioids, antidepressants, and gabapentin are commonly used, as well as TENS units, spinal cord stimulators, and biofeedback methods *(Barash: Clinical Anesthesia, ed 8, p 1618)*.

812. (D) IV regional anesthesia (IVRA, or Bier blocks after August Bier, who first described the technique) is simple to perform and is usually done only on an upper extremity. A small 20- or 22-gauge IV catheter is placed in the extremity to be blocked, then the limb is raised, and an Esmarch bandage is wrapped around the extremity to remove as much blood from the limb as possible, followed by the inflation of a tourniquet to 250 to 300 mm Hg, or 2.5 times the patient's systolic pressure, and injection of a local anesthetic into the limb. An IV line is always placed in another site (not below the tourniquet) in case sedation is needed for tourniquet pain, or in case local anesthetic toxicity develops when the tourniquet is eventually released. Typically, a minimum of 40 to 45 minutes of tourniquet time is needed to have enough local anesthetic to diffuse into the tissues to prevent serious systemic local anesthetic toxicity from developing when the tourniquet is deflated. For safety, the tourniquet is deflated for about 5 seconds and then reinflated for 45 seconds while one looks for signs of toxicity. This should be repeated four to five more times. Postoperative analgesia is lost once the tourniquet is deflated and the local anesthetic diffuses from the nerves. Tourniquet times less than 60 to 90 minutes are used to prevent pain and nerve damage from the tourniquet. Lidocaine 0.5% at a dose of 1.5 to 3 mg/kg is the most commonly administered local anesthetic because of its relative safety and effectiveness. About a 10-minute period is needed for surgical anesthesia to develop. Bupivacaine is not recommended for Bier blocks because of reports of CV toxicity and death that have occurred after the tourniquet was released *(Miller: Miller's Anesthesia, ed 8, p 1732)*.

813. (D) Both phenylephrine and epinephrine will prolong a spinal anesthetic when administering lidocaine. The Taylor approach for spinal anesthesia uses a paramedian approach to the L5-S1 interspace—the largest interspace of the vertebral column. The sympathetic nervous system originates in the thoracic and lumbar spinal cord T1-L3; therefore, a high thoracic sensory level can cause a complete sympathetic block. The dural sac extends to S2, not S4-S5. The spinal cord extends to L3 in the infant and L1-L2 in adults *(Miller: Miller's Anesthesia, ed 8, pp 1684–1693; Barash: Clinical Anesthesia, ed 8, pp 914–942)*.

814. (A) Development of an epidural abscess is fortunately an exceedingly rare complication of spinal and epidural anesthesia. Most anesthetic-related epidural abscesses are associated with epidural catheters. When an epidural abscess is developing, prompt recognition and treatment are essential if permanent sequelae are to be avoided. Symptoms from an epidural abscess may not become apparent until several days (mean, 5 days) after placement of the block. There are four clinical stages of epidural abscess symptom progression. Initially, localized back pain develops. The second stage includes nerve root or radicular pain. The third stage involves motor and sensory deficits or sphincter dysfunction, followed by the last stage of paraplegia. Unlike an epidural hematoma, in which severe back pain is the key feature, patients with epidural abscesses will complain of radicular pain approximately 3 days after development of the back pain. Fever may develop with an abscess and is rare with a hematoma. A magnetic resonance imaging (MRI) scan is helpful in the diagnosis. Anterior spinal artery syndrome is characterized predominantly by motor weakness or paralysis of the lower extremities. Meralgia paresthetica is related to entrapment of the lateral femoral cutaneous nerve as it courses below the inguinal ligament and is associated with burning pain over the lateral aspect of the thigh. It is not a complication of epidural anesthesia *(Barash: Clinical Anesthesia, ed 8, pp 939–941).*

815. (B) CRPS is associated with trauma. The main feature is burning, with continuous pain that is exacerbated by normal movement, cutaneous stimulation, or stress, usually weeks after the injury. The pain is not anatomically distributed. Other associated features include cool, red, clammy skin and hair loss in the involved extremity. Chronic cases may be associated with atrophy and osteoporosis *(Barash: Clinical Anesthesia, ed 8, p 161).*

816. (D) Neurolytic blockade with phenol (6%-10% in glycerine) is painless because phenol has a dual action as both a local anesthetic and a neurolytic agent. The initial block wears off over a 24-hour period, during which time neurolysis occurs. For this reason, you must wait a day to determine the effectiveness of the neurolytic block. Alcohol (50%-100% ethanol) is painful on injection and should be preceded by local anesthetic injection. Unfortunately, there is no neurolytic agent that affects only sympathetic fibers *(Miller: Miller's Anesthesia, ed 8, pp 1910–1911).*

817. (B) Testicular innervation can be traced up to the T10 dermatomal level. For this reason, any operation that involves manipulation or traction on the testicles must have adequate anesthesia to prevent pain. This can be achieved with spinal or epidural anesthesia, which is associated with a T10 level of blockade *(Miller, ed 8, p 2219).*

818. (C) Blood supply to the spinal cord comes from several sources. The anterior spinal artery is derived from the vertebral arteries and runs the entire length of the spinal cord and supplies the anterior two thirds of the cord. There are segmental arteries from the aorta that join the anterior spinal artery to help supply the spinal cord. One of the larger arteries is called the artery of Adamkiewicz, which arises from the lower thoracic area (T9-T12). Damage to this artery can lead to ischemia for the lower two thirds of the spinal cord and can result in paraplegia. The posterior one third of the cord is supplied by two posterior spinal arteries that also arise from the vertebral arteries and receive some blood supply from the segmental arteries *(Miller: Miller's Anesthesia, ed 8, p 1131).*

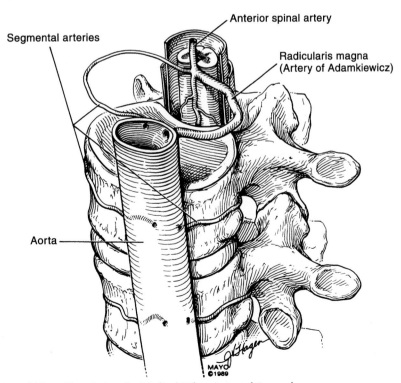

By permission of Mayo Foundation for Medical Education and Research.

819. (A) Amino ester local anesthetics undergo hydrolysis in the bloodstream and tend to have short elimination half-times. Amino amides undergo biotransformation by the liver and have longer elimination half-times. The elimination half-time for bupivacaine is 3.5 hours, for levobupivacaine is 3.5 hours, for lidocaine is 1.6 hours, for mepivacaine is 1.0 hour, for procaine is 0.1 hour, and for ropivacaine is 1.9 hours *(Miller: Miller's Anesthesia, ed 8, pp 1046–1047)*.

820. (D) To perform a sciatic nerve block, first draw a line from the posterior superior iliac spine to the greater trochanter of the femur, then draw a 5-cm line perpendicular from the midpoint of this line caudally and a second line from the sacral hiatus to the greater trochanter. The intersection of the second line with the perpendicular line marks the point of entry *(Miller: Miller's Anesthesia, ed 8, pp 1742–1743)*.

821. (C) Deep cervical plexus blocks (C2, C3, and C4) can be used for unilateral neck anesthesia for carotid endarterectomy and cervical node dissections. Complications of deep cervical plexus block include injection of the local anesthetic into the vertebral artery, subarachnoid space, or epidural space. Other nerves that may be anesthetized include the phrenic nerve (which is why bilateral deep cervical plexus blocks should be performed with caution, if at all) and the recurrent laryngeal nerve. Some local anesthetic may spread outside the deep cervical fascia and may produce blockade of the sympathetic chain, producing Horner syndrome. Inadvertent blockade of the recurrent laryngeal nerve has also been reported. The spinal accessory nerve, or cranial nerve XI, innervates the sternocleidomastoid muscle, as well as the trapezius muscle. The accessory nerve comes out cephalad to the injections *(Miller: Miller's Anesthesia, ed 8, pp 1722–1723)*.

822. (C) A retrobulbar block anesthetizes the three cranial nerves responsible for movement of the eye (cranial nerve III—oculomotor nerve, cranial nerve IV—trochlear nerve, and cranial nerve VI—abducens nerve). The ciliary ganglion (deep within the orbit and lateral to the optic nerve) and ciliary nerves are also blocked, providing anesthesia to the conjunctiva, cornea, and uvea. Branches of the facial nerve (cranial nerve VII) are not blocked by the retrobulbar block but are often separately blocked to produce akinesia of the eyelids *(Barash: Clinical Anesthesia, ed 8, pp 1383–1386)*.

823. (D) The vagus nerve innervates the airway by two branches: the superior laryngeal nerves and the recurrent laryngeal nerves. All of the muscles of the larynx are innervated by the recurrent laryngeal nerve except for the cricothyroid muscle. The superior laryngeal nerve divides into the internal and external laryngeal branches. The external laryngeal branch innervates the cricothyroid muscle. The internal laryngeal branch provides sensory fibers to the cords, epiglottis, and arytenoids *(Barash: Clinical Anesthesia, ed 8, p 768)*.

824. (C) Because of the potential for cardiotoxicity and because bupivacaine has no advantages over other local anesthetics in this setting, it is contraindicated for use in IV regional anesthesia *(Miller: Miller's Anesthesia, ed 8, p 1736)*.

825. (C)

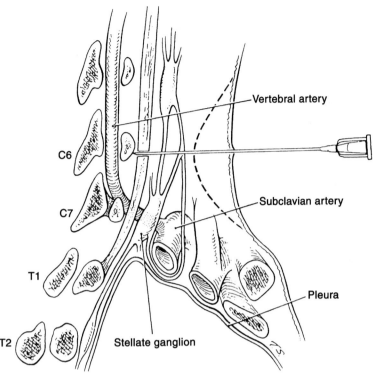

From Raj PP: Practical Management of Pain, *ed 2, St Louis, Mosby, 1992, p 785.*

The stellate ganglion usually lies in front of the neck of the first rib. The vertebral artery lies anterior to the ganglion, as it has just originated from the subclavian artery. After passing over the ganglion, it enters the vertebral foramen and lies posterior to the anterior tubercle of C6 *(Miller: Miller's Anesthesia, ed 8, p 1732).*

826. (D) The median nerve is the most medial structure in the antecubital fossa. To block this nerve, first the brachial artery is palpated at the level of the intercondylar line between the medial and lateral epicondyles, and then a needle is inserted just medial to the artery and directed perpendicularly to the skin *(Barash: Clinical Anesthesia, ed 8, p 977).*

827. (D) When an epidural catheter is placed without fluoroscopic guidance, the exact location of the needle tip relative to the anatomic structures of the back can only be surmised. If malposition of either the needle or the catheter is suspected, it is prudent to withdraw the entire apparatus and reinsert a second time, rather than pulling back on the catheter itself because of shearing. In this case, it is possible that the catheter tip has found its way into a nerve root. Under these circumstances, injection of a local anesthetic or opioid could produce pressure that could possibly lead to ischemia and neurologic damage. During placement or injection of a needle or epidural catheter, a paresthesia that is sustained is always a warning sign that should be heeded *(Barash: Clinical Anesthesia, ed 8, pp 914–915).*

828. (B) There are five nerves that innervate the ankle and foot: the posterior tibial, sural, superficial peroneal, deep peroneal, and saphenous nerves. All are branches of the sciatic nerve except for the saphenous nerve, which is a branch of the femoral nerve. These nerves are superficial at the level of the ankle and are easy to block. The posterior branch of the tibial nerve gives rise to the medial and lateral plantar nerves, which supply the plantar surface of the foot *(Barash: Clinical Anesthesia, ed 8, pp 986–998).*

829. (C) The median nerve is most frequently injured at the antecubital fossa by extravasation of IV drugs that are toxic to neural tissue, or by direct injury caused by the needle during attempts to cannulate the medial cubital or basilic veins. The median nerve provides sensory innervation to the palmar surface of the lateral three and one-half fingers and adjacent palm, and motor function to the abductor pollicis brevis, flexor pollicis brevis, and opponens pollicis muscles *(Miller: Basics of Anesthesia, ed 7, p 313).*

830. (D) Reactivation of phantom limb sensations has been reported in patients who have received both spinal and epidural anesthetics (90% in some series). In the majority of these cases (80%), phantom limb sensation persisted until the block receded. With a history of phantom limb sensations that drove this patient to attempt suicide, it is probably wise to avoid spinal and epidural anesthetics. Phenelzine (Nardil) is a monoamine oxidase (MAO) inhibitor that is occasionally used for the treatment of depression. Any anesthetic or combination of techniques that involves meperidine is contraindicated in patients receiving MAO inhibitors. The combination of meperidine and MAO inhibitors has been associated with hyperthermia, hypotension, hypertension, ventilatory depression, skeletal muscle rigidity, seizures, and coma. Because of this unfavorable drug interaction, meperidine should be avoided in patients receiving MAO inhibitors. Accordingly, the only acceptable choice in this question would be general anesthesia with propofol, succinylcholine, nitrous oxide, and fentanyl. As an interesting side point, the drug phenelzine prolongs the duration of action of succinylcholine by decreasing plasma cholinesterase activity *(Miller: Miller's Anesthesia, ed 8, p 909)*.

831. (C) The recurrent laryngeal nerve innervates all the muscles of the larynx (e.g., abductors and adductors) except the cricothyroid muscle (which tenses the vocal cords and is innervated by the external branch of the superior laryngeal nerve). With complete bilateral transections of the recurrent laryngeal nerve, both the abductor and adductor muscles are affected, and the vocal cords will adopt an intermediate position (i.e., lie within 2-3 mm of the midline). Acute complete injury to the recurrent laryngeal nerves can result in stridor and respiratory distress requiring treatment (e.g., intubation and possible tracheostomy). If a patient sustained a partial bilateral paralysis of the recurrent laryngeal nerve that affected only the abductor muscles, then the unopposed adductor muscles would bring the cords together (i.e., closed) and complete airway obstruction would ensue *(Miller: Miller's Anesthesia, ed 8, p 2526)*.

832. (D) PDPH is due to a loss of CSF through a dural puncture and characteristically has a postural component. When the patient is supine, the headache is usually gone, but may be mild in some cases. When the head is elevated, the headache may be severe, is bilateral, and may be associated with diplopia, nausea, and vomiting. The headache pain is typically frontal and/or occipital in location. Typically the onset of the headache is 12 to 24 hours after a dural puncture and lasts several days if untreated (rarely it can last for months). The other headaches listed rarely have a significant postural component *(Barash: Clinical Anesthesia, ed 8, p 938)*.

833. (C) VAN (*Vein, Artery, Nerve*) describes the anatomic relationship of the intercostal structures deep to the lower border of the ribs from the cephalad to caudal direction. The block is performed by walking off the inferior edge of the rib with the needle, typically about 5 to 7 cm from midline. The two principal risks are pneumothorax and intravascular injection of local anesthetics. Because of the close proximity of the vein and artery to the nerve, intercostal blocks have relatively high blood levels compared with other blocks (e.g., epidural, brachial plexus, brachial plexus block, infiltration), and caution with dose is needed if many levels are blocked *(Barash: Clinical Anesthesia, ed 8, p 979)*.

834. (A) The site of injection of the local anesthetic is one of the most important factors influencing systemic local anesthetic absorption and toxicity. The degree of absorption from the site of injection depends on the blood supply to that site. Areas that have the greatest blood supply have the greatest systemic absorption. For this reason, the greatest plasma concentration of local anesthetic occurs after an intercostal block, followed by caudal epidural, lumbar epidural, brachial plexus, sciatic/femoral nerve block, and subcutaneous *(Miller: Miller's Anesthesia, ed 8, p 1046)*.

835. (D) Local anesthetics are weak bases. The neutral (nonionized) form of the molecule is able to pass through the lipid nerve cell membrane, whereas the ionized (protonated) form actually produces anesthesia. Chloroprocaine has the highest pKa of local anesthetics, meaning that a greater percentage of it will exist in the ionized form at any given pH than any of the other local anesthetics. Despite this fact, 3% chloroprocaine has a more rapid onset than 2% lidocaine, presumably because of the greater number of molecules (concentration). However, if one compares onset time for 1.5% lidocaine against 1.5% chloroprocaine, the former will have a more rapid onset *(Miller: Miller's Anesthesia, ed 8, p 1039)*.

836. (B) The risk of pneumothorax is a significant limitation for supraclavicular brachial plexus blocks (traditionally the incidence is 0.5%-6%, depending on experience; with the ultrasound technique, the incidence may be lower). Furthermore, the technique is difficult to teach and describe. For these reasons, this block should not be performed in patients in whom a pneumothorax or phrenic nerve block (30%-60% of patients) would result in significant dyspnea or respiratory distress. A pneumothorax should be considered if the patient begins to complain of chest pain or shortness of breath or begins to cough during placement of a supraclavicular brachial plexus block. In some cases, symptoms of a pneumothorax may be delayed up to 24 hours *(Miller: Miller's Anesthesia, ed 8, pp 1727–1728)*.

837. (D) The femoral nerve is the largest branch of the lumbar plexus (it primarily arises from the second to fourth lumbar nerve roots). The femoral nerve divides into an anterior and a posterior division. The anterior division provides motor innervation to the sartorius muscle and cutaneous sensation to the anterior and medial aspects of the thigh. The posterior division innervates the quadriceps muscle and provides cutaneous sensation to the anterior, medial, and lateral aspects of the knee, as well as the articular aspects of the knee joint. The nerve passes under the inguinal ligament and lies just lateral to the femoral artery and vein. If the stimulating needle produces sartorius muscle contraction without patellar movement, then you are too anterior for proper femoral nerve blockade, and the needle needs to be advanced in a more posterior (i.e., deeper) direction. Proper needle placement will elicit quadriceps muscle contraction, with patellar elevation that disappears with local anesthetic injection *(Barash: Clinical Anesthesia, ed 8, pp 988–989)*.

838. (A) The obturator nerve provides variable cutaneous innervation of the thigh and can be used to supplement femoral and sciatic nerve blockade for patients having lower-extremity surgery. An obturator nerve block is achieved by placement of the needle 1 to 2 cm lateral to and 1 to 2 cm below the pubic tubercle. After contact with the pubic bone, the needle is withdrawn and walked cephalad to identify the obturator canal. Between 10 and 15 mL of local anesthetic should be placed in the canal. If a nerve stimulator is used, contraction of the adductor muscles with nerve stimulation indicates proximity to the nerve *(Miller: Miller's Anesthesia, ed 8, pp 1741–1742; Barash: Clinical Anesthesia, ed 8, pp 989–990)*.

839. (A) The most serious complication associated with a supraclavicular brachial plexus block is pneumothorax, which fortunately is rare (0.5%-5%). The most common complication is a phrenic nerve block, which is usually mild and relatively common (30%-60% of blocks). Bilateral supraclavicular blocks, however, are not recommended, due to the possibility of bilateral phrenic nerve paralysis or pneumothoraces. Other potential complications include Horner syndrome (ipsilateral eye ptosis, miosis, and anhidrosis), nerve damage or neuritis, infection, or intravascular injection *(Barash: Clinical Anesthesia, ed 8, pp 969–970; Miller: Miller's Anesthesia, ed 8, pp 1727–1728)*.

840. (A) The arm receives sensory innervation from the brachial plexus, except for the shoulder, which is innervated by the supraclavicular nerves from the cervical plexus, and the posterior medial aspect of the arm, which is supplied by the intercostobrachial nerve *(Barash: Clinical Anesthesia, ed 8, pp 969–972)*.

841. (B) The brachial plexus starts out at the root level from the ventral rami of C5-T1 with a small amount from C4 and T2. These roots at the level of the scalene muscle become the three trunks: superior, middle, and inferior. The trunks then divide into the dorsal and ventral divisions at the lateral edge of the first rib. When the divisions enter the axilla, they become the cords: posterior, lateral, and medial. At the lateral border of the pectoralis muscle, they become the five peripheral nerves: radial, musculocutaneous, median, ulnar, and axillary. The interscalene block is at the level of the roots/trunks (but spares the inferior trunk); the supraclavicular block is at the level of the trunks/divisions; the infraclavicular block is at the level of the cords; and the axillary block is at the level of the branches *(Barash: Clinical Anesthesia, ed 8, pp 966–972)*.

842. (A) The celiac plexus innervates most of the abdominal viscera, including the lower esophagus, stomach, all of the small intestine, and the large intestine up to the splenic flexure, as well as the pancreas, liver, biliary tract, spleen, kidneys, adrenal glands, and omentum. The pelvic organs (e.g., uterus, ovaries, prostate, distal colon) are supplied by the hypogastric plexus *(Barash: Clinical Anesthesia, ed 8, pp 1618–1619)*.

843. (D) The great toe is innervated mainly by the deep peroneal, posterior tibial, superficial peroneal, and, occasionally, by the saphenous nerve. All four of these nerves should be blocked for surgery on the great toe. The sural nerve is the fifth nerve for ankle blocks but covers only the lateral side of the foot, not the medial side or great toe area *(Barash: Clinical Anesthesia, ed 8, pp 996–998).*

844. (D) Frequent dosing by a patient receiving postoperative analgesia through a PCA pump suggests the need to increase the magnitude of the dose. It is important to keep in mind that a patient should be given a sufficient loading dose of opioid before initiative therapy with a PCA pump. Otherwise, the patient will be playing the frustrating game of "catch up." The most commonly used opioids in the United States for PCA pump use are morphine, fentanyl, and hydromorphone. Meperidine should not be used as the opioid for PCA pumps, since the toxic metabolite normeperidine may accumulate *(Barash: Clinical Anesthesia, ed 8, p 1602).*

845. (D) TENS produces a tingling or vibratory sensation in the area in which pads are placed. Although the exact mechanism is unclear, it is thought that TENS units produce analgesia by releasing endogenous endorphins, since its effects are partially blocked by naloxone. These endorphins have an inhibitory effect at the spinal cord level and augment descending inhibitory pathways *(Miller: Miller's Anesthesia, ed 8, pp 2339, 2991).*

846. (C) Although the more hydrophilic drugs, such as morphine, have a longer duration of action of analgesia, they also have a higher potential for inducing delayed respiratory depression through cephalad migration in the CNS, compared with the more lipid-soluble drugs listed in this question *(Miller: Miller's Anesthesia, ed 8, p 2983).*

847. (B) The thumb corresponds to dermatome C6, the second and middle fingers correspond to dermatome C7, and the fourth and little fingers correspond to dermatome C8 *(Barash: Clinical Anesthesia, ed 8, p 920).*

848. (C) Increasing the total dose (mass) of local anesthetic is more efficacious in hastening the onset and increasing the duration of an epidural anesthetic than increasing the volume or increasing the concentration (while holding the total dose constant) *(Barash: Clinical Anesthesia, ed 8, pp 930–931).*

849. (C) Alcohol and phenol are similar in their ability to cause nonselective damage to neural tissues. Alcohol causes pain when injected and sometimes is mixed with bupivacaine, whereas phenol is relatively painless. Alcohol has a slightly longer duration of analgesia (3-6 months) compared with phenol (2-3 months). Neural tissue will regenerate; therefore, neurolytic blocks are never "permanent," and neurolysis can lead to denervation hypersensitivity, which can be extremely painful *(Miller: Miller's Anesthesia, ed 8, p 1911).*

850. (D) TNS, previously called transient radicular irritation (TRI), can occur in 4% to 40% of patients after spinal anesthesia with lidocaine, in ambulatory patients undergoing surgery in the lithotomy position, or undergoing knee arthroscopy. The baricity, concentration injected (lidocaine 0.5%-5%), addition of epinephrine, presence of dextrose, or hypotension does not seem to be related to the development of TNS. The symptoms of TNS include pain or sensory abnormalities in the lower back, buttocks, or lower extremities. Although TNS has been reported with all local anesthetics, the incidence is significantly greater with lidocaine *(Miller: Miller's Anesthesia, ed 8, p 1692).*

851. (A) After the proper transducer is selected, you can adjust the frequency, depth, and gain to optimize an image. In general, higher-frequency ultrasound waves provide better image quality (i.e., better resolution) due to the higher number of cycles per second of transmitted and reflected energy used to produce the image. However, higher-frequency waves have more signal attenuation at increasing depths and cannot penetrate to deeper tissue levels. Therefore higher-frequency ultrasound is typically used for shallower structures, and lower frequencies are used for deeper structures. Usually the depth is adjusted so the structure in question is in the center, top-to-bottom, of the image. Increasing the gain increases, or amplifies, the reflected signal energy and increases the brightness of the image *(Barash: Clinical Anesthesia, ed 8, pp 732–734).*

852. (B) Younger adults have a higher incidence of PDPH than older adults or children. Women have a slightly higher incidence than men. Pregnant women have a higher incidence than nonpregnant women. Since the incidence and severity of PDPH relate to the amount of CSF leakage through the dural hole, it makes sense that the larger the needle and the more holes in the dura, the greater the incidence of PDPH. In addition, the shape of the tip of the needle is important: A cutting needle (e.g., Quincke) has a greater incidence of PDPH than a noncutting needle (e.g., Whitacre, Sprotte). The incidence of headache has been shown to be less when the dural fibers are split longitudinally than when they are cut, while the needle is held in a transverse direction. The timing of ambulation relative to dural puncture has not been shown to affect the incidence of postspinal headache. The block should wear off before ambulation is attempted *(Barash: Clinical Anesthesia, ed 8, p 938; Miller: Miller's Anesthesia, ed 8, pp 1694–1695).*

853. (A) Virtually all pain arising in the thoracic or abdominal viscera is transmitted via the sympathetic nervous system in unmyelinated type C fibers. Visceral pain is dull, aching, burning, and nonspecific. Visceral pain is caused by any stimulus that excites nociceptive nerve endings in diffuse areas. In this regard, distention of a hollow viscus causes a greater sensation of pain than does the highly localized damage produced by transecting the gut. Although the vagus nerve has a large number of afferent fibers, they do not include pain fibers *(Miller: Miller's Anesthesia, ed 8, p 2975; Barash: Clinical Anesthesia, ed 8, p 336).*

854. (A) The duration of regional blocks differs among local anesthetics, as well as among block locations. When bupivacaine with epinephrine (1:200,000) is used, epidural anesthesia may last 180 to 350 minutes; infiltration anesthesia may last 180 to 240 minutes; and major nerve blocks such as axillary block may last 360 to 720 minutes. Spinal bupivacaine without epinephrine may last 90 to 200 minutes; if epinephrine (0.2-0.3 mg) is added to the spinal block, it will last about 50% longer *(Miller: Miller's Anesthesia, ed 8, pp 1041–1044).*

855. (D) Psoas compartment block is also called the posterior lumbar plexus block and can be used for any procedure in which a lumbar plexus block is required, but most often it is used for analgesia for the proximal aspect of the thigh and hip. When combined with a sciatic block, complete leg anesthesia will result. Remembering that the femoral nerve (which innervates the quadriceps muscles) is a distal branch helps one to understand why quadriceps muscle contraction is useful in locating the plexus with a stimulating needle (1-1.5 mA). If the hamstring muscles are stimulated, the needle is too caudally located, and the needle should be aimed in a more cephalad direction. Continuous psoas catheters are commonly used for postoperative analgesia *(Barash: Clinical Anesthesia, ed 8, pp 986–987).*

856. (C) All of the nerves of the foot (with the exception of the saphenous) are derived from the sciatic nerve. The sciatic nerve distally becomes the tibial and peroneal nerves, which can be blocked at the popliteal fossa for surgery below the knee. The saphenous nerve is a branch of the femoral nerve and provides sensory innervation along the medial aspect of the lower leg between the knee and the medial malleolus, and must also be blocked for surgery below the knee *(Barash: Clinical Anesthesia, ed 8, pp 991–993).*

857. (A) The sympathectomy produced by a celiac plexus block causes hypotension by decreasing preload to the heart. This complication can be avoided by volume loading the patient with lactated Ringer solution. By blocking the sympathetic chain, unopposed parasympathetic activity may also result in increased gastrointestinal activity and transient diarrhea. Back pain is also common. Paraplegia may result from spasm of the lumbar segmental arteries that perfuse the spinal cord, direct vascular or neurologic injury, or retrograde spread of drug to the nerve roots and spinal cord. Seizure is possible with an intravascular injection. Retroperitoneal hematoma is also possible, but rare *(Waldman: Atlas of Interventional Pain Management, ed 4, pp 389–394).*

858. (D) The occiput receives sensory innervation from the greater and lesser occipital nerves (C2 and C3 spinal roots), which are terminal branches of the cervical plexus. Blockade of these nerves is usually carried out as a diagnostic step in the evaluation of head and neck pain *(Barash: Clinical Anesthesia, ed 8, pp 954–955).*

859. (C) Thoracic paravertebral blocks are used for surgical anesthesia and postoperative analgesia for breast, axillary, or chest wall surgery. The major complication is a pneumothorax. Since the paravertebral space is continuous with the epidural space medially, epidural spread may result if large volumes of local anesthetic are injected into the paravertebral. Typically 5 mL are injected at each of three sites for unilateral paravertebral blocks, and 3 mL per each of six sites (three on each side) if bilateral paravertebral blocks are performed. If the needle is directed too medially, then the intrathecal space may be entered (dural sleeves extend to the level of the intervertebral foramina) with the possibility of a total spinal if 5 to 10 mL is injected. The sympathetic chain is in the anterior part of the paravertebral space, and sympathetic blockade may develop; however, hypotension would be more likely than hypertension to develop from blocking the sympathetic chain (*Barash: Clinical Anesthesia, ed 8, pp 980–982*).

860. (C) With the unintentional injection of an epidural dose of local anesthetic into the subarachnoid space, spinal anesthesia develops rapidly. Blockade of the sympathetic fibers (T1-L2) produces hypotension, particularly if the patient is hypovolemic. Bradycardia is produced by blocking the cardiac accelerator fibers (T1-T4). Respiratory arrest is due to hypoperfusion of the respiratory centers, as well as paralysis of the phrenic nerve (C3-C5). The pupils become dilated (mydriasis) after intrathecal injection of large quantities of local anesthetics; they will return to normal size after the block recedes. Cauda equina syndrome has occasionally developed when the epidural dose was unintentionally administered into the subarachnoid space (most commonly with chloroprocaine). If one suspects an unintentional placement of the epidural dose subarachnoid, supportive methods are initially used (the basic ABCs of resuscitation). One can also aspirate CSF from the epidural catheter (if it was inserted) to help remove some of the drug, as well as to reduce the pressure in the subarachnoid space, which might help better perfuse the spinal cord and decrease the chance of cauda equina syndrome developing (*Miller: Miller's Anesthesia, ed 8, pp 1690, 1702; Barash: Clinical Anesthesia, ed 8, pp 925–926*).

861. (B) Somatic pain in the extremities is relieved with spinal anesthesia. If a patient fails to obtain pain relief despite complete sympathetic, sensory, and motor blockade, a "central" mechanism for the pain is likely or the lesion causing the pain is higher in the CNS than the level of blockade achieved by the spinal. Central pain states may include encephalization, psychogenic pain, or malingering. Persistence of pain in the lower extremities after successful spinal blockade suggests a central source or psychological source of pain (*Miller: Miller's Anesthesia, ed 8, pp 1898–1910*).

862. (D) During a seizure, both arterial hypoxemia and acidosis (metabolic and respiratory) develop due to the increased oxygen consumption from contracting muscles and hypoventilation that occurs. Administration of 100% O_2 helps to prevent and treat hypoxemia. Elevated CO_2 not only enhances cerebral blood flow and delivery of local anesthetic to the brain but also diffuses into neural tissue, causing intracellular pH to fall. Because local anesthetics are either amino esters or amino amides, lowering the pH allows more binding of hydrogen ions to the amino group, making it more ionic or protonated, which traps the local anesthetic inside the cells. Hyperventilation can reverse many of the changes that occur with acidosis (i.e., causes cerebral vasoconstriction and can decrease delivery of local anesthetic to the brain). Hyperventilation induces hypokalemia and respiratory alkalosis, both of which result in hyperpolarization of nerve membranes and elevation of the seizure threshold. Hyperventilation also raises the patient's pH (respiratory alkalosis) and converts local anesthetics into the nonionized (nonprotonated) form, which crosses the membrane more easily than the ionized form, which is detrimental. Benzodiazepines and/or propofol are used to suppress the seizure activity (*Miller: Miller's Anesthesia, ed 8, pp 1048–1050*).

863. (D) Para-aminobenzoic acid is a metabolite of the ester-type local anesthetics. Local anesthetics may be placed into two distinct categories based on their chemical structure: amino esters or amino amides. The amides (two *i*'s in the name), which are ropivacaine, lidocaine, etidocaine, prilocaine, mepivacaine, and bupivacaine, are metabolized in the liver. The ester local anesthetics (one *i* in the name) are cocaine, procaine, chloroprocaine, tetracaine, and benzocaine. These drugs are metabolized by the enzyme pseudocholinesterase found in the blood. Para-aminobenzoic acid is a metabolic breakdown product of ester anesthetic and is responsible for allergic reactions in some individuals (*Barash: Clinical Anesthesia, ed 8, p 569*).

864. (D) Peripheral nerve axons are always enveloped by a Schwann cell. The myelinated nerves may be enveloped many times by the same Schwann cell. Transmission of nerve impulses (i.e., action potentials) along nonmyelinated nerves occurs in a continuous fashion, whereas transmission along myelinated nerves occurs by saltatory conduction from one node of Ranvier to the next. Myelination speeds transmission of neurologic impulses; it also renders nerves more susceptible to local anesthetic blockade. An action potential is associated with an inward flux of sodium that occurs after a certain membrane threshold has been exceeded *(Miller: Miller's Anesthesia, ed 8, pp 1031–1035)*.

865. (C) The needle insertion site for an interscalene block is C6 (i.e., lateral to the cricoid cartilage). Local anesthetics usually spread to C5, C6, and C7, which supply much, but not all, of the cutaneous innervation to the shoulder. With low-to-moderate volume blocks, there will be sparing of the C3-C4 nerve roots, which supply some of the innervation to the anterior shoulder. Of note, C8 and T1 may also be spared, often resulting in the need for ulnar nerve supplementation if this block is used for a hand operation. Complete anesthesia for shoulder arthroscopy may require a supplemental superficial cervical plexus, with use of low-to-moderate volumes of a local anesthetic *(Barash: Clinical Anesthesia, ed 8, pp 967–968)*.

866. (B) Hand washing is one of the most important techniques to prevent infections, especially when alcohol-based antiseptic solutions are used with sterile gloves. Although soap and water remove bacteria, they do not effectively kill organisms. Antiseptic solutions with alcohol appear to be better than nonalcoholic antiseptics (e.g., povidone-iodine). Nail length does not appear to be a risk factor for infections, because the majority of bacterial growth occurs along the proximal 1 mm of nail adjacent to the subungual skin. Universal use of gowns and gloves does not appear to be better than gloves alone in preventing infections in intensive care units (ICUs) and presumably is less important than adequate hand washing and use of sterile gloves *(Miller: Miller's Anesthesia, ed 8, pp 1702, 3048–3051; Anesthesiology 126:585–601, 2017)*.

867. (A) In patients taking low-molecular-weight heparin (LMWH) (e.g., enoxaparin, dalteparin, tinzaparin), caution should be exercised before proceeding with an epidural or spinal anesthetic, because of the risk of producing an epidural or spinal hematoma. The amount of time between the last dose of the LMWH and the relative safety of starting a central neuraxial block depends on the dose of the LMWH. At the lower doses, used for thromboprophylaxis, the LMWH should be held at least 10 to 12 hours before the block. At the higher doses, used to treat an established DVT, one should wait at least 24 hours after the last dose of LMWH before the block *(Miller: Miller's Anesthesia, ed 8, pp 1702, 2344–2345)*.

868. (B) NSAIDs, ticlopidine, and clopidogrel exert effects on platelet function. NSAIDs are not a problem if given alone before epidural or spinal anesthesia; however, before having a neuraxial block placed, patients taking ticlopidine should wait 14 days, and patients taking clopidogrel should wait 7 days, because of the increased risk of spinal hematoma formation. Keep in mind that caution is always needed and that the ASRA statement "Careful preoperative assessment of the patient to identify alterations of health that might contribute to bleeding is crucial" is important *(Miller: Basics of Anesthesia, ed 7, p 282, Table 17-1; Barash: Clinical Anesthesia, ed 8, pp 570–571)*.

869. (D) Adding sodium bicarbonate to local anesthetic solutions hastens the onset of action of the local anesthetics, especially when the local anesthetic solution contains epinephrine (which is produced at a lower pH). By raising the pH, more of the local anesthetic is in the nonionized, more lipid-soluble state. Raising the pH too much (i.e., >6.05-8) would cause precipitation of the local anesthetic. Some studies have shown that alkalization of the local anesthetic may decrease the duration of a peripheral block, especially if epinephrine was not added. It also seems to decrease pain with skin infiltration. Pain on injection can also be decreased by a slow injection of the local anesthetic *(Miller: Miller's Anesthesia, ed 8, p 1040)*.

870. (C) This figure shows the anatomic structures that must be traversed by the spinal needle during the performance of a subarachnoid block. The structures include the skin, subcutaneous tissue, supraspinous ligament, interspinous ligament, ligamentum flavum, the epidural space, and, finally, the dura (posteriorly). If you were to continue to advance the spinal needle, you would encounter the dura (anteriorly) while exiting the subarachnoid space, the posterior longitudinal ligament, the periosteum of the vertebral body, and, finally, bone *(Barash: Clinical Anesthesia, ed 8, p 926).*

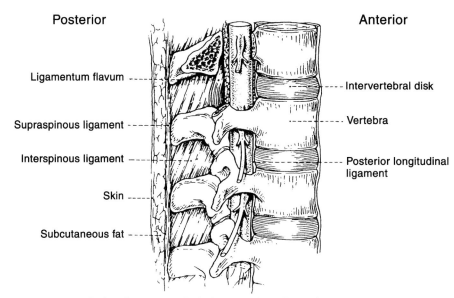

Posterior   Anterior

Ligamentum flavum

Supraspinous ligament

Interspinous ligament

Skin

Subcutaneous fat

Intervertebral disk

Vertebra

Posterior longitudinal ligament

From Cousins MJ, Bridenbaugh PO: Neural Blockade in Clinical Anesthesia and Management of Pain, *ed 2, Philadelphia, JB Lippincott, 1988, pp 255–263.*

871. (D) In the epidural space, bupivacaine (as well as levobupivacaine) is four times more potent than lidocaine, so 0.5% bupivacaine is similar to 2% lidocaine for analgesia. The duration of the bupivacaine block will be longer because bupivacaine has a long duration of action and lidocaine has an intermediate duration of action. In addition, motor block would be less for bupivacaine compared with lidocaine, since there is a greater difference between sensory and motor block for bupivacaine compared with lidocaine *(Miller's Anesthesia, ed 8, pp 1702, 2344–2345).*

872. (D) Drugs with α-adrenergic agonist activity (phenylephrine, 2-5 mg; epinephrine, 0.2-0.5 mg; clonidine, 75-150 mg) possess some analgesic activity but less than opioids and local anesthetics. In addition, these intrathecal α-adrenergic agonists may reduce systemic/vascular uptake of local anesthetics, thereby enhancing their effects, including hypotension. Clonidine alone, when administered neuraxially, is an effective analgesic. Neostigmine has some mild analgesia properties, but experience is limited. Opioids (e.g., fentanyl, sufentanil, hydromorphone, and morphine) added to the spinal solution enhance surgical anesthesia and provide postoperative pain relief. Fentanyl or sufentanil is commonly added for short surgical procedures (outpatient), whereas hydromorphone or morphine can be used when longer postoperative analgesia is desired for inpatients *(Miller: Miller's Anesthesia, ed 8, pp 1693, 2983).*

873. (B) For topical anesthesia, lidocaine, tetracaine, cocaine, dibucaine, and benzocaine are effective, as well as the combination of lidocaine and prilocaine, or Eutectic Mixture of Local Anesthetics (EMLA) cream. For IV regional anesthesia or Bier blocks, many drugs have been used. Ester local anesthetics are not used for IV regional blocks because they can be broken down in the bloodstream (by plasma ester hydrolysis), which can shorten the drug's duration of action and can also cause thrombophlebitis of the vein (reported with chloroprocaine). Because CV collapse has been reported with bupivacaine, it should not be used for IV regional anesthesia. Lidocaine and prilocaine are used for Bier blocks because of their relative safety. For infiltrative and epidural anesthesia, almost all local anesthetics can be used (with the exception of cocaine and benzocaine, which are used only topically) *(Miller: Miller's Anesthesia, ed 8, pp 1041–1044, 1736).*

874. (A) Procaine and 2-chloroprocaine have a short duration of action; lidocaine, mepivacaine, and prilocaine have an intermediate duration of action; and etidocaine, bupivacaine, levobupivacaine, tetracaine, and ropivacaine have a long duration of action. For similar sensory anesthesia, a higher concentration of local anesthetic is needed for the short duration of local anesthetics compared with both the intermediate- and long-duration agents, because they are less potent *(Miller: Miller's Anesthesia, ed 8, pp 1710–1711)*.

875. (B) Under sevoflurane general anesthesia, an increase in the T-wave amplitude of 25% (usually in lead II), an increase in heart rate of 10 beats/min, or a systolic blood pressure increase of greater than 15 mm Hg is considered a positive dose response to an epinephrine-containing local anesthetic solution. As always, slow incremental dosing is safer than a large bolus dose *(Miller: Miller's Anesthesia, ed 8, p 2721)*.

876. (D) All of the choices listed are potential complications of stellate ganglion blockade except an increase in heart rate. The stellate ganglion supplies sympathetic fibers to the upper extremity and head and some to the heart. Loss of the cardiac acceleratory fibers may slow the heart rate, not speed it up. Other potential complications of stellate ganglion blockade include accidental injection of the local anesthetic into a vertebral artery, resulting in seizure, phrenic nerve paralysis, and inadvertent cervical epidural *(Miller: Miller's Anesthesia, ed 8, p 1732)*.

877. (C) Spinal hematomas can have catastrophic consequences, and knowledge of the waiting time after cessation of the various antiplatelet and anticoagulant drugs is paramount. American Society of Regional Anesthesia (ASRA) has published guidelines for anticoagulants and neuraxial anesthesia. Ticlopidine should be stopped 14 days, clopidogrel for 7 days, and abdiximab for 8–48 hours before the administration of a spinal or epidural anesthetic. No delay is needed for a patient taking aspirin or NSAIDs *(Miller: Basics of Anesthesia, ed 7, p 282)*.

878. (A) Postdural puncture headaches (PDPHs) (spinal headaches) usually develop within 12 to 72 hours after a dural puncture but may develop immediately or take months to develop. The most characteristic symptom is a postural component in which the headache occurs in the upright position and is usually completely gone when the patient is in the supine position. The headache is typically frontal and/or occipital in location. Other symptoms include nausea, vomiting, anorexia, visual disturbances (blurred vision, double vision, photophobia), and occasionally hearing loss (routinely found with auditory testing) *(Barash: Clinical Anesthesia, ed 8, pp 938–939)*.

879. (C) TAP block is used to provide abdominal wall analgesia. The subcostal (T12), ilioinguinal (L1), and iliohypogastric (L1) nerves are the nerves primarily blocked. Ultrasound is often used to locate the proper plane where the local anesthetic is injected, since the nerves are too small to visualize. After visualization of the three abdominal wall muscles—the external oblique, the internal oblique, and the transversus abdominis muscles—the needle is inserted. The local anesthetic is injected into the muscle plane between the internal oblique and the transversus abdominis muscles (which is where these nerves travel), and not the muscle, for effective analgesia. Typically 20 to 30 mL of local anesthetic (e.g., 2 mg/kg of bupivacaine) is needed for adequate spread of local anesthetic *(Barash: Clinical Anesthesia, ed 8, pp 983, 1596)*.

880. (A) Five nerves are blocked when performing an ankle block. The saphenous, superficial peroneal, and sural nerves are all sensory below the ankle, and electrical stimulation would have no effect. Stimulation of the posterior tibial nerve causes flexion of the toes by stimulating the flexor digitorum brevis muscles and abduction of the first toe by stimulating the abductor hallucis muscles. The posterior tibial nerve also is sensory to most of the plantar part of the foot. Stimulation of the deep peroneal nerve causes extension of the toes by stimulating the extensor digitorum brevis muscles. The deep peroneal nerve has a small sensory branch for the first interdigital cleft. For practical reasons, many anesthesiologists perform a purely infiltration block of these nerves. If a nerve stimulator is used, it is mainly to find the posterior tibial nerve, which can be difficult to anesthetize if small volumes of local anesthetic are administered. The posterior tibial nerve can be difficult to stimulate in diabetic patients with diabetic neuropathy *(Barash: Clinical Anesthesia, ed 8, pp 996–998)*.

881. (C) Peripheral nerve stimulation is a common technique when performing axillary nerve blocks. The desired motor response from the nerve can be seen with 0.5 mA or less. The musculocutaneous nerve elicits elbow flexion. The radial nerve elicits extension of all the digits, the wrist, and the elbow, as well as supination of the forearm. The ulnar nerve elicits flexion at the wrist and fourth and fifth digits, as well as adduction (not abduction) of the thumb. The median nerve elicits flexion at the wrist and second and third digits, as well as opposition of the thumb and pronation of the forearm *(Barash: Clinical Anesthesia, ed 8, p 971)*.

882. (C) Unilateral numbness or paresthesia in the upper extremity during extension of the neck usually represents nerve root impingement at the vertebral foramina. C6 nerve distribution is the thumb. Specifically, unilateral degenerative changes restrict the foramen to such a degree that it compresses and irritates the nerve root traversing the vertebral foramen when the head is extended. Treatment ranges from NSAIDs to steroids and may require surgical intervention if there is muscle weakness. Lhermitte sign, named after Jean Lhermitte, occurs when head flexion causes shooting sensations down the back and into the lower limbs. It is a sign of posterior column disease *(Miller: Miller's Anesthesia, ed 8, p 1725)*.

883. (C) Although a successful interscalene block causes ipsilateral phrenic nerve paralysis in almost 100% of patients, identifying the phrenic nerve means that you are anterior to the brachial plexus and that you should reposition your needle. You should redirect the needle in a posterior direction *(Miller: Miller's Anesthesia, ed 8, pp 1725–1727)*.

884. (C) With an intravascular injection, the main symptoms would most likely be CNS toxicity (e.g., seizures), as blood flow is directly to the brain. The Bezold-Jarisch reflex (hypotension and bradycardia) has been reported in awake, sitting patients undergoing shoulder surgery with an interscalene block. This may be related to intracardiac mechanoreceptors being stimulated by the decreased venous return in the sitting position. This leads to decreased sympathetic tone and increased parasympathetic tone. Breathing is still present with this reflex. Block of the stellate ganglion would produce Horner syndrome, which is not associated with breathing abnormalities. Injection into the intrathecal space is uncommon, but possible (especially if the needle is not pointed in the caudal direction), and would lead to a total spinal block with little local anesthetic injected (e.g., hypotension, bradycardia, and respiratory paralysis that would lead to cyanosis) *(Miller: Miller's Anesthesia, ed 8, pp 1725–1727)*.

885. (C) The pipecoloxylidide local anesthetics (mepivacaine, bupivacaine, ropivacaine, and levobupivacaine) are chiral drugs, which means that they have an asymmetric carbon atom (i.e., have a left or S and a right or R hand configuration). Mepivacaine and bupivacaine are produced as racemic mixtures (50% S:50% R). The pure S forms show reduced neurotoxicity and reduced cardiotoxicity (e.g., ropivacaine and levobupivacaine). Clinical studies suggest that the pure S forms have a slight decrease in potency and a shorter duration of action compared with racemic mixtures. Lidocaine is an achiral compound (i.e., has no chiral carbon atom) *(Barash: Clinical Anesthesia, ed 8, pp 1189–1190)*.

886. (A) Nerves to the lower extremity emerge from the L1-S4 nerve roots. The upper roots (mainly L1-L4) form the lumbar plexus, which gives rise to the genitofemoral (L1-L2), lateral femoral cutaneous (L2-L3), obturator (L2-L4), and the femoral (L2-L4) nerves. A branch from the lumbar plexus (L4), along with the sacral plexus (L4-S3), gives rise to the sciatic nerve. Branches of the sciatic nerve include the common peroneal (branches to make the superficial and deep) and the tibial, and the sural nerves *(Miller: Miller's Anesthesia, ed 8, p 1736)*.

887. (D) Anesthetic-related nerve injuries to the brachial plexus are rare and poorly understood. The only way to minimize nerve injury is to minimize trauma to neural fibers. Although ultrasound-guided technique is promising, currently there is no clinical evidence for this *(Neal et al: Upper extremity regional anesthesia: Essentials of our current understanding, 2008, Reg Anesth Pain Med 34:134–170, 2009; Miller: Miller's Anesthesia, ed 8, p 1049)*.

888. (C) Local anesthetic systemic toxicity (LAST) is a multisystem phenomenon, but the most crucial manifestation involves the heart (atrioventricular conduction block, arrhythmias, myocardial depression, and cardiac arrest). In this case of CV collapse, treatment consists of getting help with the initial focus of airway management and CV support (i.e., basic and advanced cardiac life support). BUT AVOID the use of vasopressin, calcium channel blockers, β-blockers, or local anesthetics. Epinephrine doses should be reduced to less than 1 μg/kg. Lipid emulsion therapy should be started; the initial bolus of 20% Intralipid is 1.5 mL/kg (lean body mass) over 1 minute, followed by a continuous infusion of 0.25 mL/kg/min. Repeat the bolus one or two times for persistent CV collapse, and double the continuous infusion rate if the blood pressure remains low. Continue the infusion for at least 10 minutes after CV stability is attained. The upper limit of 20% Intralipid is 10 mL/kg over 30 minutes. Failure to respond with the above treatment should prompt consideration for cardiopulmonary bypass. Although propofol is formulated as a lipid emulsion and as such would bind bupivacaine to some degree, the cardiac depressant effects of propofol would far overshadow any therapeutic benefit of binding bupivacaine. Also see explanation for Question 722 *(Barash: Clinical Anesthesia, ed 8, p 1155)*.

889. (A) When performing an interscalene block, the needle is usually inserted where the line extending lateral to the cricoid cartilage (C6 level) intersects the interscalene groove. The needle is inserted perpendicular to the skin and is slowly advanced in a medial, caudal, and slightly posterior direction. The caudal direction is used to decrease the chance of injecting the local anesthetic into the vertebral artery, or obtaining a spinal or epidural block. Injecting into the vertebral artery may lead to an immediate convulsion, since the local anesthetic would go directly to the brain. The phrenic nerve is routinely blocked (100% of the time) and, in healthy patients, rarely leads to symptoms. However, in patients with borderline respiratory insufficiency, respiratory compromise can result. Occasionally the recurrent laryngeal nerve is blocked. Unilateral paralysis rarely is clinically significant, but if contralateral recurrent paralysis existed preoperatively, then complete airway obstruction may develop. The vagus nerve can also be blocked but is rarely clinically significant *(Miller's Anesthesia, ed 8, pp 1725–1728)*.

890. (D) Epidural hematomas are rare complications of spinal anesthesia (1:220,000) and epidural anesthesia (1:150,000). However, in the presence of LMWH, the incidence is much higher: 1:40,000 with spinal anesthesia and 1:3000 with continuous epidural catheter. Clinical symptoms include radicular back pain, bowel and bladder dysfunction, and sensory or motor deficits. An MRI is the diagnostic test of choice, and prompt (<8 hours) decompressive laminectomy is the treatment of choice. Epidural abscesses typically progress slowly compared with epidural hematomas and are also associated with fever. See also explanation for Question 814 *(Miller: Miller's Anesthesia, ed 8, pp 2344–2345)*.

891. (C) Peripheral nerves are classified according to the fiber size and physiologic properties, such as the presence or absence of myelin, conduction velocity, location, and function. All type A fibers are myelinated. These fibers are subclassified into four groups based on their diameter, location, and function. A-alpha (Aα) and A-beta (Aβ) fibers are 6 to 22 μm in diameter and have conduction velocities of 30 to 120 m/sec. Aα fibers are efferent to the skeletal muscles. Aβ fibers are afferent from the skin and joints to provide touch and proprioception sensations. A-gamma (Aγ) fibers are 3 to 6 μm in diameter, have conduction velocities of 15 to 35 m/sec, and are efferent to the muscle spindles to provide muscle tone. A-delta (Aδ) fibers are 1 to 4 μm in diameter and have conduction velocities of 5 to 25 m/sec and are afferent fibers, which provide sharp localized pain and temperature and touch sensations. B fibers are myelinated, preganglionic sympathetic nerve fibers that are less than 3 μm in diameter, have medium conduction velocities 3 to 15 m/sec, and are involved with various autonomic nervous system control. C fibers are nonmyelinated, postganglionic sympathetic nerves that are 0.3 to 1.3 μm in diameter and have slow conduction velocities of 0.1 to 2 m/sec. C fibers are afferent sensory nerves involved with nonlocalized pain, temperature, and touch sensations *(Miller: Miller's Anesthesia, ed 8, pp 1013–1014)*.

892. (C) Overdose of intrathecal opiates would not be a sign of an intradural mass lesion. Granulomas at the tip of intrathecal catheters used with intrathecal drug delivery systems are gaining increased attention. Granulomas are more frequently associated with high concentrations and doses of either morphine (>10 mg/day) or hydromorphone (>10 mg/day). Most patients who will develop granulomas receive the intrathecal medications for more than 6 months. Presenting symptoms may include loss of drug effect, new pain or paresthesias, or neurologic deficits. Patients should be routinely screened for signs and symptoms of granuloma formation at scheduled intrathecal pump refill appointments. In suspicious cases, patients should undergo prompt diagnostic imaging, and neurosurgical consultation should be considered *(Miller: Miller's Anesthesia, ed 8, pp 1911–1912)*.

893. (C) In an unconscious patient, a unilateral dilated pupil would be a matter of grave concern. In an awake patient with a normal neurologic examination, however, it is less worrisome. An inferior alveolar nerve block involves injection of about 2 mL of 2% lidocaine around the inferior alveolar nerve just behind the molars in the lower jaw. Even a grossly misdirected needle probably could not reach the stellate ganglion, but were it possible, the result would be a Horner syndrome (miosis, not mydriasis, ptosis, anhidrosis, and vasodilation over the face). Blockade of the ciliary ganglion could cause mydriasis on the ipsilateral side, but reaching the ciliary ganglion, located between the optic nerve and lateral rectus muscle about 1 cm from the posterior limit of the orbit, would be almost impossible with a needle directed toward the mandible. Glycopyrrolate administered systemically does not cause mydriasis, as it is not capable of crossing the blood-brain barrier. Lidocaine instilled directly into the eye does not produce mydriasis, but phenylephrine does. Care must be taken not to spray local anesthetic (with or without vasoconstrictor) into the eyes while applying topical anesthesia to the nares (*Brunton: Goodman & Gilman's The Pharmacologic Basis of Therapeutics, ed 12, pp 176–189, 295, 1775–1777*).

894. (C) The un-ionized form of the local anesthetic traverses the nerve membrane, whereas the ionized form actually blocks conduction. About three nodes of Ranvier must be blocked to achieve anesthesia. The presence of myelin enhances the ability of a local anesthetic to block conduction, as does rapid firing. The local anesthetic blocks nerve transmission by inhibiting the voltage-gated sodium ion channels (*Barash: Clinical Anesthesia, ed 8, p 564–565*).

895. (D) PDPHs typically appear within 12 to 48 hours of a dural puncture, but may be immediate and occasionally have become delayed for several days or months after a dural puncture. The headaches are characterized by dull or throbbing frontal or occipital pain, which worsens with sitting and improves with reclining. Postspinal headaches may be associated with neurologic symptoms such as diplopia, tinnitus, and reduced hearing acuity. Very rarely, a subdural hematoma will develop. The etiology of postspinal headaches is believed to be due to a reduction in CSF pressure and resulting tension on meningeal vessels and nerves (which results from leakage of CSF through the needle hole in the dura mater). Factors associated with an increased incidence of postspinal headaches include pregnancy, needle size (larger needles leave bigger holes than smaller needles), type of needle used to perform the block (cutting Quincke needles are more commonly associated with PDPH than pencil-point Whitacre or bullet-shaped Sprotte needles), and the number of dural punctures. They occur more frequently in young adults, compared with children and elderly persons. Conservative therapy for a postspinal headache includes bed rest, analgesics, and oral and IV hydration. If conservative therapy is not successful after 24 to 48 hours, an epidural "blood patch" with 10 to 20 mL of the patient's blood can be performed. An epidural blood patch usually provides prompt relief of the postspinal headache (*Barash: Clinical Anesthesia, ed 8, pp 938–939*).

896. (B) Radio-frequency needles are placed along the posterior elements of a vertebra, and the epidural space is avoided. For spinal cord stimulation therapy, a trial is performed first; if it is successful, permanent implantation is performed. When a spinal cord stimulator is inserted, a Touhy epidural needle is advanced into the epidural space. After confirmation of proper needle placement with anteroposterior and lateral fluoroscopic views, the stimulation electrode is passed through the needle and threaded to the desired vertebral level. The needle is then removed and the leads attached to the external programmer. Vertebroplasty involves the injection of 2 to 6 mL of cement (polymethylmethacrylate) into a vertebral body to help treat vertebral compression fractures (*Waldman: Atlas of Interventional Pain Management, ed 4, pp 839–844*).

897. (A) Many drugs have been used to treat neuropathic pain, including analgesics (NSAIDs and opioids), first-generation antiepileptic drugs (e.g., carbamazepine and phenytoin), second-generation antiepileptic drugs (e.g., gabapentin, pregabalin), topical agents (e.g., lidocaine, capsaicin), antiarrhythmics (e.g., mexiletine), and tricyclic antidepressants (e.g., amitriptyline, nortriptyline, desipramine), as well as other antidepressants (e.g., duloxetine, venlafaxine). Duloxetine (Cymbalta) is a selective serotonin and norepinephrine reuptake inhibitor (SNRI) that is used for major depressive disorders, generalized anxiety disorders, fibromyalgia, and neuropathic pain. Mexiletine is an orally effective amine analog of lidocaine and may be effective in decreasing neuropathic pain when other drugs have failed. Gabapentin, a structural analog of γ-aminobutyric acid (GABA), works by increasing the synthesis of the inhibitory neurotransmitter GABA. Carbamazepine (Tegretol) is an anticonvulsant with specific analgesic properties for trigeminal neuralgia. Carbamazepine seems to reduce polysynaptic responses by an unknown mechanism (*Barash: Clinical Anesthesia, ed 8, pp 1620–1621*).

898. (E)

899. (B)

900. (A)

901. (C)

(Hebl: Mayo Clinic Atlas of Regional Anesthesia and Ultrasound-Guided Nerve Blockade, ed 1, pp 260–269).

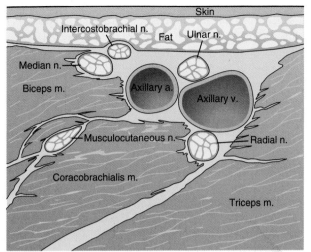

Modified from Hebl J: Mayo Clinic Atlas of Regional Anesthesia and Ultrasound-Guided Nerve Blockade, *New York, Oxford University Press, 2010, Figure 12B.*

902. (A)

903. (B)

904. (E)

905. (D)

906. (C) In the normal adult, breathing and coughing can be done exclusively by the diaphragm, which is innervated by the phrenic nerve (C3-C5). The heart rate is dependent on intrinsic pacemaker activity of the sinoatrial node, which can be affected by the autonomic nervous system's sympathetic nervous system's cardiac accelerator fibers (T1-T4), as well as the parasympathetic nervous system's vagus nerve (cranial nerve X). The first stage of labor pain is related to uterine contractions and dilation of the cervix (T10-L1). The second stage of labor is related to both uterine pain (T10-L1) and birth canal pain, which is conducted by the pudendal nerve (S2-S4). The greater splanchnic (T5-T9) and the lesser splanchnic (T10-T12) nerves supply sympathetic fibers to the celiac plexus, which inhibits much of the gastrointestinal tract *(Miller: Miller's Anesthesia, ed 8, pp 347–349, 1688, 2339).*

907. (A)

908. (A)

909. (C)

910. (E)

911. (B)

912. (B)

913. (E)

914. (D) When an awake intubation is needed, local anesthetics can be applied topically or injected to anesthetize the airway. The sensory nerve supply to the upper airway is predominantly by three cranial nerves: the trigeminal nerve (cranial nerve V), the glossopharyngeal nerve (cranial nerve IX), and the vagus nerve (cranial nerve X). Branches from the trigeminal nerve provide sensory supply to the mucous membranes of the nose as well as the superior and inferior portions of the hard and soft palate. The glossopharyngeal nerve provides sensory innervation of the posterior third of the tongue, the vallecula, and the anterior surface of the epiglottis (lingual branch), the pharyngeal walls (pharyngeal branch), and the tonsils (tonsillar branch). The vagus nerve gives rise to the internal and external branches of the superior laryngeal nerve as well as the recurrent laryngeal nerve. The sensory innervation of the mucosa of the larynx above the vocal cords comes from the internal branch of the superior laryngeal nerve, and the sensory innervation of the mucosa of the larynx below the vocal cords comes from the recurrent laryngeal nerve. With the exception of the cricothyroid muscle, the recurrent laryngeal nerve provides motor innervation of all the intrinsic muscles of the larynx. The cricothyroid muscle is supplied by the external branch of the superior laryngeal nerve. The muscles of the pharynx are supplied through the pharyngeal plexus from motor fibers from the spinal accessory nerve (cranial nerve XI) *(Barash: Clinical Anesthesia, ed 8, pp 794–796).*

CHAPTER 11

Cardiovascular Physiology and Anesthesia

915. An oximetric pulmonary artery (PA) catheter is placed in a 69-year-old man who is undergoing surgical repair of an abdominal aortic aneurysm under general anesthesia. Before the aortic cross-clamp is placed, the mixed venous O_2 saturation decreases from 75% to 60%. Each of the following could account for the decrease in mixed venous O_2 saturation **EXCEPT**
  A. Hypovolemia
  B. Bleeding
  C. Congestive heart failure (CHF)
  D. Sepsis

916. Postoperatively a 64-year-old man develops heparin-induced thrombocytopenia (HIT), type II (antibody proven), after anticoagulation for aortic valve replacement with 25,000 units of heparin. The same patient requires an elective tricuspid valve replacement soon thereafter because of trauma from a transvenous pacemaker. The best option for cardiopulmonary bypass anticoagulation for this patient with the second operation would be
  A. Defer until disappearance of antibodies; use heparin
  B. Cardiopulmonary bypass with lepirudin in place of heparin
  C. Cardiopulmonary bypass with tirofiban in place of heparin
  D. Anticoagulation with fondaparinux

917. Which of the following is the **MOST** sensitive indicator of left ventricular myocardial ischemia?
  A. Wall-motion abnormalities on the echocardiogram
  B. ST segment changes in lead V_5 of the electrocardiogram (ECG)
  C. Appearance of V waves on the pulmonary capillary wedge pressure tracing
  D. Decrease in cardiac output as measured by the thermodilution technique

918. Oxygen consumption (V_{O_2}) is measured in a 70-kg subject on a treadmill at 2500 mL per minute. This corresponds to:
  A. 1 metabolic equivalent (MET)
  B. 5 METs
  C. 10 METs
  D. 15 METs

919. Accidental injection of air into a peripheral vein would be **LEAST** likely to result in arterial air embolism in a patient with which of the following anatomic cardiac defects?
  A. Patent ductus arteriosus
  B. Eisenmenger syndrome
  C. Tetralogy of Fallot
  D. Tricuspid atresia

920. Each of the following could be placed on the x-axis of the curve shown in the figure **EXCEPT**

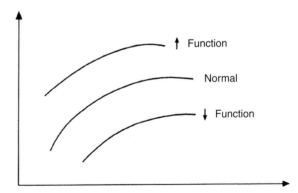

  A. Stroke volume
  B. Left ventricular end-diastolic pressure
  C. Left ventricular end-diastolic volume
  D. Left atrial pressure

921. The ECG rhythm strip below represents

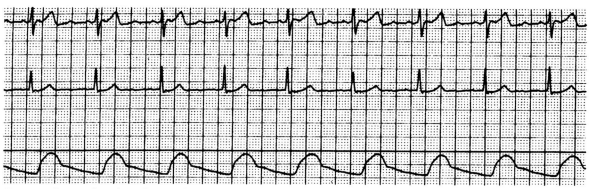

From Mark JB: Atlas of Cardiovascular Monitoring, *New York, Churchill Livingstone, 1998.*

    A. Atrial flutter
    B. Third-degree heart block
    C. Sinus tachycardia second-degree heart block
    D. Junctional rhythm

922. A 71-year-old man is undergoing revascularization of three coronary vessels on cardiopulmonary bypass at 28° C. After the last graft is sewn into the aorta, the arterial pressure measured from a left radial artery is 47 mm Hg and the PA pressure is 6 mm Hg. Thirty minutes later, the arterial pressure is 52 mm Hg and PA pressure is 31 mm Hg. The **MOST** likely explanation for this is
    A. Malposition of the aortic cannula
    B. Malposition of the venous cannula
    C. Faulty ventricular venting
    D. PA catheter migration

923. A 78-year-old patient is anesthetized for right hemicolectomy with isoflurane and nitrous oxide. Vecuronium is administered to facilitate muscle relaxation. At the end of the operation, the neuromuscular blockade is reversed with neostigmine 4 mg and glycopyrrolate 0.8 mg. The rhythm below is noted shortly after administration of these drugs. The patient's blood pressure is 90/60. The **MOST** appropriate course of action at this point is

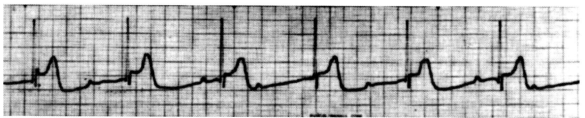

From Jackson JM, Thomas SJ, Lowenstein E: *Anesthetic management of patients with valvular heart disease,* Semin Anesth 1:244, 1982.

    A. DC cardioversion
    B. Isoproterenol drip
    C. Atropine
    D. Transcutaneous pacemaker

924. While on cardiopulmonary bypass during elective coronary artery revascularization, the patient is noted to have bulging sclerae. Mean arterial pressure (MAP) is 50 mm Hg, temperature is 28° C, and there is no ECG activity. The **MOST** appropriate action to take at this time is to
    A. Administer mannitol, 50 g IV
    B. Decrease the cardiac index
    C. Check the position of the aortic cannula
    D. Check the position of the venous return cannula

925. The wave designated by the arrow is produced physiologically by

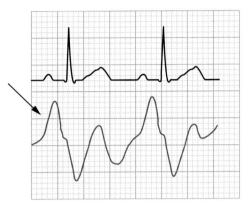

From Szocik J, Teig M, Tremper KK: Anesthetic monitoring. In: MC Pardo, RD Miller, eds, Basics of Anesthesia, *ed 7, Elsevier, 2018, p 355.*

    A. Atrial filling
    B. Bulging of tricuspid valve into right atrium
    C. Contraction of atrium against closed valve
    D. Pressure transmitted from carotid artery

926. Anastomosis of the right atrium to the PA (Fontan procedure) is a useful surgical treatment for each of the following congenital cardiac defects **EXCEPT**
    A. Tricuspid atresia
    B. Hypoplastic left heart syndrome
    C. Pulmonary valve stenosis
    D. Truncus arteriosus

927. By what percentage is tissue metabolic rate reduced during cardiopulmonary bypass at 30° C?
    A. 10%
    B. 25%
    C. 50%
    D. 75%

928. Effective inflation of an intra-aortic balloon catheter should occur at which of the following times?
    A. Immediately after P wave on ECG
    B. Immediately after closure of aortic valve
    C. During opening of the aortic valve
    D. During systolic upstroke on arterial tracing

929. Afterload reduction is beneficial during anesthesia for noncardiac surgery in patients with each of the following conditions **EXCEPT**
    A. Aortic insufficiency
    B. Patent ductus arteriosus
    C. Tetralogy of Fallot
    D. CHF

930. Administration of protamine to a patient who has not received heparin can result in
    A. Anticoagulation
    B. Hypercoagulation
    C. Profound bradycardia
    D. Hypertension

931. The primary determinants of myocardial O_2 consumption, from most to least important, are
    A. Preload > afterload > heart rate
    B. Heart rate > preload > afterload
    C. Afterload > preload > heart rate
    D. Heart rate > afterload > preload

932. Cardiac tamponade is associated with
    A. Pulsus alternans
    B. Pulsus tardus
    C. Pulsus parvus
    D. Pulsus paradoxus

933. Which of the following drugs should **NOT** be administered via an endotracheal tube?
    A. Lidocaine
    B. $NaHCO_3$
    C. Atropine
    D. Naloxone

934. The MAP in a patient with a blood pressure of 180/60 mm Hg is
    A. 90 mm Hg
    B. 100 mm Hg
    C. 110 mm Hg
    D. 120 mm Hg

935. Hypothyroidism and hyperthyroidism could develop in patients receiving which of the following antidysrhythmic drugs?
    A. Amiodarone
    B. Verapamil
    C. Procainamide
    D. Lidocaine

936. Calculate the systemic vascular resistance (SVR; in dyne-sec/cm^5) from the following data: cardiac output 5.0 L/min, central venous pressure (CVP) 8 mm Hg, mean arterial blood pressure 86 mm Hg, mean pulmonary arterial blood pressure 20 mm Hg, pulmonary capillary wedge pressure 9 mm Hg, heart rate 85 beats/min, patient weight 100 kg.
    A. 750
    B. 1000
    C. 1250
    D. 1500

937. A 57-year-old man with a history of Brugada syndrome is scheduled for appendectomy. The greatest anesthetic concern for this patient would be
A. Airway
B. Response to nondepolarizing muscle relaxants
C. Risk of malignant hyperthermia
D. Dysrhythmias

938. A 65-year-old female patient with sepsis is undergoing an emergency exploratory laparotomy. After induction of anesthesia and tracheal intubation, the patient's blood pressure is noted to be 65 systolic with a heart rate of 120 beats/min. Cardiac output determined by a thermodilution PA catheter is 13 L/min. Of the following vasopressors the **LEAST** appropriate choice would be
A. Dobutamine
B. Vasopressin
C. Norepinephrine
D. Phenylephrine

939. A 61-year-old man develops this rhythm after thoracotomy and right upper lobe resection. Cardioversion is planned, the image below is taken from the biphasic defibrillator, and the device is set to deliver 200 J.

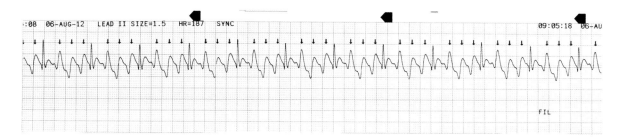

The **MOST** appropriate step would be
A. Select a different lead
B. Deliver shock
C. Reduce energy and deliver shock
D. Set to asynchronous mode and shock

940. The **MOST** important pathophysiologic difference between pericardial effusion and cardiac tamponade is
A. Type of fluid (e.g., transudate, exudate, blood)
B. Quantity of fluid
C. Pressure
D. Inflammation

941. A healthy 59-year-old, 60-kg woman with a normal preoperative ECG develops wide complex tachycardia under general anesthesia for breast biopsy. Blood pressure is 81/47 mm Hg, and heart rate is 220 beats/min and regular. The **MOST** appropriate therapy would be
A. Electrical cardioversion
B. Administration of lidocaine, 60 mg IV
C. Administration of procainamide, 20 mg/min IV
D. Administration of amiodarone, 300 mg IV

942. Although β-adrenergic receptor blockade is the best treatment for reentrant tachydysrhythmia associated with Romano-Ward syndrome, these dysrhythmias can also be effectively treated with
A. Lidocaine
B. Procainamide
C. Left stellate ganglion blockade
D. Right stellate ganglion blockade

943. A 64-year-old patient with an axial flow left ventricular assist device (VAD; e.g., HeartWare) is scheduled for laparoscopic cholecystectomy under general anesthesia. Monitoring which of the following parameters is likely to be difficult in this patient?
A. Blood pressure with blood pressure cuff
B. Blood pressure with arterial line
C. PA pressure with PA catheter
D. Temperature with esophageal temperature probe

944. In a normal person, what percentage of the cardiac output is dependent on the "atrial kick"?
A. 25%
B. 35%
C. 45%
D. 55%

945. This arterial waveform is consistent with

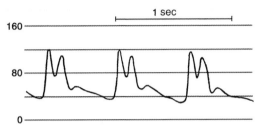

A. Aortic regurgitation
B. Aortic stenosis
C. Cardiac tamponade
D. Hypovolemia

946. Using transesophageal echocardiography (TEE), the midesophageal short axis view at 45 degrees shows a valve shaped like the "Mercedes Benz" sign. Which valve is examined in this view?
A. Tricuspid valve
B. Pulmonic valve
C. Mitral valve
D. Aortic valve

947. The left ventricular pressure-volume loop shown in the figure depicts

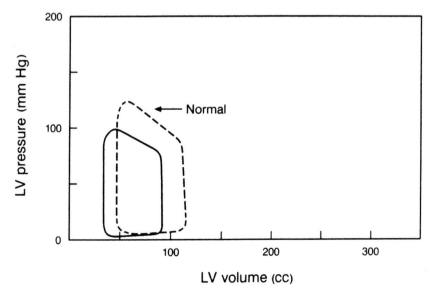

A. Mitral stenosis
B. Mitral regurgitation
C. Aortic stenosis
D. Acute aortic insufficiency

948. A 54-year-old patient is undergoing a three-vessel coronary artery bypass graft (CABG) under general anesthesia. After induction, the pulmonary capillary wedge pressure is 15 mm Hg and PA pressures are 26/13 mm Hg. Suddenly, new 30-mm Hg V waves appear on the monitor screen. Systemic blood pressure is 120/70 mm Hg, heart rate is 75 beats/min, and PA pressure is 50/35 mm Hg. Which of the following drugs should be administered to the patient?
   A. Nitroglycerin
   B. Nitroprusside
   C. Esmolol
   D. Dobutamine

949. A 62-year-old patient scheduled for elective repair of an abdominal aortic aneurysm develops a wide complex regular tachycardia (heart rate 150 beats/min) during induction of anesthesia. Blood pressure is 110/78 mm Hg. Which of the following drugs would be **MOST** useful in the management of this dysrhythmia?
   A. Esmolol, 35 mg IV
   B. Amiodarone, 150 mg IV over 10 minutes
   C. Adenosine, 6 mg rapidly over 3 seconds
   D. Verapamil, 5 to 10 mg IV

950. A 47-year-old patient with known hypertrophic obstructive cardiomyopathy (HOCM) is anesthetized with propofol and nasally intubated. After induction, his blood pressure rises to 180/120 mm Hg and heart rate rises to 110. One millimeter ST depression is noted on leads I, II, and AVF. Which of the following interventions would be most appropriate at this time?
   A. Esmolol 30 mg IV
   B. Start sodium nitroprusside infusion
   C. Start nitroglycerin infusion
   D. Deepen the volatile anesthetic with desflurane

951. With pacemakers, the concept of upper tracking rate (UTR) is relevant with which type(s) of device?
   A. VDD
   B. DDI
   C. AAI
   D. All of the above

952. Calculate the cardiac output from the following data: patient weight 70 kg, hemoglobin concentration 10 mg/dL, arterial blood gases on 100% O_2: PaO_2 450 mm Hg, $PaCO_2$ 32 mm Hg, pH 7.46, SaO_2 99%. Mixed venous blood gases are: PvO_2 30 mm Hg, $PaCO_2$ 45 mm Hg, pH 7.32, SvO_2 60%.
   A. 1.5 L/min
   B. 2.5 L/min
   C. 3.5 L/min
   D. 4.5 L/min

953. Normal resting myocardial O_2 consumption is
   A. 2.0 mL/100 g/min
   B. 3.5 mL/100 g/min
   C. 8 mL/100 g/min
   D. 15 mL/100 g/min

954. A 22-year-old man with HOCM is undergoing an elective cholecystectomy under general anesthesia. Immediately after induction with propofol, 2.5 mg/kg IV, the arterial blood pressure decreases from 140/82 to 70/40 mm Hg. What would be the most appropriate drug for treatment of hypotension in this patient?
   A. Ephedrine
   B. Epinephrine
   C. Isoproterenol
   D. Phenylephrine

955. A 65-year-old patient with moderate aortic stenosis develops a sudden increase in heart rate during an appendectomy under general anesthesia. The ventricular rate is 190 beats/min and is irregularly irregular, arterial blood pressure is 70/45 mm Hg, and there is 2-mm ST segment depression in lead V_5 of the ECG. Which of the following would be the **MOST** appropriate treatment for myocardial ischemia in this patient?
   A. Electrical cardioversion
   B. Esmolol
   C. Phenylephrine
   D. Verapamil

956. All of the following are **TRUE** concerning purely vasospastic angina **EXCEPT**
   A. Chest discomfort occurs most often at rest
   B. Pain may awaken the patient in the morning
   C. β-blockers suppress episodes
   D. Transient ST segment elevation occurs with the discomfort

957. Normal resting coronary artery blood flow is
   A. 10 mL/100 g/min
   B. 40 mL/100 g/min
   C. 75 mL/100 g/min
   D. 120 mL/100 g/min

958. Each of the following is associated with an increased incidence of PA rupture in patients with PA catheters **EXCEPT**
   A. Pulmonary hypertension
   B. Presence of PA atheromas
   C. Old age
   D. Anticoagulation

959. Allergic reactions to protamine can occur with each of the following **EXCEPT**
  A. Diabetes treated with NPH insulin
  B. Diabetes treated with regular insulin
  C. Diabetes treated with PZI insulin
  D. Previous vasectomy

960. A 66-year-old patient is undergoing a three-vessel coronary artery bypass operation. Anticoagulation is achieved with 20,000 units of heparin. How much protamine should be administered to this patient to completely reverse the heparin after cardiopulmonary bypass?
  A. 100 mg
  B. 200 mg
  C. 300 mg
  D. 400 mg

961. The graph below represents

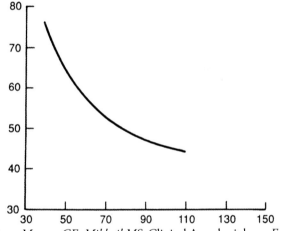

From Morgan GE, Mikhail MS: Clinical Anesthesiology, *East Norwalk, NJ, Appleton & Lange, 1992, p 301.*

  A. Diastolic time (as percentage of cardiac cycle) as a function of heart rate
  B. Stroke volume as a function of end-diastolic pressure
  C. Cardiac index as a function of end-diastolic pressure
  D. Cardiac output as a function of ventricular end-diastolic volume

962. A 72-year-old woman is undergoing cardiopulmonary bypass for aortic and mitral valve replacement. The surgery is uneventful; however, in the intensive care unit, blood is noted to ooze from the PA catheter and venous access sites. Mediastinal chest tube output is 500 mL/hr. A thromboelastogram is obtained and shown in the figure. What is the **MOST** likely cause of profuse bleeding in this patient?
  A. Fibrinolysis
  B. Excess heparin
  C. Thrombocytopenia
  D. Factor VIII deficiency

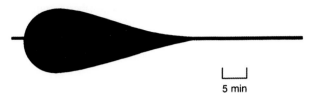

From Spiess BD, Ivankovich AD: Thromboelastography: car-diopulmonary bypass. In: Effective Hemostasis in Cardiac Surgery, *Philadelphia, Saunders, 1988, p 165.*

963. A 69-year-old man with an axial flow left VAD is anesthetized for kidney stone removal from the left ureter. The patient is "dry," and blood pressure falls precipitously to a mean pressure of 51 mm Hg with no pulsatility on the arterial tracing. In addition to a fluid bolus, each of the other interventions would be useful **EXCEPT**
  A. Increase pump speed from 7800 to 8500 rpm
  B. Ephedrine
  C. Phenylephrine
  D. Trendelenburg position

964. The dose of adenosine necessary to convert paroxysmal supraventricular tachycardia (PSVT) to normal sinus rhythm should be initially reduced
  A. In patients receiving theophylline for chronic asthma
  B. In patients with a history of arterial thrombotic disease taking dipyridamole
  C. In patients with a history of chronic renal failure
  D. In chronic alcoholics

965. A 56-year-old male patient is anesthetized for elective coronary revascularization. A urinary catheter is placed after induction and coupled to a temperature transducer. A PA catheter is inserted, and the temperature probe on the distal portion of the catheter is also connected to a transducer. The reason for measuring the temperature of both the bladder and the blood in the pulmonary vasculature is
  A. Both are necessary for determining cardiac output by the thermodilution technique
  B. Bladder temperature is more accurate prebypass; PA catheter temperature is more accurate postbypass
  C. PA catheter temperature is more accurate prebypass; bladder temperature is more accurate postbypass
  D. It is helpful in determining the likelihood of temperature "after-drop" following discontinuation of cardiopulmonary bypass

966. Which of the following would be the best intraoperative TEE view to monitor for myocardial ischemia?
    A. Midesophageal four-chamber view
    B. Transgastric midpapillary left ventricular short axis view
    C. Midesophageal long axis view
    D. Midesophageal two-chamber view

967. Select the **TRUE** statement regarding cardiopulmonary resuscitation (CPR) and defibrillation by a health care provider in patients experiencing sudden cardiac arrest.
    A. Defibrillation times one should always precede CPR
    B. CPR should always be carried out for 2 minutes before defibrillation
    C. Two minutes of chest compressions alone (no ventilation) should be carried out before first shock
    D. If arrest less than 1 minute (witnessed), deliver one biphasic shock, then five cycles of CPR

968. Which of the following medications blocks angiotensin at the receptor?
    A. Losartan (Cozaar)
    B. Terazosin (Hytrin)
    C. Lisinopril (Prinivil, Zestril)
    D. Spironolactone (Aldactone)

969. Untoward effects associated with administration of sodium bicarbonate during massive blood transfusion include each of the following **EXCEPT**
    A. Hyperkalemia
    B. Paradoxical cerebrospinal fluid acidosis
    C. Hypercarbia
    D. Hypernatremia

970. Useful therapy for hypercyanotic "tet spells" in patients with tetralogy of Fallot might include any of the following **EXCEPT**
    A. Esmolol
    B. Morphine
    C. Phenylephrine
    D. Isoproterenol

971. Sildenafil (Viagra) belongs to the same class of drugs as which of the following?
    A. Yohimbine
    B. Hydralazine
    C. Enalapril
    D. Milrinone

972. What is the minimal time after angioplasty and placement of a drug-eluting stent (DES) that dual antiplatelet therapy (DAPT) should be continued before considering stopping it for elective surgery?
    A. 3 months
    B. 6 months
    C. 1 year
    D. 18 months

973. Bivalirudin is used as an anticoagulant for cardiopulmonary bypass primarily in patients with
    A. Heparin resistance
    B. Protamine allergy
    C. HIT type I
    D. HIT type II

974. Which of the following anatomic sites is associated with the **LEAST** incidence of central line infection?
    A. Internal jugular vein
    B. External jugular vein
    C. Subclavian vein
    D. Femoral vein

975. The effects of clopidogrel (Plavix) can be reversed with
    A. Fresh frozen plasma
    B. Factor VIII concentrate
    C. Aprotinin
    D. None of the above

976. A disadvantage of port access coronary artery bypass surgery utilizing the da Vinci robot versus "standard" coronary artery revascularization with cardiopulmonary bypass is
    A. Need for hypothermic cardiac arrest
    B. Greater incidence of intraoperative hypoxia
    C. Greater incidence of trauma to sternum
    D. Increased transfusion requirements

977. A right-sided double-lumen tube will be used to separate ventilation of the right and left lungs for a left pneumonectomy. The plan for placement is to insert the distal tube into the trachea with a laryngoscope and then to advance the distal tube into the right mainstem bronchus under bronchoscopic guidance. After insertion of the tube with the laryngoscope, CO_2 is seen on infrared spectrometer and the scope is passed through the bronchial port until it exits the tube inside the lumen of the patient's airway. A structure is seen that appears to be the carina. The scope is then passed into the right branch, and the structure in the picture below is visualized. The scope is located in the

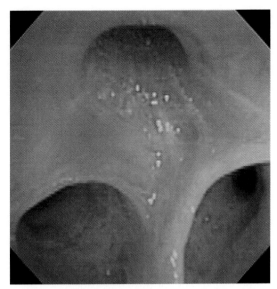

A. Right mainstem bronchus
B. Left mainstem bronchus
C. Lingular segment
D. Right upper lobe

978. Which of the following maneuvers (after assuring proper tube placement) is **LEAST** likely to raise the PaO$_2$ during one-lung ventilation with a double-lumen endotracheal tube?
A. Continuous positive airway pressure (CPAP) to the nondependent lung
B. Positive end-expiratory pressure (PEEP) to the dependent lung
C. Continuous infusion of epoprostenol (Flolan) via central line
D. Raising MAP from 60 to 85 mm Hg

979. Which of the following drugs or interventions will cause the **LEAST** increase in heart rate in the transplanted denervated heart?
A. Glucagon
B. Atropine
C. Isoproterenol
D. Norepinephrine

980. A patient with known Wolff-Parkinson-White (WPW) syndrome develops a wide complex tachycardia during a hernia operation under general anesthesia. Vital signs are stable, and pharmacologic treatment is desired. Which of the following drugs is **MOST** likely to be successful in controlling heart rate in this patient?
A. Verapamil
B. Esmolol
C. Adenosine
D. Procainamide

981. A 63-year-old patient with a DDD-R pacemaker is scheduled for right hemicolectomy. The indication for pacemaker implantation was sick sinus syndrome, and the pacemaker has been reprogrammed to the asynchronous (DOO) mode at a rate of 70 for surgery. After induction, the patient's native heart rate rises to 85 beats/min with blood pressure 130/90 mm Hg. Which of the following actions would be **MOST** appropriate?
A. Turn off pacemaker for duration of case
B. Administer lidocaine
C. Administer esmolol
D. Observe

982. The main advantage of milrinone is that it lacks which side effect, compared with amrinone, for long-term use?
A. Tachycardia
B. Hypothyroidism
C. Thrombocytopenia
D. Hyperglycemia

983. Systemic inflammatory response syndrome (SIRS) differs from sepsis in that patients with SIRS have
A. A normal temperature
B. A heart rate less than 90 beats/min
C. A normal white blood cell count
D. No documented infection

984. Arrange the percutaneous insertion sites from nearest to farthest for placement of a PA catheter.
A. Left internal jugular, right internal jugular, antecubital, femoral
B. Right internal jugular, left internal jugular, antecubital, femoral
C. Right internal jugular, left internal jugular, femoral, antecubital
D. Left internal jugular, right internal jugular, femoral, antecubital

985. A PA catheter capable of continuously monitoring S$\bar{v}$O$_2$ is placed in a patient for coronary artery bypass surgery. Just before instituting cardiopulmonary bypass, the S$\bar{v}$O$_2$ falls from 85% to 71%. Which of the following could account for this change in S$\bar{v}$O$_2$?
A. Cooling the patient to 27° C
B. Transfusion of two units of packed red blood cells
C. Epinephrine, 25 µg IV
D. Myocardial ischemia

986. Which of the following terms refers to myocardial relaxation or diastole?

A. Inotropy
B. Chronotropy
C. Dromotropy
D. Lusitropy

987. A 31-year-old female with primary pulmonary hypertension is scheduled for a mastectomy. Pharmacologic agents that might be useful in reducing pulmonary vascular resistance (PVR) include each of the following **EXCEPT**

A. Prostaglandin I_2 (epoprostenol)
B. Oxygen
C. Nitrous oxide
D. Milrinone

988. PVR as a function of lung volume is the **LEAST** at which volume?

A. Total lung volume
B. Residual volume
C. Functional residual capacity (FRC)
D. Expiratory reserve volume

989. A 45-year-old patient with hypertrophic cardiomyopathy is anesthetized for skin grafting after suffering third-degree burns on his legs. As skin is harvested from his back, his heart rate rises and his systolic blood pressure falls to 85 mm Hg. Which of the following interventions is **LEAST** likely to improve this patient's hemodynamics?

A. Administration of esmolol
B. Fluid bolus
C. Dobutamine infusion
D. Administration of sufentanil

990. A 59-year-old patient is scheduled for right knee replacement. The patient has a long history of CHF with 87% oxygen saturation while breathing room air in the holding area. Rales are audible throughout both lung fields with the patient upright. The **MOST** appropriate plan would be

A. Arterial line and spinal with isobaric bupivacaine
B. Arterial line, etomidate induction, sevoflurane, intraoperative TEE
C. Arterial line, CVP line, ketamine induction, N_2O narcotic anesthetic, furosemide, milrinone
D. Cancel the case

991. You are called to the postanesthesia care unit to see a patient who had undergone a general anesthetic for a debridement of an infected sternum after aortic valve surgery 3 weeks earlier. The patient has a heart rate of 110 and a respiratory rate of 24 and is confused. The blood pressure is 85/40 mm Hg.

Under the current sepsis guidelines, this patient meets the criteria for:

A. Septic shock
B. SIRS syndrome
C. Sepsis
D. Severe septic shock

992. You made an infusion of dopamine by mixing 200 mg of dopamine in 250 mL of sodium chloride (NS) or 5% dextrose injection (D_5W). What is the infusion pump rate when infusing dopamine at a rate of 5 µg/kg/min for this 70-kg patient?

A. 10 mL/hr
B. 16 mL/hr
C. 20 mL/hr
D. 26 mL/hr

993. A 79-year-old patient returns to the operating room with cardiac tamponade after three-vessel coronary artery grafting. In addition to gentle positive-pressure ventilation, which of the following permutations in hemodynamics would be **MOST** beneficial in this scenario?

A. Increased preload, slow heart rate, increased afterload
B. Normal preload, slow heart rate, decreased afterload
C. Normal preload, fast heart rate, decreased afterload
D. Increased preload, fast heart rate, increased afterload

994. Which of the following treatments would be the **LEAST** useful in treatment of the rhythm shown below?

A. Procainamide
B. Magnesium
C. Overdrive pacing
D. Unsynchronized cardioversion

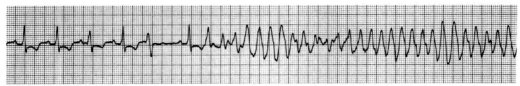

From Miller RD: Miller's Anesthesia, *ed 6, Philadelphia, Saunders, Figure 78-12.*

DIRECTIONS (Questions 995 through 997): Each group of questions consists of several numbered statements followed by lettered headings. For each numbered statement, select the ONE lettered heading that is most closely associated with it. Each lettered heading may be selected once, more than once, or not at all.

995. P wave flattening, widening of the QRS complex, peaked T wave

996. Depressed ST segments, flat T wave, U wave present

997. Normal or increased PR interval, short QT interval
  A. Hypokalemia
  B. Hyperkalemia
  C. Hyponatremia
  D. Hypercalcemia

DIRECTIONS (Questions 998 through 1001): Each group of questions consists of several numbered statements followed by lettered headings. For each numbered statement, select the ONE lettered heading that is most closely associated with it. Each lettered heading may be selected once, more than once, or not at all.

How long does the antiplatelet effect of each of the following medications last?

998. Clopidogrel

999. Ticlopidine

1000. ASA

1001. Ibuprofen
  A. 3 days
  B. 7 days
  C. 21 days
  D. Life of platelet

Cardiovascular Physiology and Anesthesia

Answers, References, and Explanations

915. (D) The normal mixed venous O_2 saturation is 75%. Physiologic factors that affect mixed venous O_2 saturation include hemoglobin concentration, arterial PaO_2, cardiac output, and O_2 consumption. Anemia, hypoxia, decreased cardiac output, and increased O_2 consumption decrease mixed venous O_2 saturation. During sepsis with adequate volume resuscitation, the cardiac output is increased and maldistribution of perfusion (distributive shock) results in an elevated mixed venous O_2 saturation. *(Miller: Miller's Anesthesia, ed 8, pp 1386–1387; Barash: Clinical Anesthesia, ed 8, pp 375, 1642).*

916. (A) Type II HIT is a serious, life-threatening condition. The clinical diagnosis is made by demonstrating a decrease in platelet count to 100,000/mm^3 or half the preoperative value 5 to 10 days after administration of heparin. Patients with HIT are prone to paradoxical thrombosis and must be closely monitored. Serologically, patients demonstrate antibodies to the platelet factor 4 (PF4)/heparin antigen.

If surgery involving cardiopulmonary bypass is contemplated, waiting until antibody titers become undetectable is the best choice. For emergency operations, various strategies for anticoagulation exist that include direct thrombin inhibitors, bivalirudin, and argatroban. Other options are use of danaparoid (factor Xa inhibitor) or use of unfractionated heparin plus a drug to prevent thrombosis such as tirofiban (glycoprotein IIb/IIIa inhibitor), or epoprostenol (prostacyclin [PGI$_2$]). Fondaparinux is not used for cardiopulmonary bypass anticoagulation. There is also the option of performing plasmapheresis to remove antiplatelet antibodies if time allows *(Miller: Miller's Anesthesia, ed 8, pp 2017–2022; Miller: Basics of Anesthesia, ed 7, p 389).*

917. (A) All of the choices listed in this question occur during myocardial ischemia. However, of the choices listed, presence of left ventricular wall-motion abnormalities is the most sensitive indicator *(Barash: Clinical Anesthesia, ed 8, pp 748–749).*

918. (C) One MET is equal to the amount of energy expended during 1 minute at rest, which is roughly 3.5 mL of oxygen per kilogram of body weight per minute (3.5 mL/kg/min). For a 70-kg (150 lb) person, one MET would equal 250 mL O_2 per minute, so 2500 mL would correspond to 10 METs *(Miller: Basics of Anesthesia, ed 7, p 190).*

919. (A) The anesthetic management of patients with CHD requires thorough knowledge of the pathophysiology of the defect. In general, congenital heart defects can be categorized into those that result in left-to-right intracardiac shunting and into those that result in right-to-left shunting. The main features in congenital heart defects that result in right-to-left intracardiac shunting are a reduction in pulmonary blood flow and arterial hypoxemia. The more common congenital heart defects that result in right-to-left intracardiac shunting include tetralogy of Fallot, Eisenmenger syndrome, Ebstein malformation of the tricuspid valve, pulmonary atresia with a ventricular septal defect, tricuspid atresia, and patent foramen ovale. Meticulous care must be taken to avoid infusion of air via intravenous solutions, because this can lead to arterial air embolism. Patients with congenital cardiac defects that result in left-to-right intracardiac shunting, such as patent ductus arteriosus, are at minimal risk for arterial air embolism, because blood flow through the shunt is primarily from the systemic vascular system to the pulmonary vascular system *(Barash: Clinical Anesthesia, ed 8, pp 1106–1107).*

920. (A) The Frank-Starling curve relates left ventricular filling pressure to left ventricular work. Left ventricular end-diastolic volume, left ventricular end-diastolic pressure, left atrial pressure, PA occlusion pressure, and, in some instances, CVP can reflect left ventricular filling pressure. Left ventricular work can be represented on the y-axis by left ventricular stroke work index, stroke volume, cardiac output, cardiac index, and arterial blood pressure *(Miller: Miller's Anesthesia, ed 8, pp 476–477).*

921. (A) The rhythm strip in the question depicts atrial flutter. The importance of examining more than one lead is emphasized in this question. The lower tracing looks like a junctional rhythm, but upon examination of the upper tracing, discrete P waves (actually F waves) corresponding to a rate of about 300/min are easily discerned. An atrial rate of 300 is common, often with 2:1 conduction, yielding a ventricular rate of 150/min. In the rhythm presented here, the ventricular rate is around 75/min, corresponding to a 4:1 conduction *(Miller: Miller's Anesthesia, ed 8, p 1441).*

922. (D) During cardiopulmonary bypass, it is common for a PA catheter to migrate distally 3 to 5 cm into the PA. In fact, PA catheter migration during cardiopulmonary bypass is so common that withdrawing the catheter 3 to 5 cm before the initiation of cardiopulmonary bypass may be routinely indicated. Distal catheter migration into a wedge position is often detected by noting an increase in the measured PA pressure. PA catheter migration during cardiopulmonary bypass has been implicated in cases of PA rupture. Although catheter migration is the most likely explanation for a rise in PA pressure during cardiopulmonary bypass, the anesthesiologist must also consider inadequate ventricular venting as a potential cause of increasing PA pressures during cardiopulmonary bypass, particularly if the PA pressure does not decline after withdrawal of the PA catheter from a presumed wedge position. Ventricular distention during cardiopulmonary bypass is detrimental because it can increase myocardial oxygen demand at a time when there is no coronary blood flow. Malposition of the aortic cannula may result in unilateral facial blanching. Malposition of the venous cannula may result in facial or scleral edema or may manifest as poor blood return to the cardiopulmonary bypass circuit *(Barash: Clinical Anesthesia, ed 8, p 1095).*

923. (C) Anticholinesterase drugs may have significant cholinergic side effects, including sinoatrial and atrioventricular (AV) node slowing, bronchoconstriction, and peristalsis. There is a high incidence of transient cardiac dysrhythmias after administration of these drugs. The cardiac effects vary from clinically unimportant atrial and junctional bradydysrhythmias and ectopic ventricular foci, to clinically important dysrhythmias such as high-grade heart block, including complete heart block and cardiac arrest. The rhythm strip in this question is that of a low-grade heart block with a junctional rhythm. The most appropriate treatment of this rhythm is administration of atropine *(Butterworth: Morgan & Mikhail's Clinical Anesthesiology, ed 5, pp 224–228).*

924. (D) Incorrect positioning of the aortic perfusion and venous return cannulae is a possible complication associated with cardiopulmonary bypass. Improper positioning of the aortic cannula would tend to result in unilateral facial blanching, whereas facial edema (e.g., bulging sclerae) reflects venous congestion and may be caused by improper positioning of the venous return cannula. Incorrect positioning of the venous return cannula can occur when the cannula is inserted too far into the superior vena cava, which causes obstruction of the right innominate vein. If the venous cannula is inserted too far into the inferior vena cava, venous return from the lower regions of the body can be impaired and abdominal distention can occur. If this happens, the vena caval cannula should be withdrawn to a more proximal position, and the adequacy of the venous return from the patient to the cardiopulmonary bypass machine should be confirmed. A properly positioned venous return cannula will bleed back with nonpulsatile flow when the proximal end is lowered below the patient *(Miller: Miller's Anesthesia, ed 8, pp 2035–2036).*

925. (C) There are three waves—"a," "c," and "v"—and two descents—"x" after the "a" wave and "y" after the "v" wave—in the CVP trace. "Wave a" corresponds to the contraction of the atrium (follows the P wave on the ECG). Because there is no valve between the atrium and the CVP line, when the atrium contracts, the pressure increases in the CVP trace. If there are no P waves on the ECG (e.g., nodal rhythm), there are no "a waves." If the atrium contracts against a closed tricuspid valve (i.e., when the ventricle contracts at the same time, as in junctional rhythms), you will see large "a waves." "A waves" can also be large when the atrium has hypertrophied and atrial pressures are elevated, as seen with tricuspid stenosis, pulmonary stenosis, or pulmonary hypertension. When the atrium stops contracting, pressure decreases in the atrium (the "x" descent). When the ventricle contracts, there is a bulging of the tricuspid valve into the right atrium, causing the "c wave" (c stands for cuspid valve). The "v wave" develops as the right atrium is passively filled with blood during atrial diastole and the tricuspid valve is closed. The "y descent" develops when the left ventricular pressure decreases with ventricular diastole until the tricuspid valve opens and blood flows passively into the empty right ventricle.

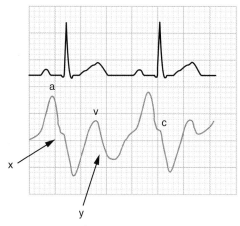

From Szocik J, Teig M, Tremper KK: Anesthetic monitoring. In: MC Pardo, RD Miller, eds, Basics of Anesthesia, ed 7, Elsevier, 2018, p 355.

926. (D) The Fontan procedure (usually modified Fontan) is an anastomosis of the right atrial appendage to the PA. This procedure is most frequently performed to treat congenital cardiac defects, which decrease PA blood flow (e.g., pulmonary atresia and stenosis, and tricuspid atresia). The Fontan procedure is also used to increase pulmonary blood flow when it is necessary to surgically convert the right ventricle to a systemic ventricle (e.g., hypoplastic left heart syndrome). Truncus arteriosus occurs when a single arterial trunk, which overrides both ventricles (which are connected via a ventricular septal defect), gives rise to both the aorta and PA. Surgical treatment of this defect includes banding of the right and left pulmonary arteries and enclosure of the associated ventricular septal defect *(Miller: Miller's Anesthesia, ed 8, p 2809).*

927. (C) For each degree Celsius that body temperature is lowered, tissue metabolic rate declines approximately 5% to 8%. A core temperature of 28° to 30° C would correspond roughly to a 50% reduction in metabolic rate *(Barash: Clinical Anesthesia, ed 8, pp 1092–1093).*

928. (B) By deflating just before ventricular systole, an intra-aortic balloon pump (IABP) is designed to reduce aortic pressure and afterload, thereby enhancing left ventricular ejection and reducing wall tension and oxygen consumption. By inflating in diastole, just after closure of the aortic valve, diastolic aortic pressure and coronary blood flow are increased. Thus proper timing of inflation and deflation is crucial to correct functioning of an IABP. The P wave on the ECG is a late diastolic event, and inflating the IABP just after the P wave would minimize augmentation of diastolic coronary blood flow. In addition, inflation of the device that late in diastole would risk having the balloon inflated during ventricular systole, which would dramatically increase ventricular afterload and worsen the myocardial oxygen supply and demand balance. Similarly, the midpoint of the QRS complex represents the electrical activation of the ventricles, which heralds the end of ventricular diastole, a time when the balloon should be deflating before ventricular ejection *(Barash: Clinical Anesthesia, ed 8, p 1102).*

929. (C) Afterload reduction during anesthesia is beneficial in all of the conditions listed in this question except tetralogy of Fallot. In tetralogy of Fallot, blood is shunted through a ventricular septal defect from the pulmonary circulation to the systemic circulation because of right ventricular outflow obstruction. A decrease in SVR would augment this right-to-left shunt through the ventricular septal defect, which would reduce pulmonary vascular blood flow and exacerbate systemic hypoxemia *(Butterworth: Morgan & Mikhail's Clinical Anesthesiology, ed 5, pp 426–427).*

930. (A) Protamine is a basic compound isolated from the sperm of certain fish species and is a specific antagonist of heparin. The dose of protamine is 1.3 mg for each 100 units of heparin. If protamine is administered to a patient who has not received heparin, it can bind to platelets and soluble coagulation factors, producing an anticoagulant effect. There is no evidence that protamine has negative inotropic or chronotropic properties. Some persons (e.g., diabetics taking NPH insulin) may be allergic to protamine.

Hypotension may occur when protamine is administered rapidly, because it induces histamine release from mast cells *(Kaplan: Kaplan's Cardiac Anesthesia, ed 7, pp 1270–1272).*

931. (D) The primary goal in the anesthetic management of patients with coronary artery disease is to maintain the balance between myocardial O_2 supply and demand. Myocardial O_2 consumption (i.e., myocardial O_2 demand) is determined by three factors: myocardial wall tension, heart rate, and myocardial contractile state. Myocardial wall tension is directly related to the end-diastolic ventricular pressure or volume (preload) and SVR (afterload). In general, myocardial work in the form of increased heart rate results in the greatest increase in myocardial O_2 consumption. Also, for a given increase in myocardial work, the increase in myocardial O_2 consumption is much less with volume work (preload) than with pressure work (afterload) *(Stoelting: Pharmacology and Physiology in Anesthetic Practice, ed 4, p 754).*

932. (D) Pulsus paradoxus describes an inspiratory fall in systolic arterial blood pressure of greater than 10 mm Hg, often seen in cardiac tamponade. This inspiratory decline in systolic blood pressure represents an exaggeration of the normal small drop in blood pressure seen with inspiration in spontaneously breathing patients. In cardiac tamponade, ventricular filling is limited by the presence of blood, thrombus, or other material in the pericardial space. During inspiration in the spontaneously breathing patient, negative intrathoracic pressure enhances filling of the right ventricle. Because total cardiac volume is limited by the pressurized pericardium in tamponade cases, as the right ventricle fills with inspiration, left ventricular preload and blood pressure decline. Pulsus paradoxus is occasionally seen in cases of severe airway obstruction and right ventricular infarction. Pulsus parvus and pulsus tardus describe, respectively, the diminished pulse wave and delayed upstroke in patients with aortic stenosis. Pulsus alternans describes alternating smaller and larger pulse waves, a condition sometimes seen in patients with severe left ventricular dysfunction. A bisferiens pulse is a pulse waveform with two systolic peaks, seen in cases of significant aortic valvular regurgitation *(Miller: Miller's Anesthesia, ed 8, pp 2073–2074).*

933. (B) The word ALONE is an acronym for five drugs that can be administered down the endotracheal tube: *A*tropine, *L*idocaine, *O*xygen, *N*aloxone, *E*pinephrine. In addition, vasopressin may be administered down the endotracheal tube. Although preoperatively clear antacids (e.g., Bicitra) have been administered orally to raise gastric pH in patients at high risk for aspiration with induction of general anesthesia to decrease the severity of acid aspiration, should aspiration occur, bicarbonate should not be instilled down the endotracheal tube because it would worsen the aspiration and might produce an alkaline burn to the lung *(Barash: Clinical Anesthesia, ed 8, pp 1669–1670).*

934. (B) Mean arterial pressure can be calculated using the following formula:

$$MAP = BP_D + 1/3(BP_S - BP_D)$$

Where MAP (mm Hg) is the mean arterial pressure, BP_D (mm Hg) is the diastolic blood pressure, and BP_S (mm Hg) is the systolic blood pressure *(Barash: Clinical Anesthesia, ed 8, p 716).*

935. (A) Amiodarone is a benzofuran derivative with a chemical structure similar to that of thyroxine, which accounts for its ability to cause either hypothyroidism or hyperthyroidism. Altered thyroid function occurs in 2% to 4% of patients when amiodarone is administered over a long period. Amiodarone prolongs the duration of the action potential of both atrial and ventricular muscle without altering the resting membrane potential. This accounts for its ability to depress sinoatrial and AV node function. Thus amiodarone is effective pharmacologic therapy for both recurrent supraventricular and ventricular tachydysrhythmias. In patients with WPW syndrome, amiodarone increases the refractory period of the accessory pathway. Atropine-resistant bradycardia and hypotension may occur during general anesthesia because of the significant antiadrenergic effect of amiodarone. Should this occur, isoproterenol should be administered or a temporary artificial cardiac pacemaker should be inserted *(Miller: Miller's Anesthesia, ed 8, p 1175).*

936. (C) SVR can be calculated using the following formula:

$$SVR = (MAP - CVP)/CO \times 80$$

where SVR is the systemic vascular resistance, MAP (mm Hg) is the mean arterial pressure, CVP (mm Hg) is the central venous pressure, CO (L/min) is the cardiac output, and 80 is a factor to convert Wood units to dyne-sec/cm^5. Calculation of SVR from the data in this question is as follows:

$$SVR = (86 - 8)/5 \times 80 = 1248 \, dyne\text{-}sec/cm^5$$

(Miller: Miller's Anesthesia, ed 8, p 1387).

937. (D) Brugada syndrome is a rare autosomal dominant genetic disease of the heart due to abnormal electrical activity of the heart muscle and is associated with characteristic ECG findings of right bundle branch block and ST segment elevation in the anterior leads (V1-V3). It appears more frequently in Southeast Asian males. Most patients with this disease are asymptomatic; however, patients may present with blackouts due to transient arrhythmias (e.g., ventricular tachycardia, ventricular fibrillation [VF], atrial fibrillation), or may present with sudden death. The abnormal heart rhythms may develop during rest, after heavy meals (increased vagal tone), after excessive alcohol ingestion, or during a febrile illness. Echocardiography, stress testing, and cardiac magnetic resonance imaging (MRI) are usually normal in these patients. Drugs to avoid (Class I: convincing evidence/opinion) include some antiarrhythmic drugs (e.g., flecainide, procainamide). Class IIa drugs (evidence/opinion is less clear) include propofol (especially prolonged propofol infusions), bupivacaine, procaine, some psychotropic drugs (e.g., amitriptyline, desipramine, nortriptyline), acetylcholine, and cocaine. Class IIb drugs (evidence/opinion is conflicting) include some antiarrhythmic drugs (e.g., amiodarone, lidocaine, propranolol, verapamil), some psychotropic drugs (e.g., carbamazepine, doxepin, phenytoin), and some analgesics (e.g., ketamine, tramadol). There is no cure for this disease, but an implantable cardiac defibrillator (ICD) may be implanted in patients to decrease the chance of death. If an anesthetic is needed in a patient with Brugada syndrome, the following recommendations have been made: continuous ECG monitoring, turn off an ICD if the patient has one implanted and if electrocautery is to be used, defibrillation pads attached to the patient before induction, have antiarrhythmics that are safe for patients with Brugada syndrome readily available (e.g., isoproterenol, quinidine), have cooling equipment available since increased body temperature is a risk factor for arrhythmias. Thiopental and inhalation anesthetics appear to be safe, and propofol as an induction dose may be safe (but avoid prolonged propofol infusions). Lidocaine for local anesthesia (with or without lidocaine) also appears to be safe *(Fleisher: Anesthesia and Uncommon Diseases, ed 6, p 33; Miller: Miller's Anesthesia, ed 8, pp 1106–1107; www.brugadadrugs.org).*

938. (A) The etiology of hypotension can be placed into two broad categories: decreased cardiac output and decreased SVR, or both. In this case cardiac output is greater than normal, as one often sees in early sepsis. Treatment of this hypotension should be carried out with pharmacologic agents with strong α-agonist properties. Of the choices in this question, phenylephrine is the only drug that is a pure α-agonist. Dopamine in high doses has strong activity, but significant $β_1$ activity and some $β_2$ activity as well. Norepinephrine likewise possesses strong α activity, with some $β_1$ activity. Vasopressin is a potent vasoconstrictor useful in the management of septic shock. Any of the aforementioned pharmacologic agents could be used to support pressure in patients with sepsis in conjunction with definitive treatment for the septic source. Because dobutamine is predominantly a $β_1$ agonist, it would be an extremely poor choice for a patient with a high cardiac output in the face of a low SVR *(Barash: Clinical Anesthesia, ed 8, pp 1639–1640).*

939. (A) The rhythm depicted is atrial flutter with 4:1 heart block. The atrial flutter waves (F waves) are occurring at approximately 300 per minute, and the ventricular rate is approximately 75 per minute. The screen shows arrows indicating when the synchronous shock would be given. Ideally, the shock should occur during ventricular contraction (depolarization), that is, with QRS complex. This will effectively "reset" the heart and allow the normal P wave to be manifested. The current display shows the shock synchronized with the flutter waves. Shocking on a flutter wave that is not occurring during ventricular repolarization would not be a problem, but a shock during repolarization would be tantamount to an R on T phenomenon and might induce ventricular tachycardia or even VF. It would be far preferable to change to a different lead in which the R wave is synchronized with the QRS, and then apply the shock.

Most atrial flutter can be terminated with a setting as low as 50 J. Delivering 200 J with the first attempt to convert to normal sinus rhythm is unwarranted in most cases. Delivering an asynchronous shock is ill advised since it too could induce an unstable rhythm through the R on T mechanism *(Miller: Miller's Anesthesia, ed 8, p 1441; Hines: Stoelting's Anesthesia and Co-Existing Disease, ed 7, p 163).*

940. (C) Patients with pericardial disease may develop an increase in the amount of fluid (normally 15-30 mL) in the pericardial sac. Normally the pressure in the pericardial sac is 5 mm Hg less than the CVP and approximates pleural pressure. When the fluid pressure becomes elevated and impairs cardiac filling, cardiac tamponade is said to develop. If the amount of fluid increases acutely, as little as 100 mL may cause tamponade. If the increase in fluid develops slowly, an increase in volume of 2 L may develop before tamponade is produced. The type of fluid does not affect pressure. Inflammation may cause an increase in fluid, but it is the pressure that causes the tamponade *(Miller: Miller's Anesthesia, ed 8, pp 2073–2074; Hines: Stoelting's Anesthesia and Co-Existing Disease, ed 7, pp 226–227).*

941. (A) An unstable patient with a wide complex tachycardia is presumed to be ventricular tachycardia, and this rhythm represents a medical emergency that requires immediate synchronized cardioversion *2015 American Heart Association Guidelines Update for Cardiopulmonary Resuscitation and Emergency Cardiovascular Care, Circulation 132:S315–S367, 2015; Miller: Miller's Anesthesia, ed 8, p 3191).*

942. (C) Romano-Ward syndrome is a rare congenital abnormality characterized by prolonged QT intervals on the ECG. Jervell-Lange-Nielsen syndrome is a congenital syndrome characterized by prolonged QT intervals on the ECG in association with congenital deafness. An imbalance between the right and left sides of the sympathetic nervous system may play a role in the etiology of these syndromes. This imbalance can be temporarily abolished with a left stellate ganglion block, which shortens the QT intervals. If this is successful, surgical ganglionectomy may be performed as permanent treatment *(Hines: Stoelting's Anesthesia and Co-Existing Disease, ed 7, p 167).*

943. (A) The use of mechanical circulatory support is becoming more frequent because of advances in technology and a relative scarcity of organs available for transplant. Mechanical circulatory support can be used as bridge therapy for patients awaiting cardiac transplantation or as a bridge to recovery from a viral cardiomyopathy or from cardiogenic shock after myocardial infarction (MI). In other patients, it can be destination therapy. Currently, the HeartMate VE (vented electrical) is the only mechanical device approved for destination therapy in the United States. Various versions of these devices can be used to support the right (not approved for destination therapy), the left, or both ventricles. Axial (continuous) flow is nonpulsatile and nonphysiologic. These pumps are connected in parallel to the heart. Specifically, on the left side, blood is taken from the apex of the heart and returned to circulation via the aorta. In this configuration, little or no blood exits the aortic valve during systole. Measuring blood pressure with a cuff is not accurate in most patients and may be impossible. Pulse oximeters do work with some patients, but this, too, requires pulsatile flow. Measurement of blood pressure with an arterial line is easily done, just as it is in patients on cardiopulmonary bypass undergoing open-heart operations *(Miller: Miller's Anesthesia, ed 8, pp 2066–2067).*

944. (A) In a normal heart, approximately 15% to 20% of the cardiac output is produced by atrial systole "atrial kick." In pathologic conditions, such as aortic stenosis, the "atrial kick" may contribute more substantially to cardiac output *(Kaplan: Kaplan's Cardiac Anesthesia, ed 7, p 152).*

945. (A) The figure in this case shows a bisferiens pulse, recognized by its two systolic peaks. A bisferiens pulse can be seen in patients with significant aortic regurgitation. In aortic regurgitation, the left ventricle ejects a large volume of blood in systole, with a rapid diastolic runoff, as blood flows both to the periphery and back into the left ventricle. The first systolic peak of the bisferiens pulse represents the wave of blood ejected from the left ventricle. The second systolic peak represents a reflected pressure wave from the periphery. In contrast, patients with aortic stenosis display a delayed pulse wave with a diminished upstroke (pulsus tardus and pulsus parvus), whereas patients with cardiac tamponade show an exaggerated inspiratory decline in systolic blood pressure (pulsus paradoxus). Patients with hypovolemia may demonstrate systolic blood pressure variation, particularly during mechanical ventilation *(Miller: Miller's Anesthesia, ed 8, p 1358).*

946. (D) There are two recognized levels of training for perioperative TEE (basic and advanced). For basic training, the anesthesiologist "should be able to use TEE for indications that lie within the customary practice of anesthesiology" and "must be able to recognize their limitations in this setting and request assistance, in a timely manner, from a physician with advanced training." Anesthesiologists with advanced training in TEE "should, in addition to the above, be able to exploit the full diagnostic potential of the TEE in the perioperative period." The basic TEE examination should include at least 8 of the 28 cross-section views used in the comprehensive TEE examination. Each valve can be visualized in multiple TEE views. The midesophageal aortic valve short axis view (ME AV SAX) is ideal for the determination of aortic valve morphology (cusp number, stenosis, associated masses, etc.). The midesophageal long axis view (ME-LAX) provides a longitudinal view of the left ventricular outflow tract (LVOT), aortic valve, mitral valve, and, with color flow Doppler, can assess valve competence. The midesophageal 4-chamber (ME 4C) view is easily recognized and gives an excellent view of both atria, both ventricles, and the atrial and ventricular septae. The ME 4C view also displays long axis images of the tricuspid and mitral valves, whereas a long axis view of the pulmonic valve can be seen with the midesophageal right ventricular inflow-outflow tract (ME-RVOT) view. Both the tricuspid and pulmonic valves can be visualized in the ME AV SAX view, although at most only two leaflets of each of these valves are displayed, and they do not resemble a "Mercedes Benz" symbol in this orientation *(Barash: Clinical Anesthesia, ed 8, pp 731–766; Miller: Miller's Anesthesia, ed 8, pp 1396–1428).*

947. (A) Mitral stenosis in adults occurs almost exclusively in individuals who had rheumatic fever during childhood. Mitral stenosis causes pathophysiologic changes both proximal and distal to the abnormal valve. In general, the left ventricle is "protected" or unloaded; that is, it is not exposed to excessive volume or pressure loads and therefore is rarely associated with abnormalities in left-sided myocardial contractility. In contrast, proximal to the valve, a diastolic pressure gradient develops between the left atrium and left ventricle in order to force blood across the stenotic valve orifice, which results in elevated left atrial pressures and decreased left atrial compliance and function. The elevated left atrial pressures are reflected back into the pulmonary vascular system, causing an increase in PVR and eventually poor right ventricular function. The left ventricular pressure-volume loop in patients with mitral stenosis demonstrates low-to-normal left ventricular end-diastolic volumes and pressures and a corresponding reduction in stroke volume *(Miller: Miller's Anesthesia, ed 8, pp 2050–2052).*

948. (A) Ischemia of the posterior wall of the left ventricle and posterior leaflet of the mitral valve can cause prolapse of the posterior leaflet and retrograde blood flow into the left atrium during systole. This can be manifested as V (ventricular) waves on the pulmonary capillary wedge pressure tracing, even before ST segment depression can be seen on the ECG *(Miller: Miller's Anesthesia, ed 8, p 1377).*

949. (B) The patient described in this question has a wide complex tachycardia of undetermined origin. As this patient appears to be hemodynamically stable and has an uncertain rhythm, amiodarone 150 mg IV over 10 minutes, repeated as needed to a maximum dose of 2.2 g IV over 24 hours is recommended *(Miller: Miller's Anesthesia, ed 8, pp 1391–1393).*

950. (A) Hypertrophic cardiomyopathy, formerly called idiopathic hypertrophic subaortic stenosis, occurs in about 1 in 500 people. It is the most common genetic cardiovascular disease (autosomal dominant with variable penetrance) characterized by left ventricle hypertrophy in the absence of other reasons for hypertrophy (e.g., aortic stenosis or systemic hypertension). Most commonly, the intraventricular septum and the anterior wall of the left ventricle are hypertrophied (some patients having concentric hypertrophy). Most patients are asymptomatic during their lifetime, some develop severe heart failure, and some develop cardiac arrhythmias and sudden death. There are three types of hypertrophic cardiomyopathy: obstructive (peak LVOT pressure gradients >30 mm Hg), nonobstructive (peak pressure gradients <30 mm Hg), and latent (exercised-induced pressure gradients >30 mm Hg). Because the hypertrophied muscle needs a more prolonged relaxation interval to allow the coronary arteries to supply blood to the cardiac muscle, myocardial ischemia may develop in the absence of coronary artery disease, when tachycardia develops. Factors that increase outflow obstruction include increasing myocardial contractility (e.g., beta adrenergic stimulation such as light anesthesia or beta sympathomimetics drugs or inotropic drugs), decreasing the size of the ventricle such as decreased preload (e.g., hypovolemia, tachycardia, venodilators such as nitroglycerin, positive-pressure ventilation), and decreasing afterload, which makes emptying of the ventricle easier and produces a smaller ventricular volume (e.g., arterial vasodilators such as sodium nitroprusside, and hypotension). Factors that decrease outflow obstruction include decreasing myocardial contractility (e.g., beta adrenergic blockers such as the rapidly acting esmolol, volatile anesthetics such as sevoflurane and isoflurane, which work slowly, and calcium channel blockers), increasing ventricular size, such as increasing preload (e.g., increased intravascular volume, and bradycardia induced by fentanyl or sufentanil), and increasing afterload, making the ventricle size larger (hypertension and alpha adrenergic agonists such as phenylephrine). Be cautious with desflurane, since rapid increases in desflurane concentration may cause sympathetic stimulation, which can worsen the obstruction *(Hines: Stoelting's Anesthesia and Co-Existing Disease, ed 7, pp 215–219; Miller: Basics of Anesthesia, ed 7, pp 435–436; Miller's Anesthesia, ed 8, pp 2056–2057).*

951. (A) The generic pacemaker code NASPE/BPEG (North American Society of Pacing and Electrophysiology/British Pacing and Electrophysiology Group) has five positions for pacemaker designation: I = paced chamber(s), II = sensed chamber(s), III = response(s) to sensing, IV = programmability, V = multisite pacing.

UTR is applicable only to devices programmed to pace the ventricle based on depolarization (tracking) of the atrium, i.e., a triggering function. The purpose of UTR is to prevent a rapid (paced) ventricular rate in response to a rapid atrial rate, such as PSVT, atrial fibrillation, or atrial flutter. When the sensed atrial depolarization exceeds the UTR, the pacemaker (depending on model) will switch to the DDI mode (atrial tachy response). This would effectively stop the rapid supraventricular impulses from driving the ventricles, unless these impulses could cross the native AV node.

With other models, exceeding the UTR will result in the pacemaker creating a type II heart block. This would modulate the number of atrial contractions that ultimately drive the ventricle.

UTR is applicable only to DDD and VDD pacemakers. AAI does not require UTR because it (1) does not pace the ventricle and (2) responds only with inhibition, not triggering *(Miller: Miller's Anesthesia, ed 8, pp 1467–1476).*

952. (D) The Fick equation can be used to calculate cardiac output ($\dot{Q}$) if the patient's O_2 consumption ($\bar{v}o_2$), arterial O_2 content (CaO_2), and mixed venous O_2 content ($C\bar{v}O_2$) are determined. The downfalls of this type of $\dot{Q}$ measurement are threefold: (1) sampling and analysis errors in $\bar{v}o_2$, (2) changes in Q while samples are being taken, and (3) accurate determination of $\bar{v}o_2$ may be difficult because of cumbersome equipment. The Fick equation is as follows:

$$\dot{Q} = \frac{\dot{V}O_2}{(CaO_2 - C\bar{v}O_2) \times 10}$$

$$\dot{V}O_2 = 250 \text{ mL/min } (\approx 4 \text{ mL/kg})$$

$$CaO_2 = 1.36 \times \text{hemoglobin concentration} \times SaO_2 + (0.003 \times PaO_2)$$

$$1.36 \times 10 \text{ mg/dL} \times 0.99$$

$$13.5 \text{ mL } O_2/\text{dL of blood}$$

$$C\bar{v}O_2 = 1.36 \times \text{hemoglobin concentration} \times S\bar{v}O_2 + (0.003 \times PvO_2)$$

$$1.36 \times 10 \text{ mg/dL} \times 0.60$$

$$8.16 \text{ mL } O_2/\text{dL of blood}$$

$$\dot{Q} = \frac{250 \text{ mL/min}}{(13.5 \text{ mL/dL} - 8.16 \text{ mL/dL}) \times 10^*} = 250/53.4 = 4.68 \text{ L/min}$$

*The factor 10 converts O_2 content to mL O_2/L of blood (instead of mL O_2/dL of blood) *(Miller: Miller's Anesthesia, ed 8, pp 478–479).*

953. (C) Myocardial preservation is achieved during cardiopulmonary bypass primarily by infusing cold (4° C) cardioplegia solutions containing potassium chloride 20 mEq/L. This rapidly produces hypothermia of the cardiac muscle and a flaccid myocardium. In the normal contracting muscle at 37° C, myocardial O_2 consumption is approximately 8 to 10 mL/100 g/min. This is reduced in the fibrillating heart at 22° C to approximately 2 mL/100 g/min. Myocardial O_2 consumption of the electromechanically quiescent heart at 22° C is less than 0.3 mL/100 g/min *(Hemmings: Pharmacology and Physiology for Anesthesia, ed 1, p 383; Miller: Miller's Anesthesia, ed 8, p 2038).*

954. (D) All of the drugs listed in this question except phenylephrine will increase the inotropic state of the myocardium, which can increase left ventricular outflow obstruction and decrease cardiac output. Phenylephrine, because it is a pure α-adrenergic receptor agonist, has minimal direct effects on myocardial contractility *(Miller: Basics of Anesthesia, ed 7, p 436).*

955. (A) The classic signs and symptoms of critical aortic stenosis (angina, syncope, and CHF) are related primarily to an increase in left ventricular systolic pressure, which is necessary to maintain forward stroke volume. These elevated pressures cause concentric left ventricular hypertrophy. With severe disease, the left ventricular chamber becomes dilated, and myocardial contractility diminishes. The primary goals in the anesthetic management of such patients undergoing noncardiac surgery are to maintain normal sinus rhythm and avoid prolonged alterations in heart rate (especially tachycardia), SVR, and intravascular fluid volume. Supraventricular tachycardia (especially new-onset atrial fibrillation) should be terminated promptly by electrical cardioversion in this patient, because of concomitant hypotension and myocardial ischemia *(Miller: Miller's Anesthesia, ed 8, pp 3191–3193).*

956. (C) Vasospastic angina (previously called Prinzmetal's angina, variant angina, coronary artery vasospasm) is based on the documentation of transient ischemic ST segment elevation (>0.1 mV), ST segment depression (>0.1 mV), or new negative U waves during rest (i.e., rest angina), although one third of patients experience symptoms during exercise. It often affects women <50 years of age. The discomfort may often awaken the patient from sleep in early morning, when sympathetic activity is increasing. The symptoms promptly respond to nitroglycerin. If symptoms are suggestive but documentation of angina is not obtained by an ECG, cardiac angiography with a provocative test (acetylcholine, ergot alkaloids, or hyperventilation) can confirm the diagnosis of coronary artery spasm ($>90\%$ constriction of the coronary artery). β-blockers are contraindicated in patients with vasospastic angina, since they can worsen the clinical attacks by blocking the beta 2 receptors that produce some vasodilatory effects, leaving unopposed alpha-adrenergic vasoconstrictor effects. Long-acting calcium channel blockers (nifedipine, diltiazem, amlodipine) and nitrates (isosorbide dinitrate, isosorbide mononitrate) are often used to help decrease the vasospasm. Some patients have associated vasospastic disorders such as Raynaud phenomenon or migraine headaches, suggesting a more generalized vasospastic disorder. Patients should stop smoking and avoid cocaine use. Stress and cold weather can also induce spasms. Vasoconstricting medications such as ephedrine, phenylephrine, sumatriptan, and caffeine may induce the angina *(Beltrame JF et al: International standardization of diagnostic criteria for vasospastic angina, Eur Heart J 38:2565–2568, 2017; Goldman, Schafer: Goldman-Cecil Medicine, ed 25, p 431; Papadakis, McPhee: Current Medical Diagnosis & Treatment 2018, pp 371–372; www.heart.org- Prinzmetal's angina).*

957. (C) Resting coronary artery blood flow is approximately 225 to 250 mL/min or about 75 mL/100 g/min, or approximately 4% to 5% of the cardiac output. Resting myocardial O_2 consumption is 8 to 10 mL/100 g/min, or approximately 10% of the total body consumption of O_2 *(Barash: Clinical Anesthesia, ed 8, p 282).*

958. (B) PA rupture is a disastrous, but fortunately rare, complication associated with the use of PA catheters. The hallmark of PA rupture is hemoptysis, which may be minimal or copious. Efforts should be made to separate the lungs. This can be achieved by endobronchial intubation with a double-lumen endotracheal tube. The presence of atheromas in the PA is not associated with an increased risk of PA rupture. Atheromatous changes are usually minimal or absent in the middle and distal portions of the PA (i.e., in the segments where the tip of the PA catheter typically resides) *(Miller: Miller's Anesthesia, ed 8, pp 1372–1373).*

959. (B) Anaphylactic and anaphylactoid reactions to protamine occur in less than 5% of all allergic reactions during anesthesia, and when they occur, usually do so within 5 to 10 minutes of exposure. These reactions can occur in patients who have been exposed to protamine (e.g., diabetics taking NPH or PZI insulin, both of which contain protamine as a protein modifier; regular insulin does not contain protamine). Since protamine is derived from salmon sperm, patients with seafood allergies, as well as men who have had a vasectomy (who may develop circulating antibodies to spermatozoa), may develop a reaction. The likelihood of reactions may be reduced with prior administration of H_1 blockers, H_2 blockers, and corticosteroids. Protamine should be avoided in patients who have a history of previous anaphylactic reactions to protamine *(Hines: Stoelting's Anesthesia and Co-Existing Disease, ed 7, p 580).*

960. (B) Twenty thousand units of heparin are equal to 200 mg. Heparin is commonly neutralized by administration of 1.0 to 1.5 mg of protamine for each milligram (or 100 units) of heparin. Protamine is a basic protein that combines with the acidic heparin molecule to produce an inactive complex that has no anticoagulant properties. The half-life of heparin is 1.5 hours at 37° C. At 25° C, metabolism of heparin is minimal *(Miller: Miller's Anesthesia, ed 8, p 2017)*.

961. (A) Unlike most organs of the body where perfusion is continuous, coronary perfusion is somewhat intermittent. It is determined by the difference between aortic diastolic pressure and left and right ventricular end-diastolic pressures. During systole, left ventricular pressure increases to or above systemic arterial pressure, resulting in almost complete occlusion of the intramyocardial portions of the coronary arteries. Thus perfusion of the left ventricular myocardium occurs almost entirely during diastole, resulting in a decrease in left ventricular coronary perfusion as heart rate increases. In contrast, the right ventricle is perfused during both systole and diastole, because right ventricular pressures remain less than that of the aorta. An increase in heart rate results in a relatively shorter diastolic period *(Butterworth: Morgan & Mikhail's Clinical Anesthesiology, ed 5, pp 362–365)*.

962. (A) The thromboelastograph is a viscoelastometer that measures the viscoelastic properties of blood during clot formation. The coagulation variables measured from a thromboelastogram are (1) the R value (reaction time; normal value 7.5-15 minutes) and K value (normal 3-6 minutes), which reflect clot formation time; (2) MA (maximum amplitude; normal value 50-60 mm), which represents maximum clot strength; and (3) A_{60} (amplitude 60 minutes after the MA; normal value MA—5 mm), which represents the rate of clot destruction (i.e., fibrinolysis). The MA is determined by fibrinogen concentration, platelet count, and platelet function. The thromboelastogram depicted in the figure of this question is consistent with fibrinolysis *(Miller: Miller's Anesthesiology, ed 8, p 1878)*.

963. (A) VADs are implanted in patients with end-stage heart failure in whom medical management has failed or is beginning to fail. VADs can be left sided only (LVAD), right sided only (RVAD), or biventricular (BiVAD). VADs may be implanted until the patient recovers (bridge to recovery), until the patient can receive a heart transplant (bridge to transplantation), or as the final method of treating heart failure (destination therapy). Patients can survive for long periods of time with LVAD therapy; the current record is just over 5 years. "Destination LVADs" have been implanted in patients ineligible for heart transplant, whose status improved to the extent they were subsequently reclassified and received heart transplantation.

   LVADs are in relatively widespread use, and patients are presenting to the operating room for other noncardiac-related operations. Treatment of hypotension may be a problem after induction of anesthesia. LVADs require adequate preload to function properly. The decrease in SVR, as well as venodilation associated with induction and maintenance of general anesthesia, can be treated in several ways. Phenylephrine and ephedrine are α_1 agonists and increase SVR. Ephedrine may also increase inotropy and be beneficial on that basis in the face of right ventricular dysfunction. Fluids and Trendelenburg position are also likely to help raise the MAP. An LVAD with inadequate preload will not perform better by increasing the rpm. Such an increase could simply make the device "suck down" and may actually worsen performance. The suck-down effect results in a completely empty left ventricle with myocardium being drawn over the inflow cannula. This greatly impairs preload to the LVAD and can result in hemodynamic collapse *(Miller: Miller's Anesthesia, ed 8, p 2067; Kaplan: Kaplan's Cardiac Anesthesia, ed 7, pp 1059–1060, 1503–1504)*.

964. (B) Adenosine in doses of 6 mg IV (repeated, if needed, 1-2 minutes later, with 12 mg) can be very effective in the treatment of supraventricular tachycardias, including those associated with WPW syndrome (unless atrial fibrillation with a wide complex WPW occurs, where adenosine may increase the heart rate). The drug is rapidly metabolized such that it is not influenced by liver or renal dysfunction. Its effects, however, can be markedly enhanced by drugs that interfere with nucleotide metabolism such as dipyridamole. Administration of the usual dose of adenosine to a patient receiving dipyridamole may result in asystole. If adenosine is used in patients receiving dipyridamole, or the patient has a central line, the initial dose is 3 mg. Methylxanthines, such as caffeine, theophylline, and amrinone, are competitive antagonists of this drug, and doses may need to be adjusted accordingly *(Miller: Miller's Anesthesia, ed 8, pp 3195–3197)*.

965. (D) Temperature of the thermal compartment can be measured accurately in the PA, distal esophagus, tympanic membrane, or nasopharynx. These temperature monitoring sites are reliable, even during rapid thermal perturbations, such as cardiopulmonary bypass. Other temperature sites, such as oral, axillary, rectal, and urinary bladder, will estimate core temperature reasonably accurately, except during extreme thermal perturbations. During cardiac surgery, the temperature of the urinary bladder is usually equal to the PA when urine flow is high. However, it may be difficult to interpret urinary bladder temperature, because it is strongly influenced by urine flow. The adequacy of rewarming after coronary artery bypass is thus best evaluated by considering both the core and urinary bladder temperatures (*Stoelting: Pharmacology and Physiology in Anesthetic Practice, ed 4, p 694*).

966. (B) The transgastric midpapillary short axis view images the myocardium supplied by all three major coronary arteries: left anterior descending (LAD), left circumflex (CX), and right coronary (RCA) arteries. Thus this view is preferred for the purpose of ischemia monitoring. The midesophageal four-chamber view displays the anterolateral (LAD or CX) and inferoseptal (LAD or RCA) walls only, whereas the long axis view displays the anterior septal (LAD) and inferolateral (CX or RCA) walls. Two-chamber views display the anterior (LAD) and inferior (RCA) walls (*Kahn et al: Intraoperative echocardiography. In Kaplan: Essentials of Cardiac Anesthesia for Cardiac Surgery, ed 2, p 252*).

967. (D) The most frequent initial rhythm in a witnessed sudden cardiac arrest is VF. Delays in either starting CPR or defibrillation reduce survival from SCA. Current recommendations for health care providers in any facility with an automated external defibrillator (AED) readily available is AED use within moments of the cardiac arrest. If an AED is not readily available, then CPR is started until the AED arrives at the scene. Recall that one cycle of CPR is 30 compressions and two breaths. It is no longer recommended to deliver a three-shock sequence with biphasic defibrillators, because it is unlikely for the second or third shock to work after a failed first shock, and the second and third shocks may be harmful. After the shock, continue CPR for five cycles, then check for a pulse. If VF persists, repeat one shock and add epinephrine or vasopressin before or after a shock, when an IV or intraosseous (IO) line is available. With monophasic defibrillators, it may be acceptable to deliver three-shock sequences, but all adult shocks should be 360 J. With out-of-hospital cardiac arrest unwitnessed by emergency medical service (EMS) personnel, five cycles of CPR (about 2 minutes) should be performed before checking the ECG and attempting defibrillation, especially when the response interval is greater than 4 minutes, because shock effectiveness appears more successful after CPR (*Part 1: Executive Summary: 2010 International Consensus on Cardiopulmonary Resuscitation and Emergency Cardiovascular Care Science with Treatment Recommendations, Circulation 122:S250–S275, 2010*).

968. (A) The renin-angiotensin-aldosterone system is important in controlling blood pressure and blood volume. Renin helps to convert angiotensinogen to angiotensin I. Angiotensin-converting enzyme (ACE) helps to convert angiotensin I to angiotensin II. Angiotensin II has many pharmacologic actions, including potent vasoconstriction action, as well as stimulating aldosterone release from the adrenal gland. Losartan is an angiotensin receptor blocker (ARB) and is commonly used to treat hypertension. Patients taking ARBs, as well as patients who are on ACE inhibitors, are more prone to develop hypotension during anesthesia. In addition, the hypotension that develops may be more difficult to treat. That is why ARBs are commonly discontinued the day before surgery. Terazosin is an α_1 blocker, lisinopril is an ACE inhibitor, spironolactone is a competitive antagonist to aldosterone, and amlodipine is a calcium channel blocker. Note: The endings of many generic drug names indicate the drug class (e.g., ARBs end in -*sartan*, α_1 blockers end in -*osin*, ACE inhibitors end in -*pril*, and calcium channel blockers end in -*dipine*) (*Miller: Miller's Anesthesia, ed 8, p 377*).

969. (A) Hemodynamically unstable cardiac dysrhythmias can result in hypoperfusion and metabolic acidosis. If severe metabolic acidosis is confirmed on arterial blood gases, intravenous sodium bicarbonate should be administered. Adverse effects associated with administration of sodium bicarbonate are well documented and include severe plasma hyperosmolality, paradoxical cerebrospinal fluid acidosis, hypernatremia, and hypercarbia, particularly in patients who are not adequately ventilated. Bicarbonate lowers potassium by lowering the extracellular hydrogen ion concentration, which results in lowering, not raising, the potassium concentration (*Barash: Clinical Anesthesia, ed 8, p 1672*).

970. (D) Hypercyanotic attacks primarily occur in infants 2 to 3 months of age and are frequently absent after 2 to 3 years of age. These attacks usually occur without provocation, but can be associated with episodes of excitement, such as crying or exercise. The mechanism for these attacks is not known. It is believed, however, that hypercyanotic attacks occur as a result of spasm of the infundibular cardiac muscle or a decrease in SVR; both will exacerbate the right-to-left intracardiac shunt. Phenylephrine, an α-adrenergic receptor agonist, is the drug of choice for treatment of hypercyanotic attacks, because presumably phenylephrine increases SVR, which reduces the intracardiac right-to-left shunt and improves arterial oxygenation. Esmolol is also effective, presumably because it reduces spasm of the infundibular cardiac muscle. Isoproterenol, with its β-mimetic effects, reduces afterload and therefore increases right-to-left shunting, and may exacerbate infundibular spasm. Because hypovolemia may increase sympathetic stimulation, adequate hydration with IV fluids may be helpful *(Yao: Yao and Artusio's Anesthesiology, ed 8, p 771)*.

971. (D) Sildenafil (Viagra) is used for erectile dysfunction. Erection of the penis involves the local release of nitric oxide (NO), which increases cyclic guanine monophosphate (cGMP) in the corpus cavernosum. Sildenafil has no direct effects, but inhibits phosphodiesterase type 5 (PDE5), which breaks down cGMP. The net effect is increasing cGMP. Yohimbine is an α-adrenergic blocker. Nitroglycerin and hydralazine are both direct-acting smooth muscle relaxants. Enalapril is an ACE inhibitor. Milrinone is an inhibitor of phosphodiesterase type 3 (PDE3) *(Hemmings: Pharmacology and Physiology for Anesthesia, ed 1, p 413)*.

972. (C) After a DES is placed, DAPT (ASA + clopidogrel) is started to decrease the chance of stent thrombosis. Because stent thrombosis may develop months after a DES is placed, a minimum of 1 year of DAPT is recommended before stopping the drugs before elective surgery. With newer-generation (drug-eluting) stents, with better pharmacologic platforms like everolimus, the ACC/AHA guidelines for DAPT may be revised in the near future. If surgery is planned within 1 year of angioplasty and stent placement, consideration for using a bare-metal stent is recommended (where a minimum of 1 month of antiplatelet therapy is recommended) *(Miller: Miller's Anesthesia, ed 8, p 1185)*.

973. (D) HIT can be either nonimmune (type I) or immune (type II). HIT type I is a transient and clinically insignificant condition in which heparin binds to platelets, causing a shortening of the platelet's left span and a modest decrease in the platelet count. However, HIT type II can be a serious condition, in which antibodies are formed (in 6%-15% of patients who are receiving unfractionated heparin for >5 days) to a complex of heparin and a platelet protein factor 4. This heparin-platelet factor 4 antibody complex binds to endothelial cells, which then stimulates thrombin production, with a net result of both thrombocytopenia (>50% reduction in the platelet count) and venous and/or arterial thrombosis (<10% of cases). In patients with HIT, heparin should be avoided. In the setting of a thrombotic event or a patient with HIT needing anticoagulation (e.g., CABG), a direct thrombin inhibitor, such as hirudin, lepirudin, bivalirudin, or argatroban, should be used.

  Allergy to protamine can also be an indication for direct thrombin inhibitors, but HIT type II is a stronger reason for using bivalirudin (or other) than protamine allergy. Furthermore, heparinase, an enzyme derived from a gram-negative bacterium (*Flavobacterium heparinum*), can also be used to neutralize the effects of heparin. *(Barash: Clinical Anesthesia, ed 8, pp 451–452; Hines: Stoelting's Anesthesia and Co-Existing Disease, ed 7, p 497)*.

974. (C) Density of bacterial skin contamination and propensity to develop thrombosis in a cannulated vein are risk factors for the development of catheter-related bloodstream infections (CRBSIs). These risk factors are likely highest for femoral lines. In mostly observational studies, the risk of CRBSI was found to be lowest for subclavian central venous access. The Centers for Disease Control and Prevention recommends use of subclavian central lines when clinically possible *(Miller: Miller's Anesthesia, ed 8, p 1366)*.

975. (D) Clopidogrel exerts its antithrombotic action by noncompetitively and irreversibly inhibiting the specific platelet adenosine diphosphate (ADP) receptor named P2Y12. Because the P2Y12 receptor is permanently affected, the duration of action of clopidogrel is for the life of the platelets. No drug reverses these effects, and only platelet transfusion can reverse the effects of clopidogrel *(Miller: Miller's Anesthesia, ed 8, p 1873)*.

976. (B) Port access robotic surgery is a less invasive technique for coronary artery revascularization in selected patients. Access is gained to the heart through a left-sided minithoracotomy. This obviates the need for a sternotomy but does require one-lung ventilation and may result in hypoxia before initiation of cardiopulmonary bypass and after cessation. Hypothermic cardiac arrest is not required for robotic surgery *(Miller: Miller's Anesthesia, ed 8, pp 2586–2588).*

977. (D) One technique for placement of double-lumen tubes is simply to advance the tube such that the tip of the distal lumen is just above the carina, and then to place it exactly (the distal tube including cuff) into the right mainstem bronchus under direct vision using the bronchoscope. If the tube is initially advanced too far into the right mainstem bronchus (as it was in this question), a structure resembling the carina will be visualized. The "real" carina separates the left and right lungs, and if the bronchoscope is pushed into either the right or the left mainstem bronchi, a secondary "carina" will be visualized. In both cases, the secondary carina has only two branch points. On the left, the branches lead to the left upper lobe and left lower lobe. On the right, the branches lead to the right upper lobe and the right middle lobe. If the three lumens are seen after branching right from the "carina," the "carina" in question is not the true carina but is, in fact, the branching point for the right upper and right middle lobes (see figure above) *(Barash: Clinical Anesthesia, ed 8, pp 1043–1045).*

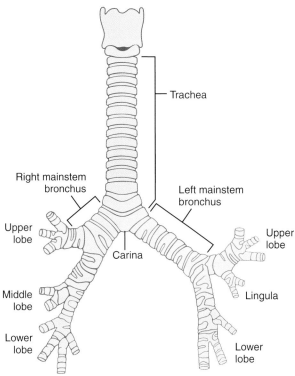

From Stoelting RK, Dierdorf SF: Anesthesia and Co-Existing Disease, *ed 4, New York, Churchill Livingstone, 2002.*

978. (C) During one-lung ventilation, $\dot{V}/\dot{Q}$ abnormalities increase. After a few minutes of one-lung ventilation, hypoxic pulmonary vasoconstriction (HPV) develops, which helps decrease blood flow to the nondependent lung. Most patients will have adequate Pa_{O_2} when the dependent lung is ventilated with 100% oxygen, using a tidal volume (V_T) of 8 to 10 mL/kg and adjusting the respiratory rate to achieve a Pa_{CO_2} of 40 mm Hg. In patients who develop hypoxemia with these settings, correction of poor hemodynamics, as well as checking the position of the double-lumen tube, is done first, then adding CPAP to the nondependent lung, adding PEEP to the dependent lung, or having the surgeon clamp the PA to the lung about to be removed, will help decrease the $\dot{V}/\dot{Q}$ mismatch. Occasionally, intermittent inflation of the nondependent lung with 100% oxygen will be needed. Epoprostenol and NO would inhibit HPV and might lead to an increase in shunt and a decrease in Pa_{O_2} *(Miller: Miller's Anesthesia, ed 8, pp 1969–1970).*

979. (B) The transplanted heart is essentially denervated and initially has an intrinsic rate of about 110 beats/min. About 25% of patients eventually develop a bradycardia that will require implantation of a permanent cardiac pacemaker. If bradycardia does develop, drugs that exert their effect by blocking the parasympathetic branches of the autonomic nervous system (e.g., atropine) will have no effect. Direct-acting drugs such as glucagon, isoproterenol, epinephrine, and norepinephrine will still be effective. Isoproterenol is commonly used for increasing heart rate in cardiac transplant recipients. Epinephrine and norepinephrine may have exaggerated β-mimetic effects on the heart rate because the increase in blood pressure will not lead to a reflex slowing of the heart rate via the baroreceptor reflexes (i.e., efferent vagus nerve). Drugs with both direct and indirect effects, such as ephedrine, evoke a less intense response. Implanted mechanical pacemakers work normally in heart transplant recipients since the cardiac leads are placed directly into the myocardium *(Miller: Miller's Anesthesia, ed 8, p 2066; Barash: Clinical Anesthesia, ed 8, pp 1480–1481).*

980. (D) Patients with WPW syndrome have an accessory pathway known as the bundle of Kent, which connects the atria with ventricles without passing through the AV node. AV nodal reentrant tachycardia (AVNRT) is the most common tachydysrhythmia associated with WPW syndrome and comprises 95% of arrhythmias associated with this syndrome. Greater than 90% of the time, conduction is orthodromic; that is, conduction passes through the AV node and the His-Purkinje system. Such conduction results in narrow, complex tachycardia, and any of the drugs mentioned in this question could be used to control rate. AVNRTs that travel through the accessory pathway (<10% of AVNRTs) are manifested as wide complex tachycardias (antidromic conduction) and are not amenable to treatment with β-blockers, calcium channel blockers, adenosine, or digoxin, and can, in fact, be made worse with these drugs. Intravenous procainamide, a class Ia antidysrhythmic agent, is the only useful pharmacologic agent among the drugs listed in the question. If pharmacologic therapy fails, electrical cardioversion is indicated to control rate *(Hines: Stoelting's Anesthesia and Co-Existing Disease, ed 7, p 160).*

981. (C) The DOO setting is the simplest dual-chamber pacing mode. Because of concerns about electromagnetic interference from an electrical surgical unit (ESU) (i.e., the Bovie), pacemakers may be temporarily programmed into the asynchronous mode for surgery, and then reprogrammed to the presurgical mode in the recovery room. With the VOO or DOO modes, the possibility of an R-on-T phenomenon exists if the native heart rate exceeds the programmed rate or when there are frequent premature ventricular contractions (PVCs) or premature atrial contractions (PACs). In the latter case, repolarization (from a PAC or PVC) may occur at the precise moment that the pacemaker is discharging (R wave). Turning off an implanted pacemaker would be extremely difficult in the middle of an operation. Furthermore, a slow rhythm could occur, wherein pacing were again necessary. Intravenous lidocaine would be useless in this setting, as would switching the volatile agent from isoflurane to desflurane. At concentrations greater than 1 minimum alveolar concentration (MAC), desflurane can actually increase heart rate further. Administration of esmolol would slow the heart rate down below 70, so that the pacemaker could again "lead" *(Miller: Miller's Anesthesia, ed 8, pp 1464–1467).*

982. (C) Milrinone and amrinone (inamrinone) are PDE3 inhibitors that increase cyclic adenosine monophosphate (cAMP) levels in cardiac and smooth muscle cells. They both produce positive inotropic effects and vasodilation (arterial and venous). Unlike milrinone, amrinone rapidly produces clinically significant thrombocytopenia, especially after prolonged use *(Hemmings: Pharmacology and Physiology for Anesthesia, ed 1, pp 390–391).*

983. (D) SIRS can result from a variety of severe clinical insults, including cardiopulmonary bypass. The diagnosis of SIRS requires the presence of two or more of the following four conditions: temperature greater than 38° C or less than 36° C; heart rate greater than 90 beats/min; respiratory rate more than 20 breaths/min or a $PaCO_2$ of less than 32 mm Hg; a leukocyte count greater than 12,000 or less than 4000/mm^3 or greater than 10% immature (band) forms. Sepsis is SIRS plus a documented infection *(Kaplan: Kaplan's Cardiac Anesthesia, ed 7, pp 231–232).*

984. (C) When a PA catheter is placed from the right internal jugular vein, the right atrium typically is reached at 20 to 25 cm, the right ventricle at 30 to 35 cm, the PA at about 40 to 45 cm, and the wedge position at 45 to 55 cm. Add about 5 to 10 cm from the left internal jugular vein and the left and right external jugular veins, 15 cm from the femoral veins, and 30 to 35 cm from the antecubital veins *(Miller: Miller's Anesthesia, ed 8, pp 1371–1372).*

985. (D) The $S\bar{v}O_2$ reflects the overall ability of cardiac output to adequately meet metabolic needs and is thus a comprehensive measure of cardiac performance. There are several factors that can influence $S\bar{v}O_2$. These factors are easily understood by rearranging the Fick equation as follows:

$$S\bar{v}O_2 = SaO_2 \frac{\dot{V}O_2}{CO \times O_2 \text{ Content}}$$

Thus SO_2 can be reduced by a decrease in SaO_2, CO, and hemoglobin, and an increase in O_2. In the present case, labetalol reduces cardiac output through its negative inotropic effect. These factors must be accounted for when interpreting SO_2 measurements *(Miller: Miller's Anesthesia, ed 8, p 1387)*.

986. (D) Inotropy refers to the force and velocity of ventricular contractions when preload and afterload are held constant. Chronotropy refers to the heart rate. Dromotropy refers to the conduction of impulses along conductive tissue. Bathmotropy refers to muscular excitation in response to a stimulus. Lusitropy refers to myocardial relaxation or diastole. A decrease in lusitropy is seen with the aging myocardium *(Miller: Miller's Anesthesia, ed 8, p 485)*.

987. (C) PA hypertension is defined as a mean PA pressure of greater than 25 mm Hg at rest or greater than 30 mm Hg with exercise. Epoprostenol, also called prostacyclin (PGI_2), and Flolan, as well as alprostadil (PGE_1), are usually administered by a continuous IV infusion centrally, producing both pulmonary and systemic vasodilation, but because systemic hypotension is common, their use is limited. Recently inhaled epoprostenol and alprostadil have been described to reduce the systemic side effects. Because hypoxia produces pulmonary vasoconstriction, oxygen therapy is often administered to reduce the magnitude of pulmonary vasoconstriction that may develop. Inhaled NO in concentrations from 1 to 80 ppm (typically 20-40 ppm) produces smooth muscle relaxation and reduces PA pressures. Because NO is so rapidly metabolized, it has minimal systemic effects. Milrinone is a phosphodiesterase inhibitor that reduces PVR while having some inotropic effects. (If right ventricle failure is severe, norepinephrine or epinephrine may be preferred as an inotrope, even though PA pressures will increase.) Milrinone is usually administered IV, but recently, inhaled milrinone has been described to reduce systemic side effects. Inhaled volatile anesthetics tend to decrease PA resistance. On the other hand, NO tends to increase PVR and is not recommended to be used in patients with pulmonary hypertension *(Hines: Stoelting's Anesthesia and Co-Existing Disease, ed 7, p 193; Miller: Basics of Anesthesia, ed 7, p 436)*.

988. (C) PVR is the sum of the resistance of small and large blood vessels and is least at the FRC. When the lung volume increases above FRC, PVR increases due to alveolar compression of the small intra-alveolar blood vessels. When the lung volume decreases below FRC, PVR increases due to the mechanical tortuosity or kinking of the large extra-alveolar blood vessels. PVR also increases in areas of atelectasis, when hypoxia causes pulmonary vasoconstriction (HPV) *(Miller: Miller's Anesthesia, ed 8, pp 681–687)*.

989. (C) Hypertrophic cardiomyopathy is characterized by LVOT obstruction and is caused by asymmetric hypertrophy of the intraventricular septal muscle. The compensatory mechanism to maintain cardiac output is left ventricular hypertrophy. Events that increase outflow obstruction include increased myocardial contractility (e.g., β stimulation), decreased ventricular preload (e.g., hypovolemia, venodilation, tachycardia with reduced time to fill the ventricle, positive-pressure ventilation), and decreased afterload (e.g., vasodilation). Perioperative management is aimed at preventing an increase in outflow obstruction. Hypotension often responds by increasing preload (fluid administration) and/or increasing afterload (α-adrenergic stimulation with phenylephrine). β-Blockade (e.g., esmolol) can help slow a fast heart rate and allow more time for ventricular filling, as well as decreasing contractility. If the patient has a painful catecholamine response to surgery, narcotics may be helpful. Drugs with β-adrenergic activity such as ephedrine, dopamine, and dobutamine are contraindicated, because they increase myocardial contractility and heart rate, which causes more LVOT obstruction *(Miller: Basics of Anesthesia, ed 7, p 436)*.

990. (D) CHF is one of the six major risk factors for patients undergoing elective major noncardiac surgery. The other major risk factors are high-risk surgery, ischemic heart disease, cerebrovascular disease, insulin-dependent diabetes mellitus, and preoperative serum creatinine of greater than 2 mg/dL. As this is an elective case, patients with CHF need to be optimally managed before surgery. This patient does not appear to be optimally managed, and surgery should be canceled *(Miller: Basics of Anesthesia, ed 7, p 435)*.

991. (C) New diagnostic criteria for sepsis are based on the quick sequential organ failure assessment score (qSOFA) *(Singer M et al: The Third International Consensus Definitions for Sepsis and Septic Shock (Sepsis-3), JAMA 315(8):801–810, 2016)*.

- If a patient exhibits 2 of the 3 criteria below (a SOFA score >2), that is associated with an in-hospital mortality of 10%.
- Lactate is not included in SOFA scoring.
- SIRS is not a specific diagnostic term with the new guidelines.
- Septic shock is defined as the need for vasopressor support to maintain a MAP of 65mm Hg and a lactate >2 in the absence of hypovolemia.
- Severe sepsis has been abandoned.
- qSOFA (Quick SOFA) Criteria
- Respiratory rate ≥22/min
- Altered mentation
- Systolic blood pressure ≤100 mm Hg

992. (D) Dopamine can be mixed in either D_5W or normal saline (NS) solution. A mixture of 200 mg of dopamine in 250 mL of D_5W would yield a concentration of 800 μg/mL (200 mg/250 mL = 0.8 mg/mL = 800 μg/mL). At an infusion rate of 5 μg/70 kg/60 min, one would need 5 μg × 70 kg × 60 min = 21,000 μg/hr. 21,000 μg/hr ÷ 800 μg/mL = 26 mL/hr

993. (D) Patients with stenotic heart valves (mitral stenosis, aortic stenosis) tend to do better with slow normal heart rates, because it takes time for the heart chambers to fill during diastole (mitral stenosis) or empty during systole (aortic stenosis). Tachycardia in patients with aortic stenosis may be especially harmful, because tachycardia leads to myocardial ischemia and ventricular dysfunction, due to the thick ventricular walls. With cardiac valves that are insufficient (e.g., aortic insufficiency), faster heart rates are helpful, because regurgitation occurs during diastole and faster rates decrease diastolic time. Patients with aortic insufficiency also benefit from a lower SVR, which promotes a better cardiac output (high SVR increases the amount of regurgitation during diastole). Too low of an SVR in these patients may lead to decreased coronary artery filling, because filling occurs during diastole. With hypertrophic cardiomyopathy, a high SVR helps to decrease the outflow obstruction, but a fast heart rate increases outflow obstruction. Patients with cardiac tamponade have a fixed ejection fraction that is very dependent on high filling pressures, and the cardiac output is very much dependent on the heart rate. A high SVR helps to maintain blood pressure in the face of the decreased cardiac output *(Miller: Basics of Anesthesia, ed 7, pp 436–437)*.

994. (A) The figure shows torsades de pointes ("twisting of the points") in a patient who had a QTc interval of 450 msec and was having an acute MI. This condition can be induced by drugs (e.g., quinidine, procainamide, and phenothiazines such as droperidol), electrolyte abnormalities (e.g., hypokalemia, hypomagnesemia), and acute cardiac ischemia or infarction. If a prolonged QT interval is present, the shortening of the QT interval is performed as time permits (e.g., correction of electrolyte abnormalities). In the past, isoproterenol was used (shortens QT interval), but overdrive atrial or ventricular pacing is the more definitive treatment. Magnesium sulfate has also been used and is recommended by many as the first-line emergency drug. If the patient does not have a prolonged QT interval, standard drugs used for ventricular tachycardia can be used. If the patient becomes hemodynamically unstable, unsynchronized shocks (defibrillation doses) should be delivered *(Miller: Miller's Anesthesia, ed 8, pp 3197–3198)*.

995. (B)

996. (A)

997. (D) The ECG recording is a reflection of cardiac muscle electrical activity, and, although it is primarily used to diagnose arrhythmias or cardiac ischemia, the changes that occur may be related to electrolyte disturbances. Both hyperkalemia and hypokalemia are associated with impaired myocardial contractility, conduction disturbances, and cardiac arrhythmias. With hyperkalemia, the earliest changes are narrowing and peaking of the T wave (7-9 mEq/L). More severe degrees of hyperkalemia (>7 mEq/L) produce widening of the QRS complex that can merge with the T wave, producing a sine wave pattern, decrease in P-wave amplitude, and an increase in the PR interval. The terminal event would be VF or asystole.

The earliest changes with hypokalemia include T-wave flattening or inversion, appearance of U waves, and ST segment depression. With severe hypokalemia, the PR interval may become prolonged and the QRS complex may widen, then arrhythmias develop.

Hypocalcemia prolongs the QT interval (ST portion), whereas hypercalcemia shortens the QT interval. Hypernatremia and hyponatremia do not produce characteristic changes in the ECG *(Barash: Clinical Anesthesia, ed 8, p 1719)*.

998. (B)

999. (C)

1000. (D)

1001. (A) Patients with cardiovascular disease often present for noncardiac surgery, both elective and emergent. Many patients receive antiplatelet therapy, and knowledge of the duration of action is important. Nonsteroidal anti-inflammatory drugs such as ibuprofen reversibly inhibit cyclooxygenase and prevent the synthesis of thromboxane A_2, as well as PGI_2, but the former effects predominate clinically. Aspirin antiplatelet effects last for the life of the platelet (7-10 days).

Thienopyridine derivatives, which include clopidogrel (Plavix) and ticlopidine (Ticlid), inhibit platelet aggregation by interference with fibrinogen binding. The antiplatelet effects from ticlopidine therapy last 14 to 21 days, while clopidogrel's duration of action is shorter (7 days) *(Miller: Basics of Anesthesia, ed 7, p 388)*.

Index

Note: Page numbers followed by f indicate figures and t indicate tables.